SECON

THE FAMILY MEDICINE BOARD REVIEW BOOK

Multiple Choice Questions & Answers

The Family Medicine Board Review Book

Multiple Choice Questions & Answers

SECOND EDITION

Editor-in-chief
Robert A. Baldor, MD, FAAFP
Professor and Founding Chair
Department of Family Medicine
UMass Chan Medical School - Baystate
Greenfield/Springfield, Massachusetts

Contributing Editors
Daniel Baldor, MD, MPH
Department of Surgery, General Surgery Residency
UMass Chan Medical School
Worcester, Massachusetts

Kathleen A. Barry, MD
Associate Professor
Department of Family Medicine & Community Health
UMass Chan Medical School
Worcester, Massachusetts

Chandra Hartman, MD, FAAFP
Program Director
BFMC Greenfield Family Medicine Residency
Associate Professor, Department of Family Medicine
UMass Chan Medical School - Baystate
Greenfield, Massachusetts

Nathan J. Macedo, MD, MPH
Associate Program Director
BFMC Greenfield Family Medicine Residency
Assistant Professor, Department of Family Medicine
UMass Chan Medical School - Baystate
Greenfield, Massachusetts

Jeannette M. Tokarz, MD
Director of Outpatient Pediatrics
BFMC Greenfield Family Medicine Residency
Baystate Medical Practices Greenfield Family Medicine
Greenfield, Massachusetts

Emma Wood, DO
Director of Osteopathic Medicine
BFMC Greenfield Family Medicine Residency
Assistant Professor, Department of Family Medicine
UMass Chan Medical School - Baystate
Greenfield, Massachusetts

SECOND EDITION

THE FAMILY MEDICINE BOARD REVIEW BOOK

Multiple Choice Questions & Answers

Robert A. Baldor, MD, FAAFP

Professor and Founding Chair
Department of Family Medicine
UMass Chan Medical School - Baystate
Greenfield/Springfield, Massachusetts

Wolters Kluwer

Philadelphia • Baltimore • New York • London
Buenos Aires • Hong Kong • Sydney • Tokyo

Acquisitions Editor: Joe Cho
Development Editor: Cindy Yoo
Editorial Coordinator: Venugopal Loganathan
Editorial Assistant: Kristen Kardoley
Marketing Manager: Kirsten Watrud
Production Project Manager: Kirstin Johnson
Manager, Graphic Arts & Design: Stephen Druding
Manufacturing Coordinator: Bernard Tombac
Prepress Vendor: TNQ Technologies

Second edition

9 8 7 6 5 4 3 2 1

Printed in Mexico

Library of Congress Cataloging-in-Publication Data

ISBN-13: 978-1-975213-46-6

Cataloging in Publication data available on request from publisher.

shop.lww.com

QUADM0823

Dedication

I would once again like to dedicate this ABFM board review book to all my fellow family physicians! The COVID-19 pandemic has stressed our health care to the point of breaking! We have been lauded for our ability to care for patients in a myriad of settings from public health clinics and offices to hospitals and emergency departments. Frequently when the call went out for "all hands-on deck," it was ***you*** who responded—providing care with competence and compassion. Thank you for a job well done!

Although we are over the crisis brought on by the SARS-CoV-2 coronavirus, we are struggling with resultant insults—lack of staff, financial strains, and increasing patient needs and demands. I have found that in a world of patient portals, tweets, and other social media influences, the doctor-patient relationship remains paramount to being a successful family physician. In 1925, Francis W. Peabody closed a lecture by noting that "the secret of the care of the patient is in caring for the patient." While these words still resonant within family medicine today, it has become apparent that we also need to care for our colleagues and ourselves. I hope this book helps decrease your stress as you prepare for your ABFM exam, and I encourage you to continue to look for ways to modify your nonpatient work to minimize hassles and "stupid stuff." If not a member, consider joining the American Academy of Family Physicians. The AAFP is the one organization that truly understands our daily work and advocates for meaningful practice transformation and support.

I would also like to recognize those who helped write this book, especially my colleagues at the newly established BFMC Greenfield Family Medicine Residency. This program was established to help address the shortage of family physicians in Western Massachusetts. Drs. Chandra Hartman, Nate Macedo, and Emma Wood are young, energetic, and forward-looking family physicians serving as role models for medical students and residents. Dr. Jeanette Tokarz, a pediatrician in our practice, has been generous with her time in providing a wonderful educational experience in caring for children and updating that section of this book. My former colleague at UMass/Worcester, Dr. Katie Barry, managed the women's health topic and I'm proud that my middle son, Danny, a newly trained surgeon had the time to update the surgery chapter.

This dedication would not be complete without a "shout-out" to all of my amazing children—Anthony, Jocelyn, Daniel, John, Angelina, and Ella! My children are my joy and motivation. Each has a special place in my heart, and I'm truly amazed, and proud at all they have accomplished in life—whether for work, for school, or on the playing field! I always save the best for last and that is to recognize Carol—my wife and partner. Her patience and support are remarkable, and I could not have completed this text (or any other task!) without knowing that she is by my side with love and understanding....

Robert A Baldor, MD, FAAFP

Preface

The Family Medicine Board Review Book is a directed review of important topics that typically appear on the American Board of Family Medicine (ABFM) in-training, board certification, and recertification examinations. This material is not intended to be an exhaustive review but, instead, should direct the examinee to areas of weakness that may need further review and study.

Family medicine is a broad field, and to provide a complete, comprehensive review of all topics that may be covered is impractical. Courses are available that attempt to provide this type of review; however, this book is more abbreviated and focuses on topics that are commonly found on the ABFM board examinations.

Adequate preparation for any test is the key to success. Given this, we all know the importance of practice tests and the benefits of testing our knowledge base before the actual examination. This review book is structured for the examinee with an established foundation of knowledge within the field of family medicine. Its primary purpose is to identify areas of weakness that can be improved upon, and to that end, each answer has a suggested *Additional Reading* section to assist readers with further study on identified areas of weakness as they prepare for the board examination.

The ABFM restructures the examination on a yearly basis; therefore it is important to visit its website (www.theabfm.org) to get updates on the structure of each examination. I hope that you will find this book interesting and, most of all, beneficial in your studies for the ABFM examination. If you have any suggestions to help improve this material, please contact me with your suggestions at robert.baldor@umassmed.edu. Our goal is to help you prepare for and then pass your board examination!

The ABFM Board Certification Process

Introduction

To be certified as a diplomate of the American Board of Family Medicine (ABFM) requires completion of an accredited family medicine residency, obtaining a full unrestricted medical license, and passing a certification examination. Below I have outlined the requirements for taking the ABFM certification examinations depending on whether you are still in training, seeking initial certification, or maintaining ABFM certification.

Residency *In-Training* Examination

The "in-training examination" is for current family medicine residents enrolled in an accredited training program. Individual registration is not required because the registration is handled by the residency office. Your Residency Director should have all the necessary details. The test is administered annually to each resident during each year of residency training. All residents receive the same test. However, there are no pass or fail ratings; instead, the results are scored based on the level of training. The examination is given in the fall, and most residency programs make any necessary arrangements to relieve residents of clinical responsibilities for the examination day. The purpose of the in-training examination is to assess the resident's knowledge base as they progress through training and to objectively evaluate the residency education program. Scores are reported to each resident with a comparison of the results with those of their respective peers in training. The in-training examination scores are also reported to the residency director, so that they may not only track the individual resident's educational development but also look for areas of weakness across the residency training program.

The Initial Board Certification Examination

To obtain board certification, not only must candidates successfully complete the initial board certification examination, but their Program Director must also verify that the resident has successfully met all of the Accreditation Council for Graduate Medical Education (ACGME) program requirements, and the candidate must hold a current valid, full, and unrestricted license to practice medicine in the United States or Canada.

The residency program can assist in the process of initial certification; however, recertification is the responsibility of each physician. The examination is held in testing centers throughout the country on various dates twice a year (usually each fall and spring). As stated by the ABFM, "The American Board of Family Medicine Certification and Recertification Examinations are tests of cognitive knowledge and problem-solving abilities relevant to Family Medicine. Appropriate subject areas of the following disciplines are included: Internal Medicine, Surgery, Obstetrics, Community Medicine, Pediatrics, Psychiatry and Behavioral Sciences, Geriatrics and Gynecology. Elements of the examinations include but are not limited to diagnosis, management, and prevention of illness."

Continuing Certification

Following the initial board certification as a family medicine specialist, the diplomate must participate in the continuing certification process to maintain their certification status. This process is required for all specialties (not just for family medicine) by the American Board of Medical Specialties to continuously assess the competence of physicians and their knowledge base and skill set. The continuing certification process emphasizes the importance of ongoing participation in assessment activities between recertification examinations, rather than just relying on a periodic recertification examination every several years.

The ABFM certification is how the Board continually assesses its diplomates, through a required process that encourages clinical excellence and benefits both physicians and their patients. Although "cognitive expertise" is verified by the successful completion of the certification examination, the ABFM's recertification program stresses the importance of ongoing participation in activities between examination periods that evaluate each of the following components:

- **Professionalism:** Fulfillment of this component requires an active, valid, full, and unrestricted license to practice medicine in any state or territory of the United States or any province of Canada and continuous compliance with the ABFM Guidelines for Professionalism, Licensure, and Personal Conduct.
    - It is the responsibility of the physician to inform the ABFM in writing of any compliance issues related to the Guidelines for Professionalism, Licensure, and Personal Conduct. Medical license status changes are required to be reported to the ABFM as well through the medical license page in the application or the physician portfolio, by letter or email immediately following any change in licensure status. Any medical license currently, or previously, held by the physician that is not currently active, valid, full, and unrestricted (ie, inactive, volunteer, retired, etc.) may not meet the Guidelines and must be reported.
    - The ABFM reviews periodic American Medical Association Disciplinary Action Reports and also requests individual physician records from the Federation of State Medical Boards to confirm licensure status as needed.
- **Self-assessment:** Fulfillment of this component requires completion of a number of knowledge self-assessment (KSA) activities during the certification stage. The purpose of these activities is to enhance knowledge and skills in areas that are of greatest use in

each diplomate's practice. Diplomates may attempt an activity as many times as necessary to achieve successful completion. These activities are accessed through the *Track Your Progress* page in your Physician Portfolio.

- The KSA is an assessment of the diplomate's knowledge in a particular domain. Each domain consists of core competencies that must be mastered. To successfully complete the assessment, 80% of the questions in each competency must be answered correctly. If not answered correctly, a review mode, with a critique and reference for each incorrectly answered question, can be accessed before inputting new answers to the missed questions. A KSA module can take from 2 to 8 hours to complete, and continuing medical education (CME) credits are awarded for successfully completing each KSA.
- The clinical self-assessment (CSA) presents patient care scenarios related to the KSA. Simulated patients evolve in response to therapeutic interventions, investigations, and the passage of time, providing an opportunity for diplomates to demonstrate proficiency in patient management skills. Four CME credits are awarded for successfully completing each CSA.

KSA topics have included the following:

- Asthma
- Care of the elderly
- Coronary artery disease
- Depression
- Diabetes
- Childhood illness
- Health behavior
- Heart failure
- Hypertension
- Maternity care
- Pain management
- Well-child care

- **Lifelong learning:** This refers to the continuing medical education (CME) requirement. All ABFM diplomates must meet the CME requirement before being allowed to take the examination.
  - Candidates may verify their CME either through membership in the American Academy of Family Physicians (AAFP) or by manual entry of CME activities on the ABFM website. The specific ABFM CME requirements are listed at the end of this overview.
- **Performance improvement**: Fulfillment of this component requires completion of the required number of performance improvement (PI) activities during the certification stage. The ABFM-developed PI activities are called *Performance in Practice Modules* (PPMs) and are Web-based, quality improvement modules in health areas that generally correspond to the KSAs.
  - PPM activities require physicians to assess their care of patients using evidence-based quality indicators. After a physician enters data from 10 patients into the ABFM online activity, feedback is provided for each of the quality indicators. The performance data are used by the physician to choose an indicator for which a quality improvement plan will be designed. Using a menu of interventions available from various online sources, the physician designs a plan of improvement, submits the plan, and implements the plan in practice. After a minimum of 1 week, the physician again assesses the care provided to 10 patients in the chosen health area and enters the data into the ABFM website. The physician is then able to compare pre- and postintervention performance and compare their results with those of their peers. Evidence of improvement is not required to satisfy this certification requirement.

There are approved alternative performance improvement activities as well, and the ABFM recognizes that many physicians already participate in quality improvement activities. The self-directed option for PI credit allows physicians to implement customized quality improvement efforts that are relevant to the physician's work context, regardless of whether you are providing continuing care. Processes for approval of these activities are found on the ABFM website.

Finally, there is recognition that many ABFM diplomates do not provide continuous patient care, and the PI requirement can also be met by completing alternative means. The *Methods in Medicine Module* (MIMM) is one example, addressing cultural competency; additional activities have been developed in collaboration with the American Board of Pediatrics. This *Hand Hygiene Module* provides for effective strategies and proven intervention tools to enhance hand hygiene. This activity includes published guidelines from the CDC and WHO that introduce practice-proven improvement strategies and tips for creating a culture of safety.

The Recertification Examination

The recertification examination is held annually in testing centers throughout the country on various dates twice a year (usually each fall and spring). Registration for the board recertification examination is done by contacting the ABFM, and a formal application (www.theabfm.org/cert/index.aspx) must be submitted. However, before sitting for the recertification examination, family physicians must have completed the Maintenance of Certification (MC-FP) process as outlined above. Applicants must have successfully completed Part I (the applicant holds a current, valid, full, and unrestricted license to practice medicine in the United States or Canada), Part II (completed the required number of KSAs and provided evidence that they have met the required CME hours), and Part IV (completion of the PPM practice quality improvement exercises). Successfully passing the recertification examination is required to complete Part III.

Summary

Once you have inquired about the certification/recertification examination (as noted above), you will receive registration information from the ABFM, including selection of your preferred testing site location. Computer-based testing vendors are used by the ABFM to administer the examination with hundreds of locations in the United States and Canada and numerous international locations as well. It is important to register early to ensure that you get your first choice of location. The examination is offered in the spring and fall, but typically the fall examination has limited seating and is primarily for those physicians who were unable to take the spring examination and for off-cycle residents who did not complete training in time to take the spring examination. Additionally, candidates who are unsuccessful on the spring administration can apply to retake the examination in the fall. There is no limit to the number of times a candidate may take the examination, provided qualifications are met with each reapplication.

Before the test, you will receive additional material that includes your assigned testing site and a registration number. Make sure you bring the information including your registration number and photo identification along with an additional form of identification to the test site on the day of the test. Failure to do this may prevent you from taking the test, or it may delay you in the on-site registration process. This is not required for in-training residency examinations.

More information can be obtained by contacting the ABFM office or accessing their website: https://www.theabfm.org/moc/index.aspx.

The American Board of Family Medicine, Inc.
1648 McGrathiana Parkway Suite 550
Lexington, KY 40511-1247
Phone: 859-269-5626 or 888-995-5700
Fax: 859-335-7501 or 859-335-7509

ABFM Continuing Medical Education Requirements

You earn CME credit by participating in Continuing Medical Education activities through ABFM, AAFP, AMA, and other organizations. 150 hours of CME must be reported for every 3 years of the certification cycle (50 hours/year on average).

Division I credits: A minimum of 50% (75 hours) of the total required 150 hours of CME must be met by the following types of Division I experiences:

1. CME conferences or workshops carrying AMA Category I CME or AAFP prescribed CME credit
2. Scientific sessions provided by medical schools approved by the Liaison Committee on Medical Education
3. Multimedia or home study correspondence courses with examinations that qualify for AMA Category I CME or AAFP prescribed CME credit upon completion
4. Other CME activities carrying AMA Category I CME or AAFP prescribed CME credit, such as documented point-of-care learning and participation in quality improvement projects
5. An educational program of a university or college having a defined curriculum, designated faculty, and accreditation from a recognized institutional accrediting organization or an agency recognized by the U.S. Department of Education, which is designed to enhance a participant's instructional, research, administrative, or clinical knowledge and skills necessary for professional development as an educator, administrator, or clinician in Family Medicine. Fifty (50) CME credits per year, on an hour-for-hour contact basis, to a maximum of 90 credits, may be received.
6. Full- or part-time faculty development fellowships offered by ACGME-accredited residency programs leading to a postgraduate degree or certificate that prepares physicians for future faculty positions in academic medicine, or provides ongoing professional development for current faculty, may receive CME credit on an hour-for-hour contact basis to a maximum of 90 credits.

Division II credits: A maximum of 50% (75 hours) of the 150 required CME hours may be composed of the following Division II activities:

A. Teaching medical students and/or other physicians
B. Individual medically related educational activities not formally accredited may be claimed as follows:
   1. Use of audiotapes, videotapes, films, sound slides, etc. Participation in telephone, television, or radio networks
   2. Programmed medical materials such as teaching machines or computer programs
   3. Medical reading and journal club participation
C. Review of manuscripts for publication in a peer-reviewed medical journal
D. Publication of a review or research article in a peer-reviewed medical journal may receive 10 credits per article

Preparing for the Examination

Just when we thought that the standardized examinations we had to pass in high school, college, and medical school were behind us, the American Board of Family Medicine (ABFM) requires an in-training examination (in some cases referred to as the *in-service examination*) yearly during residency training, and we must pass a board examination at the end of that residency training to receive board certification. Additionally, ABFM diplomates can also take a recertification examination every 10 years to maintain their board certification. For many, the board examination process is a stressful time. In addition to using this book to review your family medicine knowledge, it is always helpful to review some basic examination-taking strategies. The following are some general guidelines for preparing for your examination.

Examination Formats

The *in-training examination* consists of 240 multiple-choice questions and uses a content outline that is identical to the blueprint for the ABFM certification examination. The examination includes four to eight pictorial items, which may be radiographs, electrocardiograms, pictures of dermatologic conditions, or other images. The entire computer-based examination contains single-best-answer multiple-choice questions, with each question having four or five answers to choose from. The study questions and answers that are provided in this book will help you to study covered topics in a similar format. There is no penalty for guessing; therefore if you reach the end of the examination and are short of time, make sure you have answered all the questions.

The *initial certification* and *recertification* examinations are full-day computer-based exams that contain multiple-choice (one best answer) questions. There are four sections with scheduled (optional) breaks between each section. The four sections of the examination are all 100 minutes long, and each consists of 80 multiple-choice questions, for a total of 320 questions. Additionally, all candidates should be prepared to choose one "module topic," which they will select during the examination application process. The module topic areas include ambulatory family medicine, child and adolescent care, geriatrics, women's health, maternity care, emergent/urgent care, hospital medicine, and sports medicine. The second section of the examination covers the specific module topic that was selected.

The ABFM website can be accessed at www.theabfm.org and is an excellent resource for more detailed information.

The Examination Day

The certification and recertification examinations are given at specific computer-based examination centers across the United States and may involve traveling to reach the location. Ensure that you have identified the site and are familiar with the surrounding traffic patterns and parking locations. On arrival, you are photographed and fingerprinted for access to and from the examination site. You must have two forms of identification (one with a photo) when you check in.

Adequate sleep is imperative as you prepare for any examination, and this examination is no exception. It is a good idea to arrange your call schedule to allow plenty of sleep the week before the examination so that you arrive well rested. On the morning of the examination, eat a light breakfast and consider bringing a lunch for the board and recertification examinations. Find a quiet place to enjoy your snacks or meal and relax during the scheduled lunch break. Bring along aspirin, ibuprofen, or acetaminophen to take should a headache occur during the examination. Cough drops and allergy medication (nonsedating) should be remembered. Calculators and watches are not allowed and beeping electronic devices or cellular phones should be left at home. Earplugs may help mute unwanted noises that distract you.

The examinations require you to sit for extended periods. Bring a lightweight jacket or sweater, in case it gets cold, and loose-fitting clothing with comfortable shoes. Also, do not forget your glasses. You are *not* allowed to take any additional materials into the examination room for the certification/recertification examination. Personal items are to be left in a secure locker provided by the examination site. The examination site may offer hard candy or mints, and you are given a small white erasable board with a magic marker for making notes or doing calculations.

Make sure you use the bathroom before entering the examination room; having to leave requires you to raise your hand, and the proctor must log you out from your computer, allow you to leave the room, and then get your fingerprint when you return; needless to say, this can waste valuable examination-taking time. While in the examination room, you are seated at a small, isolated cubicle with fellow examination-takers (who might even be high school students taking their SATs!) on your left and right. A proctor is seated behind a glass enclosure and observes all who are taking the examination. Finally, it is important to recognize that you are monitored by video cameras during the examination.

Test-Taking Skills

Anxiety is a natural response when faced with a test situation. The important thing is to not let anxiety affect your performance. Relaxation techniques, such as stretching or deep breathing exercises, can be used.

Answer the easiest questions first. Start with the first question of each section and answer all the questions you can with reasonable certainty. If there is a difficult question, skip over it and return when you have finished the section. The computerized examination format allows you to flag questions that you are unsure about, so that you can return to them later.

Check your pace and be mindful of the time. On the computer, you should see the time in a small box on the screen. Pay attention to these reminders and adjust your pace as necessary. A good rule of thumb is to plan for a minute per question. Do not spend excessive amount of time on any one question, which could put you at risk for not being able to answer easy questions at the end of the test because you ran out of time.

A strategy that can be helpful when taking examinations is to read the answers first. If you do not have a good understanding of the test question, you cannot answer it correctly based on your knowledge. Reading the answers can activate your knowledge about the question, and when you then read the question, the "activated knowledge" has an impact on your understanding of the question.

A common test-taking error is failing to read ALL of the questions and/or ALL of the answers before actually marking your response. General skimming of the question can lead to premature closure and result in a wrong answer. Self-assessment is important, because you may not even realize that you tend to skim the question or fail to read all the choices. Be mindful of making such errors when you answer the questions in this book and mark any such errors on your study grid.

Being lured by a distracter is another common error. One strategy to address this is to *read the actual question to be answered* before reading through the background information/vignette. For example, there may be a sentence or two leading up to the question, "What is the best treatment?" If you read the question first, you become aware that the question is about treatment, so that you begin to think about treatment decisions as you read the question, rather than being distracted by other information presented in the question. Avoid reading extra meaning into the questions. The American Board of Family Medicine does not structure questions to try to outsmart the test-taker. Questions are designed to be fair, without any hidden agendas. Therefore, take questions literally and do not look for hidden meanings.

As you read questions, try to identify keywords. Typical keywords to look for include the specific symptoms that are present, the duration of the symptoms, and current treatments. Be mindful of other keywords that are sometimes ignored such as age and diagnoses other than those related to chief complaint. Other "nonmedical" terms (eg, season, social issues, and miscellaneous adjectives) can also be important to consider.

Guess if you do not know the answer but use what you know (partial knowledge) to narrow down the choices and resist the following: being lured by an unknown distracter; choosing on the basis of "technical words" that must be right; or using "tricks" rather than actual knowledge (ie, two are same, one of those must be right). Consider similarities and differences between answers—use these to either serve as a memory trigger to help recall the forgotten information or make a guess by choosing the outlier. However, this is a last-ditch effort because there may be more similarities and differences between options other than that which discriminates the correct answer.

You are penalized only for an incorrect or unanswered question; therefore, all questions should be answered even if they require a guess. Also, it is important to remember that if the answer uses absolute terminology, such as always, never, all, or none, it usually is a false response. Very little in the world of medicine is absolute.

If time allows, review your work. Sometimes you will want to consider changing a previously answered question. If this is based on being cued from another question, a clerical error, or realizing the question was misread, you have a good chance of changing to the correct answer. However, if this is just based on a "reconsideration of the original answer," you have a 50:50 chance of being correct because this is usually just changing one guess to another. So only change an answer if you realized that you misread the question, or you have new knowledge through spontaneous recall, or another question gave you content information or jogged your memory, or you noticed you made a clerical error.

Using This Book

Although most who sit for the American Board of Family Medicine (ABFM) examinations pass, that should not be taken for granted. A poor score could result in not becoming board-certified or losing board certification status. This book is meant as a study guide to help you identify areas of weakness. Although this book addresses topics previously covered by ABFM tests, it is not an exhaustive review of all information and not meant to be used as a reference to support medical practice. Hence, the answers are not formally referenced but are rather followed by an *Additional Reading* suggestion to help you learn more about the topic.

Adopt a structured study program that is started 6 to 8 weeks before the examination. Use this book as a study review tool for 2 hours at night during the weekdays (reserving the weekends for family, friends, and rest). Answer a topic section (or 20 questions) at one sitting, then take a break. Use the study grid found at the back of this book as a way of tracking your progress. Many questions are marked with one of the broad ABFM knowledge categories (eg, cardiovascular, musculoskeletal)—every time you get a question wrong, place a mark in the category so that you can identify your areas of weakness. During the week before the test, focus on key areas of weakness, addressing those categories that are addressed more frequently in the examination. For example, if you are having trouble with the cardiovascular or respiratory systems categories, that is a concern because each of these areas is covered by a significant portion (10%-12%) of the examination versus 1% to 2% for other areas such as hematology. Additionally, be aware of any test-taking errors that you are consistently making and be mindful of those as a way of enhancing your performance.

Finally, best wishes on a successful certification/recertification examination outcome!

Contents

Adult Medicine

CHAPTER 1

As the American Board of Family Medicine (ABFM) certifying examination is for family physicians, the focus is on the primary care management of various medical conditions. To help focus your studying for the ABFM exam, this chapter is subdivided into 10 key areas of concentration that compose the exam. Although the ABFM will report your examination based on how well you do for each major organ system (cardiovascular, pulmonary, nephrology, and so forth), many conditions, such as infections, cancers, or other exposures, are not easily characterized as primarily affecting a single organ system; such questions are grouped at the end in Section XI (*Nonspecific System*). The questions in each section are to remind you of the key areas to review. If you are struggling with a question, find the suggested "Additional Reading" to review. The majority of these readings were selected specifically as easy-to-access primary care–focused resources for you to use to solidify and expand your knowledge on the general topic area as you prepare for the exam.

Section I. Cardiovascular Disease

Questions related to cardiovascular disease (CVD) account for about 10% of the ABFM certifying examination. As you study for the examination, ensure that you have a good overview of the following CVD topics:

1. CVD risk factor screening
   - Understand the commonly accepted CVD risk factors and recommended screening strategies based on age and comorbid conditions.
   - Appreciate the use of the American Heart Association/American College of Cardiology risk calculators.
   - Appreciate risk factor targets for intervention.
   - Appreciate the use of nonpharmacologic treatments.
2. Hypertension (HTN)
   - Appreciate the workup for a patient with newly diagnosed HTN and understand secondary causes and when/how to evaluate and treat.
   - Appreciate the use of nonpharmacologic treatments (eg, dietary approaches to stop hypertension diet).
   - Know the commonly accepted first-line medications for HTN (Eighth Joint National Committee guidelines).
   - Appreciate side effects/contraindications of common medications.
   - Appreciate the complications of long-standing HTN, including when to screen for abdominal aortic aneurysm (AAA).
3. Coronary artery disease (CAD)
   - Know the workup for chest pain based on age, diverse populations, and comorbid conditions (exercise treadmill testing, stress echocardiogram, nuclear scanning, and so forth).
   - Understand the use of first-line medications for CAD.
   - Recognize the diagnostic criteria for acute coronary syndrome, including the use of serum markers and electrocardiogram changes.
   - Learn the treatment of acute coronary syndrome, including the appropriate use of thrombolytics.
   - Know the medication management for post–myocardial infarction (MI) care.
4. Congestive heart failure (CHF)
   - Understand the cardiac workup for dyspnea/fatigue.
   - Recognize the diagnostic criteria for CHF and the New York Heart Association severity classification.
   - Know the commonly accepted medications for CHF.
5. Dysrhythmias
   - Understand the workup for palpitations/presyncope/syncope.
   - Recognize the diagnostic criteria for common conduction abnormalities.
   - Understand the use of anticoagulants in atrial fibrillation (warfarin, novel oral anticoagulants).
   - Know the treatments for the rate control of atrial fibrillation.
   - Learn the indications for pacing and implantable defibrillators.
6. Peripheral vascular disease (PVD)
   - Understand the commonly accepted PVD risk factors and recommended screening strategies based on age and comorbid conditions.
   - Appreciate the common signs and symptoms of PVD.
   - Understand the workup for intermittent claudication.
   - Appreciate the use of nonpharmacologic treatments.
   - Know the medical treatment of PVD.
   - Understand the indications for surgical intervention.

Each of the following questions or incomplete statements is followed by suggested answers or completions. Select the ONE BEST ANSWER in each case.

1. According to the 2020 American Heart Association (AHA) guidelines for cardiopulmonary resuscitation (CPR), the compression rate for adults should be one of the following:

A) At least 80 compressions per minute
B) 80 to 100 compressions per minute
C) 100 compressions per minute
D) 100 to 120 compressions per minute
E) 120 compressions per minute

The answer is D: The updated 2020 AHA CPR guidelines call for faster and more forceful compressions than the compression rate suggested in the 2010 recommendations. The new standard is to compress the chest at least 2 in on each push, at a rate of 100 to 120 compressions per minute. The perfect pace is that of the Bee Gees' song "Stayin' Alive." The purpose of compressions is to squeeze the heart to circulate blood to the brain. When compressions are done faster than 120 times a minute, the heart is not given adequate time to refill, resulting in less blood being pumped out with a lessened chance for survival with intact neurologic function.

It is also recommended that untrained responders perform "compression-only" CPR, sometimes known as CCR. However, medical professionals and trained lay people are still urged to give the victim two "rescue breaths" in between each series of 30 chest compressions. Those changes apply only to adult victims who experience cardiac arrest; respirations are still recommended for children and for adults with a near-drowning or a drug overdose event. The rationale behind the changes is that an adult who has been breathing normally will still have enough oxygen in the bloodstream to maintain the heart and brain, so long as compressions circulate that oxygen.

Additional Reading: https://cpr.heart.org/en/resuscitation-science/cpr-and-ecc-guidelines

2. A diet of high levels of which of the following is associated with an increased risk for developing atherosclerotic cardiovascular disease (ASCVD)?

A) Polysaccharides
B) Trans-fatty acids
C) Polyunsaturated fatty acids
D) Monounsaturated fatty acids

The answer is B: Dietary fats are related to the development of ASCVD, and the type of fat appears to be more important than the amount of fat consumed. Recent studies have highlighted concerns over the amounts of trans fats in our diets. Fatty acids can be divided into four categories: saturated, monounsaturated, polyunsaturated, and trans fats. Saturated fatty acids and trans fats are associated with an increased ASCVD risk. Monounsaturated and polyunsaturated fatty acids are associated with a decreased risk.

Margarines and partially hydrogenated vegetable oils contain larger amounts of trans fats and are present in many manufactured foods, such as prepared breads and cookies. Fast food restaurants where oils are maintained at high temperatures for a sustained period of time to fry meats and French fries also contain significant levels of trans fats.

Polysaccharides are complex carbohydrates, which consist of several sugar molecules bonded together. Traditional diets are high in carbohydrates and are associated with low rates of coronary heart disease. Intact fruits, vegetables, legumes, and whole grains are the most appropriate sources of carbohydrate. Most of them are rich in nonstarch polysaccharides (dietary fiber) that reduce total and low-density lipoprotein cholesterol.

Additional Reading: Dietary fatty acids. *Am Fam Physician.* 2009;80(4):345-350.

3. Patients with an inherited antithrombin III deficiency are at increased risk for developing which one of the following problems?

A) Aplastic anemia
B) Myelogenous leukemia
C) Venous thrombosis
D) Idiopathic thrombocytopenia purpura

The answer is C: Antithrombin III is a non–vitamin K-dependent protease that inhibits coagulation by neutralizing the enzymatic activity of thrombin (factors IIa, IXa, and Xa). Inherited antithrombin III deficiency is the result of an autosomal dominant mutation in which a patient has inherited one copy of the *SERPINC1* (also called *AT3*) gene on chromosome 1q25.1, which encodes for the antithrombin III protein. The condition is seen in less than 0.5% of the population; however, in patients with thrombosis, the mutation is found more frequently. Homozygous deficiency is usually lethal in utero.

The condition leads to an increased risk for venous and arterial thrombosis, which typically occurs in young adulthood. In the proper clinical setting, antithrombin III activity is measured, and when found to be low, antithrombin antigen is measured to look for mutations. However, testing is unreliable if the patient is anticoagulated with heparin or warfarin.

Additional Reading: Recurrent venous thromboembolism. *Am Fam Physician.* 2022;105(4):377-385.

4. You had seen a healthy 49-year-old African American man for a sprained ankle 2 weeks ago and noted an elevated blood pressure (BP). Other than a multivitamin, he takes no medications. His family history is remarkable for hypertension (HTN), and his paternal grandfather had a stroke at the age of 64 years. He has come today for a follow-up of his BP, and although his ankle has healed, his BP remains elevated at 168/96 mm Hg. Based on the most recent Eighth Joint National Committee (JNC 8) guidelines, which one of the following is recommended as a first choice for treating his HTN?

A) Lisinopril
B) Metoprolol
C) Amlodipine
D) Losartan

The answer is C: The JNC 8 guidelines recommend either a calcium channel blocker or a thiazide diuretic as the first-line medication choices for African American patients.

Additional Reading: Common questions about the initial management of hypertension. *Am Fam Physician.* 2015;91:172-177.

5. A 49-year-old White man has recently undergone a mechanical aortic valve replacement, as he was experiencing dyspnea on exertion from progressive stenosis of a congenital bicuspid aortic valve. Which of the following medications should he be taking?

A) Apixaban (Eliquis)
B) Rivaroxaban (Xarelto)
C) Warfarin (Coumadin)
D) Aspirin
E) None of the above

The answer is C: The only drug currently approved for use as an anticoagulant for a mechanical valve is warfarin. The other two novel oral anticoagulant agents, apixaban and rivaroxaban, are approved for use in atrial fibrillation for stroke prevention but not for mechanical valves. Patients who have a porcine valve replacement without atrial fibrillation do not require chronic anticoagulation after an initial 3 months of anticoagulation. Aspirin is an antiplatelet agent and not an anticoagulant.

Additional Reading: Is a novel anticoagulant right for your patient? *J Fam Pract*. 2014;63:22-28.

6. Which of the following is NOT considered a risk factor for myocardial infarction (MI)?

A) Obesity
B) Type A personality
C) Male sex
D) Alcohol use disorder
E) Sedentary lifestyle

The answer is D: Many studies have been published associating alcohol with reduced cardiovascular mortality, and alcohol has been shown to slightly increase high-density lipoprotein cholesterol (HDL-C) levels. The benefits may be due to wine, especially red wine, which contains flavonoids and other antioxidants found in grapes. The linkage reported in many of these studies may be due to other lifestyle factors such as increased physical activity and diets high in fruits and vegetables and lower in saturated fats, rather than alcohol consumption. No direct comparison trials have been done to determine the specific effect of wine or other alcohol on the risk of developing heart disease or stroke.

The American Heart Association does not recommend drinking wine or any other form of alcohol to reduce cardiovascular risks. Although it is not recommended to start drinking alcoholic beverages to reduce risk, a modest intake of alcohol is OK. This means an average of one to two drinks per day for men and one drink per day for women. (A drink is one 12 oz beer, 4 oz of wine, or 1.5 oz of 80-proof spirits.) Excessive drinking has been linked with hypertension (HTN), obesity, stroke, breast cancer, suicide, and accidents.

Risk factors for MI include the following:

- HTN
- Hyperlipidemia—particularly high total cholesterol, high LDL-C, and low HDL-C
- Cigarette smoking
- Diabetes mellitus
- Obesity (increased weight for height)
- Male sex
- Family history of coronary artery disease
- Sedentary lifestyle
- Type A personality
- Increased age
- Postmenopausal status
- Homocysteinemia

Additional Readings:
1. Myocardial infarction. In: Domino F, ed. *The 5-Minute Clinical Consult*. Wolters Kluwer; 2022.
2. www.heart.org/HEARTORG/HealthyLiving/HealthyEating/Nutrition/Alcohol-and-Heart-Health_UCM_305173_Article.jsp#V3vCiDbmrIU

7. Which of the following drugs is indicated for all patients in the treatment of congestive heart failure (CHF) related to systolic dysfunction?

A) Isosorbide
B) Diltiazem
C) Lisinopril
D) Nifedipine
E) Verapamil

The answer is C: All patients with CHF associated with systolic dysfunction (ejection fraction < 40%) will benefit from an angiotensin-converting enzyme inhibitor (ACEI; eg, ramipril, enalapril, lisinopril) or, if intolerant, from an angiotensin receptor blocker (ARB) (losartan, candesartan) along with a β-blocker (carvedilol, long-acting metoprolol succinate) unless hemodynamically unstable or suffering from resting dyspnea with congestion.

An aldosterone antagonist (spironolactone) is indicated for patients with resting dyspnea or for patients who are symptomatic from a recent myocardial infarction. Diuretics are indicated for symptomatic patients to maintain appropriate fluid balance. Symptomatic African Americans benefit from an isosorbide-hydralazine combination (BiDil). Digoxin is recommended only for patients who remain symptomatic despite diuretics, ACEIs, and β-blockers or for those in atrial fibrillation.

Updated 2022 American Heart Association guidelines, released April 2022, recommend the following classes of medications to treat people for heart failure with reduced ejection fraction (HFrEF), also called systolic failure as the left ventricle loses its ability to contract normally.

- Diuretics, which are recommended for patients with fluid retention.
- Angiotensin receptor–neprilysin inhibitors are a new class of drugs that inhibit angiotensin and neprilysin. This combined effect allows an optimization of the heart failure treatment by acting on both pathways of the renin-angiotensin-aldosterone and of the natriuretic peptides. Entresto (valsartan/sacubitril) is recommended and if not feasible, the use of an ACEI is recommended.
- ARBs are recommended for individuals with an intolerance or potential adverse reaction to ACEI medicines.
- Mineralocorticoid receptor antagonists (spironolactone, eplerenone) or β-blockers are also recommended as in the prior guideline.
- Sodium-glucose cotransporter-2 inhibitors are now also recommended for people with symptomatic chronic HFrEF regardless of the presence of type 2 diabetes.

Additional Readings:
1. Drugs for chronic heart failure. *Med Lett Drugs Ther*. 2021;63(1626):89-96.
2. *ACC, AHA, HFSA Issue Heart Failure Guideline*: https://www.acc.org/About-ACC/Press-Releases/2022/04/01/15/22/ACC-AHA-HFSA-Issue-Heart-Failure-Guideline

8. Side effects of hydroxymethylglutaryl coenzyme-A (HMG-CoA) reductase inhibitors (statins) include all of the following except:

A) Memory loss
B) Liver injury
C) Rhabdomyolysis
D) Increased diabetes risk
E) Cataracts

The answer is E: HMG-CoA reductase inhibitors (statins) are used for the treatment of moderate to severe hypercholesterolemia. These drugs (rosuvastatin, fluvastatin, atorvastatin, pitavastatin, lovastatin, pravastatin, and simvastatin) inhibit HMG-CoA reductase, the rate-limiting enzyme in cholesterol production. Statins decrease total cholesterol and low-density lipoprotein cholesterol levels and can increase the high-density lipoprotein cholesterol level.

The U.S. Food and Drug Administration issued a statement in 2015 related to side effects advising the following:

- Routine monitoring of liver enzymes (once considered standard procedure) was no longer needed because such monitoring had not been found to be effective in predicting or preventing the rare occurrences of serious liver injury associated with statin use. However, liver enzyme testing should still be performed before statin treatment is started and then as needed if there are symptoms of liver damage.
- Cognitive (brain-related) impairment, such as memory loss, forgetfulness, and confusion, has been reported by some statin users. The reports span all statin products and all age groups, but these experiences are rare, with those affected often reporting feeling "fuzzy" or unfocused in their thinking. In general, the symptoms were not serious and were reversible within a few weeks after the patient stopped using the statin. Some people affected in this way had been taking the medicine for a day; others had been taking it for years.
- Treatment with statins may increase the risk of the development of type 2 diabetes mellitus; hence, blood sugar levels may need to be assessed after instituting statin therapy. However, the heart benefit of statins outweighs this small increased risk.
- Some drugs are metabolized through the same pathways as statins, which increases both the amount of statin in the blood and the risk of myopathy, characterized by unexplained muscle weakness or pain. This appears to be primarily a concern for lovastatin.

Although not addressed in that advisory, the rare risk of developing rhabdomyolysis from high-dose statin therapy is around 1.5 for each 100,000 people taking statins. The most common signs and symptoms of rhabdomyolysis include severe muscle aching throughout the body, muscle weakness, and dark or cola-colored urine.

Routine eye examination for the detection of lens opacities was an initial recommendation, but studies have not found any causation between cataracts and statin use, and such examinations are no longer recommended.

Additional Reading: www.fda.gov/ForConsumers/ConsumerUpdates/ucm293330.htm

9. A 19-year-old female college soccer player presents with anxiety and difficulty sleeping following the discovery of a heart murmur on her preplacement physical. A male athlete at her school recently died while playing football because of undiagnosed idiopathic hypertrophic cardiomyopathy, and she is afraid she will die in a similar manner. Other than the murmur, her physical examination is normal, and her electrocardiogram shows no abnormalities. An echocardiogram revealed mild mitral valve prolapse (MVP). She is anxious, sleepless, and fearful of physical activity. Which one of the following would be most appropriate at this point?

A) An exercise tolerance test
B) Reassurance regarding the benign course of her condition
C) Prescribing an anxiolytic such as diazepam (Valium)
D) Referral to a cardiologist
E) Referral for group psychotherapy

The answer is B: Much of the psychological distress caused by the diagnosis of MVP is related to lack of information and fear of heart disease, which, as in this case, may be reinforced by the death of a friend or relative. A clear explanation of MVP, along with printed material, is a powerful aid in relieving the patient's emotional distress. The American Heart Association publishes a helpful booklet about this condition, which can be given to this patient. It is important to avoid reinforcing illness behavior with unnecessary testing, medications, or referrals to specialists.

Additional Reading: Mitral valve prolapse. In: Domino F, ed. *The 5-Minute Clinical Consult*. Wolters Kluwer; 2022.

10. A 34-year-old White man with a history of Wolff-Parkinson-White (WPW) syndrome calls your office to report that he feels fine, but his heart is racing again. You suggest that he go to the emergency department (ED) at the nearest hospital to be assessed. The ED physician calls to let you know that while the patient is alert and is in no acute distress, his pulse rate is 220 beats per minute. His blood pressure is 134/76 mm Hg, and his oxygen saturation is also normal at 98%. An electrocardiogram (ECG) reveals a regular, wide-complex tachycardia consistent with WPW. The ED physician has decided to use pharmacologic conversion for his initial treatment. Which one of the following would be the treatment of choice?

A) Verapamil (Calan)
B) Procainamide
C) Adenosine (Adenocard)
D) Digoxin

The answer is C: In hemodynamically stable patients, following vagal maneuvers, adenosine is considered first-line therapy for most supraventricular tachycardic arrhythmias, including WPW syndrome, in the acute phase. In patients with WPW syndrome, adenosine, calcium channel blockers, or digoxin may be used acutely, but they should not be used long-term because these atrioventricular (AV) nodal blocking agents can force conduction down the accessory pathway, predisposing the patient to ventricular fibrillation.

Because atrial tachycardia is not dependent on the AV node, these treatments do not terminate this arrhythmia but can be diagnostic by slowing the rate, allowing for better exposure of atrial activity on the ECG.

If the patient is clinically unstable (eg, altered mental status, chest pain, acute heart failure, hypotension, shock), immediate direct-current cardioversion is indicated. However, even in these cases, the high effectiveness and fast onset of adenosine may merit its use as first-line treatment, with cardioversion used only if adenosine is ineffective.

Supraventricular tachycardia (SVT) can occasionally result with a wide QRS complex; thus, it can be difficult to distinguish it from ventricular tachycardia (VT). In the acute setting, ventricular tachycardia should be assumed, particularly in patients who are hemodynamically unstable. Adenosine is safe and effective for diagnosis and treatment in undifferentiated regular wide complex tachycardia. If the underlying rhythm is SVT with aberrancy, it will be slowed or converted to sinus rhythm. If it is ventricular tachycardia, the rhythm will likely be unaffected, and procainamide, amiodarone, or sotalol should be administered. If the patient remains unstable, cardioversion is indicated.

Additional Reading: Diagnosis and management of common types of supraventricular tachycardia. *Am Fam Physician*. 2015;92(9):793-802

11. A 49-year-old long-distance truck driver presents to an urgent care center complaining of shortness of breath, which he states started suddenly when he was driving home from work. Which one of the following symptoms is more closely associated with a pulmonary embolism (PE) diagnosis than the others?

A) Rhonchi
B) Chest pain
C) Orthopnea
D) Wheezes

The answer is B: Chest pain is common in patients with a pulmonary embolus. When evaluating a patient with shortness of breath, the presence of orthopnea is more likely with heart failure (HF); wheezing with asthma or chronic obstructive pulmonary disease and rhonchi are relatively nonspecific, heard in various cardiopulmonary conditions from HF to interstitial lung disease. A commonly used prediction score for pulmonary embolism (PE) is as follows:

Clinical Finding	Score
Alternative diagnosis less likely than PE	3
Signs and symptoms of deep vein thrombosis	3
Pulse rate > 100 bpm	1.5
Previous PE or deep vein thrombosis	1.5
Surgery in the previous 4 wk or immobilization in the previous 4 d)	1.5
Cancer	1
Hemoptysis	1
Total score	

The pretest probability for a PE is based on the total score: <2 is low; 2 to 6 is intermediate; and ≥7 is high.

Additional Reading: Diagnosis of deep venous thrombosis and pulmonary embolism. *Am Fam Physician*. 2012;86(10):913-919.

12. You are seeing a 71-year-old man with a history of hypertension (HTN) and mild congestive heart failure (CHF) who presents complaining of gradually progressive dyspnea on exertion (DOE) over the past few weeks. At his baseline, he is able to walk several blocks but now feels winded after only a block and has been having some associated chest pain. He denies palpitations, syncope/near syncope, cough, orthopnea, or paroxysmal nocturnal dyspnea. He is compliant with his medications, which include a mini-dose aspirin, lisinopril 20 mg, furosemide 20 mg, and potassium chloride 10 mEq daily. His cardiac examination reveals a regular rate and rhythm, normal S1 and S2, and no S3, but he has an S4 and a 2/6 mid-systolic murmur at the left-upper sternal border that radiates to the carotids. His presentation is most consistent with which one of the following conditions?

A) Acute coronary syndrome
B) Mitral regurgitation
C) Mitral stenosis
D) Mitral valve prolapse
E) Aortic stenosis

The answer is E: Aortic stenosis occurs when there is obstruction in the blood flow through the aortic valve. The causes for aortic stenosis include previous rheumatic fever with associated damage to the valves, excessive calcification of the valves leading to narrowing, or congenital causes (eg, bifid aortic valve). Men are more commonly affected than are women.

Cardiac output is usually maintained until the stenosis is severe. The classic symptoms of angina, exertional syncope, and dyspnea generally follow an extended latent period during which the patient is asymptomatic. Symptomatic patients should be advised to avoid strenuous activity. Physical findings include a harsh systolic ejection murmur found at the left sternal border. Radiation to the carotids, although not specific, is sensitive and, if not present, essentially rules out aortic stenosis. A palpable left ventricular heave and delayed carotid pulse upstroke are characteristics. Some patients may present with findings of CHF.

The survival of patients with aortic stenosis is nearly normal until the onset of severe symptoms (the classic triad is angina, dyspnea, and syncope), which can result in sudden death. Three quarters will die within 3 years after the onset of symptoms. Echocardiography is recommended, and severe cases should be referred for possible valve replacement.

Additional Reading: Aortic stenosis: diagnosis and treatment. *Am Fam Physician*. 2016;93(5):371-378.

13. You are seeing a 57-year-old obese White man with type 2 diabetes, who is treated with metformin 500 mg bid. You are asked to complete a preoperative evaluation before scheduling him for elective knee replacement surgery, as he is unable to climb up a flight of stairs without pain. He denies chest pain and dyspnea on exertion and sleeps through the night without difficulty. A metabolic panel several months ago revealed normal renal function, and his last A1c level was 6.9%. He has no other significant health problems.

Based on current guidelines, which one of the following diagnostic studies would be appropriate before surgery, because the results could alter the perioperative care for this patient?

A) Pulmonary function tests (PFTs)
B) Chest radiography
C) Electrocardiogram (ECG)
D) A hemoglobin A1c level
E) None of the above

The answer is E: Preoperative testing (chest radiography, ECG, laboratory testing, urinalysis) is often performed before surgical procedures. A preoperative evaluation before noncardiac surgery requires knowledge of the cardiovascular risk from the procedure and the functional status of the patient along with assessment of other clinical factors that can increase risk. This patient is undergoing a low-risk procedure, and he is at a low risk for complications; thus, none of the listed diagnostic studies are indicated.

The Revised Cardiac Risk Index (also called the modified Goldman index) is a validated way to estimate the risk of developing cardiac complication after noncardiac surgery. A patient is assigned 1 point for each of the following:

1. ***High-risk procedure***: intraperitoneal, intrathoracic, suprainguinal vascular surgical procedures
2. ***Ischemic heart disease***: previous myocardial infarction *or* positive exercise test *or* current anginal chest pain, current nitrate therapy *or* a pathologic Q wave on ECG
3. ***Congestive heart failure (CHF)***: pulmonary edema or paroxysmal nocturnal dyspnea *or* current bilateral rales, S3 gallop *or* chest x-ray with pulmonary vascular redistribution
4. ***Cerebrovascular disease***: history of transient ischemic attack, stroke
5. ***Diabetes***: requiring treatment with insulin
6. ***Renal insufficiency***: preoperative creatinine level >2.0 mg/dL

Score	Risk Index Class	Postoperative Cardiac Complication Risk
0	I	0.4%
1	II	0.9%
2	III	6.6%
3 or more	IV	11.0%

Patients who fall into class III or IV are considered at high risk and should undergo perioperative screening. Patients with signs or symptoms of active cardiovascular disease should be evaluated with an ECG. Chest radiography is reasonable for patients at risk for postoperative pulmonary complications (eg, chronic obstructive pulmonary disease and CHF) if the results would change perioperative management, while PFTs are not helpful.

This patient has been diagnosed with diabetes, and an A1c test is only recommended if the result would change perioperative management, which is unlikely. However, a random glucose test is suggested for patients at high risk of undiagnosed diabetes mellitus. Electrolyte and creatinine testing is indicated for those with chronic diseases or those who are on medications associated with electrolyte abnormalities or renal failure. A urinalysis is recommended only for patients undergoing invasive urologic procedures and those undergoing implantation of foreign materials. Finally, a complete blood count is indicated for those at risk for anemia or if significant perioperative blood loss is anticipated.

Additional Reading: Preoperative testing before noncardiac surgery: guidelines and recommendations. *Am Fam Physician*. 2013;87(6):414-418.

14. According to the U.S. Preventive Services Task Force (USPSTF), which one of the following patients should undergo (grade B recommendation) screening to look for an asymptomatic abdominal aortic aneurysm (AAA)?

A) Men aged 55 to 65 years who have ever smoked
B) Men aged 65 to 75 years who have ever smoked
C) Men aged 65 to 75 years who have never smoked
D) Women aged 65 to 75 years who have ever smoked

The answer is B: Cigarette smokers are five times more likely than nonsmokers to develop an AAA. The risk is associated with the number of years the patient has smoked and declines with cessation. Although women tend to develop AAA in their 60s, the USPSTF concludes that the current evidence is insufficient to assess the balance of benefits and harms of screening for women who have ever smoked (grade I recommendation). Whites are at greater risk than African Americans. Hypertension is less of a risk factor than cigarette smoking.

Additional Reading: https://www.uspreventiveservicestaskforce.org/uspstf/recommendation/abdominal-aortic-aneurysm-screening

15. Which one of the following drugs used in the treatment of congestive heart failure (CHF) has been shown to increase survival?

A) Digoxin
B) Furosemide
C) Spironolactone
D) Enalapril
E) Carvedilol

The answer is E: All these medications are useful in the treatment of CHF (related to systolic failure); however, only β-blockers (carvedilol, metoprolol) have been shown to reduce mortality in select patients—especially in patients with idiopathic dilated cardiomyopathy. With slower heart rates, diastolic function and ventricular filling improve. The ejection fraction may improve over 6 to 12 months, giving rise to improved exercise capacity. Randomized controlled trials have shown significant reduction in all-cause mortality and cardiac events in patients taking carvedilol with mildly symptomatic CHF and an ejection fraction less than or equal to 35%. The following drug classes are useful in the treatment of CHF:

- *Diuretics* have been shown to be useful in decreasing fluid overload in patients with mild CHF. Thiazide diuretics inhibit sodium chloride reabsorption at the distal tubule; however, they are not usually effective in patients with advanced symptoms. In those situations, the loop diuretics (eg, furosemide and bumetanide) are indicated; these agents inhibit solute reabsorption in the loop of Henle.
- *Aldosterone antagonists* (spironolactone, eplerenone), also known as potassium-sparing diuretics, are also used in the treatment of CHF. The main action of aldosterone is to increase sodium reabsorption by the kidneys, which increases the excretion of potassium. Aldosterone receptor antagonists block the effects of aldosterone, resulting in a diuretic effect by decreasing sodium reabsorption and water retention by the kidneys. Electrolytes should be monitored because of changes in serum potassium, as well as in sodium, magnesium, and calcium.
- *Angiotensin-converting enzyme (ACE) inhibitors* (captopril, enalapril, lisinopril, ramipril) serve as preload and afterload reducers by blocking (1) the production of angiotensin II, a potent vasoconstrictor, and (2) the release of aldosterone. ACE inhibitors are effective in the treatment of CHF and have been shown to increase survival in affected patients. Electrolytes should be monitored because of the possibility of hyperkalemia and renal insufficiency (especially in patients with renal artery stenosis). ACE inhibitors have also been shown to be beneficial in promoting renal blood flow in diabetes.
- *Angiotensin receptor blockers* (losartan, valsartan, candesartan) have similar effects to those of ACE inhibitors, although conclusive trials have not been reported regarding equal effectiveness.
- *Digoxin* has been shown to be effective in severe CHF and in CHF complicated by atrial fibrillation. Its mechanism of action involves the energy-dependent sodium-potassium pump, leading to increased intracellular calcium and a positive inotropic effect. Elderly patients and those taking other medication (eg, quinidine and amiodarone) are at increased risk for toxicity and routine monitoring of digoxin levels. Potassium levels should also be monitored closely, as hypokalemia can precipitate arrhythmias in patients taking digoxin.
- *Vasodilators* (eg, hydralazine and isosorbide dinitrate) can be used if patients are unable to tolerate ACE inhibitors. These work by decreasing preload as a result of vasodilation.

Additional Readings:
1. Drugs for chronic heart failure. *Med Lett Drugs Ther*. 2021;63(1626):89-96.
2. *ACC, AHA, HFSA Issue Heart Failure Guideline*. https://www.acc.org/About-ACC/Press-Releases/2022/04/01/15/22/ACC-AHA-HFSA-Issue-Heart-Failure-Guideline

16. A 67-year-old White man is being monitored the day after spinal surgery, and the nurses report that his cardiac monitor shows a supraventricular tachycardia (SVT) and that he is hemodynamically unstable. Which one of the following is the most appropriate treatment?

A) Carotid massage
B) Synchronized cardioversion
C) Adenosine
D) Verapamil
E) Digoxin

The answer is B: SVT is characterized by a rapid regular rhythm with a heart rate between 100 and 200 beats per minute. The electrocardiogram (ECG) demonstrates a narrow QRS complex and abnormal P waves. Although patients may be asymptomatic, some will complain of chest pain, palpitations, and shortness of breath. Hemodynamically unstable patients with SVT require immediate treatment with electrical synchronized cardioversion.

Vagal stimulation can be attempted for those patients who are stable with various physical maneuvers. Carotid massage can be performed by extending the neck with the head turned away from the side being massaged. Gentle pressure is applied beneath the angle of the jaw in a circular motion for about 10 seconds. This maneuver is contraindicated for patients with previous cerebrovascular accidents or carotid bruits.

The Valsalva maneuver is one of the more common ways to stimulate the vagus nerve. The patient is instructed to bear down as if having a bowel movement. Alternatively, the patient can attempt to blow through an occluded straw for several seconds. Valsalva maneuvers increase intrathoracic pressure and stimulate the vagus nerve activation. Finally, placing a cold ice bag on the face for about 10 seconds creates a physiologic response similar to that which occurs if a person is submerged in cold water (diver's reflex).

If these measures are unsuccessful, medications, including adenosine, verapamil, diltiazem, or a β-blocker, can be used. Untreated SVT may lead to heart failure.

Additional Reading: Clinical Manifestations, Diagnosis, and Evaluation of Narrow QRS Complex Tachycardias. In: *UpToDate*. 2022.

17. Many medications used to treat heart failure will reduce B-type natriuretic peptide (BNP) concentrations; thus, patients with stable chronic failure on such medications may have normal BNP levels. However, some medications will increase BNP levels. Which one of the following medications can increase BNP levels?

A) Lisinopril
B) Valsartan
C) Spironolactone
D) Digoxin

The answer is D: BNP is one of four human natriuretic peptides. The first was identified in 1983 and named atrial natriuretic peptide, and a closely related peptide was discovered in pig brains in 1988 and hence named brain-type natriuretic peptide. BNP was subsequently found in cardiac tissues, with levels correlating with congestive heart failure (CHF) symptoms. BNP levels increase with increasing left ventricular dysfunction.

High ventricular filling pressures stimulate the release of atrial natriuretic peptide and BNP. Both peptides have diuretic, natriuretic, and antihypertensive effects by inhibiting the renin-angiotensin-aldosterone system. In addition, BNP may provide a protective effect against the detrimental fibrosis and remodeling that occur in progressive heart failure (HF).

Medications used to treat HF, including angiotensin-converting enzyme inhibitors (lisinopril), angiotensin receptor blockers (valsartan), and aldosterone antagonists (spironolactone), can reduce BNP concentrations. Therefore, many patients with chronic stable HF will have BNP levels in the normal diagnostic range (BNP < 100 pg/mL [100 ng/L]). However, digoxin and some β-blockers appear to increase natriuretic peptide concentrations.

BNP is stored as a precursor (proBNP) in secretory granules in the ventricles and to a lesser extent in the atria. After proBNP is secreted in response to volume overload and resulting myocardial stretch, it is cleaved to the 76-peptide, biologically inert N-terminal fragment NT-proBNP and the 32-peptide, biologically active hormone BNP. The two fragments are secreted into the plasma and can be evaluated for use in the management of CHF.

Patients presenting with acute shortness of breath can have a nonspecific history, physical and chest x-ray findings, and confounding comorbidities that make it difficult to differentiate between cardiac and noncardiac etiologies. The primary value of BNP and NT-proBNP testing in such situations is to assist in the differential diagnosis of acute dyspnea and possible CHF.

Additional Reading: The role of BNP testing in heart failure. *Am Fam Physician*. 2006;74(11):1893-1900.

BNP levels less than 100 pg/mL have a 90% negative predictive value and if more than 500 pg/mL have a 90% positive predictive value for the diagnosis of CHF in patients with acute dyspnea. For intermediate levels (100-500 pg/mL), underlying LV dysfunction, renal insufficiency, cor pulmonale, or acute pulmonary embolism need to be considered as well.

18. Which of the following is not considered a first-line medication for the treatment of hypertension in the general, non-Black, population, according to the Eighth Joint National Committee (JNC 8) guidelines?

A) Metoprolol
B) Lisinopril
C) Hydrochlorothiazide
D) Losartan
E) Amlodipine

The answer is A: β-Blockers, such as metoprolol, are no longer considered first-line antihypertensive medications in JNC 8 guidelines. A Cochrane review concluded that although β-blockers provided modest improvements in cardiovascular outcomes for hypertensive patients, there was no associated mortality benefit. JNC 8 guidelines recommend the use of one or more agents from the following four classes—angiotensin-converting enzyme (ACE) inhibitors, angiotensin receptor blockers (ARBs), calcium channel blockers, or thiazide-type diuretics as initial choices for the general, non-Black, population. These agents should be titrated to the target dose before adding a second agent, although initiating two medications simultaneously may be considered for patients with markedly elevated blood pressure or multiple comorbidities. ACE inhibitors (eg, lisinopril) and ARBs (eg, losartan) should not be prescribed concurrently because of the increased risk for renal complications.

Additional Reading: Common questions about the initial management of hypertension. *Am Fam Physician*. 2015;91(3):172-177.

19. A 66-year-old White man with chronic atrial fibrillation has been on warfarin (Coumadin) daily since he was diagnosed 3 years ago. You have been monitoring the international normalized ratio (INR) regularly and the laboratory calls to inform you that his INR is 7.5 today. Your nurse calls the patient, and he states that he has had no obvious bleeding and feels well. You decide to do which of the following?

A) Stop warfarin and repeat INR in 24 hours.
B) Stop warfarin, give vitamin K, and repeat INR in 24 hours.
C) Stop warfarin and repeat INR in 3 days.
D) Stop warfarin and give vitamin K and fresh frozen plasma with daily INRs.

The answer is A: Warfarin is highly protein-bound to albumin and inhibits the formation of clotting factors II, VII, IX, and X. The INR is the patient's prothrombin time (PT) divided by the mean of the normal PT, with this ratio expressed as the INR.

After starting warfarin, a steady state is typically achieved in 2 weeks. A dosage of 4 to 5 mg/d is typical, although the required dosage is variable. Guidelines recommend that the INR be checked at least four times during the first week of therapy. The risk of bleeding is greatest in the first 6 to 12 weeks of treatment, so monitoring the INR weekly is appropriate during that time. The frequency is decreased depending on the stability of the INR; however, the maximum time between tests should be no more than 6 weeks, and most recommend monthly.

Patients with stable INR values who have changes by more than 0.2 below or 0.4 above the goal INR should be evaluated for the cause of the change. These can range from laboratory error, noncompliance, drug or dietary interactions to a change in the patient's health. If no reversible cause is found, a change in dosage should be considered, with a second INR within 2 weeks. Close follow-up with repeated testing is needed because the patients who have the most variation in results are most likely to develop bleeding or thromboembolism.

In patients who are stable with no signs of bleeding, recommendations for treatment are less aggressive than in the patient who is at an increased risk for bleeding. The following guidelines have been suggested to manage such patients with an elevated INR:

- For an INR value that is above the target but <4.5, it is reasonable to decrease or hold a warfarin dose with daily monitoring and resume at the lower dosage once the INR is within the therapeutic range.
- For INR 4.5 to 10 (as in this patient), it is recommended to hold the next one to two doses of warfarin, repeat the INR in 24 hours, and resume at a lower dosage once INR is within the therapeutic range.
- For an INR > 10, it is recommended to hold warfarin and administer vitamin K (2.5-5 mg orally as one dose), repeat the INR, and repeat vitamin K that may be necessary because the half-life of warfarin is longer than the half-life of vitamin K. Oral vitamin K is effective and may have fewer risks than the parenterally administered form. Warfarin is resumed at an appropriate dose when INR is within the therapeutic range.

Additional Reading: Updated guidelines on outpatient anticoagulation. *Am Fam Physician*. 2013;87(8):556-566.

20. You are seeing a 47-year-old patient for a second visit as her blood pressure has been elevated for the past few months. She has working hard on decreasing the salt in her diet and has been walking daily, but her values remain elevated today (148/94). She has diabetes, which has been well controlled with metformin (last hemoglobin A1c level was 7.1%). A drug from which one of the following classes of medications would be the most appropriate to prescribe for the treatment of hypertension in this diabetic patient?

A) α-Blocker
B) Angiotensin-converting enzyme inhibitor (ACEI)
C) β-Blocker
D) Calcium channel blocker (CCB)
E) Diuretic

The answer is B: Eighth Joint National Committee guidelines recommend treating diabetics without renal insufficiency like in any other patient (initial therapy with thiazide diuretic, an ACEI or angiotensin receptor blocker (ARB), or a CCB); however; most would choose an ACEI (eg, captopril, enalapril, lisinopril, or ramipril), or an ARB for those who cannot tolerate an ACEI, to slow diabetic-associated renal disease progression. ACEIs function as afterload reducers by inhibiting the renin-angiotensin-aldosterone system and are the recommended first-line agents for any patient (with or without diabetes) who have chronic kidney disease.

ACEIs block the conversion of angiotensin I to angiotensin II, resulting in a decrease in aldosterone production, which leads to increased sodium and water excretion. Hemodynamic effects include decreased vascular resistance and increased renal blood flow. Side effects include headache, nausea, dizziness, and, in up to 20% of patients, an irritating nonproductive cough. Acute renal failure has been precipitated in patients with renal artery stenosis (RAS); thus, patients with preexisting renal disease or RAS require close monitoring of renal function when ACEIs are administered. Angioneurotic edema can occur at any time during therapy.

Additional Reading: Treatment of hypertension in patients with diabetes mellitus. In: *UpToDate*. 2022.

21. Which one of the following potentially severe complications can be seen with the use of warfarin that is unrelated to bleeding complications?

A) Hepatitis
B) Pancreatitis
C) Peripheral neuropathy
D) Pulmonary fibrosis
E) Skin necrosis

The answer is E: Warfarin is an anticoagulant that works by the inhibition of vitamin K-dependent clotting factors (II, VII, IX, and X). The medication is used in stroke prophylaxis for patients with prior neurologic events, atrial fibrillation, mechanical heart valves, or previous deep vein thrombosis or pulmonary embolism.

Most complications are related to bleeding; however, other side effects, including nausea, vomiting, fever, burning of the feet, and rashes, can occur. The most worrisome complication unrelated to excessive bleeding is skin necrosis, which usually occurs within the first week of therapy. Some cases may be severe enough to require surgical debridement or even amputation.

Additional Reading: Warfarin-induced skin necrosis. *J Am Acad Dermatol*. 2009;61(2):325-332.

22. You are seeing a 78-year-old White woman who has not been feeling well. She is complaining of feeling light-headed and dizzy, especially when she gets up from bed or after sitting. She was recently placed on amitriptyline to treat postherpetic neuralgia and you suspect that she is suffering from orthostatic hypotension. Which one of the following statements about orthostatic hypotension is true?

A) It can cause syncope.
B) The condition results from volume overload.
C) It is defined as a decrease in systolic blood pressure (SBP) that occurs when changing from a standing position to a sitting position.
D) It is commonly associated with a decrease in the heart rate.
E) It is rarely associated with antidepressant medications.

The answer is A: Orthostatic hypotension is defined as a decrease in SBP of at least 20 mm Hg or at least 10 mm Hg in the diastolic blood pressure, which occurs when the patient rises from a supine position to an upright position. The patient should lie flat for 3 to 5 minutes and have a baseline blood pressure (BP) recorded. They are then asked to stand and BP recorded after a minute and repeated in 3 minutes. The upright readings are compared with the baseline pressures. A compensatory increase in the pulse rate is seen, because the cardiac output is increased to address the fall in BP.

Causes of orthostatic hypotension include volume depletion, medications (eg, tricyclic antidepressants and antihypertensive agents), and autonomic dysfunction (as seen in diabetic patients). Elderly patients are at an increased risk, and syncope may result. Treatment involves discontinuation of offending pharmacologic medications and, if not possible, increasing the fluids and instructing the patient to be careful when changing positions until the BP stabilizes and the dizziness has passed.

Additional Reading: Orthostatic hypotension: a practical approach. *Am Fam Physician*. 2022;105(1):39-49.

23. A 71-year-old White man presents with complaint of leg pain when walking. He walks his dog daily, but after going about 50 yards he must stop because of an achy pain in his legs. After resting for a while, the pain resolves, and he is able to resume walking. You suspect intermittent claudication and obtain an ankle-brachial index (ABI). This patient's ABI was 0.75, consistent with which of the following?

A) A normal reading
B) Mild arterial insufficiency
C) Moderate arterial insufficiency
D) Severe arterial insufficiency

The answer is B: The ABI is used to diagnose intermittent claudication of the lower extremities. Claudication results from atherosclerosis in the arteries supplying the blood flow to the muscles of the legs. As blood flow is limited to the muscles in response to an increased demand with exercise, there is subsequent ischemic pain. Once the demand has diminished with rest, the pain resolves, only to return with resumption of activity. Pain typically is felt in one or both calves but can also occur in the feet, thighs, or hips and buttocks. The pain is usually of an achy or crampy nature, which resolves after a few minutes of rest, reoccurring again after walking the same distance. The condition is exacerbated by walking rapidly or uphill because the leg muscles demand more blood flow for these activities.

The ABI is useful to evaluate the patency of the blood flow to the lower extremities. It is a comparison of the systolic blood pressure (SBP) at the ankle with that of the brachial artery in the arm. The test involves obtaining the brachial (arm) SBP, then placing the blood pressure cuff around the lower leg and inflating the cuff above the brachial SBP. The ankle SBP is obtained by placing a Doppler probe over the dorsalis pedis or posterior tibial arteries and listening for the pulse to return as the cuff is slowly deflated. The ABI is calculated by dividing the ankle SBP by the brachial SBP, reported in percent.

The normal ankle SBP is ≥90% of the brachial SBP, whereas arterial insufficiency results in a reading lower than 90%. Readings between 90% and 70% are seen with mild insufficiency, readings between 70% and 50% with moderate insufficiency; and readings below 50% with severe insufficiency. This patient has a reading of 0.75 (75%) consistent with mild insufficiency.

Additional Reading: Lower extremity peripheral artery disease: diagnosis and treatment. *Am Fam Physician*. 2019;99(6):362-369.

24. Which one of the following sequences represents how a typical anteroseptal myocardial infract (MI) progresses on a patient's electrocardiogram?

A) ST segments elevate, T waves invert, Q waves develop, and T waves peak
B) Q waves develop, T waves peak, ST segments elevate, and T waves invert
C) T waves invert, Q waves develop, ST segments elevate, and T waves peak
D) T waves peak, ST segments elevate, Q waves develop, and T waves invert
E) T waves peak, Q waves develop, ST segments elevate, and T waves invert

The answer is D: The typical progression of electrocardiographic (ECG) changes seen with an MI begins with peaked T waves, followed by ST-segment elevation. Next Q waves develop and finally T waves invert. In anteroseptal infarction, ECG changes are usually noted in leads V1 through V3. Q waves indicate a transmural infarct.

Additional Reading: ECG tutorial: myocardial infarction. In: *UpToDate*. 2022.

25. For which of the following patients with a deep vein thrombosis (DVT) is a comprehensive evaluation recommended?

A) A 45-year-old woman with an idiopathic DVT
B) A 55-year-old man who developed a calf DVT after a 6-hour car ride
C) A 62-year-old executive who developed a DVT after a recent transatlantic flight
D) A 69-year-old smoker with a history of non–small cell cancer of lung and a left calf DVT
E) A 75-year-old man with an idiopathic right thigh DVT

The answer is A: A comprehensive evaluation is indicated in younger patients (<50 years) with an idiopathic DVT, patients with recurrent thrombosis, and patients with a family history of thromboembolism. Other than patient A, there is a likely reason for each of the above patients to have developed a DVT, and patient E is older than the recommendations suggested for a comprehensive workup, even though he has an idiopathic event.

A comprehensive workup would include measuring protein S, protein C, antithrombin III (ATIII), factor V Leiden, prothrombin 20210A mutation, antiphospholipid antibodies, and homocysteine levels, and in addition to the above indications, when venous thrombosis is detected in an unusual site or if a patient suffers from warfarin-induced skin necrosis.

Additional Reading: Diagnosis of deep venous thrombosis and pulmonary embolism. *Am Fam Physician*. 2012;86(10):913-919.

26. A 76-year-old White man presents with complaints of palpitations and chest pain, which he characterizes as a mild nonexertional discomfort. He has a history of type 2 diabetes and is on an angiotensin-converting enzyme inhibitor for his well-controlled hypertension. He reports that he keeps busy with hobbies and plays golf twice a week. On examination, you detect an irregular heart rhythm, and his electrocardiogram is demonstrated atrial fibrillation with a rapid ventricular response. After his heart rate is brought under control with metoprolol, what is the best recommendation for anticoagulation therapy in this situation?

A) He should be on aspirin to prevent strokes.
B) He should be on clopidogrel (Plavix) to prevent strokes.
C) He should be on anticoagulation with a direct oral anticoagulant (DOAC) after considering his CHA2DS2-VASc score.
D) No anticoagulation is recommended because his heart rate is well controlled on metoprolol.

The answer is C: Guidelines including those from the American College of Cardiology (ACC) and American Heart Association (AHA) recommend that patients with nonvalvular atrial fibrillation, who are at low risk of stroke, be treated with antiplatelet therapy with aspirin or clopidogrel daily, whereas patients at higher risk should be anticoagulated (warfarin or a novel oral anticoagulant).

	Condition	Points
C	Congestive heart failure (or left ventricular systolic dysfunction)	1
H	Hypertension (HTN): blood pressure consistently above 140/90 mm Hg (or treated HTN on medication)	1
A_2	Age ≥75 y	2
D	Diabetes mellitus	1
S_2	Prior stroke, transient ischemic attack, or thromboembolism	2
V	Vascular disease (eg, peripheral artery disease, myocardial infarction [MI], and aortic plaque)	1
A	Age 65-74 y	1
Sc	Sex category (ie, female)	1

This patient's score is 4 (older than 75 years, with HTN and diabetes), so anticoagulation with a DOAC or warfarin would be recommended. In 2019, AHA/ACC guidelines were updated to preference DOACs over warfarin in nonvalvular atrial fibrillation (AF) (AF without moderate to severe mitral stenosis or mechanical valve) as in this patient.

Once a decision is made that anticoagulation is indicated, it needs to be balanced with the risk of bleeding. Various scales have been developed to estimate such risk. The Outpatient Bleeding Risk Index (OBRI) is a well-accepted validated tool used to predict the risk of bleeding in patients taking warfarin. The OBRI includes four risk factors, each counting as 1 point:

1. Age above 65 years
2. History of stroke
3. History of gastrointestinal bleeding
4. Presence of one or more of the following: recent MI, severe anemia (hematocrit < 30%), diabetes, or renal impairment

Score	Risk Category	Bleeding Risk
0	Low	3%
1-2	Intermediate	12%
3-4	High	48%

This patient's OBRI score is 2 (age > 65 y, diabetes), placing him at intermediate risk, and he should be considered for anticoagulation.

Additional Reading: Management of atrial fibrillation: updated guidance from the AHA, ACC, and HRS. *Am Fam Physician.* 2020;101(2):123-124.

27. Your patient is being treated for an acute deep vein thrombosis with heparin and has developed rectal bleeding. The best way to reverse the anticoagulation effects associated with heparin therapy is to administer which one of the following treatments?

A) Cryoprecipitate
B) Vitamin K
C) Protamine sulfate
D) Fresh frozen plasma
E) Platelets

The answer is C: Heparin is an anticoagulant that works by binding to and activating antithrombin III, a potent anticoagulant that prevents thrombin generation and fibrin formation. Heparin is used to treat and prevent thrombosis and can be administered either intravenously or subcutaneously. The major side effect is bleeding, and in most cases, bleeding can be controlled by stopping the intravenous (IV) heparin administration. However, if necessary, the best way to rapidly reverse heparin's anticoagulant effect is by administering protamine sulfate.

Another relatively common complication (seen in up to 10% of patients) is heparin-induced thrombocytopenia. This condition can lead to a paradoxical life-threatening arterial thrombosis. Discontinuation of the heparin usually reverses the thrombocytopenia.

The partial thromboplastin time (PTT) is used to determine the time it takes blood to clot and should be monitored when IV heparin is administered. The goal for heparin anticoagulation is usually 1.5 to 2.0 times the normal value, and the change from an increase or decrease in heparin dosing is usually detected 4 hours later. Low-molecular-weight heparin has a similar anticoagulation effect, but PTT and thrombin times are minimally affected, and laboratory monitoring is not required.

Patients should not take aspirin while taking heparin; intramuscular injections should also be avoided. Long-term use of heparin is associated with an increased risk of osteoporosis.

Additional Reading: Drugs for treatment and prevention of venous thromboembolism. *Med Lett Drugs Ther.* 2022;64(1655):113-120.

28. A 31-year-old White man presents with episodes of fleeting chest pain, and he is worried that he has a heart problem because his older sister has recently been diagnosed with mitral valve prolapse (MVP). This heart disorder is typically associated with which one of the following conditions?

A) Obesity
B) Syncope
C) Rheumatic heart disease
D) A myxomatous transformation of the valve leaflet
E) A diastolic click that disappears with Valsalva maneuver

The answer is D: MVP, which is also called systolic click syndrome, Barlow syndrome, or floppy valve syndrome, is a relatively common finding that is associated with myxomatous transformation of the valve leaflet. Myxomatous transformation is seen histologically as the disruption and loss of the normal valvular architecture, with an increase in ground substance but no associated inflammatory reaction. MVP is usually asymptomatic but may cause chest pain, palpitations, or dyspnea. The condition usually affects healthy, young, 15- to 30-year-old, thin women.

MVP produces a mid-systolic click, followed by a late systolic murmur, and becomes louder with Valsalva maneuver, although the presence of both click and murmur is not necessary for the diagnosis. A high-pitched late systolic crescendo-decrescendo murmur heard best at the apex may also be present. In patients with MVP, cardiac arrhythmias, including premature ventricular contractions, paroxysmal supraventricular tachycardia, and ventricular tachycardia, may cause palpitations and may need treatment (usually with β-blockers). Such symptoms often cause anxiety about the condition, but it is considered benign, although, in rare cases, it can progress to mitral insufficiency because of rupture of the chordae tendineae and may require valve replacement.

Additional Reading: Mitral valve prolapse. In: Domino F, ed. *The 5-Minute Clinical Consult*. Wolters Kluwer; 2022.

29. A 53-year-old White male smoker, with a history of hypertension, presents with complaints of chest pain. Which of the following statements would be most consistent with a diagnosis of angina?

A) He reports that the pain typically lasts 1-2 hours.
B) He reports associated chest wall tenderness.
C) He reports no pain radiating to his jaw or left arm.
D) He reports associated nausea and feels like vomiting.

The answer is D: "Angina" is a term used for chest pain caused by reduced blood flow to the heart muscles and is a symptom of coronary artery disease. Angina pectoris is typically described as substernal chest pain or pressure that lasts from 2 to 10 minutes and rarely as much as 30 minutes. Symptoms are usually precipitated by physical exertion or stress and are relieved with rest. It may radiate to the neck, jaw, or left arm, and patients often report associated shortness of breath, dizziness, nausea, and vomiting with diaphoresis. Atypical presentations can include epigastric pain, indigestion, right-arm pain, and light-headedness. Symptoms that occur without associated chest pain are referred to as anginal equivalents.

Pain is usually relieved with sublingual nitroglycerin, and medical treatment is with the prescription of nitrates, β-blockers, and calcium channel blockers. An electrocardiogram may have ST-segment depression or T-wave inversion, but in many cases it is normal. An exercise stress test can be used to clarify the diagnosis. Angina is classified based on classic symptoms:

Stable: Intensity, character, and frequency of episodes are predictable; angina occurs in response to a known amount of exercise or stress.

Unstable: Intensity, frequency, and duration vary and are unpredictable; pain is precipitated by a lesser amount of exercise, or the angina is longer in duration. Angina at rest or new-onset angina is considered unstable.

Variant: Pain may occur at rest and is secondary to spasm of the coronary arteries, rather than from atherosclerotic narrowing of the arteries.

Additional Reading: Pathophysiology and clinical presentation of ischemic chest pain. In: *UpToDate*. 2022.

30. A 57-year-old Hispanic woman has presented to the emergency department with complaints that she is light-headed and that her heart is racing. Her electrocardiogram is consistent with a supraventricular tachycardia (SVT). Which of the following is the best medication to use in the emergent treatment of SVT?

A) Digoxin
B) Diltiazem
C) Verapamil
D) Adenosine
E) Isoproterenol

The answer is D: Treatments for stable patients, who are experiencing an SVT (also referred to as regular *narrow QRS tachycardias*), include inducing a vagal response with various maneuvers. These include asking the patient to "bear down" or cough; carotid sinus massage; and placing an ice bag on the face or swallowing ice-cold water. Unilateral carotid sinus massage is done at the angle of the jaw on one side for 3 to 5 seconds. Patients with a history of carotid artery disease are at increased risk for the dislodgment of plaque, which may lead to stroke.

Adenosine (Adenocard) and verapamil (Isoptin) administered intravenously are also effective if the previously mentioned measures fail to succeed. Adenosine is preferred because of its rapid onset of action and short half-life. In unstable patients, low-energy electrical cardioversion is the treatment of choice, and many patients can be subsequently treated with radiofrequency ablation.

Additional Reading: Diagnosis and management of common types of supraventricular tachycardia. *Am Fam Physician*. 2015;92(9):793-802.

31. A 47-year-old car salesman presents to your office with complaints that his heart seems to be skipping and he is having some associated shortness of breath. He reports that he had been celebrating an excellent month of sales and had been drinking excessively the night before. On cardiac examination, you hear an irregular heartbeat and find a rapid pulse rate of 132 beats per minute. Which one of the following is the most likely diagnosis?

A) Atrial fibrillation
B) Ventricular fibrillation
C) Ventricular tachycardia
D) Premature ventricular contractions

The answer is A: Atrial fibrillation is the most commonly diagnosed cardiac arrhythmia. On auscultation, the rhythm is considered "irregularly irregular," and the electrocardiogram is characterized by the absence of P waves with an irregular ventricular response. The atrial rate can range from 400 to 600 beats per minute, whereas the ventricular rate usually ranges from 80 to 180 beats per minute. Causes include thyrotoxicosis, rheumatic or ischemic heart disease, hypertension, pericarditis, and excessive alcohol intake. Once symptoms are controlled, the major concern is the associated risk for a stroke secondary to cardiac embolism.

The rapid ventricular response of atrial fibrillation is treated with rate-controlling medications. β-Blockers (eg, metoprolol) and calcium channel blockers (eg, diltiazem) are first-line agents for rate control. They can be administered intravenously for medical conversion of atrial fibrillation with a rapid ventricular response and orally to maintain a slower rhythm. Unstable patients may need electrical cardioversion. Patients with long-standing atrial fibrillation (longer than 6 months) have less chance for successfully being converted back to a normal sinus rhythm than those who have new or relatively new onset.

Anticoagulation therapy with warfarin for 4 weeks before and after cardioversion can decrease the risk of stroke and is recommended before any attempt at cardioversion because the risk of embolism during cardioversion is 1% to 7%. The CHADS 2 score, as previously described, is a useful clinical prediction tool for estimating the risk of stroke in patients with nonrheumatic atrial fibrillation to help guide decisions on whether to treat the patient with long-term warfarin therapy.

Controlled trials demonstrate no reductions in either mortality or stroke rates in those patients managed with simple rate control and anticoagulation compared with those receiving cardioversion with rhythm maintenance using antiarrhythmic medications.

Additional Readings:
1. Newly detected atrial fibrillation: AAFP updates guideline on pharmacologic management. *Am Fam Physician*. 2017;96(5):332-333.
2. Management of atrial fibrillation: updated guidance from the AHA, ACC, and HRS. *Am Fam Physician*. 2020;101(2):123-124.

32. You are seeing a tall, thin young man for a preparticipation basketball examination and find that he also has pectus excavatum. You consider that he may have Marfan syndrome. Which one of the following is a characteristic of this syndrome?

A) Café au lait spots
B) Webbing of the neck
C) Arm span less than height
D) Decreased mobility of joints
E) Aortic dilatation with possible rupture

The answer is E: Marfan syndrome is caused by a mutation of the *FBN1* gene affecting the connective tissues. People with Marfan syndrome tend to be tall and thin with an arm span that exceeds their height. Scoliosis can be severe and may require bracing or surgery. A high-arched palate, pectus excavatum, and hyperextensibility of the joints are commonly seen as well. The syndrome is inherited in an autosomal dominant fashion, although up to 25% of cases develop from spontaneous mutations and the degree to which people are affected varies.

Myopia is the most common ocular finding, and displacement of the lens from the center of the pupil is a characteristic feature seen in approximately 60% of the affected individuals. Patients are at an increased risk for retinal detachment, glaucoma, and early cataract formation. A formal ophthalmologic evaluation with a slit lamp examination should be obtained. Cardiac problems are the most concerning and include aortic regurgitation, MVP, mitral regurgitation, and aortic dilatation. The most common cause of cardiovascular death is subsequent aortic dissection and rupture. Patients should be evaluated with an electrocardiogram to determine any heart rate or rhythm irregularities and an echocardiogram to evaluate the valves and the aorta.

Café au lait spots are seen with neurofibromatosis.

Webbing of the neck is a clinical feature of Turner syndrome.

Additional Reading: Marfan syndrome. In: Domino F, ed. *The 5-Minute Clinical Consult*. Wolters Kluwer; 2022.

33. Which of the following statements regarding enoxaparin (Lovenox) is true?

A) It is not a cost-effective medication when used in an outpatient setting.
B) The incidence of thrombocytopenia is the same as with heparin.
C) It must be given intravenously.
D) It does not require laboratory monitoring.
E) It is safe to use in patients with renal failure.

The answer is D: The two types of heparins used as anticoagulants are unfractionated heparin (UFH) and low-molecular-weight heparin (LMWH). UFH has been used for the prevention and/or treatment of thrombosis for many years. LMWH is derived from UFH but has a more predictable dose response and fewer side effects. Because of these clinical advantages, LMWHs have gradually replaced UFH for most indications. Enoxaparin was the first LMWH approved for treating deep vein thrombosis (DVT). In patients with a DVT, subcutaneous administration of a dosage of 1 mg/kg twice daily or 1.5 mg once daily of heparin is as effective as continuous infusion of UFH in preventing complications and reducing the risk of recurrence.

Outpatient management of DVT using LMWH for short-term anticoagulation until warfarin is at a therapeutic level is considered safe and cost-effective. LMWH is typically given in combination with warfarin for 4 to 5 days. Laboratory monitoring is not required. Candidates for outpatient therapy must be hemodynamically stable, without renal failure, and not at high risk for bleeding. In addition, thrombocytopenia is seen less often than with UFH. Dalteparin (Fragmin), another LMWH, is primarily used for DVT prophylaxis.

Additional Reading: Anticoagulation: updated guidelines for outpatient management. *Am Fam Physician*. 2019;100(7):426-434.

34. A 73-year-old White smoker with a history of diabetes and known cardiovascular disease presents to your office complaining of bilateral leg pain that occurs after walking about 100 yards. He reports that rest improves his symptoms but then recurs when he goes about the same distance again. You obtain ankle-brachial indices (ABIs) and make a diagnosis of intermittent claudication. Which of the following would be most appropriate at this time?

A) A magnetic resonance imaging of the pelvic girdle
B) An ultrasonography of the lower extremities
C) An electromyography (EMG) of the lower extremities
D) An arteriography of the lower extremities
E) No diagnostic testing

The answer is E: The ABI is used to diagnose intermittent claudication of the lower extremities. Claudication results from atherosclerosis in the arteries supplying the blood flow to the muscles of the legs. As blood flow is limited to the muscles in response to an increased demand with exercise, there is subsequent ischemic pain. Once the demand has diminished with rest, the pain resolves, only to return with resumption of activity. If the pain or discomfort occurs with varying distances, a workup for other causes is necessary.

Patients who experience significant restriction in their activities may be considered for surgery; however, their overall health status should be considered first. The ABI is the simplest method to estimate blood flow to the lower extremities; an EMG and other imaging tests are not necessary, although an arteriogram is useful if surgery is a consideration.

Pressure is normally higher in the ankle than in the arm, with normal ABI ratios ranging from 1.0 to 1.4. A value below 0.9 is considered diagnostic of peripheral artery disease, and values above 1.4 suggest a noncompressible calcified blood vessel.

Additional Reading: Lower extremity peripheral artery disease: diagnosis and treatment. *Am Fam Physician*. 2019;99(6):362-369.

35. You have diagnosed a 63-year-old Black man diabetic with intermittent claudication. He is only able to walk about 50 yards before he has to stop due to achy pain on his calves. He is not interested in surgery and is asking about medications that would help. All of the following medications have been recommended, except which one?

A) Aspirin
B) Pentoxifylline (Trental)
C) Clopidogrel (Plavix)
D) Cilostazol (Pletal)

The answer is B: The American College of Chest Physicians recommends the use of aspirin (75-100 mg daily) for all patients with intermittent claudication. Clopidogrel (Plavix) is recommended for patients who cannot take aspirin. Cilostazol (Pletal) is recommended only for patients with disabling intermittent claudication who do not respond to risk factor modification and exercise, and who are not surgical candidates. The guidelines also recommend against the use of pentoxifylline (Trental), prostaglandins, and anticoagulants for patients with intermittent claudication.

American College of Cardiology/American Heart Association guidelines for the management of peripheral arterial disease recommend statins, antiplatelet therapy, risk factor modification, and supervised exercise training (30-45 minutes at least three times per week) for all patients with peripheral arterial disease. They recommend a trial of cilostazol for patients with lifestyle-limiting claudication.

Additional Reading: Effective therapies for intermittent claudication. *Am Fam Physician*. 2011;84(6):699-704.

36. A 71-year-old White woman has been brought to the emergency department by her husband after she fell at home. She has a bruise on her left elbow, and the left side of her cheek has an abrasion. She is alert and reports that she does not know what happened. She was walking to the bathroom and the next thing that she knew she was on the floor. Her husband reports that he heard her fall and when he got to her, she was able to talk. She denies chest pain and had no incontinence during the episode. All of the following factors would place this patient in a low-risk category, indicating no need to admit her for observation and a workup, except which one?

A) A normal electrocardiogram (ECG)
B) A normal cardiac examination
C) A family history of sudden death
D) Orthostatic vital signs

The answer is C: The causes of syncope are varied, and a workup needs to be pursued to determine the underlying cause. Patients with syncope have an increased risk of death from any cause, and when it is secondary to a cardiac condition, the risk of death is doubled. Neurogenic syncope and orthostatic syncope do not confer an increased risk of cardiovascular morbidity or death. Although the workup can be pursued on an outpatient, patients at a high risk for death should be admitted for observation and workup. The following factors help with risk stratification:

High risk (hospital admission recommended if any of the following are present):

- History suggests an underlying arrhythmia (eg, palpitations and syncope during exercise)
- Comorbid conditions (eg, electrolyte abnormalities and significant anemia)
- A family history of sudden death
- Older age
- Structural heart condition or coronary artery disease
- ECG findings suggestive of an arrhythmia (eg, bifascicular block, sinus bradycardia, abnormal QT interval, and ST-segment elevation leads V1 through V3 [Brugada syndrome])

Low risk (evaluation as an outpatient if all of the following are present):

- Younger than 50 years
- No known cardiovascular disease
- Normal ECG
- Unremarkable cardiovascular examination
- Symptoms consistent with neurogenic or orthostatic syncope

Additional Reading: Syncope: evaluation and differential diagnosis. *Am Fam Physician*. 2017;95(5):303-312.

37. Mr. Jones, a 69-year-old retired firefighter, presents with achy lower leg pain that he has noted for several months, which is now interfering with his sleep. His wife told him to keep his feet elevated, as it helps her swollen ankles, but it seems to make his pain even worse. He has a history of smoking and is on metoprolol and lisinopril to control his hypertension. His blood pressure is 138/86 mm Hg today, and his pulse rate is 78 beats per minute. A recent metabolic panel was normal, except for an elevated glucose of 156 mg/dL. You ask him to get undressed so that you can perform an examination, and while he is doing so, you consider that the most likely diagnosis based on his symptoms is which one of the following?

A) Diabetic neuropathy
B) Severe claudication
C) Thromboangiitis obliterans
D) Spinal stenosis

The answer is B: Claudication results from atherosclerosis in the arteries supplying the blood flow to the muscles of the legs. As blood flow is limited to the muscles, there is subsequent ischemic pain. Typically, the symptoms begin as intermittent pain occurring with activity, such as walking, which resolves after a few minutes of rest, reoccurring again after walking the same distance. As the disease progresses, the distance that the patient can walk without pain is shortened. Eventually, ischemic pain may occur at rest, beginning in the most distal parts of a limb as a severe, unrelenting pain aggravated by elevation and often interfering with sleep. If intermittent claudication is the only symptom, the extremity may appear normal, but the pulses are reduced or absent.

The location of the pain is correlated with the location of the occluding atherosclerotic plaque. Disease in the aortoiliac region frequently causes claudication symptoms in the buttocks, hips, and calves. On examination, the femoral pulses are reduced or absent. Impotence can also be a complaint for older male patients, depending on the location and extent of occlusion. Occlusion in the femoropopliteal arteries results in more distal symptoms, typically in the calf, and pulses below the femoral pulse are significantly decreased or absent altogether.

Diabetic neuropathy typically presents with pain and numbness in the legs and feet, often described as uncomfortable tingling ('pins and needles'), burning, or oversensitivity. There is a reduced sensation of touch on exam.

Thromboangiitis obliterans (Buerger disease) is a rare condition of the arteries and veins in the arms and legs. Symptoms include tingling or numbness in the hands or feet, which can be exacerbated by activity and relieved by rest from claudication. The skin will show discoloration (pale, reddish, or blue-tinted hands or feet) and overtime ulcers can develop on the fingers and toes.

Spinal stenosis is often asymptomatic; when symptoms do occur, they slowly worsen over time. Spinal stenosis in the lower back can cause low back discomfort and pain or cramping in one or both legs with prolonged standing or walking. Symptoms typically get better with forward bending or sitting.

Additional Reading: Lower extremity peripheral artery disease: diagnosis and treatment. *Am Fam Physician.* 2019;99(6):362-369.

38. Angioneurotic edema is associated with the use of which one of the following medication classes?

A) Angiotensin-converting enzyme (ACE) inhibitors
B) β-Blockers
C) Loop diuretics
D) α-Receptor blockers
E) Calcium channel blockers

The answer is A: Angioneurotic edema, also known as angioedema or Quincke edema, is the rapid swelling of the dermis, subcutaneous tissue, and mucosal and submucosal tissues. Patients should be observed because upper airway swelling can rapidly progress, resulting in laryngeal obstruction. The reaction is different from urticaria because the swelling is more pronounced and not just limited to the upper dermis as seen with urticarial hives.

Acquired angioedema is usually caused by allergy but also occurs as a medication side effect. It occurs in about 0.1% of patients on an ACE inhibitor but can also occur with angiotensin receptor blockers and, rarely, with other medications. Although the reaction usually develops within the first week of therapy, it can occur at any time. It is typically characterized by repetitive episodes of swelling of the face, lips, and tongue, but edema of the limbs and genitals can also be seen. Some patients will complain of abdominal pain from edematous swelling of the gastrointestinal mucosa.

Additional Reading: Drugs for chronic heart failure. *Med Lett.* 2015;57(1460):9-13.

39. A 63-year-old White man returns to the emergency department 2 weeks after being discharged following a 2-day admission for an acute myocardial infarction (AMI). He is complaining of substernal chest pain similar to that he had at the time of his AMI. He also notes that he has had a low-grade fever and that his joints have felt achy as well. His creatine kinase and troponin levels are normal. The most likely diagnosis to explain this presentation is which of the following?

A) Costochondritis
B) Dressler syndrome
C) Meigs syndrome
D) Non–ST-segment elevation myocardial infarction
E) Pneumonia

The answer is B: Dressler syndrome is a type of pericarditis, likely triggered by an autoimmune response after damage to the heart tissues or to the pericardium following a myocardial infarction (MI), surgery, or trauma. Symptoms include chest pain, which can be similar to the pain experienced during the AMI. The syndrome can occur several days to weeks after the original cardiac event. In addition to the chest pain, the condition is characterized by fever, pleurisy, and diffuse joint pains. On examination, a pericardial friction rub can be heard, and on the chest radiograph, pericardial and pleural effusions can be seen.

Chest pain following a recent MI is disconcerting, and the differential diagnosis includes Dressler syndrome. Typically, in Dressler syndrome, there is minimal or no increase in cardiac enzymes. Treatment is focused on anti-inflammatory medications such as aspirin and nonsteroidal anti-inflammatory drugs such as ibuprofen; refractory cases are treated with colchicine or corticosteroids.

Additional Reading: Acute pericarditis: diagnosis and management. *Am Fam Physician.* 2014;89(7):553-560.

40. A 77-year-old White man presents to the emergency department with complaints of dyspnea on exertion and some mild orthopnea. His blood is drawn for a B-type natriuretic peptide (BNP) assay. What level would be consistent with a diagnosis of congestive heart failure (CHF) to explain his symptoms?

A) 10 pg/mL
B) 150 pg/mL
C) 200 pg/mL
D) 500 pg/mL

The answer is D: BNP is released by myocytes in heart failure (HF) as a result of the accompanying ventricle wall stretching. This blood test reliably correlates with the presence or absence of left ventricular dysfunction on an echocardiogram. A BNP level of 100 pg/mL or less is unlikely to support the diagnosis of CHF, whereas a level above 500 pg/mL is an indication that HF is likely present. Intermediate values require further evaluation to determine whether HF is present.

Additional Readings:
1. Brain natriuretic peptide levels for ruling out heart failure. *Am Fam Physician.* 2011;83(11):1333-1334.
2. Heart failure with preserved ejection fraction: diagnosis and management. *Am Fam Physician.* 2017;96(9):582-588.

41. Digoxin can be useful in which one of the following settings?

A) Congestive heart failure (CHF) following a recent myocardial infarction
B) CHF due to diastolic dysfunction
C) CHF with atrial fibrillation
D) Idiopathic hypertrophic subaortic stenosis
E) Emergent treatment of ventricular flutter

The answer is C: Digoxin is a purified cardiac glycoside extracted from the foxglove plant *Digitalis lanata*. Digoxin slows the heart rate by blocking the number of electrical impulses that pass through the atrioventricular node into the ventricles, and it has inotropic effects that strengthen ventricular contractions. Digoxin decreases the symptoms of heart failure, increases exercise tolerance, and is associated with a decrease in the rate of hospitalization from CHF, but it does not prolong survival. The primary use of digoxin is to treat patients with both atrial fibrillation and heart failure. Low-dose digoxin (level 0.5-0.9 ng/mL) is recommended for symptomatic patients with class III and IV heart failure.

The most common adverse effects include nausea and cardiac arrhythmias, with confusion and visual disturbances also being reported. In patients with normal systolic function but with decreased ventricular compliance (diastolic dysfunction) that gives rise to CHF, the use of digoxin is not recommended. Digoxin should also not be used in patients with idiopathic hypertrophic subaortic stenosis. There is no evidence that any drug improves clinical outcomes in patients who have heart failure with preserved systolic function.

Additional Reading: Drugs for chronic heart failure. *Med Lett Drugs Ther*. 2021;63(1626):89-96.

42. Which of the following medications has been shown to improve survival following a myocardial infarction (MI)?

A) Hydrochlorothiazide
B) Metoprolol
C) Morphine
D) Nitroglycerin
E) Warfarin

The answer is B: β-Blockers, such as metoprolol, have been shown to reduce mortality when used during an acute MI and for long-term management post MI. Administration of intravenous β-blockers within the first 24 hours of infarction, followed by oral therapy, has been found to reduce the mortality rate within the first week of infarction. Initiation of a β-blocker after an MI, with continuation of therapy, reduces total mortality, nonfatal MI, and sudden death, regardless of the patient's age, sex, infarct location, initial heart rate, or presence of a ventricular arrhythmia. The greatest benefit occurs in the elderly, those with large anterior infarctions, arrhythmias, or left ventricular dysfunction.

Additional Reading: Myocardial infarction. In: Domino F, ed. *The 5-Minute Clinical Consult*. Wolters Kluwer; 2022.

43. Still murmur is best characterized by which of the following statements?

A) It is common in the elderly and of no physiologic consequence.
B) It is associated with severe aortic regurgitation.
C) It is benign and usually disappears over time.
D) It should always be assessed with an echocardiogram.
E) Atrial fibrillation of flutter is usually an associated rhythm.

The answer is C: Still murmur can occur at any age, although it is most common among children 2 to 7 years of age and disappears before the onset of puberty. It is rare in adulthood. It is characterized as a humming or musical-sounding systolic murmur that is loudest at the left sternal border. It is a benign murmur, and no workup is necessary.

The murmur associated with severe chronic aortic regurgitation is known as an Austin Flint murmur and may be mid-diastolic or presystolic. The murmur occurs when there is backflow of blood from the aorta into the left ventricle and flow into the left ventricle from the left atrium. The regurgitated stream often prevents the full opening of the mitral valve, thus obstructing flow into the ventricle.

Additional Reading: Heart murmurs in children: evaluation and management. *Am Fam Physician*. 2022;105(3):250-261.

44. A 20-year-old cross-country runner is brought to the emergency department following a syncopal episode while on a training run. On physical examination, she appears healthy and is in no acute distress. On cardiac auscultation, the patient has a palpable bifid carotid pulse and a systolic ejection murmur, which is heard best along the left sternal border and becomes louder with a Valsalva maneuver. Which of the following is the likely diagnosis?

A) Bicuspid aortic valve
B) Rheumatic heart disease
C) Hypertrophic obstructive cardiomyopathy
D) Mitral valve prolapse (MVP)

The answer is C: Hypertrophic obstructive cardiomyopathy is an autosomal dominant disorder that is characterized by an enlarged cardiac septum, which obstructs blood flow from the left ventricle. Symptoms include dizziness, light-headedness, palpitations, chest pain, dyspnea, or syncope with physical exertion. The most important complication of the disease is sudden death. The condition has an annual incidence of 4% to 6% in children. Signs include bifid pulses and a systolic ejection murmur along the left sternal border, which becomes louder with movements that decrease venous return (afterload), such as standing or Valsalva maneuver. Movements that increase venous return (afterload), such as squatting, reduce the murmur. The electrocardiogram usually shows evidence of left ventricular hypertrophy and septal Q waves in the lateral leads. Diagnosis is accomplished by echocardiography.

A bicuspid aortic valve is a common cardiac valve anomaly, occurring in 1% to 2% of the general population. It is twice as common in men as in women. This is usually an asymptomatic condition until later in life when calcification results in aortic stenosis.

Rheumatic fever is a delayed inflammatory sequela of group A streptococcal infection that affects multiple organ systems. This includes the heart; however, rheumatic heart disease is largely restricted to developing countries. Symptoms from aortic or mitral valve abnormalities due to rheumatic fever typically present later in life.

MVP is often asymptomatic. On exam, one may hear a midsystolic click, followed by a late systolic murmur, that becomes louder with Valsalva maneuver.

Additional Reading: Cardiomyopathy. In: Domino F, ed. *The 5-Minute Clinical Consult*. Wolters Kluwer; 2022.

45. Niacin is used to treat patients with lipid abnormalities. Which of the following is an effect of niacin use?

A) Increased high-density lipoprotein cholesterol (HDL-C) levels
B) Increased high-density lipoprotein cholesterol (LDL-C) levels
C) Increased triglyceride levels
D) Hypoglycemia
E) Decreased uric acid levels

The answer is A: Niacin, also known as nicotinic acid, is one of the B vitamins (B3). Prescription or niacin supplements are primarily used to treat lipid disorders and pellagra (niacin deficiency). Insufficient niacin in the diet can cause nausea, skin and mouth lesions, anemia, headaches, and tiredness. In the United States, it is primarily used to treat hyperlipidemia. It lowers LDL-C and triglyceride levels, while increasing HDL-C levels. Side effects include flushing, pruritus, hepatotoxicity, elevated glucose and uric acid levels, and gastrointestinal irritation. Doses range from 500 mg/d to a maximum of 3 g/d. Aspirin taken approximately 45 minutes before the administration of niacin may help to decrease flushing episodes. Liver function tests should be periodically monitored when patients are taking the medication.

Additional Reading: What about niacin? *Med Lett Drugs Ther*. 2011;53(1378):94.

46. Which of the following interventions can distinguish atrial flutter from sinus tachycardia?

A) Administration of adenosine
B) Administration of diltiazem
C) Administration of isoproterenol
D) Carotid sinus massage

The answer is D: Atrial flutter is the second-most common tachyarrhythmia, after atrial fibrillation. Atrial flutter is a rapid, regular rhythm caused by an ectopic focus that gives rise to atrial rates from 280 to 350 impulses per minute. Usually, impulses are only transmitted to the ventricles every second or third impulse, resulting in a pulse rate of around 150 bpm. Rapid atrial flutter can be difficult to distinguish from sinus tachycardia; however, carotid sinus massage or other Valsalva maneuvers can slow the rate so that the characteristic atrial flutter "saw tooth" waves can be seen.

Flutter waves are best seen in the inferior leads (II, III, aVF) and in V1. The RR interval may be regular, reflecting a fixed-ratio atrioventricular (AV) block (2:1, 3:1), or may be variable, reflecting a Wenckebach pattern. Treatment consists of verapamil, diltiazem, β-blockers, or digoxin, which slows conduction through the AV node. Electric cardioversion (low energy) is indicated for patients who are unstable and show signs of heart failure.

Additional Reading: Diagnosis and management of common types of supraventricular tachycardia. *Am Fam Physician.* 2015;92(9):793-802.

47. Which of the following β-blockers is indicated in the treatment of chronic mild to moderate CHF?

A) Acebutolol
B) Atenolol
C) Metoprolol
D) Propranolol
E) Timolol

The answer is C: Metoprolol, bisoprolol, and carvedilol are β-blockers that have been shown to slow the progression of heart failure (HF) and have been shown to reduce mortality and hospitalization in patients with New York Heart Association (NYHA) class II to IV HF by 30% to 40%. Unless there is a contraindication, those with HF and systolic dysfunction (EF ≤ 40%) should take both an ACE inhibitor and a β-blocker, and a diuretic if volume overloaded. An angiotensin receptor blocker is used for individuals who cannot tolerate an angiotensin-converting enzyme inhibitor. Addition of an aldosterone antagonist can be beneficial for patients with symptomatic HF or for patients with left ventricular dysfunction after a myocardial infarction.

β-Blockers are also useful in treating diastolic HF. With diastolic HF, the heart does not have enough time to relax and fill the left ventricle with blood before pumping it out to the rest of the body. β-Blockers slow the pulse rate and allow more time for the left ventricle to fill, thus increasing the ejection fraction.

Hydralazine and isosorbide dinitrate have been effective in Blacks when added to standard therapy for HF. Digoxin can decrease symptoms and lower the rate of hospitalization for HF but has not been shown to decrease mortality. There is no evidence that any drug improves clinical outcomes in patients with HF with preserved systolic function.

β-Blockers are started at a low dose and increased gradually to the highest dose tolerated. Full clinical benefits may not occur for 3 to 6 months or more. β-Blockers should be used cautiously, if at all, in patients with symptomatic asthma or severe bradycardia.

HF may involve the left heart, the right heart, or the biventricular. The NYHA classification is a subjective grading scale used for classifying patients with HF:

NYHA I: asymptomatic
NYHA II: symptomatic with moderate exertion
NYHA III: symptomatic with mild exertion and may limit activities of daily living
NYHA IV: symptomatic at rest

Additional Readings:
1. Drugs for chronic heart failure. *Med Lett Drugs Ther.* 2021;63(1626):89-96.
2. *ACC, AHA, HFSA Issue Heart Failure Guideline*: https://www.acc.org/About-ACC/Press-Releases/2022/04/01/15/22/ACC-AHA-HFSA-Issue-Heart-Failure-Guideline

48. You are treating a patient in the emergency department who presents with mild confusion and chest pain. His electrocardiogram (ECG) is consistent with an acute myocardial infarction (AMI). Which one of the following factors would be considered a contraindication for administering streptokinase to treat this acute situation?

A) Mental confusion
B) A blood pressure of 164/96
C) Chest pain that started 5 hours ago
D) ECG with 2 mm of ST elevation in two adjacent precordial leads (STEMI)

The answer is A: Fibrinolytic therapy is a proven treatment for the management of AMI and is indicated in patients with evidence of ST-segment elevation myocardial infarction (STEMI) or new left bundle branch block, who are seen within 12 hours of the onset of symptoms. Efficacy declines as the duration of ischemia continues, and the goal is a door-to-needle time of less than 30 minutes. The majority of those suffering from an STEMI have a complete occlusion of a coronary artery due to a clot (thrombus). Streptokinase is the most commonly used thrombolytic agent to treat an AMI. It works by converting plasminogen into the natural fibrinolytic agent plasmin, which breaks down the fibrinogen and fibrin, lysing clots.

Percutaneous coronary intervention is the preferred method for reperfusion for most patients with STEMI because there are better outcomes (lower mortality and less recurrent ischemia) with fewer complications such as intracranial hemorrhage that occurs with thrombolytic use. However, not all facilities have proper resources to be able to offer timely percutaneous coronary intervention.

The criteria for thrombolysis include cardiogenic chest pain of at least 30 minutes' duration and associated electrocardiographic changes of 1 to 2 mm of ST elevation in two adjacent precordial leads. Absolute contraindications to thrombolytics include the following:

- Intracranial bleed, stroke, or cerebrovascular events within 1 year
- Intracranial neoplasm
- Unclear mental status
- Active gastroesophageal bleeding
- Aortic dissection
- Acute pericarditis

Relative contraindications include the following:

- Surgery within the past 3 weeks or major surgery within the past 3 months
- More than 10 minutes of cardiopulmonary resuscitation
- Arterial puncture in a noncompressible region within the past 2 weeks
- Uncontrolled hypertension (systolic blood pressure >180 mm Hg or diastolic blood pressure > 110 mm Hg)
- Pregnancy
- Bleeding diathesis
- Active peptic ulcer disease

Additional Reading: Fibrinolytic therapy in acute ST elevation myocardial infarction: initiation of therapy. In: *UpToDate*. 2022.

49. Many patients are taking β-blockers for various cardiac conditions, including hypertension, heart failure, and tachycardias. Which one of the following signs is indicative of a therapeutic effect?

A) Constricted pupils
B) Peripheral cyanosis
C) Peripheral edema
D) A pulse rate between 60 and 70 bpm

The answer is D: β-Blockers (eg, propranolol, metoprolol, labetalol, and nadolol) are considered negative inotropic and chronotropic agents; hence, the therapeutic effect will result in a low heart rate. Thus, these agents should be used cautiously in patients with bradycardia or heart block. β-Blockers improve survival after a myocardial infarction by reducing myocardial oxygen demand from a lower heart rate and a decreased contractility. Once considered first-line treatment of hypertension (HTN), the Eighth Joint National Committee guidelines now consider β-blockers as third-line or adjunctive therapies for treating hypertension.

β-Blockers should be used cautiously in patients with asthma, and chronic obstructive pulmonary disease as nonselective β-blockers can induce bronchoconstriction and in diabetics because they may blunt the physiologic response to hypoglycemia. Other side effects can include fatigue, impotence, impaired glucose tolerance, and rebound tachycardia and hypertension if the drug is abruptly discontinued.

Additional Reading: High blood pressure: ACC/AHA releases updated guideline. *Am Fam Physician*. 2018;97(6):413-415.

50. Sudden cardiac death is a concern for patients with which one of the following electrocardiographic findings?

A) Sinus arrhythmia
B) First-degree atrioventricular block
C) Prolonged QT interval
D) Right bundle branch block
E) Premature ventricular contractions

The answer is C: Abnormal rhythms can be caused by a prolongation of the QT interval due to medications (typically psychotropic), electrolyte abnormalities (hypokalemia, hypomagnesemia), myocarditis, nutritional deficiencies, and other metabolic disorders. *Torsades de pointes* and ventricular fibrillation are the fatal arrhythmias usually associated with a prolonged QT interval resulting in a sudden cardiac death. The QT interval is measured on the electrocardiogram and is corrected for the pulse rate—expressed as the QTc.

QTc Intervals (ms)		
	Men	Women
Normal	<430	<450
Borderline	431-450	451-470
Prolonged	>450	>470

Gene mutations are associated with cardiac ion channel abnormalities that can result in a "long QT syndrome," an inherited congenital condition associated with arrhythmias, and an increased risk for sudden death. This syndrome should be suspected in patients with recurrent syncope during exertion and those with family histories of sudden, unexpected death. Men are more commonly affected by the long QT syndrome, with an average age of 32 years for death. Arrhythmias can be induced by vigorous exercise or significant emotional stress, but they also can occur during sleep.

Additional Reading: Sudden arrhythmia death syndrome: importance of the long QT syndrome. *Am Fam Physician*. 2003;68:483-488.

51. A 32-year-old White woman presents with complaints of fever, night sweats, chest pain, and achy muscles and joints. You note painless erythematous lesions on the palms of her hands and splinter hemorrhages on the fingernails. She has a history of abusing intravenous drugs and admits to having injected a "couple of times" over the past few days. Her presentation is mostly likely consistent with which of the following diagnosis?

A) Syphilis
B) Lyme disease
C) Human immunodeficiency virus infection
D) Bacterial endocarditis
E) Hepatitis C

The answer is D: Bacterial endocarditis is an infection caused by bacteria that enter the bloodstream and settle in the heart lining or on a heart valve. The aortic and mitral valves are the most affected and can lead to valve damage and congestive heart failure. However, the tricuspid valve is most commonly involved with intravenous drug abuse. Various neurologic deficits can be seen in individuals with cardiac vegetation, which may result in infected embolic strokes or microabscesses. Other physical findings can include splenomegaly and conjunctival hemorrhages.

Almost all patients will have a fever, which is often low grade and intermittent. A heart murmur is also always heard. The following classic clinical signs are often noted:

- Petechiae: small (1-2 mm) red/purple spots on the skin, caused by minor bleeding from broken capillary blood vessels
- Splinter (subungual) hemorrhages: dark-red, linear lesions in the nail bed
- Janeway lesions: maculae on the palms or soles
- Osler nodes: tender subcutaneous nodules on finger pads
- Roth spots: retinal hemorrhages with small, clear centers

Infections are usually caused by gram-positive bacteria, primarily *Staphylococcus aureus*, *Streptococcus viridans*, or *Streptococcus pneumoniae*. Blood cultures can determine the causative agent, although up to 20% of patients with clinical endocarditis may have negative blood cultures, particularly if they have recently taken antibiotics. Nonspecific laboratory findings can be seen, including anemia, hypergammaglobulinemia, and a positive rheumatoid factor. The patient's erythrocyte sedimentation rate may be elevated. Urinalysis frequently shows proteinuria and microscopic hematuria consistent with glomerulonephritis. Echocardiography is the best diagnostic test for bacterial endocarditis because a transesophageal echocardiography will detect vegetations in >90% of cases.

Additional Reading: Infectious endocarditis: diagnosis and treatment. *Am Fam Physician*. 2012;85(10):981-986.

52. You are seeing a 47-year-old White woman with chronic osteoarthritis (OA), for which she takes a daily naproxen. Over the past few months, her blood pressure (BP) has been elevated, and you have encouraged her to diet and exercise. Additionally, you advised her to decrease the use of naproxen, but she has been unable to function without it and is back in the office for a follow-up visit. On examination, today, her blood pressure is 152/94 mm Hg, and her pulse rate is 76 beats per minute. Which of the following classes of antihypertensive medications can be used safely with nonsteroidal anti-inflammatory drugs (NSAIDs), without ongoing monitoring of renal function, potassium levels, and blood pressure?

A) Angiotensin-converting enzyme inhibitors
B) β-Blockers
C) Calcium channel blockers (CCBs)
D) Diuretics

The answer is C: All NSAIDs in doses adequate to reduce inflammation and pain can increase blood pressure in normotensive and hypertensive individuals. The average increase in BP is only 2 to 3 mm Hg but varies considerably. The hypertensive effect is dose-dependent and likely relates to the inhibition of COX-2 in the kidneys, which reduces sodium excretion and increases intravascular volume. In addition, NSAID use can reduce the effect of antihypertensive medications except for calcium channel blockers. Thus, when taking NSAIDs while using other antihypertensive medications, renal function, potassium levels, and BP should be monitored regularly.

Additional Reading: Evaluation and management of the patient with difficult-to-control or resistant hypertension. *Am Fam Physician*. 2009;79(10):863-869.

53. A 47-year-old White woman presents with complaints of swelling and pain in her left lower calf. She has been healthy; however, she suffers from a smoker's cough. She smokes a pack per day and has been unable to quit. On examination, she has pitting edema in the lower part of the left leg, and the leg measures 4 cm greater than her right leg in diameter. She has tenderness to palpation of the calf but no obvious varicosities. Given her presentation what is the probability that she has a deep vein thrombosis (DVT) based on the Wells criteria?

A) No probability of DVT
B) Low probability of DVT
C) Moderate probability of DVT
D) High probability of DVT

The answer is D: The Wells criteria are a validated scoring system to determine the pretest probability of a DVT. A point is given for each of the following findings:

- Localized tenderness in deep vein system
- Swelling of the entire leg
- Calf swelling 3 cm greater than the other leg (measured 10 cm below tibial tuberosity)
- Pitting edema greater in the symptomatic leg
- Collateral nonvaricose superficial veins
- Paralysis, paresis, or recent orthopedic casting of lower extremity
- Recently bedridden (more than 3 days) or major surgery within past 4 weeks
- Active cancer or cancer treated within 6 months

Additionally, an alternative diagnosis needs to be considered, and if it is more likely than a DVT to explain the patient's symptoms, 2 points would be subtracted from the total. The diagnosis includes Baker cyst, cellulitis, muscle damage, superficial venous thrombosis, postphlebitic syndrome, inguinal lymphadenopathy, or external venous compression.

The Wells DVT Risk Score Interpretation depends on the point total:

Probability of DVT	Points
Low	−2 to 0
Moderate	1 to 2
High	3 to 8

The patient in this case has a total of 3 points (localized tenderness, left calf swelling >3 cm larger than the right, and pitting edema), placing her at high risk for a DVT.

Although a D-dimer assay is useful in the workup of a DVT, with a high sensitivity (up to 97%), it has poor specificity (as low as 35%); thus, it is used to rule out a DVT, not to confirm the diagnosis of DVT. A negative D-dimer rules out DVT in patients with low to moderate risk (Wells DVT score <2), whereas those with a moderate to high risk of DVT (Wells DVT score >2) require a diagnostic duplex ultrasonography study (as do all patients with a positive D-dimer assay). This patient should have a duplex scan, regardless of the D-dimer result.

Additional Reading: D-dimer versus ultrasonography for DVT: use prediction rule. *Am Fam Physician*. 2013;88(5):337.

The D-dimer assay is useful to rule out a DVT, but has low specificity and cannot confirm the diagnosis of DVT (Duplex ultrasound indicated)

54. A permanent pacemaker should be considered for placement for which one of the following arrhythmias?

A) Asymptomatic bradyarrhythmia
B) Atrial fibrillation
C) Atrial flutter
D) Mobitz I atrioventricular (AV) block
E) Mobitz II AV block

The answer is E: A permanent pacemaker should be considered for placement in the patient with a Mobitz II AV block. Additionally, a pacemaker would be indicated for those with symptomatic bradyarrhythmia and is often necessary for a complete (third-degree) heart block. Atrial fibrillation and flutter are not treated with pacing unless there is associated symptomatic bradycardia.

First-degree heart block is associated with a prolonged PR interval on the electrocardiogram (ECG), indicating slowing of the electrical signals between the atria and ventricles. This is typically asymptomatic and does not require any treatment; however, it can be associated with disabling symptoms that may benefit from permanent pacing, particularly if the PR interval is longer than 0.3 second.

Second-degree heart block is divided into two types: Mobitz type I and Mobitz type II.

- In Mobitz type I (also known as Wenckebach block), the electrical signals are delayed more and more with each heartbeat, until the heart skips a beat. On the ECG, the delay is shown as progressively lengthening PR intervals, until a QRS wave does not follow the next P wave. This type of AV block does not usually require permanent pacing because progression to a higher degree of block is not common.
- In Mobitz type II, the pattern is less regular than in Mobitz type I. Some signals move between the atria and ventricles normally, whereas others are blocked; thus, on ECG, the QRS wave follows the P wave at a normal PR interval, but at other times, the signal is blocked and the P wave is not followed by a QRS wave. Mobitz type II is less common than type I, and a pacemaker is indicated to maintain the heart rate.

Third-degree heart block is also called complete heart block or complete AV block, because none of the electrical signals from the AV node reach the ventricles. With a complete heart block, a slow junctional rhythm is seen on the ECG, and while P waves are present, they occur independently from the QRS waves. Complete heart block can result in sudden cardiac arrest and death, and a temporary pacemaker might be necessary until a permanent pacemaker can be placed.

Additional Reading: Indications for permanent cardiac pacing. In: *UpToDate*. 2022.

55. A 64-year-old White man is being seen for follow-up of his hypertension. You recently added metformin for his newly diagnosed diabetes to the lisinopril that he has been taking to control his blood pressure (BP). His fasting laboratory work includes an A1c level of 6.9%; a total cholesterol of 216 mg/dL, with a low-density lipoprotein cholesterol (LDL-C) of 166 mg/dL and a high-density lipoprotein cholesterol of 45 mg/dL. His BP is 148/88 mm Hg and you decide to add hydrochlorothiazide to his treatment regimen and consider whether he needs a medication for his cholesterol. You decide on which one of the following?

A) Refer him to a diabetologist to further determine treatment
B) To calculate his cardiovascular risk to decide on whether to start treatment
C) To avoid other medications today but to repeat a lipid panel in 6 months
D) To also prescribe a statin today

The answer is D: The 2013 American Heart Association/American College of Cardiology guidelines defined four patient groups for which statin therapy is recommended. This patient falls into one of the four groups (no. 3), and he should also have a statin prescribed at this visit—no further evaluation is necessary. The four groups include those with the following:

1. Atherosclerotic cardiovascular disease (ASCVD): acute coronary syndromes; a history of myocardial infarction and angina; coronary or other arterial revascularization; previous stroke or transient ischemic attack; peripheral arterial vascular disease.
2. An LDL-C level ≥190 mg/dL.
3. Diabetes patients between the ages of 40 and 75 years, whose LDL-C level is 70 to 189 mg/dL.
4. Patients with an LDL-C level between 70 and 189 mg/dL, without clinical ASCVD or diabetes but who have an estimated 10-year ASCVD risk ≥7.5%. A risk calculator can be found at http://cvdrisk.nhlbi.nih.gov/calculator.asp.

Additional Reading: 2013 ACC/AHA guideline on the treatment of blood cholesterol to reduce atherosclerotic cardiovascular risk in adults: a report of the American College of Cardiology/American Heart Association Task Force on Practice Guidelines. *Circulation*. 2014;129(25 suppl 2):S1-S45.

56. Which one of the following tests is considered routine (recommended) in the initial evaluation of a patient with newly diagnosed hypertension (HTN)?

A) Chest x-ray
B) Thyroid-stimulating hormone (TSH)
C) Uric acid level
D) 24-hour urine protein
E) Electrocardiogram (ECG)

The answer is E: Although the initial management of hypertension (BP > 140/90) should consist of lifestyle modifications (maintaining a normal body weight, DASH diet, sodium restriction, limitation of alcohol consumption, and a regular exercise program), the initial evaluation of a patient with HTN should include a thorough history and several tests to rule out common secondary causes and to look for comorbid conditions. These include the following:

Routine tests
- Complete blood count
- Chemistry panel, including fasting glucose, potassium, creatinine, and blood urea nitrogen (BUN)
- Cholesterol panel (total cholesterol and low-density lipoprotein cholesterol/low-density lipoprotein cholesterol)
- 12-lead ECG
- Urinalysis

Optional tests
- Creatinine clearance
- 24-hour urinary protein
- Uric acid
- Glycosylated hemoglobin
- TSH
- Limited echocardiography
- Chest x-ray

Additional Reading: Initial evaluation of the hypertensive adult. In: *UpToDate*. 2022.

57. A 43-year-old administrative assistant presents with pain and swelling in her right lower leg. She notes that she has been working overtime since last week typing up a long report, which has required prolonged hours sitting at her keyboard. Her D-dimer level was 300 mg/mL, and she was diagnosed with a small isolated distal deep vein thrombosis (DVT) confined to the calf veins below the knee in her right calf by a duplex ultrasonogram. She does not smoke, and other than a sedentary lifestyle with a body mass index of 29, she is otherwise healthy. Appropriate management at this time would include which one of the following?

A) Treat as an outpatient by prescribing aspirin.
B) Treat as an outpatient by prescribing clopidogrel.
C) Treat as an outpatient by administration of low-molecular-weight heparin.
D) Treat as an outpatient by performing a second scan next week.
E) Treat as an inpatient by administration of IV heparin.

The answer is D: The classic presentation of a DVT includes swelling, pain, warmth, and redness in extremity. DVT refers to a clot formation, usually in the lower extremity veins. Predisposing conditions include lack of activity; previous DVT; recent surgery; smoking; and hypercoagulable states, including antithrombin III deficiency, protein C or S deficiency, lupus, cancer, and estrogen use.

An isolated distal DVT is located below the knee and is confined to the calf veins (peroneal, posterior, anterior tibial, and muscular veins), with no proximal component. The physical examination may be normal. In this situation, a positive Homans sign is not a reliable predictor, and a diagnosis is usually made with Doppler ultrasound (duplex) studies, which is operator-dependent and does not detect thrombi below the knee well. The gold standard test is contrast venography.

The treatment of isolated distal DVT varies, but a select minority can avoid anticoagulation because patients with an isolated distal DVT are at lower risk of embolization than those with proximal DVT, and distal DVTs can resolve spontaneously without therapy. Those who are considered to be at high risk for extension to the proximal veins should be anticoagulated and include patients with the following:

- An unprovoked DVT
- A D-dimer level > 500 mg/mL
- Large thrombosis (>5 cm long, >7 mm width) involving multiple veins
- Thrombosis close to the proximal veins
- Persistent/irreversible risk factors such as active cancer
- Prior DVT or pulmonary embolism
- Prolonged immobility
- Inpatient at the time of diagnosis

It appears that when left untreated one-third of those with symptomatic isolated distal DVT will extend into the proximal veins, usually within the first 2 weeks after diagnosis. Thus, patients (like the woman in this case) can be followed with weekly ultrasonography for 2 to 3 weeks to look for extension of the lower extremity clot into the proximal veins, rather than initially treating with an anticoagulant.

Additional Reading: Deep vein thrombophlebitis (DVT). In: Domino F, ed. *The 5-Minute Clinical Consult*. Wolters Kluwer; 2022.

58. A 49-year-old White woman presents complaining of generalized weakness for the last couple of months. She has a history of difficult-to-control hypertension (HTN), for which you have prescribed chlorthalidone 25 mg, lisinopril (Zestril) 40 mg, amlodipine (Norvasc) 10 mg, and doxazosin (Cardura) 8 mg, daily. Other than her ill-defined weakness complaint, the history is benign. Her cardiac examination is normal, and you do not hear any abdominal or carotid bruits; her pulses are palpably normal as well. However, her blood pressure (BP) is elevated at 160/109 mm Hg. Follow-up laboratory work reveals a normal complete blood count and chemistry panel, except for a serum potassium level of 3.1 mmol/L (N 3.5-5.5). Which one of the following would be best for confirming the most likely diagnosis in this patient?

A) A renal artery duplex scan
B) A 24-hour urine collection for metanephrines
C) A fasting cortisol
D) A plasma aldosterone/renin ratio

The answer is D: Difficult-to-control or "resistant" HTN is defined as BP that remains elevated above goal despite administration of a three-drug regimen that includes a diuretic. Causes include nonadherence to medication, alcohol abuse, long-term nonsteroidal anti-inflammatory drug use, and other medications. Secondary HTN can be caused by relatively common problems such as chronic kidney disease, obstructive sleep apnea, or primary hyperaldosteronism, which is likely in this woman. It is more common in women and often asymptomatic. Although many patients will not be hypokalemic, this is a key finding. Screening can be done with a morning plasma aldosterone/renin ratio. If the ratio is 20 or more and the aldosterone level is >15 ng/dL, then primary hyperaldosteronism is likely and referral for confirmatory testing should be considered.

Additional Reading: Secondary hypertension: discovering the underlying cause. *Am Fam Physician*. 2017;96(7):453-461.

59. Which of the following statements about treadmill exercise testing is true?

A) Women have a low incidence of false-positive results.
B) A positive result requires >3 mm of ST-segment depression.
C) It is contraindicated in patients with symptomatic severe aortic stenosis.
D) The appearance of a bundle branch block on electrocardiogram (ECG) represents no concern.
E) It is useful to document ECG changes for patients who experience angina at rest.

The answer is C: Exercise stress testing is used to evaluate chest pain in patients with suspected cardiovascular disease. The sensitivity ranges from 56% to 81%, and the specificity ranges from 72% to 96%. Given this relatively low sensitivity and specificity, a patient with a high pretest likelihood of ischemic heart disease still has a high probability of cardiovascular disease even in the face of a normal (negative) test, and a patient with a low probability of ischemic heart disease still has a low chance of significant disease even if the test is positive. The optimal use of diagnostic testing is for those patients with moderate pretest probabilities.

In the standard exercise stress test (Bruce protocol), the patient is asked to exercise for 3-minute intervals on a motorized treadmill device while being monitored for changes in heart rate and blood pressure (BP), symptoms, ECG response (specifically ST-segment displacement), dysrhythmias, and exercise capacity. A positive test is defined as an ST-segment depression of at least 1 mm below baseline. Women tend to have a higher incidence of false-positive results.

Contraindications to exercise stress testing include the following:

- Symptomatic severe aortic stenosis
- Myocardial infarction (MI) within the preceding 4 to 6 weeks (except for a submaximal exercise stress test [65% of predicted maximum heart rate] performed before discharge for patients with a recent MI)
- Angina at rest
- Rapid ventricular or atrial arrhythmias
- High-grade atrioventricular (AV) block or bradyarrhythmia
- Uncompensated congestive heart failure
- Recent acute noncardiac illness
- Uncontrolled BP (systolic > 200 or diastolic > 110 mm Hg)
- Active myocarditis/pericarditis
- Acute pulmonary embolism
- Systemic illness

Criteria for stopping an exercise stress test include the following:

- Predicted heart rate is achieved
- Complaints of excessive fatigue, claudication, or dyspnea
- Premature ventricular contractions that increase in frequency or ventricular tachycardia (VT)
- High-grade AV block appears on ECG
- Significant ST changes seen on ECG (>3 mm depression)
- Severe angina
- Elevated BP (systolic >220 mm Hg or diastolic > 120 mm Hg) during exercise
- Decrease in systolic blood pressure (SBP) with exercise
- Appearance of a bundle branch block

A poor prognosis is associated with a failure to complete stage 2 of a Bruce protocol or to achieve a pulse rate of >120 bpm, ST-segment depression of >2 mm or if seen with a heart rate of <120 bpm, or if present in multiple leads or if lasting >6 minutes into recovery. Additional poor prognostic signs include a poor SBP response to exercise, angina with exercise, or exercise-induced VT.

Additional Reading: Exercise stress testing: indications and common questions. *Am Fam Physician*. 2017;96(5):293-299.

60. A 71-year-old Black man presents to the emergency department with shortness of breath, hemoptysis, and chest pain. Further tests include an electrocardiogram with findings of right-axis deviation, an S1-Q3-T3 pattern, and a right bundle branch block. The most likely diagnosis is which one of the following?

A) An acute myocardial infarction
B) Bronchogenic carcinoma
C) Community-acquired pneumonia
D) Pulmonary embolism (PE)
E) Pericarditis

The answer is D: A pulmonary embolus is a clot that lodges in the pulmonary vasculature and may give rise to a pulmonary infarction. In most cases, the clot originates in the leg or pelvic veins, with the most dangerous thrombi originating from the iliofemoral vein. Other rare causes of emboli include fat emboli after fractures and amniotic fluid emboli.

Risk factors for PE include malignancy, hereditary impaired coagulation, estrogen therapy, obesity, congestive heart failure, orthopedic or pelvic surgery, and prolonged anesthesia. Signs and symptoms include tachypnea, cough, hemoptysis, chest pain, and fever. Diagnosis is based on the clinical history and supportive tests, including a ventilation-perfusion scan and pulmonary arteriogram. Chest radiographs are usually normal; however, a homogeneous, wedge-shaped density based in the pleura and pointing to the hilum (Hampton hump) is highly suggestive of PE.

Arterial blood tests show hypoxia (PO_2 < 60 mm Hg), and although electrocardiographic findings are often nonspecific (T-wave abnormalities and sinus tachycardia), a right-axis deviation, S1-Q3-T3 pattern, and a right bundle branch block may be observed.

The Wells criteria risk-stratifies patients for PE and provides an estimated pretest probability, which can assist in deciding on what further testing is required for diagnosing PE (ie, D-dimer or computed tomographic angiography). In a 2-tier model, if the patient's risk for a PE is determined to be "unlikely," obtain a high-sensitivity D-dimer test; if that is negative, consider stopping workup, and if positive, obtain the angiogram. If the risk is determined to be "PE likely," obtain the angiogram without a D-dimer. The criteria are listed below:

Factor	Points
Clinical signs and symptoms of deep vein thrombosis (DVT)	3
PE is no. 1 diagnosis or equally likely	3
Heart rate > 100 bpm	1.5
Immobilization for at least 3 d or surgery in the previous 4 wk	1.5
Previous, objectively diagnosed PE or DVT	1.5
Hemoptysis	1
Malignancy with treatment within 6 mo or palliative care	1
Total score	

PE unlikely: 0 to 4 points (12.1% incidence of PE).
PE likely: >4 points (37.1% incidence of PE).

Treatment involves anticoagulation for 3 to 6 months with oral warfarin. Thrombolytic therapy is not indicated for the routine treatment of patients with PE, unless the patient has hypotension and continuing hypoxemia while receiving high fractions of inspired oxygen.

Additional Reading: Diagnosis of deep venous thrombosis and pulmonary embolism. *Am Fam Physician*. 2012;86(10):913-919.

61. You are seeing a 42-year-old mother for complaints of vaginitis, and she asks you to prescribe an antibiotic before she sees her dentist next week for a filling of a recently diagnosed dental cavity. She reports that her dentist wanted her to ask you as she has a history of mitral valve prolapse (MVP), for which you had assessed with an echocardiogram a couple of years ago. When you review her most recent echocardiogram, you note no evidence of regurgitation of the valve. She currently has no urinary symptoms or signs of infection. Which of the following would you advise her?

A) She needs to take amoxicillin and gentamycin 1 day before and 1 day after the procedure.
B) She needs to take amoxicillin 1 hour before the procedure.
C) She needs to take vancomycin before, during, and 1 day after the procedure.
D) She needs no prophylaxis.

The answer is D: Evidence to support antimicrobial prophylaxis for prevention of endocarditis is weak, and the 2007 American Heart Association guideline clarifies patients who should receive prophylactic treatment. This patient would not need any antibiotics before having her cavity filled.

The following conditions place patients in a high risk for endocarditis:

- A prosthetic heart valve
- A history of infectious endocarditis
- An unrepaired cyanotic congenital heart condition, including palliative shunts and conduits
- Completely repaired congenital heart defects with prosthetic material or device, during the first 6 months after the procedure
- Repaired congenital heart disease with residual defects at the site or adjacent to the site of the prosthetic patch or prosthetic device
- Valve regurgitation due to a structurally abnormal valve in a transplanted heart

In addition to the patient factors, consideration is made for what procedure the patient is scheduled to undergo. The following procedures place the patient at high risk of developing endocarditis and are indications for antibiotic prophylaxis:

- Dental procedures that involve manipulation of gingival tissue or the periapical region of teeth or perforation of the oral mucosa; this includes routine dental cleaning for high-risk individuals
- Procedures of the respiratory tract, which involve incision or biopsy of the respiratory mucosa
- Gastrointestinal (GI) or genitourinary (GU) procedures in patients with ongoing GI or GU tract infection
- Procedures on infected skin, skin structure, or musculoskeletal tissue
- Surgery to place prosthetic heart valves or prosthetic intravascular or intracardiac materials

Antibiotic prophylaxis is not recommended for low-risk individuals for the following common procedures:

- Routine dental work
- GI/GU scoping procedures
- Vaginal delivery
- Ear or body piercing or tattooing

Additional Reading: Prevention of infective endocarditis: guidelines from the American Heart Association. *Circulation*. 2007;116:1736-1754.

62. Which of the following statements about premature ventricular complexes (PVCs) is correct?

A) They are narrow QRS complexes seen on an electrocardiogram (ECG) that are not preceded by P waves.
B) In most cases, they worsen with exercise.
C) Treatment with antiarrhythmics improves survival.
D) The first-line medication to treat symptomatic PVCs is a β-blocker.
E) Ethyl alcohol use is not associated with PVCs.

The answer is D: PVCs are also known as ventricular premature beats and are triggered from the ventricular myocardium in various situations. PVCs are common and occur in patients without any structural heart disease and those with various forms of cardiac disease. They typically are asymptomatic, although the most common symptom reported is palpitations or a feeling of "skipped beats." On ECG, they occur as wide QRS complexes, without a preceding P wave. PVCs may not be recorded on a routine ECG; thus, 24- or 48-hour ambulatory (Holter) monitoring should be performed. The 24 Holter monitoring is also used to quantify the frequency of PVCs and to evaluate if they are monomorphic or multimorphic. If PVCs are frequent, electrolyte abnormalities and heart disease should be excluded.

An exercise treadmill stress test is used to evaluate the response of the PVCs to exercise (with a normal heart, PVCs usually disappear with exercise) and to determine if sustained or nonsustained ventricular tachycardia (VT) can be induced with exercise, as well as to screen for underlying ischemia. For those with frequent ventricular premature beats or more repetitive forms (couplets or nonsustained VT), further evaluation and management is based on the presence or absence of underlying structural heart disease and/or symptoms; thus, an echocardiography should be performed.

There is no clear evidence that suppressing PVCs with antiarrhythmics improves overall survival; thus, such agents are not indicated in patients who have no related symptoms and have not had a major arrhythmic event. Initial treatment for symptomatic patients is focused on avoiding known stimulants or triggers (eg, caffeine, alcohol, exogenous catecholamines, and sympathomimetic amines). However, if symptoms persist despite avoidance of known triggers, a β-blocker or, less commonly, a calcium channel blocker is considered the first-line drug for treatment.

Patients with frequent, repetitive, or multiform PVCs and underlying heart disease are at increased risk for sudden death because of cardiac arrhythmia (particularly ventricular fibrillation). Without underlying cardiac disease, bigeminy and trigeminy are considered benign rhythms.

Additional Reading: Ventricular premature beats. In: *UpToDate*. 2022.

63. You are seeing a 32-year-old White man who was married a year ago and he and his wife are planning a family. He is worried about his risk for coronary artery disease because his 58-year-old father had a myocardial infarction (MI) last year. Which one of the following is not considered a risk factor for developing coronary heart disease (CHD)?

A) Age: >45 years for men and >55 years for women
B) A father who had an MI before the age of 60 years
C) Smoking tobacco
D) Having hypertension (HTN)
E) A high-density lipoprotein cholesterol (HDL-C) level <35 mg/dL

The answer is B: It is important to screen all individuals for the known CHD risk factors. This patient is not at an increased risk, as his father was >55 years of age when he had his MI. While premature CHD is a first-degree relative, family history is an important risk factor; this refers to an MI in a male before the age of 55 or in a female before the age of 65. The other risk factors that are typically screened for include the following:

- Age: men who are older than 45 years; women older than 55 years or with premature menopause without estrogen replacement
- Smoking
- HTN
- HDL-C < 35 mg/dL (a "negative risk factor" includes an HDL-C > 60 mg/dL)
- Diabetes
- Obesity
- History of cerebral or peripheral vascular disease

Additional Reading: Global risk of coronary heart disease: assessment and application. *Am Fam Physician*. 2010;82(3):265-274.

64. Which one of the following tests is used for the diagnosis of Raynaud phenomenon?

A) Allen test
B) Finkelstein test
C) Phalen test
D) Reverse Phalen test

The answer is A: Raynaud phenomenon is secondary to spasm of the arterioles that usually supply the hands but can also affect the nose and other appendages. Raynaud disease is usually idiopathic but has been associated with emotional stress, connective tissue diseases (eg, lupus, rheumatoid arthritis, and scleroderma), arterial obstructive diseases, medications (eg, ergots, β-blockers, clonidine, and methysergide), and endocrine disorders. Idiopathic Raynaud phenomenon occurs more frequently in women and frequently occurs in patients with migraines or variant angina.

Symptoms include blanching, cyanosis, and paresthesias that affect the distal extremities. Diagnosis can be determined by performing Allen test. The radial and ulnar arteries are occluded by the examiner while the patient makes a fist. The hand is then opened, and one side of the wrist is released. Blood flow to the hand should be detected by color, which is restored to the hand. If the hand remains pale and cyanotic on either of the two sides, Raynaud phenomenon should be suspected. During asymptomatic periods, the examination is entirely normal.

Treatment for mild to moderate cases should only involve avoiding triggering factors (eg, cold, stress, nicotine, and previously listed medications). The medication of choice for the treatment of severe Raynaud phenomenon includes the calcium channel blockers nifedipine and diltiazem. Other medications include reserpine, phenoxybenzamine, methyldopa, terazosin, doxazosin, and prazosin. Surgical treatment for resistant, severe cases involves sympathectomy.

Finkelstein test is used to diagnose de Quervain tenosynovitis by grasping the thumb, while the hand is deviated in the ulnar direction. The test is positive when pain is reproduced along the distal radius.

Phalen test is used to diagnose carpal tunnel syndrome. The patient holds their wrists in complete and forced flexion (pushing the dorsal surfaces of both hands together) for 30 to 60 seconds. The test is positive when symptoms (eg, paresthesias in the thumb and index finger) are reproduced. The reverse Phalen test adds to the sensitivity of the first test and is performed by having the patient in full wrist and finger extension for 2 minutes.

Additional Reading: Raynaud phenomenon. In: Domino F, ed. *The 5-Minute Clinical Consult*. Wolters Kluwer; 2022.

65. A 57-year-old man, with well-controlled type 2 diabetes presented to the emergency department with chest pain that has occurred over the past hour. His electrocardiogram (ECG) was normal. Cardiac troponins are also obtained. If levels are elevated, they can remain elevated up to how long after an acute myocardial infarction (MI)?

A) 24 hours
B) 48 hours
C) 72 hours
D) 1 week
E) 2 weeks

The answer is E: Acute coronary syndrome refers to a range of events, including unstable angina, ST-elevated MI, and non-ST-elevated MI. Symptoms of acute coronary syndrome include chest pain, referred pain, nausea, vomiting, dyspnea, diaphoresis, and light-headedness. Pain may be referred to the arms, jaw, neck, back, and the abdomen. Pain radiating to the shoulder, left arm, or both arms increases the likelihood of acute coronary syndrome.

Evaluation of the patient with acute chest pain includes obtaining an ECG to review for signs of cardiac ischemia. In acute coronary syndrome, common electrocardiographic abnormalities include T-wave tenting or inversion, ST-segment elevation or depression (including J-point elevation in multiple leads), and pathologic Q waves.

MI refers to damage to the cardiac muscle as evidenced by elevated cardiac troponin levels in the setting of acute ischemia. Cardiac troponins T and I are highly specific to myocardial cells and are the primary measure of myocardial injury. Measurement of other biomarkers, such as creatine kinase and myoglobin, is no longer recommended. Troponin is measured at presentation and 3 to 6 hours after the onset of symptoms. A troponin value above the 99th percentile of the upper reference level (which is laboratory specific) is required for the diagnosis of myocardial necrosis, and an increase or decrease of at least 20% is required for the diagnosis of acute myocardial necrosis.

Blood levels of cardiac troponins (cTnI and cTnT) begin to increase 3 to 4 hours after an MI, with levels peaking at 12 to 16 hours and staying elevated for up to 2 weeks. Nonischemic conditions, such as congestive heart failure, can also elevate troponins, and serial measurements can help differentiate these conditions. Patients with an acute MI will have a rising or falling pattern, whereas levels will remain relatively stable with chronic conditions.

Additional Reading: Acute coronary syndrome: diagnostic evaluation. *Am Fam Physician*. 2017;95(3):170-177.

66. The U.S. Preventive Services Task Force (USPSTF) has recommended the use of low- to moderate-dose statins to prevent adverse cardiovascular events in patients with all of the following, except which one of the following situations?

A) Aged between 35 and 70 years
B) Currently smoking
C) Diagnosed with dyslipidemia
D) Diagnosed with diabetes mellitus
E) Has a calculated 10-year risk of a cardiovascular event of ≥10%

The answer is A: The USPSTF recommends (grade B recommendation) that adults without a history of cardiovascular disease (ie, symptomatic coronary artery disease or ischemic stroke) use a low- to moderate-dose statin for the prevention of cardiovascular disease (CVD) events and mortality when all of the following criteria are met:

1. They are aged 40 to 75 years.
2. They have ≥1 CVD risk factors (dyslipidemia, diabetes, hypertension, smoking).
3. They have a calculated 10-year risk of a cardiovascular event of 10% or greater.

Although statin use may be beneficial for the primary prevention of CVD events in some adults with a 10-year CVD event risk of less than 10%, the likelihood of benefit is smaller because of a lower probability of disease and uncertainty in individual risk prediction. In those situations, it is suggested that clinicians may choose to offer a low- to moderate-dose statin for those with a calculated 10-year risk of a cardiovascular event of 7.5% to 10%.

For the purposes of this guideline, dyslipidemia was defined as a low-density lipoprotein cholesterol level greater than 130 mg/dL or a high-density lipoprotein cholesterol level less than 40 mg/dL.

Additional Reading: USPSTF Final Recommendation Statement. *Statin Use for the Primary Prevention of Cardiovascular Disease in Adults: Preventive Medication*. 2022. www.uspreventiveservicestaskforce.org/Page/Document/RecommendationStatementFinal/statin-use-in-adults-preventive-medication

Section II. Respiratory Disease

Questions related to respiratory disease account for about another 10% of the American Board of Family Medicine certifying examination. Although this section covers most of the topic areas, additional topics are covered in Chapter 2, Care of Children and Adolescents. As you study for the examination, ensure that you have a good overview of the following respiratory disease topics:

1. Asthma
    - Understand the common presentation and clinical findings of reactive airway disease.
    - Understand how to evaluate patients who present with wheezing, including the indications for and results of pulmonary function testing.
    - Know the diagnostic categories of asthma, based on symptoms control.
    - Appreciate the pathophysiology of asthma and its implications for treatment.
    - Know what preventive measures should be used for those with asthma.
    - Understand the appropriate use of rescue and preventive medication in the treatment of acute and chronic asthma.
2. Chronic obstructive pulmonary disease (COPD)
    - Understand the common presentation and clinical findings of COPD.
    - Know the indications for pulmonary function testing and differences between obstructive and restrictive lung disease.
    - Appreciate the pathophysiology of COPD and its implications for treatment.
    - Know the staging categories of COPD and its role in directing treatment.
    - Understand the appropriate use of medication in the treatment of COPD.
    - Know the implications of tobacco abuse and how cessation is critical to treatment.

- Know indications for use of home oxygen treatment and chronic steroid therapy.

3. Pneumonia and other respiratory tract infections
   - Understand the diagnostic and management approach to community-acquired pneumonia.
   - Know which bacteria are common, by age, and the appropriate medication to be used.
   - Know the common presenting signs and symptoms of influenza.
   - Understand the importance and methods of influenza testing and reporting.
   - Know the medications for treatment and prophylaxis for influenza, and when they are indicated.
   - Know indications for hospitalization when severity or comorbidity is present with pneumonia.
4. Allergy/rhinitis/sinusitis
   - Know the common presentation and diagnostic evaluation of allergic and nonallergic rhinitis.
   - Understand the role of lifestyle modification and which environmental changes improve clinical symptoms.
   - Know the medical management of allergic rhinitis (oral vs intranasal) and the role of allergy testing and immunotherapy.
   - Know the diagnostic criteria and evidence-based treatment methods for acute sinusitis.
5. Pulmonary embolism (PE) and deep vein thrombosis (DVT)
   - Understand the common presentation and clinical findings of DVT and PE.
   - Appreciate the timely and diagnostic evaluation of DVT and PE, including the appropriate use of scoring scales, D-dimer, and imaging.
   - Know the indications for inpatient vs outpatient care for DVT.
   - Understand the appropriate use of medication in the treatment of DVT and PE and appreciate side effects/contraindications of common medications.
   - Understand when a more detailed diagnostic evaluation is needed to rule out a thrombophilia condition or to search for an underlying malignancy.
6. Smoking and lung cancer
   - Understand the methods of prevention for lung cancer.
   - Know the statistics concerning tobacco use in all forms and their respective implications, including lung, colon, and breast cancers; heart disease; and COPD.
   - Understand effective smoking cessation techniques, including counseling, medications, and the use of ancillary services.
   - Appreciate the common types of lung cancer.

Each of the following questions or incomplete statements is followed by suggested answers or completions. Select the ONE BEST ANSWER in each case.

1. You are seeing a 33-year-old elementary school teacher who presents complaining of a nonproductive cough for the past 3 weeks. You consider that she likely has *Bordetella pertussis* infection. Which one of the following medications is considered the treatment of choice for *B pertussis* infection?

A) Azithromycin
B) Cefuroxime
C) Ciprofloxacin
D) Penicillin
E) Tetracycline

The answer is A: In studies of adults with chronic cough, up to a quarter were found to have serologic evidence of recent *B pertussis* infection. However, pertussis is rarely considered in adults because the signs and symptoms are nonspecific. Apart from a prolonged cough, there are no specific symptoms suggestive of pertussis in older individuals who have been immunized. With this in mind, pertussis should be considered in the differential diagnosis of persistent cough in previously immunized children and adults.

Administration of erythromycin or other macrolide (azithromycin or clarithromycin) may be a consideration in patients presenting with persistent cough. Prophylaxis of exposed persons before culture or serologic results that are available would be another consideration. Early treatment with a macrolide should limit the spread of infection to persons whose immunity has waned or in unimmunized children. The acellular vaccine may allow booster immunization, which can be a method of preventing *B pertussis* infection after immunity from the pertussis vaccination has waned.

Additional Reading: Pertussis: common questions and answers. *Am Fam Physician*. 2021;104(2):186-192.

2. A mother presents with her teenage son who has an episode of wheezing after she gave him an aspirin to treat a pulled muscle in the leg as a result of playing soccer. She is worried that he is allergic to aspirin. True statements regarding aspirin-induced asthma include all of the following, except which one?

A) Ibuprofen is a safe alternative to aspirin.
B) Leukotriene modifiers are considered the treatment of choice.
C) Patients will develop nasal polyps.
D) Salsalate is not considered a safe alternative to aspirin.
E) Vasomotor rhinitis is usually seen.

The answer is D: Aspirin-induced asthma is a syndrome of rhinorrhea, nasal polyps, sinusitis, conjunctival edema, and wheezing following aspirin ingestion. Cross-reactivity may be seen with other nonsteroidal anti-inflammatory drugs, including indomethacin, naproxen, ibuprofen, fenoprofen, mefenamic acid, and phenylbutazone. Safe alternatives to aspirin include salsalate and acetaminophen. Leukotriene modifiers are regarded as the treatment of choice for patients with aspirin-induced asthma.

Additional Reading: Aspirin-exacerbated respiratory disease. In: *UpToDate*. 2022.

3. Omalizumab (Xolair) can be used in the treatment of persistent asthma. True statements about this medication include all of the following, except which one?

A) It is a murine monoclonal antibody directed against circulating immunoglobulin E (IgE).
B) It can reduce corticosteroid requirements.
C) It is administered subcutaneously.
D) Its use is limited because of musculoskeletal pain.

The answer is D: Omalizumab (Xolair) is a murine monoclonal antibody directed against circulating IgE. In patients with moderate to severe persistent asthma, the use of omalizumab can improve symptoms and reduce exacerbations and may reduce corticosteroid requirements. Omalizumab is administered subcutaneously and is generally well tolerated.

Additional Readings:
1. Drugs for asthma and COPD. *Treat Guidel Med Lett*. 2013;11(132):75-86.
2. Difficult-to-treat and severe asthma: management strategies. *Am Fam Physician*. 2021;103(5):286-290.

4. Mrs Jones, a 52-year-old teacher, presents complaining that she is having trouble breathing. Which one of the following signs, if present, would make a diagnosis of pulmonary embolism (PE) more likely to explain the sudden onset of dyspnea?

A) A temperature of >38.0 °C (100.4 °F)
B) Complaints of chest pain
C) Complaints of orthopnea
D) Rhonchi heard on lung examination
E) Wheezes heard on lung examination

The answer is B: Chest pain is common in patients with PE. When evaluating a patient with dyspnea, the presence of orthopnea suggests heart failure (HF); fever suggests an infectious process; wheezing suggests asthma or chronic obstructive pulmonary disease; and rhonchi suggests HF, interstitial lung disease, or infection. These generalizations are supported by a 2008 study designed to improve the diagnosis of PE on the basis of the history, physical examination, electrocardiogram, and chest radiograph.

Additional Reading: Diagnosis of deep venous thrombosis and pulmonary embolism. *Am Fam Physician*. 2012;86(10):913-919.

5. You are evaluating a 57-year-old smoker who has been experiencing an exacerbation of his chronic obstructive pulmonary disease (COPD), with a productive cough. He is in the office and asking for an antibiotic to help with the treatment. Which one of the following infections is least likely in a patient with COPD?

A) *Haemophilus influenzae*
B) *Moraxella catarrhalis*
C) *Mycoplasma pneumoniae*
D) *S pneumoniae*

The answer is C: COPD is a disease process involving progressive chronic airflow obstruction because of chronic bronchitis, emphysema, or both. Chronic bronchitis is defined clinically as excessive cough and sputum production on most days for at least 3 months during at least 2 consecutive years. Emphysema is characterized by chronic dyspnea resulting from the destruction of lung tissue and the enlargement of air spaces. Asthma, which features airflow obstruction, airway inflammation, and increased airway responsiveness to various stimuli, may be distinguished from COPD by reversibility of pulmonary function deficits.

Acute exacerbations of COPD are treated with oxygen (in hypoxemic patients), inhaled β2-agonists, inhaled anticholinergics, antibiotics, and systemic corticosteroids. Theophylline may be considered in patients who do not respond to other bronchodilators.

Antibiotic therapy is directed at the most common pathogens, including *S pneumoniae*, *H influenzae*, and *M catarrhalis*. Mild to moderate exacerbations of COPD are usually treated with broad-spectrum antibiotics such as doxycycline, trimethoprim-sulfamethoxazole, and amoxicillin-clavulanate potassium. Treatment with extended-spectrum penicillins, fluoroquinolones, third-generation cephalosporins, or aminoglycosides may be considered in patients with severe exacerbations.

The management of chronic stable COPD includes smoking cessation and oxygen therapy. Inhaled β2-agonists, inhaled anticholinergics, and systemic corticosteroids are also used in patients with chronic stable disease. Inhaled corticosteroids decrease airway reactivity and can reduce the use of health care services for management of respiratory symptoms. Avoiding acute exacerbations helps to reduce long-term complications. Long-term oxygen therapy, regular monitoring of pulmonary function, and referral for pulmonary rehabilitation are often utilized and can improve the quality of life and reduce hospitalizations. Influenza and pneumococcal vaccines should be administered. Selected patients who do not respond to standard therapies may benefit from lung reduction surgery.

Additional Reading: Pharmacologic management of COPD exacerbations: a clinical practice guideline from the AAFP. *Am Fam Physician*. 2021;104(1).

6. Which one of the following asthma medications has been associated with an increased risk of asthma exacerbation and death from an acute asthmatic attack when used as monotherapy?

A) Short-acting β-agonists
B) Long-acting β-agonists (LABAs)
C) Inhaled corticosteroids
D) Leukotriene receptor antagonists
E) Mast cell stabilizers

The answer is B: LABAs paradoxically increase the risk of asthma exacerbation and asthma-related death when used as monotherapy. However, they do have a role in treating persistent asthma but only when prescribed in combination with inhaled corticosteroids, leukotriene receptor antagonists, or mast cell stabilizers.

Additional Reading: Drugs for asthma and COPD. *Treat Guidel Med Lett*. 2013;132:75.

7. A 10-year-old middle school student complaining of a sore throat is in the office with his father. He reports that "strep throat" has been making the rounds at his school, and he is worried that he has developed a streptococcal infection. Which one of the following signs is *least* likely to be seen in a patient with group A β-hemolytic streptococcal (GABHS) pharyngitis?

A) Fever
B) Malaise
C) Tonsillar exudates
D) Palatine petechiae
E) Rhinorrhea

The answer is E: Sore throat is one of the most common reasons for visits to family physicians. Although most patients with sore throat have an infectious cause (pharyngitis), <20% have a clear indication for antibiotic therapy (ie, GABHS infection). Viral pharyngitis is the most common cause of sore throat. Infectious mononucleosis (IM) is most common in patients 15 to 30 years of age.

Patients typically present with fever, sore throat, and malaise. On examination, there is pharyngeal redness with exudates. Posterior cervical lymphadenopathy is common in patients with IM, and its absence makes the diagnosis much less likely. Hepatosplenomegaly also may be present. If these patients are treated with amoxicillin or ampicillin, 90% develop a classic maculopapular rash.

Patients with bacterial pharyngitis generally do not have hoarse voice, rhinorrhea, cough, or conjunctivitis. Children younger than 15 years are more likely to have strep throat. Signs of strep throat may include pharyngeal erythema and swelling, tonsillar exudate, edematous uvula, palatine petechiae, and anterior cervical lymphadenopathy.

Untreated, streptococcal pharyngitis lasts 7 to 10 days. Patients with untreated streptococcal pharyngitis are infectious during the acute phase of the illness and for 1 additional week. Antibiotic therapy shortens the infectious period to 24 hours, reduces the duration of symptoms by about 1 day, and prevents most complications.

The incidence of complications with strep infection, such as rheumatic fever and peritonsillar abscess, is low. Peritonsillar abscess occurs in <1% of patients treated with antibiotics. Patients with peritonsillar abscess typically have a toxic appearance and may present with a muffled voice, fluctuant peritonsillar mass, and asymmetric deviation.

Additional Reading: Common questions about streptococcal pharyngitis. *Am Fam Physician*. 2016;94(1):24-31.

8. You are seeing a 27-year-old White woman in your office for a pink eye infection. She is planning on a trip to hike in the Rocky Mountains next month on vacation with a group of her friends. She is concerned about altitude sickness, because they are planning on hiking to the summit of Pikes Peak, which is 14,110 ft above the sea level. Which of the following statements about altitude sickness is false?

A) Most people are affected at altitudes more than 8000 ft.
B) Dehydration is usually an associated problem.
C) The most common symptom is headache.
D) Acetazolamide is used for prophylaxis.
E) A high-carbohydrate diet can help prevent symptoms.

The answer is E: As altitude increases, the partial pressure of oxygen decreases. Approximately 20% of people experience symptoms ascending to more than 8000 ft in less than 1 day, and 80% show some symptoms at altitudes higher than 12,700 ft. Symptoms include headache (most common), impaired concentration, nausea, vomiting, fatigue, dyspnea and hyperventilation, palpitations, and insomnia. Any type of physical exertion usually aggravates the symptoms, and excessive hyperventilation leads to dehydration. In severe cases, pulmonary and cerebral edema can occur. The most common manifestation is acute mountain sickness, heralded by malaise and headache.

Risk factors include young age, residence at a low altitude, rapid ascent, strenuous physical exertion, and a history of altitude illness. However, activity restriction is not necessary for those with coronary artery disease who are traveling to high altitudes. Acetazolamide (a carbonic anhydrase inhibitor) helps prevent respiratory alkalosis, which contributes to the symptoms. It is an effective prophylactic treatment started 1 day before ascent and continued until the patient acclimatizes to the final altitude. Dexamethasone is an effective alternative treatment for those with contraindications to acetazolamide (which includes a sulfa allergy). Treatment involves hydration, and usually only symptomatic measures are necessary.

Additional Reading: Acute altitude illness: updated prevention and treatment guidelines from the Wilderness Medical Society. *Am Fam Physician*. 2020;101(8):505-507.

9. You are following up a 57-year-old smoker who is being treated for lung cancer. A recent metabolic panel is normal except that his sodium level is low at 127 Meq/L. You diagnose him with the syndrome of inappropriate secretion of antidiuretic hormone (SIADH). Which type of lung cancer is he most likely to have?

A) Adenocarcinoma
B) Large cell carcinoma
C) Mesothelioma
D) Small cell (oat cell) carcinoma
E) Squamous cell carcinoma

The answer is D: Lung cancer is often associated with a paraneoplastic syndrome, which occurs as a result of cancer and is extrapulmonary. The following are some common neoplastic syndromes:

- *Squamous cell*: hypercalcemia
- *Small cell*: Cushing syndrome, SIADH with hyponatremia, myasthenic syndrome, Eaton-Lambert syndrome, peripheral neuropathy, subacute cerebellar degeneration
- *Large cell*: gynecomastia
- *Adenocarcinoma*: clubbing, thrombophlebitis, marantic endocarditis, periostitis, or hypertrophic osteoarthropathy. In addition, all of the previously mentioned lung cancers may be associated with dermatomyositis, disseminated intravascular coagulation, eosinophilia, thrombocytosis, and acanthosis nigricans.

Additional Reading: Overview of the risk factors, pathology, and clinical manifestations of lung cancer. In: *UpToDate*. 2022.

10. You are doing preparticipation physical examinations for a local college. A 20-year-old Black woman who plays basketball informs you that she wheezes and gets short of breath when she is playing sports. She states that she had asthma in her childhood and used a nebulizer when she was young—but since middle school has not had problems except when she exercises. She asks what you would recommend for preventive treatment. Your recommendation for the best preventative therapy is to prescribe which one of the following?

A) Inhale a short-acting β2-agonist before exercise.
B) Inhale a long-acting β2-agonist before exercise.
C) Inhale a steroid the morning before exercising.
D) Take a leukotriene receptor antagonist the morning before exercise.
E) Take an anxiolytic medication before exercise.

The answer is A: Exercise-induced asthma occurs mainly in patients already diagnosed with asthma. Wheezing usually begins shortly after the initiation of exercise and can be debilitating and limit participation. Short-acting β2-agonists such as albuterol, taken 10 to 20 minutes before exercise, are the recommended first-line agents for pharmacologic treatment because they can prevent bronchospasm and help control exercise-induced asthma. Cromolyn sodium (Intal) inhaled 15 to 20 minutes before exercise has also been found to be helpful. However, those with more severe symptoms would benefit from leukotriene receptor antagonists or corticosteroids with or without long-acting β2-agonists.

Other preventive measures include a slow warm-up and the avoidance of extremely warm and cold conditions.

Additional Reading: Exercise-induced bronchoconstriction: diagnosis and management. *Am Fam Physician*. 2011;84(4):427-434.

11. A 27-year-old White woman returns with ongoing complaints of a postnasal drip, congestion, and facial pressure for the past 6 weeks. She has been treated with an extended course of antibiotics, but despite this therapy, her symptoms remain. She is afebrile and otherwise looks well. The most appropriate management step at this time is which one of the following?

A) Order a magnetic resonance imaging scan of the sinuses.
B) Order a computed tomographic (CT) scan of the sinuses.
C) Order plain films of the sinuses.
D) Refer for sinus drainage.
E) Prescribe an additional 2-week course of antibiotic therapy.

The answer is B: Most sinus infections are caused by viruses and will not respond to antibiotics. Evidence-based guidelines recommend only using antibiotics in the following situations:

- Symptoms last for 10 days or more and are not improving.
- Symptoms are severe (temperature ≥ 102 °F, nasal discharge, and facial pain lasting for 3-4 days).
- Symptoms worsen with new fever, headache, or increased nasal discharge after a viral upper respiratory tract infection that lasted a few days and initially seemed to improve.

Treatment recommendations include the following:

- 5 to 7 days of antibiotics to treat a bacterial infection without encouraging resistance.
- 10 to 14 days of antibiotics to treat children.
- Avoid decongestants and antihistamines, which are not found to be helpful and may make symptoms worse.
- Nasal steroids for those with a history of allergic sinusitis.
- Nasal irrigation using a saline solution (sprays, drops, or liquid) to relieve symptoms.

Amoxicillin is considered the first-line antibiotic for most patients with acute bacterial rhinosinusitis. Trimethoprim-sulfamethoxazole (Bactrim, Septra) and macrolide antibiotics are reasonable alternatives to amoxicillin for treating acute bacterial rhinosinusitis in patients who are allergic to penicillin.

Radiographic imaging in patients with acute rhinosinusitis is not recommended, unless a complication or an alternative diagnosis is suspected. Nasal endoscopy and CT scan of the sinuses are reserved for circumstances that include a failure to respond to therapy as expected (as in this case), spread of infection outside the sinuses, questionable diagnosis, and when surgery is being considered.

Laboratory tests are rarely needed and are reserved for patients with suspected allergies, cystic fibrosis, immune deficiencies, mucociliary disorders, and similar disease states.

Additional Reading: Current concepts in adult acute rhinosinusitis. *Am Fam Physician*. 2016;94(2):97-105.

12. You are counseling a 42-year-old Hispanic man for smoking cessation. He has been smoking since he was in high school and is currently smoking one pack per day. In addition to your counseling, you also decide to prescribe medication to help him quit. Which one of the following is considered to be the most effective pharmacologic therapy for tobacco cessation?

A) Bupropion
B) Clonidine
C) Nicotine polacrilex gum
D) Nicotine transdermal patch
E) Varenicline

The answer is E: The most effective drugs available for treatment of tobacco dependence are bupropion (Zyban and among others) and varenicline (Chantix). Bupropion is a dopamine-norepinephrine reuptake inhibitor used mainly for treatment of depression, but it also has some nicotine receptor–blocking activity. Varenicline is a partial nicotine agonist that binds selectively to $\alpha 4/\beta 2$ nicotinic acetylcholine receptors; it stimulates receptor-mediated activity, relieving cravings and withdrawal symptoms during abstinence. Because varenicline binds to the $\alpha 4/\beta 2$ receptor with greater affinity than does nicotine, it also acts as an antagonist to nicotine delivery from active cigarette use, thus reducing the reward of smoking. Although varenicline is more effective, bupropion offers the benefit of mitigating the weight gain that often accompanies smoking cessation.

All nicotine replacement therapies (NRTs) deliver nicotine, which acts as an agonist at the nicotinic acetylcholine receptor, to the central nervous system in a lower dose and at a substantially slower rate than tobacco cigarettes. All of these products roughly double smoking cessation rates. Nicotine is subject to first-pass metabolism, limiting the effectiveness of oral pill formulations. Nicotine gum, lozenges, and patches are available in the United States without a prescription; these products appear to be as effective as those that require a prescription (the oral inhaler and nasal spray).

All of the NRTs appear to be about equally effective, but results may be better with the combination of a patch and a rapid-onset nicotine medication. NRTs should be started 1 to 4 weeks before the target quit date. The optimum duration of treatment is not clear; 3 to 6 months is probably the minimum, and some patients may need even longer treatment to remain abstinent.

Tobacco dependence is a chronic disease that often requires pharmacologic therapy, but counseling improves the effectiveness of any treatment for this indication. The greater the number of office visits and the longer the counseling time, the higher the smoking cessation rates have been.

Additional Reading: Interventions for tobacco smoking cessation in adults, including pregnant persons. *Am Fam Physician*. 2021;103(12):753-754.

13. You are seeing a 63-year-old smoker who was recently diagnosed with small cell carcinoma of the lung. She is complaining of weakness with difficulty climbing stairs, lifting objects, and needing to use her hands to push herself up from a sitting. The most likely diagnosis is which one of the following?

A) Tetanus
B) Myasthenia gravis
C) Parkinson disease
D) Polymyalgia rheumatica
E) Lambert-Eaton syndrome

The answer is E: Lambert-Eaton syndrome (also known as Lambert-Eaton myasthenic syndrome [LEMS]) is an uncommon neurologic disorder that results from inadequate release of acetylcholine from the presynaptic nerve endings. Often associated with a paraneoplastic syndrome (eg, small cell or oat cell carcinoma of the lung), the condition causes weakness and sometimes pain associated with the proximal muscles, paresthesia, impotence, and ptosis. Reflexes are usually reduced or absent.

This is an autoimmune disease with an attack on the voltage-gated calcium channel (VGCC) protein. VGCC is required for the release of acetylcholine. Cases of LEMS associated with lung cancer are believed to be due to increased production by the tumor of the VGCC protein, with resultant development of antibodies against the tumor cells and VGCC.

Diagnosis is made by checking the blood for the presence of anti-VGCC antibodies. An electromyography and nerve conduction velocity tests typically show characteristic findings as well.

Treatment includes immunosuppressant medication (eg, steroids and azathioprine) and plasmapheresis. Anticholinesterase medications (eg, pyridostigmine and neostigmine) are variably effective.

Additional Reading: Clinical features and diagnosis of Lambert-Eaton myasthenic syndrome. In: *UpToDate*. 2022.

14. A 24-year-old woman reports that her hay fever seems to flare up at the end of the summer and she thinks that she is allergic to goldenrod. Which one of the following is most likely triggering her symptoms at that time of year?

A) *Alternaria* molds
B) Grass pollen
C) Mites
D) Tree pollen
E) Weed pollen

The answer is E: Patients with seasonal allergies become symptomatic only after exposure to triggering pollens or molds. Many plants shed their pollen during predictable times of the year. Although many people complain of goldenrod (a weed) allergy as it blooms in the late summer, it is not a common allergen; indeed, it is often used in decorative arrangements in countries other than the United States. The culprit is usually ragweed, which also blooms at the same time. Ragweed is wind-pollinated, and a single plant can release a billion pollen grains into the air for individuals to inhale. Goldenrod, on the other hand, is insect-pollinated, whose pollen is not a significant allergen for most individuals.

Season	Allergen
Early spring	Tree pollen
Late spring	Grass pollen
Late summer to fall	Weed pollen
Summer and fall	Molds and mites

Additional Reading: Treatment of allergic rhinitis. *Am Fam Physician*. 2015;92(11):985-992.

15. The most common cause of superior vena cava syndrome is which one of the following?

A) Aortic aneurysm
B) Carcinoma of the lung
C) Constrictive pericarditis
D) Metastatic carcinoma from a distant site
E) Tuberculosis

The answer is B: Superior vena cava syndrome results from compression of the superior vena cava most commonly by a neoplastic process and occasionally by an inflammatory condition. Other causes include benign tumors, aortic aneurysm, thyroid enlargement, and thrombosis of a central venous line. Lung cancer, particularly small cell and squamous cell type, is the most commonly associated malignancy. The obstruction of venous drainage to the heart leads to dilation of collateral veins of the upper chest and neck.

Signs include plethora and swelling of the face, neck, and upper torso. Edema of the conjunctiva; shortness of breath in a supine position; and central nervous system disturbances, including headache, dizziness, stupor, and syncope, may be seen. Acute development of symptoms indicates a poor prognosis, and a potentially life-threatening complication of a superior mediastinal mass is tracheal obstruction.

The diagnosis of superior vena cava syndrome is essentially a clinical one. Chest x-rays may show widening of the mediastinum, particularly on the right, but the best confirmatory test is a chest computed tomographic scan. Treatment includes steroids, chemotherapy, and radiation to the tumor. Although the most common cause of this syndrome is metastasized carcinoma of the lung, other less common infectious causes include tuberculosis, histoplasmosis, and constrictive pericarditis.

Additional Reading: Superior vena cava syndrome. In: Domino F, ed. *The 5-Minute Clinical Consult*. Wolters Kluwer; 2022.

16. A 63-year-old man presents with increasing shortness of breath over the past few years. He is a nonsmoker and worked for many years in a factory that produced fluorescent lights. On examination, you find granulomas on the skin and on hidden conjunctiva. A chest radiograph shows evidence of parenchymal infiltrates and intra-alveolar edema with mediastinal lymphadenopathy. The most likely diagnosis is which one of the following conditions?

A) Asbestosis
B) Berylliosis
C) Coccidioidomycosis
D) Sarcoidosis
E) Tuberculosis

The answer is B: Long-term inhalation of beryllium compounds and their products can result in a disease characterized by granulomas that affect primarily not only the lungs but also the skin and conjunctivae. Beryllium is found in electronics and chemical plants, aerospace factories, beryllium-mining sites, and industries in which fluorescent lights are manufactured.

Symptoms of the disease include dyspnea with shortness of breath, cough, and weight loss. Changes that occur in the lungs include diffuse parenchymal inflammatory infiltrates with the development of intra-alveolar edema. The hallmark finding is a granulomatous reaction involving the hilar lymph nodes and pulmonary parenchyma, which is indistinguishable from sarcoidosis. Chest radiographs usually show diffuse alveolar consolidation with hilar lymphadenopathy.

Long-term exposure tends to cause a progressive decrease in pulmonary function with the development of right heart failure and cor pulmonale. The prognosis of the disease is variable and ranges from mild pulmonary symptoms to respiratory compromise and death. Treatment is usually supportive. Steroids have been used with little benefit in chronic cases but may be used for acute berylliosis. Those exposed to beryllium dust should be counseled to protect themselves with masks and should take measures to avoid exposure.

Asbestosis is a chronic lung disease caused by inhaling asbestos fibers. Asbestos is a natural mineral used in products such as insulation, cement, and brake pads. Most people with asbestosis acquired it on the job before the federal government began regulating the use of asbestos in the 1970s. A chest x-ray (CXR) may show irregular opacities with a fine reticular pattern, and calcified pleural plaques may be evident.

Coccidioidomycosis, also called Valley fever, is caused by the *Coccidioides* fungus, which is found in the soil in the southwestern United States. Often asymptomatic, patients can present with fatigue, cough, dyspnea, headache, night sweats, myalgias, and rash. The primary pulmonary disease is often self-limiting, but some patients develop complications or chronic pulmonary disease.

Sarcoidosis is an autoimmune disease and can present with dyspnea on exertion, a nonproductive cough, chest pain, and wheezing. While sarcoidosis can affect any organ, the lungs are most often involved and a CXR will show characteristic symmetric hilar and mediastinal adenopathy and pulmonary micronodules in a perilymphatic distribution.

Tuberculosis is an infection due to *Mycobacterium tuberculosis*, which usually involves the lungs. The three major CXR findings are parenchymal infiltrates, hilar adenopathy, and pleural effusion.

Additional Reading: Fibrosis, pulmonary. In: Domino F, ed. *The 5-Minute Clinical Consult*. Wolters Kluwer; 2022.

17. A 36-year-old day care worker presents with generalized malaise and "a cold that will not go away." It started a couple of weeks ago with a runny nose and a low-grade fever. She reports that she is now having "coughing fits," which are sometimes so severe that she vomits. She does not smoke and cannot remember when she last had any immunizations. On examination, you note excessive lacrimation and conjunctival injection. Her lungs are clear. Which one of the following is the most likely diagnosis?

A) Cough-variant asthma
B) Eosinophilic bronchitis
C) Gastroesophageal reflux
D) Pertussis
E) Rhinovirus infection

The answer is D: Pertussis, once a common disease in infants, declined to around 1000 cases in 1976 as a result of widespread vaccination. The incidence began to increase again in the 1980s, possibly because the immunity from vaccination rarely lasts more than 12 years. The disease is characterized by a prodromal phase that lasts 1 to 2 weeks and is indistinguishable from a viral upper respiratory tract infection. It progresses to a more severe cough after the second week. The cough is paroxysmal and may be severe enough to cause vomiting or fracture ribs. Patients are rarely febrile but may have increased lacrimation and conjunctival injection. The incubation period is long compared with a viral infection, usually 7 to 10 days.

Eosinophilic bronchitis, cough-variant asthma, and gastroesophageal reflux disease cause a severe cough not associated with a catarrhal phase. A rhinovirus infection would probably be resolving within 2 to 3 weeks.

Additional Reading: Pertussis: common questions and answers. *Am Fam Physician*. 2021;104(2):186-192.

18. You are seeing a 72-year-old White man with severe chronic obstructive pulmonary disease (COPD) for a routine follow-up. He is dyspneic with any exertion and gets short of breath climbing onto the examination table. He quit smoking a year ago after many decades of tobacco abuse. He is accompanied today by his daughter, who waits outside the room and asks about his prognosis and the best therapy to improve his longevity. You note that which one of the following has been shown to improve survival in patients with COPD?

A) Long-term antibiotic therapy
B) Inhaled corticosteroids
C) Long-acting β2-agonist
D) Smoking cessation
E) Supplemental oxygen

The answer is E: For patients with the diagnosis of severe COPD, only the administration of supplemental oxygen has been shown to positively affect survival, reduce dyspnea, and reduce pulmonary artery pressure. β2-Agonist and inhaled corticosteroids can lower the rate of exacerbations but have no direct effect on survival. Unfortunately, although smoking cessation can slow the decline in lung function, it has no effect on survival. Long-term use of antibiotics is not helpful.

Additional Reading: Chronic obstructive pulmonary disease and emphysema. In: Domino F, ed. *The 5-Minute Clinical Consult*. Wolters Kluwer; 2022.

19. You are seeing a 57-year-old White male smoker, who has recently returned from a conference in New York City and has come down with a fever and cough. He reports that there were reports of an outbreak of Legionnaire disease among his coworkers who had attended the conference from around the country. Which one of the following would be the medication of choice for the treatment of this infection?

A) Amphotericin
B) Azithromycin
C) Cefuroxime
D) Gentamicin
E) Penicillin

The answer is B: Legionnaire disease is caused by *Legionella pneumophila*. It was discovered after an outbreak in Philadelphia in 1976 that affected many American Legion members. This atypical pneumonia usually affects immunocompromised patients, diabetics, those with renal disease, smokers, and patients with chronic lung disease. Most affected individuals are middle-aged or elderly men. The *Legionella* bacteria are found in water supplies, air conditioners, showers, condensers, and aerosol nebulizers. Transmission occurs by inhalation of aerosolized bacteria.

Symptoms include a nonproductive cough that becomes productive, high fevers with relative bradycardia, pleuritic chest pain, diarrhea, and a toxic appearance. Laboratory tests usually show a moderate leukocytosis (10,000-15,000 per mm^3), hyponatremia (50% of patients), hypophosphatemia, and elevated liver function tests. Sputum smears often show many polymorphonuclear neutrophils but do not show organisms. Chest radiographs show patchy infiltrates, which may progress to consolidations in the lobes. Pleural effusions are common. Diagnosis is achieved by culture, serologies, and direct and indirect antibody assays.

The treatment of choice is typically oral erythromycin or similar macrolide antibiotics. More severe cases may require intravenous antibiotics and the addition of rifampin. Alternative medication includes clarithromycin, azithromycin, doxycycline, trimethoprim-sulfamethoxazole, tetracycline, and ciprofloxacin.

Additional Reading: *Legionnaires' Disease and Pontiac Fever*. 2021. www.cdc.gov/legionella/clinicians.html

20. You are examining a 45-year-old otherwise healthy man who presents with a productive cough and a fever. On examination, you note that he is febrile, and you detect rhonchi on auscultation of his lungs. His chest radiograph is consistent with community-acquired pneumonia. What is the most likely organism that is causing this infection?

A) *H influenzae*
B) *Klebsiella pneumoniae*
C) *Legionella pneumoniae*
D) *Mycoplasma pneumoniae*
E) *S pneumoniae*

The answer is E: Pneumonia in middle-aged adults with no underlying disease is usually caused by *S pneumoniae*, representing more than 50% of community-acquired pneumonias that require hospitalization. Other causes in this patient age group include *H influenzae*, *Legionella*, *Mycoplasma* (more commonly seen in adolescents and younger adults), and influenza viruses. *Pneumocystis carinii* and, occasionally, *Legionella* are seen in immunocompromised patients.

If the patient is older than 60 years and has other significant medical problems (eg, diabetes, chronic obstructive pulmonary disease, heart disease, and alcoholism), the most common pathogens include the previously mentioned organisms as well as *Klebsiella*, Enterobacteriaceae, *Chlamydia*, and *S aureus*. For patients with aspiration or nosocomial infections, the causative organisms include the previously mentioned organisms and the gram-negative organisms (including *Pseudomonas*) and anaerobes.

The treatments of choice for otherwise healthy patients who are being treated as an outpatient for community-acquired pneumonia include high-dose amoxicillin, doxycycline, or a macrolide.

Additional Reading: Community-acquired pneumonia in adults: rapid evidence review. *Am Fam Physician*. 2022;105(6):625-630.

21. A 27-year-old schoolteacher presents with a cough and runny nose. She reports an outbreak of "the flu" at her school. Which one of the following statements about influenza is true?

A) A maculopapular rash is often seen on the trunk and back.
B) Diagnosis requires sputum culture.
C) Immunization for healthy adults should begin at 65 years of age.
D) Influenza C is the most common cause of the epidemic flu.
E) Symptoms usually include cough and coryza.

The answer is E: Influenza is an acute viral illness characterized by fever, cough, coryza, headache, myalgias, and fatigue. Symptoms usually last 3 to 7 days, and on average, patients feel poorly enough that they require bed rest for 3 to 4 days. Residual symptoms, which typically include fatigue and a nonproductive cough, can last for several weeks. Epidemics usually occur in the winter months. The disease usually spreads through school-age children first. Those with underlying medical problems (eg, diabetes, chronic obstructive pulmonary disease, congestive heart failure, chronic renal disease, and immunodeficiencies) are at higher risk. There are three different types of influenza, but only types A and B cause epidemics:

A is the most common cause of the flu; the causative agent is an RNA orthomyxovirus.
B is usually caused by paramyxovirus, rhinovirus, or echovirus.
C is an endemic virus that occasionally causes mild respiratory disease.

Rapid influenza diagnostic tests are immunoassays that can identify the presence of influenza A and B viral nucleoprotein antigens in respiratory specimens. They may be used to help with diagnostic and treatment decisions for patients in clinical settings, such as whether to prescribe antiviral medications. However, because of the limited sensitivities, negative results of rapid influenza diagnostic tests do not exclude influenza virus infection in patients with signs and symptoms suggestive of influenza. Therefore, antiviral treatment should not be withheld from patients with suspected influenza, even if they test negative by rapid influenza diagnostic testing and further influenza testing of respiratory specimens by molecular assays may be indicated. Once influenza activity has been documented in the community or geographic area, a clinical diagnosis of influenza can be made for outpatients with signs and symptoms consistent with suspected influenza, especially during periods of peak influenza activity in the community.

Oral oseltamivir (Tamiflu), inhaled zanamivir (Relenza), and intravenous peramivir (Rapivab) are chemically related antiviral neuraminidase inhibitors; with activity against both influenza A and B viruses.

Amantadine and rimantadine are antiviral drugs in a class of medications known as adamantanes. These medications are active against influenza A viruses, but not influenza B viruses, and there is increasing resistance developing for the H3N2 and H1N1 influenza A strains. Thus, these medications are not recommended for antiviral treatment or chemoprophylaxis. For antiviral agents to be effective, they must be initiated within 48 hours of the onset of influenza symptoms. Antiviral agents reduce the duration of fever and illness by 1 day and also reduce the severity of some symptoms.

Additional Reading: *Influenza Antiviral Medications*. Centers for Disease Control and Prevention. www.cdc.gov/flu/professionals/antivirals/summary-clinicians.htm

22. Silo filler's disease is a pulmonary disease caused by the long-term inhalation of which one of the following substances?

A) Carbon dioxide
B) Carbon monoxide
C) Nitrogen dioxide
D) Nitrogen mustard
E) Nitrous oxide

The answer is C: Silo filler's disease is a pulmonary disease caused by the inhalation of nitrogen dioxide. Those affected are usually farmers who are exposed to the toxic gas, which is produced from moldy hay found in silos and grain bins. Because of the irritant effects, the gas can lead to the development of pulmonary edema, usually 10 to 12 hours after exposure to the gas. In severe cases, exposure can lead to bronchiolitis obliterans with associated respiratory failure and death. Symptoms include irritation to the mucous membranes and eyes, cough, hemoptysis, wheezing, nausea, vomiting, and dyspnea.

Chest radiographs usually show alveolar infiltrates and pulmonary edema. Bacterial superinfections can occur and can lead to serious complications. Treatment usually involves bronchodilators, intravenous fluids, mechanical ventilation, and steroids. Long-term exposure may lead to chronic bronchitis.

Additional Reading: *Diagnosing Silo-Filler's Disease*. http://nasdonline.org/1033/d000831/diagnosing-silo-filler-039-s-disease.html

23. You are assessing a 52-year-old White man who has been complaining of gradual increasing shortness of breath over the past few months and he comes in now because he is having more problems while working, as he has decreased endurance for any physical activity. You obtain a chest radiograph, which demonstrates honeycombing of the lungs. You refer him to a pulmonologist for formal pulmonary function tests (PFTs), which show both decreased vital and diffusing capacities as well as reduced total lung volumes. However, his forced expiratory volume in 1 second–to–forced vital capacity (FEV1/FVC) ratio is normal. The most likely diagnosis for these findings would be which one of the following?

A) Asthma
B) Chronic pulmonary emboli
C) Chronic obstructive pulmonary disease
D) Idiopathic pulmonary fibrosis
E) Tuberculosis

The answer is D: Idiopathic pulmonary fibrosis is a form of interstitial lung disease, which results when chronic inflammation of the lung tissue leads to fibrosis. A toxic exposure or antigenic response is thought to precipitate the inflammatory process. Affected patients may report a gradual, increasing shortness of breath; a dry cough; and generalized fatigue with lack of endurance with physical exercise.

Physical examination shows bibasilar dry rales, clubbing, and, occasionally, cyanosis. In advanced disease, chest radiographs show honeycombing, and PFTs show a restrictive pattern with reduced vital capacity, diffusing capacity for carbon monoxide, and total lung volume. In addition, there is a normal or increased FEV1-to-FVC ratio. Arterial blood gases may show mild hypoxemia, but hypercarbia is rare. The patient's erythrocyte sedimentation rate may be increased. Transthoracic or transbronchial biopsy is usually needed for a definitive diagnosis.

The treatment of idiopathic pulmonary fibrosis is controversial because of a lack of understanding of the natural history of the disease. Only 10% to 15% of patients improve with corticosteroid therapy, and a quarter of patients treated with steroid actually develop serious complications from that therapy. Indicators of good response to steroid therapy include young age, female sex, ground-glass lesions on computed tomographic scan, and active inflammation on lung biopsy samples. Azathioprine, cyclophosphamide, and other cytotoxic drugs have been used as second-line agents or in combination with steroids as first-line therapy. Although the general prognosis was poor, combined treatment improved 3-year survival rates. Selected patients with idiopathic pulmonary fibrosis have been treated with lung transplantation.

Additional Reading: Chronic dyspnea: diagnosis and evaluation. *Am Fam Physician*. 2020;101(9):542-548.

24. A 53-year-old White man is in for a "physical examination." He has been fasting overnight and wants his cholesterol checked and a test for diabetes because both his parents developed diabetes in their 50s. Additionally, he started smoking since he was a teenager and wants to get screened for lung cancer. He has no pulmonary complaints on your review of symptoms. He drinks socially and his BP has occasionally been borderline, but he is otherwise healthy. Which one of the following statements according to the U.S. Preventive Services Task Force (USPSTF) is true?

A) Yearly chest computed tomographic (CT) scans are recommended for smokers above 50 years.
B) Yearly chest CT scans are recommended for male smokers above 55 years and female smokers older than 60 years.
C) Yearly chest CT scans are recommended for smokers above 50 years, who have a 30 pack-year smoking history.
D) Yearly chest CT scans are not recommended for former smokers if they have not smoked for the past 15 years.

The answer is D: The USPSTF recommends annual screening for lung cancer with low-dose CT scan in adults aged 55 to 80 years who have a 30 pack-year smoking history and currently smoke or have quit within the past 15 years. Screening should be discontinued once a person has not smoked for 15 years or develops a health problem that substantially limits life expectancy or the ability or willingness to have curative lung surgery.

Additional Reading: https://www.uspreventiveservicestaskforce.org/uspstf/recommendation/lung-cancer-screening

25. Which one of the following statements about lung cancer is true?

A) Large cell tumors are common, arise centrally, and typically spread locally.
B) Small cell carcinoma is usually located peripherally and rarely metastasizes.
C) Oat cell tumors are usually associated with asbestos exposure.
D) Squamous cell tumors typically arise in central bronchi and may be diagnosed with sputum cytology.

The answer is D: Lung cancer caused by tobacco abuse is a significant health problem that accounts for approximately 150,000 deaths yearly in the United States. Most cases appear between 50 and 70 years of age. Unfortunately, at the time of diagnosis, only approximately 20% of patients have localized disease. The following are the most common types, with cancers subdivided into small cell or non–small cell cancers.

- *Squamous cell (epidermoid)*—30% to 35% of lung cancers. These tumors, one of the most common types seen in men, tend to arise from the central (larger) bronchi and are the most easily diagnosed with sputum cytology. Most of these tumors metastasize locally to the regional lymph nodes and are more localized at the time of diagnosis.
- *Adenocarcinoma*—25% to 35% of lung cancers. These tumors are usually located peripherally and are usually advanced at the time of diagnosis, with metastasis through the bloodstream and lymphatics.
- *Small cell (oat cell)*—approximately 15% of lung cancers. This type also tends to occur centrally and is usually widespread at the time of diagnosis.
- *Large cell*—10% to 15% of lung cancers. These tumors, less common in incidence, are usually located peripherally and metastasize through the bloodstream. Approximately 20% of patients may develop cavitary lesions.

Additional Reading: Lung, primary malignancies. In: Domino F, ed. *The 5-Minute Clinical Consult*. Wolters Kluwer; 2022.

26. A 21-year-old landscape worker presents complaining of "hay fever." He reports that in addition to itchy eyes, he is sneezing a lot and feeling congested. He reports that his nose is "like a runny faucet." His boss has given him Benadryl (diphenhydramine), which has only helped a little and makes him groggy. He is asking about other treatments. Which one of the following is the treatment of choice for chronic allergic rhinitis?

A) Immunotherapy
B) Intranasal cromolyn sodium
C) Intranasal decongestants
D) Intranasal steroids
E) Systemic nonsedating antihistamines

The answer is D: Allergic rhinitis is characterized by nasal congestion, clear rhinorrhea, mucosal thickening, and conjunctivitis with the absence of fever or sinus tenderness. Patients may exhibit a bluish discoloration below the eyelids ("allergic shiners") as a result of venous congestion. Constant nose rubbing is known as the "allergic salute" and can result in a crease across the bridge of the nose.

Treatment involves avoiding the triggering factors such as pollens, molds, cigarette smoke, animal dander, and dust mites. Many patients report symptoms related to seasons (spring, summer, or fall). The best treatment is the administration of intranasal steroids (eg, fluticasone), which have few associated side effects.

Other treatment options include montelukast (Singulair); azelastine (Astelin nasal spray); cromolyn sodium; ipratropium bromide; and second-generation (nonsedating) systemic antihistamines such as loratadine (Claritin), fexofenadine (Allegra), and cetirizine (Zyrtec).

Long-term use of topical decongestants (eg, Afrin) can lead to rebound congestion known as rhinitis medicamentosa and should be used only on a temporary basis (ie, no more than 3 days). Immunotherapy may also be an alternative treatment for debilitating symptoms.

Additional Reading: Treatment of allergic rhinitis. *Am Fam Physician*. 2015;92(11):985-992.

27. A 63-year-old smoker, who has been smoking a pack per day since he was 16 years of age, presents for follow-up after a recent bout of acute bronchitis. He reports having a productive cough for several months and states that every time he gets a cold, it settles into his chest and lasts for "ever." He also reports dyspnea on exertion. On lung examination, you hear scattered rhonchi. A chest x-ray done 3 months ago when he went to the emergency department for the last similar episode was negative except for hyperinflation and flattened diaphragms. Which one of the following would be best for making the diagnosis?

A) A chest radiograph
B) A B-type natriuretic peptide level
C) An arterial blood gas
D) Computed tomographic scan of the chest
E) Spirometry

The answer is E: This patient's presentation is consistent with chronic obstructive pulmonary disease (COPD). Patients with COPD are usually in their 60s when the diagnosis is made. Symptoms of chronic cough (sometimes for months or years), dyspnea, or sputum production are often not reported because the patient may attribute them to smoking, aging, or poor physical condition. Spirometry is the best test for the diagnosis of COPD. The presence of outflow obstruction that is not fully reversible is demonstrated by postbronchodilator spirometry showing a forced expiratory volume–to–forced vital capacity ratio of 70% or less.

Additional Reading: Chronic obstructive pulmonary disease: diagnosis and management. *Am Fam Physician*. 2017;95(7):433-441.

28. You are seeing a middle-aged woman who has had a cough for the past few weeks, and she has noted some blood-tinged sputum. Which one of the following tests should you obtain in the initial evaluation of persistent hemoptysis?

A) Computed tomographic (CT) scan of chest
B) Chest radiograph
C) Fiber-optic bronchoscopy
D) Laryngoscopy
E) Magnetic resonance imaging of chest

The answer is B: Hemoptysis is the presence of blood in the expectorate. Intrapulmonary causes include infections (eg, bronchitis, pneumonia, tuberculosis and fungal infections), neoplasm, bronchiectasis, pulmonary embolus, atrioventricular malformations, Goodpasture disease, vasculitis, trauma, or the presence of a foreign body. Extrapulmonary causes include gastrointestinal (GI) bleeding, CHF with pulmonary edema, severe mitral stenosis, and epistaxis.

Most cases of hemoptysis are self-limited and require no additional workup; however, persistent or severe hemoptysis should be evaluated. If a lower respiratory tract source is suspected, the patient should undergo a chest x-ray first, and if a mass is noted, bronchoscopy should be performed. Additionally, sputum should be sent for a Gram stain and culture, cytology, acid-fast bacillus stains, and complete blood count, prothrombin time, and partial thromboplastin time laboratory test results obtained. A high-resolution CT scan may be helpful in the diagnosis.

It is important to distinguish between GI blood loss (which has a dark red color and acidic pH) and true hemoptysis (which is typically bright red and alkaline).

Additional Reading: Etiology and evaluation of hemoptysis in adults. In: *UpToDate*. 2022.

29. The pneumococcal vaccine should be administered to all otherwise healthy individuals beginning at which of the following ages?

A) 50 years
B) 55 years
C) 60 years
D) 65 years
E) 70 years

The answer is D: Pneumococcal disease is common in young children, but older adults are at greatest risk of serious pneumococcal infections and even death. The Centers for Disease Control and Prevention (CDC) recommends vaccination with the pneumococcal conjugate vaccine for all babies and children younger than 2 years, all adults 65 years or older, and those 2 to 64 years of age who are at increased risk for pneumococcal disease as noted below. Per guidelines, the CDC recommends routine administration of pneumococcal conjugate vaccine (PCV15 or PCV20) for all adults 65 years or older who have never received any pneumococcal conjugate vaccine or whose previous vaccination history is unknown.

- If PCV15 is used, this should be followed by a dose of PPSV23 1 year later. The minimum interval is 8 weeks and can be considered in adults with an immunocompromising condition, a cochlear implant, or a cerebrospinal fluid leak.
- If PCV20 is used, a dose of PPSV23 is not indicated.

Additional Reading: *Pneumococcal Vaccination*. Center for Disease Control and Prevention. https://www.cdc.gov/vaccines/vpd/pneumo/hcp/recommendations.html

30. Which one of the following best describes Ludwig angina?

A) Substernal chest pain that does not radiate to the left arm
B) Back pain secondary to an enlarging AAA
C) A tonsillar infection that leads to chronic abscess formation
D) An infection involving the sublingual and submaxillary space
E) Ischemic pain related to insufficient blood flow to an extremity

The answer is D: Ludwig angina usually develops from a periodontal or dental infection and is one of the most common neck space infections. The condition is usually a rapidly developing, bilateral cellulitis that affects the sublingual and submaxillary space, without involvement of the lymph nodes or formation of abscesses. The infection usually rapidly arises from the second and third mandibular molars as a result of poor dental hygiene, tooth extraction, or trauma.

Symptoms include edema and erythema of the upper neck (under the chin) and floor of the mouth, trismus, drooling, dysphonia, dysphagia, and dyspnea. Fever, chills, and tachycardia are usually present. Tongue displacement upward may also occur and threaten the airway. In severe cases, the condition may be fatal.

Treatment includes protection of the airway in severe cases and intravenous antibiotics (eg, penicillin and wide-spectrum cephalosporins) in high doses to cover anaerobic organisms (*Bacteroides*). Incision and drainage may be required.

Additional Reading: Ludwig angina. In: Domino F, ed. *The 5-Minute Clinical Consult*. Wolters Kluwer; 2022.

31. Your daughter is buying a house and has been told that she should have it inspected for radon gas. You tell her that exposure to radon gas has been associated with the development of which one of the following?

A) Bladder cancer
B) Esophageal cancer
C) Lung cancer
D) Pancreatic cancer
E) Renal cell carcinoma

The answer is C: Radon gas exposure has been linked to the development of lung cancer. The highest amounts of radon exposure are associated with people who mine uranium. Radon found in the soil and in the water supply around homes represents a theoretic risk to inhabitants. Levels associated with excess lung cancer risk may be present in as many as 10% of houses in the United States. Concrete block foundations provide a better barrier against radon compared with cinder block foundations. Adequate ventilation of the home is also important to minimize radon levels.

According to the Environmental Protection Agency, the maximum limit for radon in homes is 4 pCi/L. Radon levels tend to be higher in the winter months when houses are more poorly ventilated. Radon levels <1.5 pCi/L are considered safe. When smokers reside in the affected household, the problem is potentially greater because the molecular size of radon particles allows them to readily attach to smoke particles that are inhaled.

Additional Reading: Lung, primary malignancies. In: Domino F, ed. *The 5-Minute Clinical Consult*. Wolters Kluwer; 2022.

32. A 28-year-old man with a history of human immunodeficiency virus (HIV) infection presents to your office complaining of a nonproductive cough, shortness of breath, fever, and chills. A chest radiograph shows bilateral interstitial infiltrates. The best treatment for this patient would be to recommend which one of the following?

A) Intravenous penicillin
B) Intravenous amphotericin
C) Oral azithromycin
D) Oral trimethoprim-sulfamethoxazole (TMP-SMX)
E) Observation only

The answer is D: *Pneumocystis jirovecii* (formerly *P carinii*) is an opportunistic infection that often affects patients with profound immune suppression; the abbreviation of *P carinii* pneumonia (PCP) is used to designate this infection. Before the introduction of prophylaxis for PCP and the advent of potent antiretroviral therapy for HIV, 70% to 80% of patients with acquired immunodeficiency syndrome presented with PCP.

Symptoms include fever, progressive dyspnea, nonproductive cough, and chest discomfort. Common findings on physical examination include tachypnea, tachycardia, and dry rales, although the lung may be normal at rest. Chest radiograph classically shows diffuse bilateral symmetrical infiltrates in a butterfly pattern but can be normal in early disease. Definitive diagnosis involves demonstration of the organism in tissue obtained either through inducted sputum collection or bronchoalveolar lavage.

Treatment involves TMP-SMX for 21 days; intravenous therapy is indicated if patient is unable to tolerate oral medication. Oral prednisone or intravenous methylprednisolone may also be added once tuberculosis is ruled out if the PaO_2 is <70 mm Hg. For those who cannot take TMP-SMX due to allergy or adverse effects, alternatives include dapsone, aerosolized pentamidine, or atovaquone.

Prophylactic therapy should be initiated for all patients with CD4 counts <200 cells/mm^3 or with a previous infection with PCP or oral thrush. Prophylaxis against PCP can be discontinued once the CD4 count is >200 cells/mm^3 for >3 months.

Additional Reading: *Guidelines for the Prevention and Treatment of opportunistic Infections in HIV-Infected Adults and Adolescents.* http://aidsinfot.nih.gov/contentfiles/lvguidelines

33. A 67-year-old smoker presents for a follow-up visit. You have been treating her for chronic obstructive pulmonary disease (COPD) and note clubbing of her fingers on your examination. Clubbing is thought to be a result of which one of the following conditions?

A) Chronic hypercarbia
B) Chronic hypoxemia
C) Excess amyloid production
D) Malignancy
E) Protein storage disease

The answer is B: Clubbing refers to an enlargement and softness of the nail beds and a reduction in the angle between the nail and the distal phalanx. The ratio of the anteroposterior diameter of the finger at the nail bed to that at the distal interphalangeal joint is a simple measurement of finger clubbing. If the ratio is more than 1, clubbing is present and the patient should be evaluated with a chest radiograph to look for an underlying lung condition.

The cause is thought to be related to chronic hypoxemia and causes include bronchogenic carcinoma, chronic pulmonary tuberculosis, COPD, and bronchiectasis; cyanotic congenital heart disease; subacute bacterial endocarditis; inflammatory bowel disease; and biliary cirrhosis.

Additional Reading: Evaluation of nail abnormalities. *Am Fam Physician*. 2012;85(8):779-787.

34. A 47-year-old nurse presents with complaint of a chronic cough. She is a nonsmoker who has been plagued by a nonproductive irritating cough for several months now. She worries that she has "caught" something at work, as she frequently cares for hospitalized patients with pneumonia. The most common cause of chronic cough is which one of the following?

A) Angiotensin-converting enzyme (ACE) inhibitors
B) Asthma
C) Bronchiectasis
D) Gastroesophageal reflux
E) Postnasal drip

The answer is E: Coughing is part of the body's infection protective system and helps remove particles and material from the airway. In some cases, the patient may experience a chronic cough that can be attributed to several different problems, including postnasal drip (the most common cause), gastroesophageal reflux, and bronchoconstriction as seen in cough-variant asthma patients. Other common associated conditions include the use of ACE inhibitors, chronic bronchitis seen in smokers, and bronchiectasis.

Treatment involves eliminating the underlying cause. Treatment of postnasal drip may involve the use of antihistamines and topical nasal steroids. Patients should be informed that it may take 8 to 12 weeks before their cough improves when using inhaled steroids. Treatment of gastroesophageal reflux involves the use of antacids, H_2 receptor blockers, and proton pump inhibitors. Eliminating a cough caused by ACE inhibitors usually takes several days before improvement is seen.

Additional Reading: Chronic cough: evaluation and management. *Am Fam Physician*. 2017;96(9):575-580.

35. A 21-year-old nurse's aide is seen in your office with a recent purified protein derivative tuberculin skin test that was positive when checked as part of a preemployment examination at the nursing home where she will be working. She is otherwise healthy, has no signs of disease, and has no known exposure. You obtain a chest radiograph, which is negative. The most appropriate treatment for such a patient is which one of the following?

A) Isoniazid (INH) and rifampin for 6 months
B) INH for 6 months
C) INH, rifampin, and streptomycin (or ethambutol) for 12 months
D) Streptomycin for 6 months
E) Reassurance

The answer is B: Tuberculosis is caused by *M tuberculosis*, a nonmotile acid-fast rod that is spread primarily by inhalation. The organism can affect many different systems but usually affects the lungs. There has been a recent increase in incidence, particularly in the immunocompromised and elderly populations. Symptoms include fever, fatigue, weight loss, a productive cough, dyspnea, and, occasionally, hemoptysis.

A Mantoux tuberculin skin test using purified protein derivative injected intradermally is used to screen for tuberculosis or as a diagnostic test in suspected cases. In most cases, an area of induration >10 mm (with risk factors), 15 mm (without risk factors), or 5 mm (in human immunodeficiency virus [HIV] patients) 48 hours after administration is a positive response. A negative response does not exclude the diagnosis.

Diagnosis is usually accomplished with a chest radiograph, which shows apical infiltrates and mediastinal lymphadenopathy. A calcified focus of infection seen on chest radiograph is referred to as a *Ghon complex*. An acid-fast stain of sputum shows acid-fast rods. A definitive diagnosis is achieved with a culture of early morning sputum growing *M tuberculosis*.

All patients who have a positive skin test, but no evidence of active disease and a negative chest radiograph, are diagnosed with latent tuberculosis infection, regardless of bacille Calmette-Guérin vaccination history, and should be treated with INH 300 mg/d for 6 months, or an alternative regimen if needed.

Treatment for active disease is accomplished with INH, rifampin, and pyrazinamide. In some cases, a fourth drug (eg, streptomycin or ethambutol) is necessary. Most treatment regimens require extended courses lasting at least 6 to 9 months.

Compliance is a critical factor in ensuring adequate treatment for both active and latent tuberculosis and is often followed by the local department of public health. Other sites affected by tuberculosis include the kidneys, pericardium, and spine. All patients with a new diagnosis of tuberculosis should be tested for HIV and vice versa.

Additional Reading: *Treatment Regimens for Latent TB Infection (LTBI)*. www.cdc.gov/tb/topic/treatment/ltbi.htm

36. Which one of the following tests is the most appropriate to diagnose carbon monoxide (CO) poisoning?

A) Arterial blood gas
B) Carboxyhemoglobin levels
C) Complete blood count
D) Chest radiograph
E) Lactic acid levels

The answer is B: CO poisoning is a dangerous but relatively common occurrence, especially during the winter months in cold regions of the United States. The affinity of CO for hemoglobin is 240 times greater than that of oxygen; it shifts the oxygen dissociation curve to the left, which impairs hemoglobin release of oxygen to tissues and inhibits the cytochrome oxidase system. Symptoms include headache, confusion, fatigue, and nausea; in more severe cases, seizures, rhabdomyolysis, parkinsonian-type symptoms, coma, and death may occur. In many cases, the initial symptoms are attributed to a flulike illness, and CO poisoning is overlooked.

The diagnosis is usually made by obtaining a history of exposure (usually a fuel oil furnace or exhaust fumes in a poorly ventilated enclosure) and laboratory testing, which shows elevated carboxyhemoglobin levels. Treatment involves the use of 100% oxygen and, in severe cases, hyperbaric oxygen. Prolonged exposures usually have a worse prognosis. Patients with CO poisoning necessitating treatment need follow-up neuropsychiatric examinations.

Additional Reading: Carbon monoxide poisoning. In: Domino F, ed. *The 5-Minute Clinical Consult*. Wolters Kluwer; 2022.

37. An elderly Black woman has been admitted with urosepsis and treated overnight with intravenous antibiotics. The next morning, she has become dyspneic with hypoxia and you diagnose adult respiratory distress syndrome (ARDS). The best treatment approach at this time is which one of the following?

A) β2-Agonist via nebulizer treatments
B) Intravenous administration of loop diuretics
C) Intravenous administration of corticosteroids
D) Intubation with positive end-expiratory pressure

The answer is D: ARDS is characterized by respiratory distress that is usually associated with pulmonary sepsis (46%) or nonpulmonary sepsis (33%). Risk factors include those causing direct lung injury (eg, pneumonia, inhalation injury, and pulmonary contusion) and those causing indirect lung injury (eg, nonpulmonary sepsis, burns, and transfusion-related acute lung injury). The mechanism of injury involves damage of capillary endothelial cells and alveolar epithelial cells, which leads to pulmonary edema with decreased pulmonary compliance and decreased functional residual capacity.

Symptoms include rapid onset of dyspnea, usually 12 to 48 hours after the insult, with wheezing and intercostal retractions. Laboratory tests show hypoxemia that responds poorly to oxygen administration, requiring frequent monitoring of arterial blood gases. Radiographs show diffuse or patchy alveolar and interstitial infiltrates without cardiomegaly or pulmonary vascular redistribution.

Treatment with mechanical ventilation is often required, with the use of low-volume ventilation with higher positive end-expiratory pressure values (12-18 or more cm H_2O) initially. Most patients who develop ARDS also have multiple organ failure, which is the major cause of death, with mortality rates of 50%.

Additional Reading: Acute respiratory distress syndrome: diagnosis and management. *Am Fam Physician*. 2020;101(12):730-738.

38. A 16-year-old adolescent with a history of asthma presents to your office with his mother. He is complaining of shortness of breath with wheezing over the last day. Which of the following medications is indicated in the initial treatment of this patient?

A) Albuterol nebulization
B) Cromolyn inhaler
C) Ipratropium nebulization
D) Salmeterol intramuscularly
E) Theophylline intravenously

The answer is A: Asthma is a reversible obstructive lung disorder that is characterized by reactive airways. The condition is thought to be inherited; however, some individuals may be affected without a family history. Many factors may precipitate an attack, including infections, smoke, cold weather, exercise, toxic fumes, and stress. Symptoms include wheezing, shortness of breath, tachypnea, cough (particularly in children), and tightness or pressure in the chest.

The mainstay of short-term treatment (rescue therapy) is an inhalant form of a β2-adrenergic agonist, such as albuterol. Inhaled corticosteroids and salmeterol (a long-acting β2-adrenergic agonist) are used in long-term therapy. For patients who have more severe asthmatic attacks, short courses of oral corticosteroids may be necessary, particularly with upper respiratory tract infections. Cromolyn sodium, a mast cell stabilizer; ipratropium bromide, an anticholinergic medication; and leukotriene modifiers can be used for chronic asthmatic conditions. Theophylline is reserved for refractory cases as an add-on medication.

Pulmonary function tests in patients affected with asthma usually show a normal or decreased vital capacity, decreased forced expiratory volume in 1 second, increased residual volume, increased total lung capacity, and a positive response to inhaled bronchodilators.

Additional Reading: Asthma management guidelines: focused updates for 2020. *Am Fam Physician*. 2021;104(5):446-447.

39. A 49-year-old man presents with complaints of dyspnea that tends to occur with exercise. He has been diagnosed with exercise-induced asthma in the past and currently smokes with a 35-pack-year history. He denies any other medical problems. On spirometry, his expiratory loop is normal, but he has a flattened inspiratory loop. What is the most likely diagnosis to account for this finding?

A) Asthma
B) Chronic obstructive pulmonary disease (COPD)
C) Restrictive lung disease
D) Vocal cord dysfunction

The answer is D: Vocal cord dysfunction occurs when the vocal cords move toward the midline during inspiration or expiration, leading to varying degrees of obstruction. It is often misdiagnosed as exercise-induced asthma. Precipitating factors, including exercise, psychological conditions, irritants, sinusitis, and gastroesophageal reflux disease.

Spirometry generally will show a normal expiratory loop with a flattened inspiratory loop. In asthma and COPD, the forced expiratory volume in 1 second–to–forced vital capacity (FEV1/FVC) ratio is decreased, resulting in a concave shape in the expiratory portion of the flow-volume curve. The inspiratory loops are generally normal. Patients with restrictive lung disease have a normal FEV1/FVC ratio with a reduced FVC.

Additional Reading: Vocal cord dysfunction: rapid evidence review. *Am Fam Physician*. 2021;104(5):471-475.

40. A 67-year-old obese woman with known coronary artery disease presents with chest pain that becomes worse when taking a deep breath. She does not feel well and reports a low-grade fever. Her medications include simvastatin (Zocor), lisinopril (Zestril), spironolactone (Aldactone), furosemide (Lasix), isosorbide mononitrate (Imdur), hydralazine, carvedilol (Coreg), and prn nitroglycerin. A chest radiograph is normal with no signs of pneumonia, and the workup is negative for an acute coronary event and pulmonary embolus. You make a diagnosis of pleurisy. Which one of the patient's medications could be related to this condition?

A) Carvedilol
B) Hydralazine
C) Lisinopril
D) Simvastatin
E) Spironolactone

The answer is B: Drug-induced pleuritis is one cause of pleurisy, and many drugs are associated with drug-induced pleural disease or drug-induced lupus pleuritis. Drugs known to cause lupus pleuritis include hydralazine, procainamide, and quinidine. Other drugs known to cause pleural disease include amiodarone, bleomycin, bromocriptine, cyclophosphamide, methotrexate, minoxidil, and mitomycin.

Additional Reading: Pleuritic chest pain: sorting through the differential diagnosis. *Am Fam Physician*. 2017;96(5):306-312.

41. You are assessing a 23-year-old teacher in your office with a complaint of a sore throat, and he reports that the school nurse said he should get checked for a strep throat because several of his classmates have recently been treated for strep throat. You ask your medical assistant to perform a rapid strep test. Which one of the following statements about rapid enzyme immunoassay streptococcal screening testing is true?

A) Their specificity is generally poor.
B) They are less accurate than latex agglutination tests performed in a laboratory.
C) They typically require a follow-up culture to confirm results.
D) They may be avoided if the criteria for streptococcal pharyngitis are met.

The answer is D: Rapid streptococcal in-office screening tests are quick, easy to perform, and approximately as accurate as the latex agglutination tests. Their sensitivity approaches 80%, whereas their specificity is 85% to 100%; thus, a positive test is fairly predictive of a streptococcal infection and a culture is unnecessary. If negative, cultures can be performed to confirm the results.

In adults, the use of clinical decision rules for diagnosing group A β-hemolytic streptococcal (GABHS) pharyngitis improves quality of care while reducing unwarranted treatment and overall cost. Treatment can be started or avoided without a strep test. The criteria include the following:

- Fever
- Tonsillar exudates
- No cough
- Tender anterior cervical lymphadenopathy

Patients are then assessed a point for each of the criterion:

- Those with zero or one criterion are unlikely to have streptococcal pharyngitis and do not need to be tested.
- Those with two to three criteria are at risk and should be tested.
- Those with four criteria have a high likelihood of GABHS and can be treated empirically, without testing.

Additional Reading: Diagnosis of streptococcal pharyngitis. *Am Fam Physician*. 2014;89(12):976-977.

42. Coccidioidomycosis ("valley fever") is an opportunistic infection that is usually asymptomatic; however, in severe cases requiring treatment, the drug of choice is which one of the following agents?

A) Ceftriaxone
B) Ciprofloxacin
C) Fluconazole
D) Mefloquine
E) Tetracycline

The answer is C: As noted here, coccidioidomycosis is usually asymptomatic; however, in some cases, nonspecific symptoms resembling influenza or acute bronchitis occur. Less frequently, acute pneumonia or pleural effusion can develop. Symptoms include fever, cough, chest pain, chills, sputum production, sore throat, and hemoptysis.

Physical signs may be absent or limited to scattered rales with or without areas of dullness to percussion over lung fields. Other signs can include arthritis, conjunctivitis, erythema nodosum, or erythema multiforme.

On chest radiograph the primary lung findings can resolve, leaving nodular coin lesions that may be confused with cancer, tuberculosis, or other granulomatous infections. In some cases, thin-walled cavitary lesions develop. Although dissemination does not occur from these residual areas, a small percentage of these cavities fail to heal. Hemoptysis or the threat of rupture into the pleural space may occasionally require surgery. Leukocytosis and, in some cases, eosinophilia are seen.

Treatment for mild primary coccidioidomycosis may be unnecessary in low-risk patients. Mild to moderate nonmeningeal extrapulmonary involvement should be treated with fluconazole or itraconazole. Intravenous fluconazole is preferable for severely ill patients. Amphotericin B is an alternative treatment. As with histoplasmosis, patients with acquired immunodeficiency syndrome–associated coccidioidomycosis require maintenance therapy to prevent relapse. Treatment for meningeal coccidioidomycosis must be continued for many months, probably lifelong. Surgical removal of involved bone may be necessary to cure osteomyelitis.

Additional Reading: Coccidioidomycosis (valley fever) in primary care. *Am Fam Physician*. 2020;101(4):221-228.

43. Patients often take vitamins and supplements to improve their health. However, which one of the following has been associated with an increased risk of lung cancer in smokers?

A) β-Carotene
B) Folic acid
C) Ginseng
D) Saw palmetto
E) Vitamin E

The answer is A: β-Carotene is a vitamin A precursor carried in plasma and low-density lipoprotein (LDL). It is an antioxidant that reduces oxidized LDL uptake but does not prevent LDL oxidation. Sources of dietary carotenoids include fruits, yellow-orange vegetables (eg, carrots, squash, and sweet potatoes), and deep-green vegetables (eg, spinach and broccoli). No recommended daily allowance has been established for carotenoids. Research supports the benefit of antioxidants and a carotenoid-rich diet but not β-carotene supplementation.

The Beta-Carotene and Retinol Efficacy Trial combined β-carotene and retinol supplementation in 18,314 smokers and patients with asbestos exposure. However, the study was terminated prematurely because of a significant increase in lung cancer mortality and a nonsignificant increase in coronary heart disease (CHD mortality. Additional studies have failed to demonstrate any significant beneficial effects on CHD mortality, nonfatal myocardial infarction, or stroke.

Additional Reading: *American College of Preventive Medicine*. https://www.choosingwisely.org/clinician-lists/american-college-preventive-medicine-vitamin-supplements/

44. A 13-year-old asthmatic is brought in by his mother, as he has been having more trouble with wheezing over the past few weeks, needing to use his albuterol "rescue inhaler" daily. His mother is concerned because over this last month he has been waking up a couple of times a week with symptoms as well. This has been a tough year for him and he has been treated with oral prednisone twice already, and she thinks he needs another prescription. Given the severity of his symptoms, his asthma would be classified as which one of the following?

A) Intermittent
B) Mild persistent
C) Moderate persistent
D) Severe persistent

The answer is C: This patient's symptoms are consistent with persistent asthma, with symptoms and use of his rescue inhaler more than twice a week, along with nighttime awakenings more than twice a month. Persistent asthma is further subclassified as mild, moderate, or severe. The following criteria are used to classify asthma:

Intermittent: symptoms ≤2 d/wk, nighttime awakenings less than two times per month, short-acting β-agonist use ≤2 d/wk, no interference with normal activity, and normal forced expiratory volume in 1 second (FEV1) between exacerbations with FEV1 (predicted) > 80% and FEV1/forced vital capacity (FVC) ratio >80%

Mild persistent: symptoms >2 d/wk but not daily, nighttime awakenings three to four times per month, short-acting β-agonist use >2 d/wk but not daily, minor limitations in normal activity, and FEV1 (predicted) >80% and FEV1/FVC ratio >80%

Moderate persistent: daily symptoms, nighttime awakenings more than one time per week but not nightly, daily use of short-acting β-agonist, some limitation in normal activity, and FEV1 (predicted) 60% to 80% and FEV1/FVC ratio 75% to 80%

Severe persistent: symptoms throughout the day, nighttime awakenings often seven times per week, short-acting β-agonist use several times a day, extremely limited normal activity, and FEV1 (predicted) <60% and FEV1/FVC ratio <75%

Additional Reading: Asthma. In: Domino F, ed. *The 5-Minute Clinical Consult*. Wolters Kluwer; 2022.

45. You are seeing a 17-year-old patient, who presents for a physical examination, as she will be going to college in the fall. She has been healthy, except she has struggled with her asthma. She uses her albuterol inhaler two to three times every week and occasionally misses a class as she is in the nurse's office with wheezing. You have diagnosed her with mild persistent asthma. As she leaves for college, what should you recommend for her asthma?

A) Continue current management and ensure that she has albuterol refills.
B) Prescribe a long-acting β-agonist (LABA) for daily use and continue the albuterol prn.
C) Prescribe an inhaled corticosteroid for daily use and continue the albuterol prn.
D) Prescribe a LABA and an inhaled corticosteroid for daily use and continue the albuterol prn.

The answer is C: If an asthmatic is using their rescue inhaler more than twice a week, or if they are waking up with asthma once a week or more, the asthma is not being adequately controlled and stepped therapy is recommended. Other indicators for stepped therapy are when asthma is interfering with a person's usual activities or if their peak flows are less than 80% of that person's normal measurements. Although those with intermittent symptoms are best treated with inhaled albuterol on an as-needed basis, but when symptoms become more persistent, preventative therapy should be prescribed. Inhaled corticosteroids are the mainstay of preventive treatment. A LABA should only be prescribed in combination with an inhaled corticosteroid.

For an individual who is already on an inhaled steroid for preventive treatment, step-up treatment may involve any or all of the following:

- An increase in the inhaled corticosteroid dose
- Addition of a second inhaler or medication (such as LABAs)
- A brief course of oral steroids

Anyone whose medication has been increased should be reevaluated in the next 2 to 4 weeks.

Additional Reading: Asthma. In: Domino F, ed. *The 5-Minute Clinical Consult*. Wolters Kluwer; 2022.

46. Patients with an asthma exacerbation will have abnormal arterial blood gases. When assessing a patient in the early stages of an acute exacerbation, which one of the following abnormal acid/base conditions would you expect to see in your patient?

A) Metabolic acidosis
B) Respiratory acidosis
C) Metabolic alkalosis
D) Respiratory alkalosis

The answer is D: Initial arterial blood gas findings in an acute asthma exacerbation typically include hypoxemia and hypocapnia. Primary hypocapnia results in respiratory alkalosis. Worrisome findings would be respiratory acidosis or hypercapnia, which would indicate respiratory muscle fatigue and impending respiratory failure.

Additional Reading: Asthma. In: Domino F, ed. *The 5-Minute Clinical Consult*. Wolters Kluwer; 2022.

47. Which one of the following drugs is a leukotriene antagonist/inhibitor?

A) Prednisone
B) Salmeterol
C) Terbutaline
D) Theophylline
E) Zafirlukast

The answer is E: Medications used in the treatment of asthma are divided into long-term control medications that are taken regularly and quick-relief (rescue) medications that are taken as needed to relieve bronchoconstriction rapidly. Quick-relief medications include short-acting β2-agonists and anticholinergics. Long-term control medications include anti-inflammatory agents (corticosteroids and leukotriene modifiers) and long-acting bronchodilators.

Patients whose symptoms are mild and infrequent can use a short-acting bronchodilator as needed for relief of symptoms. Patients with more frequent cough, wheeze, chest tightness, or shortness of breath should begin treatment with a long-term controller medication. Low daily doses of an inhaled corticosteroid suppress airway inflammation and reduce the risk of exacerbations. For patients who remain symptomatic despite compliance with inhaled corticosteroid treatment and good inhalational technique, addition of a long-acting β2-agonist is recommended. Patients with more severe disease may need higher doses of inhaled corticosteroids.

Corticosteroids remain the most potent and effective anti-inflammatory agents available for the management of asthma. An inhaled corticosteroid is the most effective long-term treatment for control of the disease in treating all types of persistent asthma in patients of all ages. Leukotriene modifiers (montelukast, zafirlukast) are less effective alternatives for those who cannot tolerate low-dose inhaled steroids. Leukotriene modifiers are also generally less effective than an inhaled LABA. Both of these classes are not recommended for treatment of acute asthma symptoms.

Salmeterol (Serevent) is a long-acting β2-agonist. Its mechanism of action and side effect profile are similar to those of other β2-agonists. Unlike the short-acting agents, salmeterol is not intended for use as a quick-relief agent.

Theophylline, in addition to its bronchodilator effects, has anti-inflammatory activity as well. Currently, theophylline is generally reserved as a third-line agent for use in patients who exhibit nocturnal asthma symptoms that are not controlled with high-dose anti-inflammatory medications.

Additional Readings:
1. Drugs for asthma and COPD. *Treat Guidel Med Lett*. 2013;11 (132):75-86.
2. Asthma management guidelines: focused updates for 2020. *Am Fam Physician*. 2021;104(5):446-447.

48. Which one of the following conditions is a contraindication to influenza vaccination?

A) Allergy to eggs
B) Allergy to red dye
C) Allergy to penicillin
D) Allergy to milk
E) None of the above

The answer is E: Influenza immunizations are administered yearly to help prevent outbreaks of different strains of viral influenza. Most flu shots and the nasal spray flu vaccine are manufactured using egg-based technology and contain a small amount of egg proteins, such as ovalbumin. Studies that have examined the use of these vaccines in egg-allergic patients indicate that severe allergic reactions in people with egg allergies are unlikely. A recent Centers for Disease Control and Prevention (CDC) study found the rate of anaphylaxis after all vaccines is 1.31 per 1 million vaccine doses given.

Thus, the CDC recommendations for flu vaccination of persons with egg allergy were modified for the 2016 to 2017 season:

- Persons with a history of egg allergy who have experienced only hives after exposure to eggs should receive flu vaccine. Any licensed and recommended flu vaccine that is otherwise appropriate for the recipient's age and health status may be used.
- Persons who report having had reactions to eggs involving symptoms other than hives, such as angioedema, respiratory distress, light-headedness, or recurrent emesis, or persons who required epinephrine or another emergency medical intervention, may similarly receive any licensed and recommended flu vaccine (ie, any form of inactivated influenza vaccine or recombinant influenza vaccine) that is otherwise appropriate for the recipient's age and health status. The selected vaccine should be administered in an inpatient or outpatient medical setting (including, but not necessarily limited to, hospitals, clinics, health departments, and physician offices). Vaccine administration should be supervised by a health care provider who is able to recognize and manage severe allergic conditions.

Additional Reading: *Flu Vaccine and People With Egg Allergies*. Centers for Disease Control and Prevention. www.cdc.gov/flu/protect/vaccine/egg-allergies.htm

Section III. Musculoskeletal Conditions

Questions related to musculoskeletal conditions account for about another 10% of the American Board of Family Medicine certifying examination. This section covers various common musculoskeletal conditions. Additional conditions are covered in Chapter 2, Care of Children and Adolescents, and Chapter 6, Care of the Elderly. Some find it helpful to make "flash cards" to practice the names of common orthopedic diagnostic maneuvers and conditions as well. As you study for the examination, ensure that you have a good overview of the following musculoskeletal conditions:

1. Arthritis (gout, rheumatod arthritis, osteoarthritis)
   - Appreciate the presentation and laboratory evaluation for the workup of gout.
   - Appreciate the use of nonpharmacologic treatments for gout (eg, dietary changes).
   - Know the commonly accepted first-line medications for gout and how to use maintenance medications for disease.
   - Understand the common presentation and clinical findings of RA and related conditions (American College of Rheumatology diagnostic criteria).
   - Appreciate the diagnostic evaluation of RA and the interpretation of laboratory data and x-rays.
   - Appreciate the use of nonpharmacologic treatments.
   - Understand the pharmacology of biologic and nonbiologic disease-modifying antirheumatic drugs and their appropriate use in the treatments of RA.
   - Understand the common presentation and clinical findings of OA.
   - Appreciate diagnostic evaluation of OA and the use and findings of x-rays.
   - Understand the pharmacology in the treatments of OA.
2. Back pain and fibromyalgia
   - Understand the common presentation, clinical findings, and prognosis for acute low back pain (including "red flags").
   - Appreciate the timely and cost-effective diagnostic evaluation of acute low back pain and the appropriate use of imaging.
   - Know the indications of when to expand the diagnostic evaluation and the appropriate use of emergent and nonemergent referrals to neurosurgeons.
   - Understand the use of rehabilitation services and physical modalities.
   - Understand the appropriate use of medication to treat acute and chronic low back pain.
   - Understand when to consider ankylosing spondylitis (eg, insidious onset of back pain, especially in the morning, before 40 years of age that is relieved by activity).
   - Understand the common presentation, findings, and diagnostic criteria for fibromyalgia.
   - Know the use of nonpharmacologic treatments (eg, sleep hygiene and exercise).
   - Know the commonly accepted first-line medications and treatments for fibromyalgia and related comorbidities (including complementary and alternative medicine).
   - Know the patient education aspects of treatment for fibromyalgia.
3. Common upper extremity injuries
   - Understand how to evaluate (physical examination, appropriate use of imaging) and treat pain in the arm/wrist, including the following:
   - Cubital tunnel syndrome (inflammation of the ulnar nerve through the medial aspect of the elbow)
   - Lateral epicondylitis (injury to the wrist extensor and supinator muscles: extensor carpi radialis)
   - Carpal tunnel syndrome (diagnostic evaluation, etiology, and initial treatment)
   - Potential fractures of the hand and wrist (pain in the anatomic snuff box)
   - Skier's thumb (ulnar collateral ligament sprain of the thumb)
   - Colles fracture (in the elderly after fall, "dinner fork" appearance on x-ray)
   - Understand how to evaluate (physical examination, appropriate use of imaging) and treat shoulder pain (impingement vs instability), including history, supporting physical examination findings, appropriate use of imaging, and initial treatment.
4. Common lower extremity injuries
   - Understand how to evaluate (physical examination, appropriate use of imaging) and treat pain in the lower extremity, including the following:
   - Understand use and limits of Ottawa rules for acute ankle sprain.
   - Know the difference between shin splints (pain over the distal third of the tibia that diminishes with rest) and stress fracture (pain with activity and at rest).
   - Know common presenting histories and examination findings with iliotibial band syndrome and anserine bursitis.
   - Appreciate the signs, symptoms, and workup for knee injuries, including meniscal and anterior cruciate ligament injuries.

Each of the following questions or incomplete statements is followed by suggested answers or completions. Select the ONE BEST ANSWER in each case.

1. A 47-year-old diabetic presents complaining of foot pain, which has been slowly worsening over the past few weeks. He has otherwise been feeling well. He is taking metformin for his diabetes and his last A1c level was 6.9%. On examination, there are no open lesions or sores on his feet, and sensation and pulses are intact. He has a slight hammer toe deformity of his toes and pain to palpation of the distal second metatarsal head. This situation is most likely a result of which one of the following conditions?

A) Diabetic neuropathy
B) Jones fracture
C) Gout
D) Metatarsalgia
E) Morton neuroma

The answer is D: Metatarsalgia is characterized by pain and sometimes swelling associated with the second (and, less commonly, the third) metatarsal head. The pain is secondary to synovitis that affects the joint. Patients with hammertoes are at an increased risk because of stress placed at the head of the metatarsals.

In most cases, radiographs are normal; however, more severe cases may show subluxation or dislocation of the metacarpal joint. Nonsteroidal anti-inflammatory drugs, hot soaks, and metatarsal pads may help; however, if subluxation or dislocation is present, surgery may be necessary.

Diabetic neuropathy is typically manifest by a burning sensation in the feet.

Morton neuroma usually presents with a feeling as if the patient is standing on a pebble in their shoe, with a burning sensation in the ball of your foot that may radiate into the toes.

A Jones fracture is a fairly common fracture of the fifth metatarsal.

Gout classically involves pain and inflammation at the first metatarsophalangeal joint, although other toes can be involved.

Additional Reading: Common foot problems: over-the-counter treatments and home care. *Am Fam Physician*. 2018;98(5):298-303.

2. Which of the following statements about Burner syndrome is true?

A) The mechanism of injury involves acute hyperextension of the shoulder while the neck and head are forced in the same direction.
B) Symptoms include temporary weakness, pain, paresthesias, and decreased sensation of the distal extremity.
C) The injury involves traction forces on the spinal cord's dorsal columns.
D) Most cases cause permanent neurologic deficits.
E) The condition is associated with overuse injury of the knees.

The answer is B: Burner syndrome (also known as transient brachial plexopathy) is seen mostly in football players and results from a tackling or blocking injury. The injury occurs when the contact shoulder is depressed, and the head and neck are forced in the opposite direction of contact. The traction-type forces placed on the brachial plexus lead to variable symptoms of weakness, pain, paresthesias, limited motion, and decreased sensation of the affected extremity. Diminished reflexes may also be seen.

The condition should be treated with caution, and cervical disk or bony injury should be ruled out. In most cases, the symptoms last only a few minutes; however, the athlete should not return to play until a complete evaluation can be performed and the symptoms resolve.

Additional Reading: Management of head and neck injuries by the sideline physician. *Am Fam Physician*. 2006;74(8):1357-1364.

3. A 29-year-old long-distance runner has been training for a marathon. He presents complaining of pain and mild swelling of his left lower leg that has not responded to anti-inflammatory agents or ice therapy. The pain is more noticeable at night. On examination, he has localized tenderness over his proximal left tibia and you obtain a plain film radiograph of the area, which is normal. The most likely diagnosis is which one of the following?

A) Gastrocnemius tear
B) Iliotibial band syndrome
C) Osteoid osteoma
D) Shin splints
E) Stress fracture

The answer is E: Stress fractures usually involve the proximal two-thirds of the tibia or distal fibula (5-7 cm proximal to the lateral malleolus). They occur after prolonged and repeated use, accounting for up to 10% of all sports injuries. Long-distance runners or athletes who are inadequately conditioned are frequently affected.

Symptoms include pain over the lower leg in the affected area; the pain usually improves with rest but recurs with repeated activity. Localized erythema and swelling may occur over the fracture site. Night pain is a common feature, which should alert the clinician to the possibility of a stress fracture.

Plain film radiographs are normal in many cases; however, technetium bone scans can be used to demonstrate the fracture. Bone scans are the most cost-effective means to diagnose stress fractures. Magnetic resonance imaging is also sensitive but is more expensive.

Treatment of stress fractures includes rest from exercise or competition for 6 to 8 weeks. Those who experience pain with ambulation or cannot adhere to limited activity for that amount of time should be placed in a walking cast or boot for 4 to 6 weeks. When patients resume their activity, they should begin slowly and gradually work back to their normal routines. If pain should recur, nonunion of the fracture should be suspected and an orthopedic referral obtained. The athlete may return to competition after 14 days without pain and no pain with gradual return to activity.

Additional Reading: Stress fractures: diagnosis, treatment, and prevention. *Am Fam Physician*. 2011;83(1):39-46.

4. A 13-year-old high school basketball player is brought into the office by his father. He was playing a game last night and landed with a twisting motion of his right ankle. He limped off the court and has been applying ice to the area. Overnight, it has gotten better, but he has some swelling and is limping when he walks. On examination, you suspect an ankle sprain and explain that the ligament most commonly injured with an ankle sprain is which one of the following?

A) Anterior talofibular ligament
B) Deltoid ligament
C) Fibulocalcaneal ligament
D) Posterior talofibular ligament

The answer is A: The most commonly injured ligament in ankle sprains is the anterior talofibular. Other ligaments associated with higher grades of sprain include the fibulocalcaneal and the posterior talofibular ligament. A positive drawer sign (movement of the talus forward when the ankle is held stable) indicates rupture of the anterior talofibular ligament. Ankle sprains are graded according to the following criteria:

- *Grade 1*: Mild sprain with no evidence of ligamentous tear; associated with mild pain and swelling
- *Grade 2*: Moderate sprain with evidence of partial tear of ligaments; associated with moderate swelling, ecchymosis, and difficulty ambulating
- *Grade 3*: Severe sprain with evidence of a complete tear of the ligament; associated with significant swelling, ecchymosis, ankle instability, and the inability to walk

Treatment for grades 1, 2, and 3 sprains involves rest, ice, compression, elevation; use of air casts; and nonsteroidal anti-inflammatory drugs followed by early mobilization and physical therapy, which emphasizes strengthening and proprioceptive training. Sprains not responding to conservative care over 4 to 6 weeks or with atypical symptoms require specialty referral. High-ankle sprains are much less common and involve injury to the syndesmosis. Mechanism is from dorsiflexion external rotation. Recovery time is increased with these injuries and requires initial non–weight-bearing for 1 to 3 weeks followed by graduated weight-bearing and physical therapy.

Additional Reading: Update on acute ankle sprains. *Am Fam Physician*. 2012;85(12):1170-1176.

5. Dermatomyositis is associated with which of the following?

A) Distal muscle weakness
B) Hyperlipidemia
C) Inflammatory bowel disease
D) Malignancy
E) Morbilliform rash

The answer is D: Dermatomyositis is a systemic connective tissue disease that involves inflammation and degeneration of the muscles. Women are affected more than men at a 2:1 ratio. Although the disease may occur at any age, it occurs most commonly in adults 40 to 60 years of age and in children 5 to 15 years of age. The cause is unknown. In adult cases (15% of men older than 50 years and a smaller proportion affecting women), there is an underlying malignant tumor, which may give rise to an autoimmune reaction and lead to an attack of tumor antigens with similar muscle antigens.

Symptoms include symmetric proximal muscle weakness, muscular pain, violaceous, flat-topped papules over the dorsal interphalangeal joints (Gottron papules), purple-red discoloration of the upper eyelids (heliotropic rash), polyarthralgia, dysphagia, Raynaud phenomenon, fever, and weight loss. Interstitial pneumonitis with dyspnea and cough may occur and precedes the development of myositis. Cardiac involvement may be detected when electrocardiographic tracings show arrhythmias or conduction disturbances.

Laboratory findings include increased erythrocyte sedimentation rate, positive antinuclear antibodies and/or lupus erythematosus preparation test, and elevated creatine kinase (most sensitive and useful marker) and aldolase. Diagnosis is confirmed by electromyography and muscle biopsy.

Initial treatment consists of steroids. Patients who fail to respond can be given immunosuppressive agents such as methotrexate, cyclophosphamide, and chlorambucil. After the diagnosis of dermatomyositis, an effort should be made to uncover an occult malignancy. Dermatomyositis associated with malignancy often remits once the tumor is removed.

Additional Reading: Polymyositis/dermatomyositis. In: Domino F, ed. *The 5-Minute Clinical Consult*. Wolters Kluwer; 2022.

6. A 63-year-old diabetic presents with an ulcer on the base of his right great toe. While he is having minimal pain, the ulcer is necrotic and odorous. Treatment of severely infected diabetic foot ulcers should involve which one of the following?

A) Topical antibiotics only
B) Debridement only
C) Debridement with systemic antibiotics
D) Debridement with topical antibiotics
E) None of the above

The answer is C: Oral antibiotics may be adequate for mild infections. However, if the infection is severe, debridement and systemic antibiotics are usually necessary. Topical antibiotics are not effective in the treatment of such infections.

Diabetic foot ulcers usually result from large vessel disease, microvascular disease, neuropathies, or a combination of all three. Ulcers associated with large vessel disease tend to affect the distal tips of the toes, whereas those secondary to neuropathy typically occur on the weight-bearing surfaces. Smoking and heavy alcohol abuse can increase the risk of diabetic ulcers.

Typically, ulcers develop because of the underlying neuropathy, which results in a lack of sensation, such that the patient is unaware of the ulcer until it has progressed to a severe stage. Prevention is the key to treatment. All diabetic patients should be instructed about foot care, and their feet should be examined daily to look for any signs of infection.

Cultures should be taken from the debrided ulcer base or from purulent drainage. Organisms that typically infect diabetic ulcers include *Staphylococcus*, *Streptococcus*, anaerobes, and gram-negative organisms. Severe infections may involve methicillin-resistant *S aureus* (MRSA) and *Pseudomonas* infections.

Additional Reading: Diabetes-related foot infections: diagnosis and treatment. *Am Fam Physician*. 2021;104(4):386-394.

7. You are examining a 43-year-old nurse who runs regularly for her mental and physical health. She has had pain over her left Achilles tendon for the past couple of weeks. She has been doing a "runner's stretch" regularly, but it has not helped. On examination, she has pain with palpation over the Achilles tendon above the insertion site on the calcaneus. Which of the following signs is associated with Achilles tendonitis?

A) Gynecoid pelvis
B) Hyperpronation
C) Increased Q angle
D) Lateral collateral ligament instability

The answer is B: Achilles tendonitis occurs with repeated stress to the Achilles tendon. Precipitating factors include brisk walking, running, jumping, or hiking. Although known as *Achilles tendonitis*, it is generally a *tendinosis* involving fibrosis of the tendon. Persons who exercise or compete in low-heel shoes and those who hyperpronate their feet are at an increased risk for Achilles tendonitis.

Patients report pain in the heel and leg discomfort when the Achilles tendon is used. Physical findings include pain with palpation over the Achilles tendon approximately 3 cm above the insertion site on the calcaneus.

Treatment goals are to decrease the inflammation associated with the inflamed structures and to reduce the stress on the Achilles tendon. Treatment includes nonsteroidal anti-inflammatory drugs, heel lifts, and strengthening and stretching exercises of the gastrocnemius and soleus muscles. For patients with hyperpronation, a soft navicular pad and medial wedge may help prevent excessive pronation. Eccentric Achilles strengthening exercises have been found to be helpful when there is a thickened nodule present consistent with Achilles tendinosis.

Additional Reading: Surgery is no better than nonoperative treatment for achilles tendon rupture in adults. *Am Fam Physician*. 2022;106(3).

8. A construction worker presents with pain over the lateral elbow. He reports that he has been using a hammer more often than usual, and this seems to aggravate his discomfort. Which of the following is the most likely diagnosis?

A) Biceps tendonitis
B) Carpal tunnel syndrome
C) Lateral epicondylitis
D) Rotator cuff dysfunction
E) Ulnar nerve entrapment

The answer is C: Lateral epicondylitis, commonly referred to as "tennis elbow," is usually caused by overuse, repeated trauma, strain, or exercise that involves the upper extremity and a gripping motion. Although associated with playing tennis, it may affect baseball players, golfers, and racquetball enthusiasts, as well as carpenters, assembly-line workers, and electricians, all of whom repeatedly extend the wrist and rotate the forearm.

The cause of pain originates at the extensor origin of the extensor carpi radialis brevis in the area of the lateral epicondyle. Symptoms include pain in the area of the lateral epicondyle but may also include the extensor surface of the forearm. In more severe cases, swelling and erythema may be noted. Pain is exacerbated by passively flexing the fingers and wrist with the elbow fully extended. Radiographs are usually negative; however, calcification may be noted in chronic cases. The condition should be distinguished from radial nerve entrapment syndrome (pain with middle finger extension and forearm supination with the elbow fully extended) and posterior interosseous nerve syndrome (pain located more distally over the forearm supinator muscle).

Treatment includes the use of nonsteroidal anti-inflammatory drugs, rest of the affected arm, ice therapy, and a volar wrist splint that immobilizes the wrist and prevents flexion and extension. If this treatment does not provide relief, a steroid injection of 1 mL of 1% lidocaine and 0.5 mL of corticosteroid should be attempted. Once the inflammation has been controlled, a constricting band can be used over the proximal forearm to help prevent recurrence. In addition, rehabilitation exercises should be instituted. In severe cases, orthopedic referral may be necessary for possible surgical treatment.

Additional Reading: Tennis elbow. *Am Fam Physician*. 2007;75(5):701-702.

9. You are seeing a 43-year-old woman who complains of pain in her right wrist. She has recently started work on an assembly-line constructing electronic keyboards. The work includes repetitive motions of the hand or thumb. On examination, she has pain when you palpate over her radial styloid. You suspect de Quervain tenosynovitis, based on a positive result for which one of the following tests?

A) Allen test
B) Anterior-posterior drawer test
C) Finkelstein test
D) Lachman test
E) Phalen test

The answer is C: The abductor pollicis longus and the extensor pollicis brevis share a common protective sheath that can become inflamed, giving rise to de Quervain tenosynovitis. Patients usually report pain with movement of the fibrous bands that make up the first dorsal compartment over the radial styloid. Paresthesia and pain that radiates distally into the thumb and dorsal part of the hand and index finger may occur. In most cases, the patient has a history of repetitive motions of the hand or thumb.

A positive Finkelstein test is the hallmark test finding: Pain is replicated over the radial styloid when a fist is made over the thumb and the wrist is placed in ulnar deviation. Long-standing inflammation may lead to calcification of the tendon and its sheath, and it is visible on a radiograph. Treatment options involve rest, anti-inflammatory agents, immobilization of the affected area with a thumb spica splint, and injection of the compartment with 0.5 mL of steroid and 1 mL of 1% lidocaine. The splint is to be worn for 3 weeks; surgery is rarely necessary but can be considered in refractive cases.

Allen test is used in the diagnosis of Raynaud phenomenon. The radial and ulnar arteries are occluded by the examiner while the patient makes a fist. The hand is then opened, and one side of the wrist is released. Blood flow to the hand should be detected by color, which is restored to the hand. If the hand remains pale and cyanotic on either of the two sides, Raynaud phenomenon should be suspected. During asymptomatic periods, the examination is entirely normal.

Phalen test is used to diagnose carpal tunnel syndrome. The patient holds his or her wrists in complete and forced flexion (pushing the dorsal surfaces of both hands together) for 30 to 60 seconds. The test is positive when symptoms (eg, paresthesias in the thumb and index finger) are reproduced.

The Lachman and anterior-posterior drawer tests are used to assess the integrity of the knee ligaments.

Additional Reading: De Quervain tenosynovitis. In: Domino F, ed. *The 5-Minute Clinical Consult*. Wolters Kluwer; 2022.

10. A 37-year-old farmer presents with pain and swelling of the elbow area. He denies any specific injury but notes that lifting the bales has become difficult while baling hay. On examination, he has swelling and tenderness over his posterior elbow. There is no obvious erythema. You diagnose olecranon bursitis, which is usually the result of which one of the following:

A) A subclinical infection
B) Autoimmune antibodies targeting the olecranon bursa
C) Deposition of negative birefringent crystals in the bursa
D) Repeated trauma to the elbow
E) Referred pain from the wrist

The answer is D: Olecranon bursitis (also known as *miner's elbow*) is an inflammation that affects the olecranon bursa. The inflammation is usually caused by repeated trauma to the affected area, such as repeated weight-bearing on the elbow as seen in this case with repeating lifting of heavy bales of hay. Patients usually report pain, discomfort, and swelling of the elbow area. In some cases, the bursa may harbor an infection, which may require antibiotic treatment; however, in most cases, there is no associated infection.

Treatment involves anti-inflammatories, aspiration of the fluid, and, in some cases, steroid injection followed by the use of a pressure dressing to help prevent reaccumulation of fluid. Infection should be excluded before administering steroid medication. The avoidance of trauma to the elbow should also be emphasized for treatment. Surgery may be necessary for resistant and debilitating cases.

Additional Reading: Evaluation of elbow pain in adults. In: *UpToDate*. 2022.

11. Which of the following statements is a common feature of fibromyalgia?

A) Aggravation of the condition is due to lack of sleep, trauma, or cold exposure.
B) Alcohol abuse is commonly associated.
C) Joint inflammation and erythema.
D) Men are more commonly affected than women.
E) Normal autonomic and neuroendocrine regulation.

The answer is A: Fibromyalgia is an idiopathic, chronic, nonarticular pain syndrome, with a distinct pathophysiology involving central amplification of peripheral sensory signals. Core symptoms include widespread muscle pain and tenderness, fatigue, and sleep disturbance. Nearly 2% of the general population in the United States suffers from fibromyalgia, with women of middle age being at increased risk.

The 2016 American College of Rheumatology criteria for the diagnosis of fibromyalgia in adults are met when all of the following criteria are present:

1. Generalized pain, defined as pain in at least four of five regions, is present.
2. Symptoms have been present at a similar level for at least 3 months.
3. Widespread pain index ≥7 and symptom severity scale score ≥5 *or* widespread pain index of 4 to 6 and symptom severity scale score ≥9.

4. A diagnosis of fibromyalgia is valid irrespective of other diagnoses. A diagnosis of fibromyalgia does not exclude the presence of other clinically important illnesses.

Fibromyalgia is characterized by generalized pain, tenderness, and muscle stiffness. Pain at the point of tendon insertion ("trigger points") and surrounding soft tissue may also be present. Inflammation of joints is not characteristic. Although the etiology remains unclear, characteristic alterations in the pattern of sleep and changes in neuroendocrine transmitters such as serotonin, substance P, growth hormone, and cortisol suggest that dysregulation of the autonomic and neuroendocrine system appears to be the basis of the syndrome.

The condition may be aggravated by stress (both physical and mental), lack of sleep, trauma, exposure to cold, and, sometimes, infection. Primary fibromyalgia syndrome is more likely to affect young women who are tense, depressed, or anxious. Symptoms of stiffness and pain are usually diffuse and have an "achy" quality that comes on gradually. Localized symptoms tend to occur more abruptly.

Other diseases (eg, rheumatoid arthritis, hypothyroidism, polymyositis, and polymyalgia rheumatica) must be excluded before the diagnosis is made. Myofascial pain syndrome is similar to fibromyalgia; however, the painful areas are usually regional, and men are as equally affected as women. In addition, fatigue is not a major finding.

Treatment for fibromyalgia includes low-dose tricyclic antidepressants (eg, amitriptyline), acupuncture, and muscle relaxants (eg, cyclobenzaprine). Nonsteroidal anti-inflammatory drugs, although commonly used, have not been shown to be effective. Stress-reduction counseling, exercise programs, and improved sleep habits can also be beneficial.

Additional Readings:
1. Common questions about the diagnosis and management of fibromyalgia. *Am Fam Physician*. 2015;91(7):472-478.
2. 2016 Revisions to the 2010/2011 fibromyalgia diagnostic criteria. *Semin Arthritis Rheum*. 2016;46(3):319-329. doi:10.1016/j.semarthrit.2016.08.012.

12. A 40-year-old woman complains of diffuse symmetric joint pain that is worse when she awakes in the morning but only improves slightly as the day progresses. Examination shows inflammation of the proximal interphalangeal and metacarpophalangeal (MCP) joints. Which of the following is the most likely diagnosis?

A) Lupus erythematous
B) Osteoarthritis
C) Polymyalgia rheumatica
D) Reiter syndrome
E) Rheumatoid arthritis (RA)

The answer is E: RA is a chronic, symmetric, and inflammatory condition that may involve multiple joints. Women are affected two to three times more often than men, and family members of affected individuals are at increased risk. Onset is usually between the fourth and sixth decade but may occur at any age. Synovial inflammation leads to the destruction of articular and periarticular structures and proliferation of the synovial tissue (termed *pannus*), all of which causes chronic joint pain. In 30% to 40% of patients, subcutaneous rheumatoid nodules may form at sites subject to trauma and are usually associated with more severe conditions.

Patients often complain of multiple joint pain, low-grade fever, fatigue, weight loss, and depression. Symmetric swelling of the hands (especially the proximal interphalangeal and MCP joints), wrists, elbows, shoulder, neck, and ankles is typical; however, any joint may be affected. Patients usually report morning stiffness that involves the small joints of the hands. This stiffness improves slowly as the day progresses. Carpal tunnel syndrome may also occur. Other manifestations, including vasculitis, pericarditis, and interstitial fibrosis, may be found in more severe cases.

Laboratory findings include elevated erythrocyte sedimentation rate (90% of cases), mild anemia, and a positive rheumatoid factor (85% of cases). Radiographs show periarticular osteoporosis, joint space narrowing, and joint erosion in more severe cases. However, no laboratory test, histologic finding, or radiographic feature confirms the diagnosis.

Treatment consists of nonsteroidal anti-inflammatory drugs (NSAIDs) (first-line therapy); interarticular and systemic steroids; etanercept (Enbrel) (a tumor necrosis factor α-blocker); infliximab (Remicade) and adalimumab (Humira); disease-modifying antirheumatic drugs (DMARDs); and antimalarials (primarily hydroxychloroquine, which requires eye examinations every 6 months because of the risk of vision loss), sulfasalazine, azathioprine, cyclosporine, and methotrexate with folate supplementation (which requires close monitoring of liver and renal function). Other agents (eg, penicillamine, cyclophosphamide, and gold compounds) are less widely used because of side effects. Traditional drug combinations for RA commonly include an NSAID, a DMARD, and short intermittent courses of oral corticosteroids. The use of etanercept and methotrexate has been effective and promising in the treatment of RA.

Other associated conditions include Felty syndrome (arthritis, splenomegaly, lymphadenopathy, anemia, neutropenia, and thrombocytopenia) and Sjögren syndrome (arthritis, dry eyes, and mucous membranes).

Additional Reading: Arthritis, rheumatoid (RA). In: Domino F, ed. *The 5-Minute Clinical Consult*. Wolters Kluwer; 2022.

13. A 21-year-old skier presents complaining of pain and some weakness of his right thumb, especially when trying to twist things. He had a bad fall skiing this past weekend and his right hand was jammed into the snow. You diagnose him with "gamekeeper's thumb," which is associated with a sprain of which one of the following tissues?

A) Extensor pollicis brevis tendon
B) Extensor pollicis longus tendon
C) Flexor carpi ulnaris tendon
D) Flexor retinaculum
E) Ulnar collateral ligament

The answer is E: Gamekeeper's thumb (also known as *skier's thumb*) occurs when there is a sprain or traumatic rupture of the ulnar collateral ligament in the area of the thumb metacarpophalangeal (MCP) joint. The injury occurs when there is hyperextension and hyperabduction of the thumb, usually as the result of a fall. The injury results in ulnar laxity of the MCP joint and often dorsal subluxation of the proximal thumb at the MCP joint.

Patients often complain of weakness and pain when using the thumb to pinch and to perform activities such as opening car doors or jars or turning the key in a door lock. Other physical findings include swelling, erythema, ecchymosis, and tenderness over the MCP joint of the thumb on the ulnar side. As much as 95% of the injuries to the MCP joint occur on the ulnar side.

Radiographs may show ulnar deviation of the proximal thumb and avulsion fracture of the ulnar collateral ligament at the base of the proximal phalanx. If the avulsed fragment is displaced more than 1 mm or involves more than 10% of the articular surface, surgery is indicated for repair. Also, if stress radiographs show laxity of the ulnar collateral ligament greater than 35° on an anteroposterior radiograph, patients should be referred to an orthopedist. However, in less severe cases, immobilization in a thumb spica cast for 4 to 6 weeks is indicated.

Additional Reading: Ulnar collateral ligament injury (gamekeeper's or skier's thumb). In: *UpToDate*. 2022.

14. A 60-year-old woman, whom you have recently started on hydrochlorothiazide to treat her HTN, presents with pain, swelling, and redness of the first metatarsal phalangeal joint. She has otherwise been feeling well, and no other joints are involved. She has no fever and denies any recent injury. Which one of the following is the most likely diagnosis?

A) Degenerative joint disease
B) Morton neuroma
C) Osteomyelitis
D) Podagra
E) Rheumatoid arthritis (RA)

The answer is D: Gout (known as podagra when it involves the big toe) is a condition characterized by recurrent pain associated with peripheral joints. The cause is attributed to the development of monosodium urate crystals, which cause acute arthritis. Longstanding gout can lead to chronic, deforming arthritis. The greater the degree of hyperuricemia, the more likely is the development of gouty attack, although most patients with hyperuricemia are asymptomatic.

Hyperuricemia may result from disorders of purine metabolism, which may be genetic or acquired. Disorders causing hyperuricemia include proliferative hematologic disorders, psoriasis, myxedema, parathyroid disorders, enzyme deficiencies, and renal disease; obesity and medications such as thiazide diuretics are also causative. Middle-aged and elderly men are usually affected more frequently than women; however, menopause is associated with a sharp increase in incidence in women (especially in those using thiazides and those with renal impairment).

Symptoms include severe, throbbing pain with redness, and swelling that is usually monoarticular and that affects the metatarsophalangeal joint of the great toe. However, other joints, including the ankle, knee, wrist, and elbow, may also be affected. Other symptoms include fever and malaise. Later, attacks may become more frequent and affect multiple joints with resolution between attacks less complete. Precipitating factors include trauma, overindulgence of foods (processed meats), alcohol, surgery, fatigue, stress, infection, or the administration of medications (eg, penicillin, insulin, and thiazide diuretics).

Diagnosis is usually made on the basis of history and physical examination. Absolute confirmation involves joint aspiration with the detection of needle-shaped urate crystals that are negatively birefringent under a polarizing microscope. Asymptomatic treatment of hyperuricemia is generally not treated with medication.

Treatment of gout involves the use of ice, rest, nonsteroidal anti-inflammatory drugs (eg, indomethacin, naproxen, and ibuprofen), colchicine (which may provide dramatic relief in the acute phase), and allopurinol (xanthine oxidase inhibitor) for patients who have chronically elevated uric acid levels after the acute attack has resolved (low-dose colchicine can also be used). In addition, uricosuric agents, including probenecid and sulfinpyrazone, may be helpful but should be used with caution in patients with renal problems. Prednisone may also be helpful in patients who cannot tolerate other medications.

Additional Reading: Gout. In: Domino F, ed. *The 5-Minute Clinical Consult*. Wolters Kluwer; 2022.

15. Inflammation and necrosis of the muscular tissue supplied by small- and medium-sized arteries is known as which of the following?

A) Dermatomyositis
B) Giant cell arteritis
C) Polyarteritis nodosa (PAN)
D) Polymyositis
E) Pyoderma gangrenosum

The answer is C: PAN is a condition characterized by inflammation and necrosis of the muscular tissue supplied by small- and medium-sized arteries. The cause is unknown but may be associated with an autoimmune response, medication (eg, sulfonamides, iodide, thiazides, bismuth, and penicillins), and infections. Involvement of the renal and visceral arteries is characteristic, but pulmonary arteries are usually spared. Affected individuals are usually between 40 and 50 years of age; men are more commonly affected.

Symptoms include fever, abdominal pain, peripheral neuropathy, headaches, seizures, weakness, and weight loss. Those with renal involvement may show hypertension, edema, azotemia, and oliguria. Other symptoms include angina, nausea, vomiting, diarrhea, myalgias, and arthralgias. Palpable subcutaneous lesions that sometimes necrose may be found in the area of an affected artery.

Laboratory studies show leukocytosis, proteinuria, microscopic hematuria, thrombocytosis, and an elevated erythrocyte sedimentation rate (ESR). Diagnosis is usually made with a biopsy of affected tissue, which shows necrotizing arteritis. Treatment involves avoidance of the offending agent and often long-term, high-dose steroid therapy and cyclophosphamide for severe cases and steroids alone for milder cases. The disease can be fatal if untreated.

Polymyositis is an idiopathic inflammatory myopathy with symmetrical, proximal muscle weakness. Histopathology demonstrates endomysial mononuclear inflammatory infiltrate and muscle fiber necrosis.

Dermatomyositis is clinically similar to polymyositis, an idiopathic, inflammatory myopathy associated with characteristic skin findings that include a violet or dusky red rash seen on the face and eyelids and on skin around the nails, knuckles, elbows, knees, chest, and back. The rash can be patchy with bluish-purple discolorations and is often the first sign of dermatomyositis.

Giant cell arteritis, also known as temporal arteritis, is a vasculitis of the large and medium arteries of the head and neck. Giant cell arteritis typically presents with a headache and nonspecific systemic symptoms. The temporal artery is tender to palpations, and a high ESR is detected. The diagnosis is confirmed by patchy inflammation of arterial walls, characterized by the infiltration of mononuclear cells and the presence of giant cells from a temporal artery biopsy.

Pyoderma gangrenosum causes deep leg ulcers, with necrotic tissue, and they can lead to chronic wounds. Ulcers initially present as small papules and progress to larger ulcers, causing pain and scarring.

Additional Reading: Systemic vasculitis. *Am Fam Physician*. 2011;83(5):556-565.

16. A 47-year-old White woman presents with complaints of pain in the ball of her foot, which is worse when she is wearing her shoes. It has been gradually worsening over the past few weeks. She denies injury and has otherwise been feeling well. You consider that she may have Morton neuroma and expect that on examination you will most commonly find her pain to be localized to which one of the following locations?

A) The distal third and fourth metatarsal heads
B) Interdigital nerves between the fourth and fifth metacarpal heads
C) Interdigital nerves between the third and fourth metatarsal heads
D) The lateral surface of the first tarsal
E) The sural nerve

The answer is C: Morton neuroma is a common type of forefoot pain. The condition arises from entrapment of the common interdigital nerves between the metatarsal heads. This nerve entrapment leads to inflammation, edema, pain, and the formation of perineural fibrosis and demyelination, which causes a neuroma. The most common location for the neuroma is between the third and fourth metatarsal heads; they also commonly occur between the second and third metatarsal heads.

Women are more commonly affected than men (5:1 ratio). Patients report pain, paresthesias, or occasionally a catching sensation in these locations, which may extend distally to the toes or proximally to the midfoot. Many patients report their symptoms are worse when wearing shoes. The distinguishing feature in the differential between metatarsalgia and Morton neuroma is pain between the metatarsal heads.

Radiographs are normal; however, magnetic resonance images may show the offending neuroma but are rarely necessary to make the diagnosis. Treatment involves nonsteroidal anti-inflammatory drugs, metatarsal footpads, wide shoes, and steroid injections (using a dorsal approach between the metatarsals); in severe cases, surgical excision of the neuroma is indicated, although persistent pain remains for approximately 33% of patients after surgery.

Additional Reading: Morton neuroma (interdigital neuroma). In: Domino F, ed. *The 5-Minute Clinical Consult*. Wolters Kluwer; 2022.

17. A 33-year-old computer technician presents with achy pain over his lower right leg, which is aggravated with running. He tends to jog a couple of times a week, but a month ago he really increased the intensity of his running as he wants to run in a marathon this fall with some friends. On examination he has mild pain and subtle diffuse swelling noted over his right tibia. You make a diagnosis of shin splints. Which of the following interventions would have helped him to prevent developing shin splints?

A) Change in running surfaces
B) Ice therapy after exercise
C) Running on varied surfaces like a path instead of the road
D) Stretching before exercise
E) Training for a half-marathon instead

The answer is D: Shin splints (medial tibial stress syndrome) are a common condition caused by overuse of the lower extremity muscles. The condition is caused by a periostitis of the tibia. They typically occur when an athlete's running surface (eg, hills, inclines, and stairs) is changed, when a different type of shoe is used, when an athlete's running style is altered, or when excessive training that does not allow adequate time for the muscles to recover is undertaken.

Most affected athletes report pain over the lower tibial area that may be referred to the foot or knee. Any type of movement or exercise that works these muscle groups tends to make the pain worse. In addition to pain, mild diffuse swelling or redness may be noted over the tibia.

The diagnosis is usually based on history and physical examination. The differential diagnosis includes stress fractures, exertional compartment syndrome, and tenosynovitis. Treatment involves applying ice to the area and taking nonsteroidal anti-inflammatory drugs. If the symptoms are mild, exercise can be continued; however, more severe cases require restriction of activity. If the pain is not improved with such therapy, plain radiographs and perhaps a bone scan should be performed to rule out a stress fracture.

When the pain and inflammation subside, the athlete should be instructed in stretching exercises for the muscles of the lower extremity, which can help prevent a recurrence. If shin splints are recurrent, examination to rule out excessive pronation should be performed; if present, orthotics should be used to correct hyperpronation. It is now thought that shin splints or medial tibial stress syndrome represents one end of a continuum of bony stress injury, with a focal stress fracture representing the other.

Additional Reading: Common running injuries: evaluation and management. *Am Fam Physician*. 2018;97(8):510-516.

18. A 36-year-old overweight office worker has recently taken up running on a treadmill in an attempt to lose weight; however, he has developed pain in his heel. The patient reports that his symptoms are worse when he first gets out of bed in the morning and starts to walk but slowly improve as the day progresses. The most likely diagnosis is which one of the following?

A) Achilles tendonitis
B) Anterior talotibial impingement syndrome
C) Calcaneal fracture
D) Calcaneal bone spur
E) Plantar fasciitis

The answer is E: Plantar fasciitis is caused by inflammation, fibrosis, or microtears of the plantar fascia at the attachment site to the os calcis. It is a common complaint in runners. Symptoms include pain at the attachment of the plantar fascia at the calcaneus. The pain is usually worse in the morning on standing or standing after prolonged sitting. The pain may improve early in the day but usually worsens toward the end of the day and is relieved when the patient lies or sits down.

Calcaneal spurs, visible on radiographs, may occur in chronic cases but are not responsible for evoking pain and discomfort. Treatment involves nonsteroidal anti-inflammatory drugs, stretching exercises (eg, runners stretch), heel pads (Viscoheel), orthotics, rest, and ice therapy. In more severe cases that are refractory to these measures, night splints or steroid injection (0.5 mL of steroid and 1.0 mL of 1% lidocaine) can be used. In addition, surgery may be indicated for severe cases that are unresponsive to conservative therapy.

Additional Reading: Plantar fasciitis. *Am Fam Physician*. 2019;99(12):744-750.

19. A 60-year-old woman presents with complaints of diffuse proximal muscle pain, low-grade fevers, and generalized fatigue. Her physical examination is unremarkable with no evidence of synovitis or muscle weakness. Laboratory findings include a significantly elevated erythrocyte sedimentation rate (ESR; 57 mm/h) and mild normocytic anemia. The most likely diagnosis is which one of the following?

A) Influenza
B) Dermatomyositis
C) Polymyalgia rheumatica (PMR)
D) Rheumatoid arthritis
E) Systemic lupus erythematosus

The answer is C: PMR is an inflammatory disease characterized by pain and stiffness associated with the proximal muscle groups. The condition is more common in women and usually occurs in patients older than 50 years. Symptoms include symmetric pain and morning stiffness associated with the proximal muscles such as the neck, shoulders, and hips. Patients may also report fever, generalized fatigue, anorexia, and weight loss. Laboratory findings include an elevated ESR (usually >50 mm/h and often >100 mm/h) and anemia of chronic disease. The physical examination is unremarkable with no evidence of synovitis or true muscle weakness.

Diagnosis is made on the basis of the clinical findings and confirmed with response to therapy. Treatment involves the use of orally administered corticosteroids (prednisone 10-20 mg/d); usually the patient responds immediately. As many as 25% of patients may have associated giant cell arteritis, which can lead to blindness if not treated immediately with steroids. Once the ESR returns to normal and the patient's symptoms are improved, the steroids may be slowly tapered. In some cases, it may take months to years to completely taper the medication.

Additional Reading: Recognition and management of polymyalgia rheumatica and giant cell arteritis. *Am Fam Physician.* 2013;88(10):676-684.

20. You have been treating a 54-year-old obese White man for gout, and he returns with pain and swelling in his right knee. He has been researching his pain on the Internet and wonders if perhaps he has pseudogout because his knee is bothering him, not his great toe. Which one of the following is associated with pseudogout?

A) High uric acid levels
B) Calcium pyrophosphate crystal deposition in the large joints
C) Negative birefringence seen with polarized microscopy
D) Lack of response with the use of colchicine
E) Lack of response with the use of anti-inflammatory medication

The answer is B: Pseudogout is a condition that results from the deposition of calcium pyrophosphate crystals in the large joints (principally the knees) and leads to a reactive synovitis. Affected patients are usually older than 60 years. Men and women appear to be equally affected. Pseudogout is associated with trauma, surgery, amyloidosis, hemochromatosis, and hyperparathyroidism.

Diagnosis is made by joint aspiration and examination of the fluid under a polarized microscope. Calcium pyrophosphate exhibits a positive birefringence in contrast to a negative birefringence seen with urate crystals in gout. Laboratory tests do not show elevated uric acid levels. Radiographs of the affected joints usually show degenerative changes and calcification of the surrounding cartilaginous structures.

Treatment involves the use of anti-inflammatory agents and colchicine. Intra-articular steroid injection is occasionally helpful in resistant cases.

Additional Reading: Management of gout: update from the American College of Rheumatology. *Am Fam Physician.* 2021;104(2):209-210.

21. You are seeing a 34-year-old special education teacher, who complains of pain in her lower back following an injury at school, where she hurt her back after lifting some therapy mats to store them for the night. Which one of the following has not been shown to be useful in the prevention of back pain?

A) Attending a formal "back education" school
B) Modifying the work site to minimize the risk of injury
C) Staying active with regular physical activity
D) Utilizing a back belt when lifting

The answer is D: Low back pain is common, with an annual incidence of 5%, and a lifetime prevalence of 60% to 90%. Patient education to stay active, avoid aggravating movements, and return to normal activity as soon as possible, along with a discussion of the often benign nature of acute low back pain, is effective in patients with nonspecific acute back pain. Bed rest is not helpful for nonspecific acute low back pain. Physical therapy (McKenzie method and spine stabilization) may lessen the risk of recurrence and need for health care services. Neither lumbar supports nor back belts appear to be effective in reducing the incidence of low back pain. Work site modifications, including educational interventions, have some short-term benefit in reducing the incidence of low back pain. However, their applicability to the primary care setting is unknown. Back (educational) schools may prevent further back injury for persons with recurrent or chronic low back pain, but their long-term effectiveness has not been well studied.

Additional Reading: Nonspecific low back pain and return to work. *Am Fam Physician.* 2019;100(11):697-703.

22. A 44-year-old White woman presents with complaints of numbness and tingling in her fingers, which seems to be worse in the cold weather. Other than smoking she is healthy and has been cutting back so that she is only smoking a half pack per day. You suspect Raynaud phenomenon to explain her symptoms and a positive test result on which one of the following would support this diagnosis?

A) Allen test
B) Finkelstein test
C) Phalen test
D) Reverse phalen test

The answer is A: Raynaud phenomenon is secondary to spasm of the arterioles that usually supply the hands but can also affect the nose and other appendages. It is usually idiopathic (termed *Raynaud disease*) but has been associated with emotional stress, connective tissue diseases (eg, lupus, rheumatoid arthritis, and scleroderma), arterial obstructive diseases, medications (eg, ergots, β-blockers, clonidine, and methysergide), and endocrine disorders. Idiopathic Raynaud phenomenon occurs more frequently in women and frequently occurs in patients with migraines or variant angina. Symptoms include blanching, cyanosis, and paresthesias that affect the distal extremities.

Diagnosis can be determined by performing Allen test. The radial and ulnar arteries are occluded by the examiner while the patient makes a fist. The hand is then opened, and one side of the wrist is released. Blood flow to the hand should be detected by color, which is restored to the hand. If the hand remains pale and cyanotic with either of the two sides, Raynaud phenomenon should be suspected. During asymptomatic periods, the examination is entirely normal.

Treatment for mild to moderate cases should only involve avoiding triggering factors (eg, cold, stress, nicotine, and previously listed medications). The medication of choice for the treatment of severe Raynaud phenomenon includes the calcium channel blockers nifedipine and diltiazem. Other medications include reserpine, phenoxybenzamine, methyldopa, terazosin, doxazosin, and prazosin. Surgical treatment for resistant, severe cases involves sympathectomy.

Finkelstein test is used to diagnose de Quervain tenosynovitis by grasping the thumb while the hand is deviated in the ulnar direction. The test is positive when pain is reproduced along the distal radius.

Phalen test is used to diagnose carpal tunnel syndrome. The patient holds their wrists in complete and forced flexion (pushing the dorsal surfaces of both hands together) for 30 to 60 seconds. The test is positive when symptoms (eg, paresthesias in the thumb and index finger) are reproduced. The reverse phalen test adds to the sensitivity of the first test and is performed by having the patient in full wrist and finger extension for 2 minutes.

Additional Reading: Raynaud phenomenon. In: Domino F, ed. *The 5-Minute Clinical Consult*. Wolters Kluwer; 2022.

23. A 20-year-old college student presents complaining that she has developed acne over her cheeks and bridge of her nose. She has been using an over-the-counter acne wash, but the acne has not gotten any better. On further questioning she notes some fatigue that she attributes to staying up late at night to study, and she has noticed that her joints are achy, but she has just started doing aerobics and denies any swelling or erythema of her joints. On examination, you note that what she is describing as acne is instead a diffuse slightly inflamed malar rash. Your differential diagnosis includes systemic lupus erythematosus (SLE). Which one of the following statements about autoantibody testing is true?

A) The lupus erythematosus (LE) preparation test should be used as a screening test.
B) The LE preparation test should be used as a confirmatory test.
C) A positive antinuclear antibody (ANA) test is specific for SLE.
D) The anti–double-stranded DNA test is a confirmatory test.

The answer is D: SLE is an autoimmune disorder affecting all major organ systems. Women are more commonly affected than men, and it most commonly begins between the ages of 15 and 45 years. Symptoms wax and wane and commonly include diffuse joint pain and facial rashes in a butterfly distribution. As the disease progresses, illness from affected organ systems can be profound and includes cardiac involvement (pericarditis, myocarditis, endocarditis), renal involvement (proteinuria, hypertension, uremia), pulmonary involvement (pleuritis, pleural effusions), central nervous system findings (depression, transient ischemic attacks, strokes, chorea, psychosis), and vasculitis.

Antibody testing plays an important role when assessing patients, but should not be used alone to diagnose SLE. The ANA test is the most commonly used screening test for SLE, which is sensitive but not specific and requires confirmatory testing. The presence of anti–double-stranded DNA, anti-Sm, and anti-phospholipid antibodies are more specific for diagnosing SLE. Anti–double-stranded DNA antibodies are highly specific for SLE; they are present in 70% of cases, whereas they appear in only 0.5% of people without SLE.

Because of the high rate of false-positive ANA titers, testing for SLE with an ANA titer or other autoantibody test is not recommended for patients with isolated myalgias or arthralgias in the absence of specific clinical signs. At least 4 of the 11 American College of Rheumatology criteria are present, serially, or simultaneously, during any interval of observation for the diagnosis:

1. Malar rash
2. Discoid rash
3. Photosensitivity
4. Oral ulcers
5. Nonerosive arthritis
6. Serositis or pericarditis
7. Renal disease
8. Neurologic disorder: seizures or psychosis
9. Hematologic disorder: hemolytic anemia or leukopenia or thrombocytopenia
10. Immunologic disorder: anti-DNA or anti-Sm or anti-phospholipid antibodies and others
11. ANA positivity

Additional Reading: Systemic lupus erythematosus: primary care approach to diagnosis and management. *Am Fam Physician*. 2016;94(4):284-294.

24. A 28-year-old active runner presents to your office complaining of lateral knee and hip pain. The patient reports she has been training intensely for an upcoming marathon. On physical examination, tenderness of the lateral portion of the thigh at the level of the femoral epicondyle is noted. Which of the following is the most likely diagnosis?

A) Iliotibial band (ITB) syndrome
B) Patellofemoral syndrome
C) Pes anserine bursitis
D) Stress fracture
E) Tibial plateau fracture

The answer is A: ITB friction syndrome is characterized by lateral knee pain and, occasionally, lateral hip pain. The pain is caused by inflammation of the distal portion of the ITB band or at the point in which the ITB crosses the lateral femoral epicondyle. Runners, hammer throwers, and racket sport enthusiasts are usually affected. The condition usually affects runners when there is an increase in the running distance, increased speed or hill running, change in running surface, or consistent running on a banked surface. These activities lead to increased friction of the ITB and cause inflammation. Associated conditions include genu valgum, prominent lateral epicondyle, trochanteric bursitis, leg length discrepancy, excessive foot pronation, and quadriceps weakness.

Testing may show an excessively tight ITB or gluteus maximus. Treatment involves relative rest, anti-inflammatory medication, ice massage, and electronic galvanic stimulation. Prevention is aimed at proper stretching techniques (eg, quadriceps strengthening) and measures to correct underlying abnormalities (eg, excessive pronation).

Additional Reading: Common running injuries: evaluation and management. *Am Fam Physician*. 2018;97(8):510-516.

25. You are covering the local high school football game on a Friday night. An 18-year-old running backward goes down on the field after a hard tackle and lies on his back. When you arrive at his side, he is holding his knee. He describes a "pop" followed by severe pain. Which of the following would be most helpful in the initial diagnosis?

A) An inability to walk
B) Anterior drawer test
C) Arthrogram of the knee
D) Computed tomography of the knee
E) Lachman test

The answer is E: Anterior cruciate ligament (ACL) injuries typically present after a noncontact deceleration, a "cutting" movement or hyperextension, often accompanied by a "pop," with the inability to continue sports participation and associated knee instability. The ACL is particularly prone to injury. Physical findings include effusion, positive ACL tests, and chronic quadriceps atrophy. In all cases of knee injury, it should be determined how quickly swelling occurred after the injury. If an effusion evolved within 4 hours of injury, there is a high likelihood of major osseous, ligamentous, or meniscal injury.

Various tests are used to assess the knee. The Lachman test is performed with the knee in 20° of flexion. The tibia is pulled anteriorly on a secured femur. A positive test result is indicated by increased tibial movement compared with the unaffected knee. The quality of the end point should also be noted; a soft end point indicates an ACL tear.

The anterior drawer test (although much less specific than the Lachman) is performed with the knee in 90° of flexion. Similar to the Lachman test, the tibia is drawn anteriorly, and asymmetric movement is an indicator of ACL injury.

The most specific test for ACL disruption is the pivot shift test, but this test is often difficult to perform with an acute injury because of patient guarding and apprehension.

Radiographs should be obtained in patients with suspected ACL injuries to rule out associated intra-articular fractures and possibly determine the presence of a marginal avulsion fracture off the lateral tibial plateau (Segond fracture), which helps confirm the diagnosis. Magnetic resonance imaging is not necessary to diagnose ACL disruption but is often used and may be helpful in diagnosing associated meniscal pathology.

Treatment involves rehabilitation with physical therapy and, in some cases, surgical repair.

Additional Reading: Management of ACL injuries: clinical practice guideline from the AAOS. *Am Fam Physician.* 2015;92(3):232-234.

26. A 54-year-old nurse presents to your office complaining of gradually increasing right-sided shoulder pain. The patient reports she is unable to sleep on her right side and has a difficult time raising the right arm. Physical examination shows her shoulder's passive range of motion (ROM) is significantly restricted. X-rays of the shoulder are unremarkable. Which of the following is the most likely diagnosis?

A) Adhesive capsulitis
B) Biceps muscle tear
C) Multiple myeloma
D) Osteoporosis
E) Subacromial bursitis

The answer is A: Adhesive capsulitis, or frozen shoulder, results from thickening and fibrosis of the capsule around the glenohumeral joint and causes loss of motion and pain. Frozen shoulder classically consists of shoulder pain that is slow in onset and presents without any radiographic abnormalities. Usually, the discomfort is localized to the deltoid muscle, and the patient is unable to sleep on the affected side. Loss of passive ROM, particularly glenohumeral abduction and external rotation, is hallmark of the disorder. Shoulder impingement and rotator cuff tears may have loss of active ROM but have full passive ROM.

An autoimmune cause of frozen shoulder has been proposed, and the condition may be associated with type 2 diabetes mellitus and thyroid disorders. The diagnosis is usually made clinically, and physicians should always be concerned about a possible underlying rotator cuff tear. Radiographs often appear normal but should be obtained to rule out glenohumeralosteoarthritis, which also is noted to have loss of passive ROM.

Arthrography demonstrates generalized constriction of the joint capsule, with loss of the normal axillary and subscapularis spaces. The capsule can be dilated during arthrography, converting the procedure from a diagnostic to a therapeutic one.

A carefully designed treatment plan for patients with frozen shoulder may include physical therapy, pain medication such as nonsteroidal anti-inflammatory drugs, and possible intra-articular corticosteroid injection. Surgical referral may be indicated after conservative treatment has failed, although the exact timing of surgery should be decided on an individual basis.

Additional Reading: Adhesive capsulitis: diagnosis and management. *Am Fam Physician*. 2019;99(5):297-300.

27. Charcot foot is most commonly seen in patients with which one of the following?

A) Diabetes mellitus
B) Gonorrhea
C) Neurofibromatosis
D) Primary syphilis
E) Rheumatoid arthritis

The answer is A: Charcot foot, first described in patients with tertiary syphilis, is now seen mostly in patients with diabetes mellitus. It is a condition of acute or gradual onset and, in its most severe form, causes significant disruption of the bony architecture of the foot. It often results in foot deformities and causes abnormal pressure distribution on the plantar surface, foot ulcers, and, in some cases, requires amputation.

The exact pathogenesis is unknown, but underlying sensory neuropathy is nearly universal. Arteriovenous shunting due to autonomic neuropathy is also thought to play a role. Repeated unrecognized microtrauma or an identifiable injury may be the inciting factors of Charcot foot. Approximately 50% of patients with Charcot foot remember a precipitating event such as a slip or a trip, or they may have had unrelated surgery on the foot as an antecedent event. In approximately 25% of patients, a similar problem ultimately develops on the other foot.

Clinical findings in patients with an acute Charcot process include warmth, erythema, and swelling, and the disease is often thought to be cellulitis. Pain and tenderness are usually absent because of sensory neuropathy, which is universal and is probably a component of the basic pathogenesis of the Charcot foot. However, because patients with Charcot foot may have some pain if the sensory loss is not complete, the presence of pain does not totally exclude the diagnosis. Such pain is always much less than what would be expected for the severity of the clinical and/or radiographic findings.

Although cellulitis should be considered in any patient with diabetes, missing the diagnosis of Charcot foot can be serious because failure to initiate proper treatment of the Charcot foot can lead to a total loss of function. Inappropriate treatment with antimicrobial therapy and even incision and drainage can lead to unnecessary complications. Minimal pain or the absence of pain (characteristic of a Charcot fracture) can lead patients and physicians to ignore this serious disease.

The initial radiographic findings can be normal, making the diagnosis difficult, but if a Charcot foot is strongly suspected from the clinical presentation, treatment should be initiated and serial radiographs should be taken. The proper treatment for a hot, swollen foot in a patient with sensory neuropathy is immobilization. Most cases of Charcot foot can be treated nonsurgically with pressure-relieving methods such as total contact casting, which is considered to be the gold standard of treatment.

Additional Reading: Charcot foot: clinical clues, diagnostic strategies, and treatment principles: *Am Fam Physician.* 2018;97(9):594-599.

28. A 67-year-old retired cook who has suffered with diabetes for many years presents with worsening of a lesion on the bottom of his right foot. You have been treating it with soaks and antibiotics, but it has not healed and he continues with surrounding erythema. You are concerned that the infection may now involve the bone. Which one of the following is the best imaging methodology for detecting osteomyelitis with a diabetic foot ulcer?

A) Computed tomographic scan
B) Indium scan
C) Magnetic resonance imaging (MRI)
D) Plain films
E) Technetium bone scan

The answer is C: Diabetic foot infection is defined as soft tissue or bone infection below the malleoli. Osteomyelitis is a serious complication of diabetic foot infection that increases the likelihood of surgical intervention and is the most frequent cause of nontraumatic lower extremity amputation. Diabetic foot infections are diagnosed clinically on the basis of the presence of at least two classic findings of inflammation or purulence. Most infections are polymicrobial, with the most common pathogens being aerobic gram-positive cocci, mainly *Staphylococcus* species.

Although plain films of the feet are often ordered initially, MRI is the imaging procedure of choice for osteomyelitis in diabetic foot ulcers. MRI can show abnormal bone marrow signal, soft tissue masses, and cortical destruction characteristic of osteomyelitis. Unlike plain films, MRI can detect these changes early (within days) in infection. MRI also provides the anatomic detail, necessary when surgical debridement is required.

Treatment is based on the extent and severity of the infection and comorbid conditions. Mild infections are treated with oral antibiotics, wound care, and pressure off-loading in the outpatient setting. Surgical debridement and drainage of deep tissue abscesses and infections should be performed in a timely manner.

Additional Reading: Diabetes-related foot infections: diagnosis and treatment. *Am Fam Physician*. 2021;104(4):386-394.

29. The presence of a "bamboo spine" on spine radiographs, elevated erythrocyte sedimentation rate (ESR), and a positive test for human leukocyte antigen (HLA-B27) supports the diagnosis of which one of the following conditions?

A) Ankylosing spondylitis
B) Multiple myeloma
C) Pott disease
D) Reiter syndrome
E) Rheumatoid arthritis (RA)

The answer is A: Ankylosing spondylitis is an inflammatory condition that usually affects the axial skeleton of young men. The exact cause is not known. Symptoms include low back pain or stiffness that radiates to the posterior thighs, decreased range of motion (ROM) in the back or hips, and decreased ROM of the chest wall. Sacroiliitis is usually one of the earliest manifestations. Other joints may be painful or swollen. Patients often report that the symptoms worsen with rest and improve with activity. The course of the disease is variable. Some patients may have no symptoms or only mild stiffness, whereas others may experience chronic pain and significant disabilities. Most patients with ankylosing spondylitis can remain gainfully employed.

Radiographs show periarticular destructive changes, destruction of the sacroiliac joint, development of syndesmophytes on the margins of the vertebral bodies, and bridging of osteophytes between the vertebral bodies, giving rise to the appearance of a "bamboo spine." Laboratory tests show an elevated ESR and a positive test for HLA-B27 antigen in approximately 90% of those affected. Acute anterior uveitis (iritis) occurs in approximately 20% of these patients.

Treatment includes the use of nonsteroidal anti-inflammatory drugs and physical therapy. Attacks of iritis are effectively managed with local glucocorticoids in conjunction with mydriatic agents. In severe cases, systemic steroids or immunosuppressive drugs may be used.

A hallmark finding in multiple myeloma is urinary Bence Jones proteins.

Pott disease refers to tuberculosis infection that has spread to the bones, and lytic destruction of anterior portion of the vertebral bodies is seen on x-ray.

Reiter syndrome is also referred to as reactive arthritis and, in addition to joint pains, typically has associated urethritis and conjunctivitis.

RA classically affects the metacarpophalangeal joints.

Additional Reading: Ankylosing spondylitis. In: Domino F, ed. *The 5-Minute Clinical Consult*. Wolters Kluwer; 2022.

30. It is recommended that all patients with low back pain be risk-stratified with an initial assessment to identify red flags. All of the following signs and symptoms are considered red flags in this situation, except which one?

A) Fever
B) History of cancer
C) Onset after heavy lifting
D) Onset after a fall
E) Urinary retention

The answer is C: Red flags should prompt further investigation with prompt imaging, testing, or referral to a spine specialist, whereas others are less concerning. Serious red flags include trauma (ie, injury related to a fall or motor vehicle crash), new and/or progressive motor or sensory deficit, new-onset bowel or bladder incontinence or urinary retention, loss of anal sphincter tone, saddle anesthesia, history of cancer metastatic to bone, and suspected spinal infection. Without clinical signs of serious pathology, diagnostic imaging and laboratory testing often are not required.

Additional Reading: Diagnosis and treatment of acute low back pain. *Am Fam Physician*. 2012;85(4):343-350.

Section IV. Gastroenterology

Questions related to gastroenterology account for about 5% of the American Board of Family Medicine certifying examination. As you study for the examination, ensure that you have a good overview of the following topics:

1. Dyspepsia/gastroesophageal reflux disease (GERD)
   - Understand the workup for dyspepsia/heartburn (eg, endoscopy).
   - Appreciate the use of nonpharmacologic treatments (eg, head-of-bed elevation and avoiding triggers).
   - Know the evidence-based guidelines for medications in the treatment of GERD.
   - Appreciate complications of Barrett esophagitis/GERD (eg, adenocarcinoma of the esophagus occurs secondary to chronic GERD and has become the most common esophageal cancer

in the United States; although squamous cell carcinoma was the most common and still is in many areas of the world, it is related to tobacco and alcohol).
- Know the testing indications and recommended treatment for *Helicobacter pylori*.
- Appreciate the side effects of commonly prescribed medications for GERD.

2. Inflammatory, irritable bowel disease and celiac disease
   - Understand the workup for chronic diarrhea/abdominal pain.
   - Understand the workup for chronic constipation/abdominal pain (eg, red flags).
   - Know the basic diagnostic criteria for irritable bowel disease and evidence-based treatments.
   - Know the diagnostic characteristics for ulcerative colitis versus Crohn disease.
   - Appreciate the use of markers (perinuclear antineutrophil cytoplasmic antibody, cytoplasmic antineutrophil cytoplasmic antibody) in the workup of inflammatory bowel disease.
   - Know the basics of Celiac disease signs and symptoms, evidence-based workup and treatment (gluten-free diet).
3. Hepatitis
   - Understand the risk factors for and recommended screening strategies for viral hepatitis.
   - Know the indications for hepatitis A and B immunizations.
   - Appreciate the use of serum markers in the workup of viral hepatitis.
   - Understand the indications for initiating antiviral treatment for hepatitis C and the basics of recommended therapies.
   - Appreciate the complications of long-standing hepatitis B, including when/how to screen for hepatocellular cancer and the indications for initiating antiviral treatment.
   - Understand the basics of nonalcoholic fatty liver disease and nonalcoholic steatohepatitis and its treatment.
4. Common colorectal diseases
   - Understand the risk factors and treatment strategies for *Clostridium difficile* colitis.
   - Understand the risk factors and know the recommended screening strategies for colon cancer.
   - Know the risk factors for developing cholelithiasis and acute/chronic pancreatitis.
   - Appreciate the common signs and symptoms of cholelithiasis/pancreatitis and appendicitis.
   - Understand the appropriate use of blood testing in the workup of acute abdominal pain.
   - Appreciate the appropriate imaging techniques to be used in the workup of abdominal pain.

Each of the following questions or incomplete statements is followed by suggested answers or completions. Select the ONE BEST ANSWER in each case.

1. Your recently hospitalized patient was treated for pneumonia and has now developed pseudomembranous colitis. Which one of the following organisms is responsible for this condition?

A) *C difficile*
B) *Enterococcus faecalis*
C) *Escherichia coli*
D) Methicillin-resistant *S aureus* (MRSA)
E) *Pseudomonas aeruginosa*

The answer is A: Pseudomembranous colitis is characterized by profuse, watery diarrhea; abdominal cramps; low-grade fevers; and, occasionally, hematochezia. The etiologic agent is *C difficile*, which produces a toxin that causes the lesions affecting the colon. The condition is thought to be associated with antibiotic use in the preceding 2 to 3 weeks (in some cases up to 6 weeks); however, antibiotic use is not necessary for the condition to occur.

The diagnosis may be achieved by a laboratory stool test, which isolates the *C difficile* toxin. Sigmoidoscopy or colonoscopy usually shows characteristic yellowish-white plaques. Complications include dehydration, electrolyte imbalances, intestinal perforation, toxic megacolon, and, in severe cases, death.

Recommendations for treatment include stopping any inciting antibiotics as soon as possible; providing adequate fluid and electrolyte replacements; avoiding antimotility medications; and reviewing the use of proton pump inhibitors. Antibiotic treatment is recommended for all except very mild cases that were triggered by antibiotic use; suitable treatments include metronidazole, vancomycin, and fidaxomicin.

- For mild/moderate disease, oral metronidazole (500 mg three times daily for 10 days) is recommended as the initial treatment. For patients whom oral treatment is not tolerated, fidaxomicin may be used; specific indications include first-line treatment in patients with recurrence or at risk for recurrence.
- For severe disease, vancomycin (125 mg four times daily for 10 days) or fidaxomicin (200 mg twice daily for 10 days) is recommended.

Relapse may occur in up to one-third of patients after treatment. Fecal transplantation is recommended for multiple recurrent infections. Patients with severe illness that would include colonic perforation and/or systemic inflammation and deteriorating clinical condition despite antibiotic treatment are candidates for colectomy or diverting loop ileostomy.

Additional Reading: Clostridioides difficile infection: update on management. *Am Fam Physician*. 2020;101(3):168-175.

2. A 23-year-old Hispanic man presents with his fiancée to discuss the best treatment for his Crohn disease. He has been using Rowasa enemas when he has flares of his mild disease, but she is wondering if there is a better way of treating his condition rather than using enemas, which she finds off-putting. You advise them of which one of the following?

A) Methotrexate is commonly used for patients who cannot tolerate rectally administered agents.
B) Oral agents, although effective, are associated with more severe side effects that limit their use.
C) Oral 5-aminosalicylic acid (5-ASA) products are usually well tolerated.
D) The most effective treatment is via rectal administration.

The answer is C: Therapeutic recommendations are determined by disease location, activity, and severity, and by disease-associated complications. Patients with mild disease activity and no systemic symptoms are ambulatory and able to tolerate oral diet and medications. The goals of therapy are control of symptoms, induction of clinical remission, and maintenance of remission with minimal adverse effects.

This patient is being treated with mesalamine enemas; these compounds are often used in the medical management of mild to moderate disease. There are numerous forms of this medication, which can be given orally (Apriso, Asacol, Lialda, Pentasa) or rectally (Canasa rectal suppositories; Rowasa enema suspension).

Aminosalicylic acids (5-ASA products) and sulfasalazine (Azulfidine) are also commonly used to treat Crohn disease. These agents have anti-inflammatory and immunosuppressive properties. 5-ASA products are well tolerated and are preferred to sulfasalazine because they have fewer adverse effects and do not carry the risk of pancreatitis or pneumonitis, which may occur with sulfasalazine and mesalamine products. Significant advances have been made for the treatment of more symptomatic, debilitating or severe disease.

Commonly used immunosuppressants for treatment of inflammatory bowel disease include azathioprine (Imuran) and mercaptopurine (Purinethol). Side effects also include inflammation of the liver or pancreas and bone marrow suppression. In the long term they are associated with certain infections (tuberculosis) and cancers such as lymphoma and skin cancer, but these are rare events.

Tumor necrosis factor (TNF) inhibitors (biologics) work by neutralizing TNF, an immune system protein. These agents include infliximab (Remicade), adalimumab (Humira), and certolizumab pegol (Cimzia). They are used for adults and children with moderate to severe disease and are usually administered by a gastroenterologist.

Two principal strategies are currently used for Crohn disease management. A traditional "step-up" approach begins with corticosteroids or mesalamine products and advances to immunomodulators or anti-TNF agents based on the severity of disease. A "top-down" approach begins with anti-TNF agents. The optimal treatment strategy remains unclear, although the American Gastroenterological Association has recently issued recommendations on use of these agents for the induction and maintenance of remission in moderate to severe Crohn disease:

For induction of remission:

- Thiopurines and methotrexate are no longer recommended as primary therapies. Instead, patients can be treated with steroids or anti-TNF-α agents as primary therapy.
- When treating patients with steroids, consider the addition of an immunomodulator (thiopurine or methotrexate) to maintain remission and obtain a corticosteroid-sparing effect.
- When treating patients with anti-TNF-α agents, consider the use of a thiopurine also.

For maintenance of remission:

- If steroids were used for induction, then use an immunomodulator or an anti-TNF-α agent with or without a thiopurine.
- If an anti-TNF-α agent was used for induction, then use an anti-TNF-α agent with or without a thiopurine.

Additional Reading:

1. Crohn's disease: diagnosis and management. *Am Fam Physician*. 2018;98(11):661-669.
2. *Drug Therapy for Crohn's*. AGA Institute Clinical Practice and Quality Management Committee. www.gastro.org/guidelines/2014/03/04/drug-therapy-for-crohns.

3. A 33-year-old salesman is recovering from an acute viral infection and is worried that he will have liver problems going forward. You advise him that his acute hepatitis was due to a virus, which is not associated with a chronic infection. Which one of the following forms of hepatitis did he have?

A) Hepatitis A
B) Hepatitis B
C) Hepatitis C
D) Hepatitis D

The answer is A: Hepatitis is an inflammation of the liver that is characterized by nausea, anorexia, fever, right-upper abdominal discomfort, jaundice, and marked elevation of liver function tests. The condition is usually classified into the following types:

- *Hepatitis A.* Also known as infectious hepatitis, this is due to an RNA viral infection. The disease is common and often presents subclinically. It is estimated that as much as 75% of the US population has positive antibodies to hepatitis A. The onset of clinical symptoms is usually acute, and children and young adults are usually affected. The transmission is via a fecal-oral route and has been linked to the consumption of contaminated shellfish (eg, raw oysters).

The course of the disease is usually mild, and the prognosis is usually excellent. There is neither an associated chronic state nor a carrier state. The diagnosis is made by the detection of elevated levels of immunoglobulin M (IgM) antibodies, which indicate active disease, and immunoglobulin G (IgG) antibodies, which indicate previous disease.

Most cases require no special treatment other than supportive care, and symptoms usually resolve after several weeks. The disease can be prevented by administering Ig to those who are in close contact with those affected. Immunization, especially for travelers, is recommended to specifically prevent hepatitis A.

- *Hepatitis B.* This DNA viral disease is more severe than hepatitis A and causes more complications. It affects as much as 10% of the US population. The infective Dane particle consists of a viral core and outer surface coat. The disease often develops insidiously and can affect persons of all ages. It is transmitted parenterally (through infected blood transfusions or infected needles used by intravenous drug abusers) and through sexual contact.

The symptoms are often severe and can be devastating to elderly patients or those who are debilitated. Approximately 10% of cases become chronic; up to 30% of affected patients become carriers of the virus after they are infected. The detection of the hepatitis B surface antigen (HBsAg) supports the diagnosis of acute illness, and values become positive between 1 and 7 weeks before the symptoms become evident. The hepatitis B antibody appears weeks to months after the development of the clinical symptoms. The presence of a hepatitis B surface antibody indicates previous disease and represents immunity.

Those who have received hepatitis B vaccination also have positive antibody titers if they are immune. An anticore antibody (IgM) usually develops at the onset of the illness, and the IgG anticore antibody (which develops shortly after IgM appears) can be used as a marker for the disease during the "window period," which occurs when the HBsAg disappears and before the hepatitis B surface antibodies appear.

The hepatitis B e antigen is found in those who are HBsAg-positive; its presence is associated with greater infectivity and a greater chance of progression to the chronic state.

The delta agent (hepatitis D) is a separate virus that may coexist with hepatitis B; it is usually associated with a more severe case of hepatitis B and in cases of chronic hepatitis B in which there is reactivation of the virus.

Prophylaxis of hepatitis B can be achieved with hepatitis B vaccine given at 1 and 6 months after the initial injection, for a total of 3 injections. Persons exposed to hepatitis B (eg, by needle stick) should also receive hepatitis B immunoglobulin at the time of exposure.

- *Hepatitis C.* This disease (previously known as *non-A, non-B hepatitis*, or *posttransfusion hepatitis*) accounts for as many as 40% of the cases of hepatitis in the United States. It is the main indication for liver transplant in the United States when cirrhosis is present. The disease is transmitted by infected blood and is commonly seen in intravenous drug abusers and those who had blood transfusions infected with the virus.

The disease is usually insidious in its presentation, and the severity is variable. As many as 50% of these patients may develop chronic disease, which may eventually lead to cirrhosis. The diagnosis is made by serologic means.

- *Hepatitis E*. The transmission is similar to the hepatitis A virus. The disease is found in India and Southeast Asia, Africa, and Mexico. Cases in the United States are usually related to travel to these endemic areas. Hepatitis E virus is associated with a high fatality in pregnant women.

Additional Readings:
1. Hepatitis A. In: Domino F, ed. *The 5-Minute Clinical Consult*. Wolters Kluwer; 2022.
2. Hepatitis B. In: Domino F, ed. *The 5-Minute Clinical Consult*. Wolters Kluwer; 2022.
3. Hepatitis C. In: Domino F, ed. *The 5-Minute Clinical Consult*. Wolters Kluwer; 2022.

4. A 19-year-old presents with complaints of acute diarrhea with foul-smelling flatulence. He had been camping this past weekend and drinking water from a mountain stream. You suspect a *Giardia lamblia* infection. Which one of the following statements about giardiasis is true?

A) Asymptomatic carriers do not require treatment.
B) Chlorination of drinking water kills the cyst.
C) Diagnosis can be achieved by peripheral blood smears.
D) The cyst form is responsible for symptoms.
E) Transmission occurs through fecal-oral contamination.

The answer is E: *Giardia lamblia* is the causative agent in parasitic giardiasis. Most cases are asymptomatic. However, these patients pass infective cysts and must be treated. Symptoms occur 1 to 3 weeks after infection and include foul-smelling watery diarrhea, flatulence, abdominal cramps and distension, and anorexia.

Outbreaks in day schools, nursing homes, and institutions are common. Transmission is through a fecal-oral route. The infective form is the cyst, but the trophozoites are responsible for the symptoms. Cysts are transmitted in contaminated food or water. *Giardia* cysts are resistant to chlorination; therefore, filtration is used to clear cysts from drinking water supplies. *Giardia* is sensitive to heat; thus, bringing water to a boil is effective before consumption.

Diagnosis is accomplished by detecting cysts or the parasite in the stool (usually three samples) or in duodenal contents (by using endoscopy, the swallowed-string test, or Enterotest).

Treatment includes metronidazole and furazolidone. The medication is available in suspension, making it useful for children. Close contacts should also be tested, especially when recurrent infections are found. Although *Giardia* is most commonly associated with beavers, there have been reports of sporadic transmission between infected dogs and people.

Additional Reading: *Parasites—Giardia*. Centers for Disease Control and Prevention. www.cdc.gov/parasites/giardia.

5. A 52-year-old lumberjack recently attended a wild-game feed banquet, consumed summer sausage made from bear meat and presents now with complaints of abdominal cramping, diarrhea, and muscle tenderness. The most likely diagnosis is which one of the following?

A) Ascariasis
B) Giardiasis
C) Salmonellosis
D) Shigellosis
E) Trichinosis

The answer is E: Trichinosis is a parasitic infection caused by the roundworm *Trichinella spiralis*. The condition results from eating inadequately prepared or raw pork, bear, or walrus meat that contains the encysted larva. Many cases are linked to the consumption of contaminated summer sausage.

Many patients are asymptomatic; however, some may exhibit diarrhea, abdominal discomfort, and a low-grade fever. Ocular symptoms may also occur with edema of the eyelids, photophobia, and retinal or subconjunctival hemorrhages. Muscle soreness and urticaria may also be associated with the parasitic infection.

Laboratory studies show an increasing eosinophilia with a leukocytosis. Diagnosis can be made by muscle biopsy showing the larva or cysts, serologic tests, or enzyme-linked immunosorbent assay tests.

Treatment is accomplished with thiabendazole with variable response. For severe cases, corticosteroids may be indicated. Complications include myocarditis, meningitis, and pneumonitis. The prognosis is usually good. Most cases can be avoided by thoroughly cooking pork before consumption.

Additional Reading: *Parasites—Trichinellosis*. Centers for Disease Control and Prevention. www.cdc.gov/parasites/trichinellosis.

6. You have been caring for a young man with chronic diarrhea and he has been diagnosed with Crohn disease. This condition is associated with which one of the following?

A) Inflammation is limited to the superficial layer of the bowel wall.
B) On colonoscopy the mucosal areas of ulceration have a continuous appearance.
C) The formation of fistulas.
D) The patient has a decreased risk for developing colon cancer.
E) The rectosigmoid junction is typically involved.

The answer is C: Crohn disease is characterized by a transmural inflammation of the gastrointestinal (GI) tract. It may affect any part of the GI tract but is usually associated with the terminal ileum, the colon, or both. The diagnosis is usually made with colonoscopy or flexible sigmoidoscopy with biopsy or with x-ray contrast studies (usually avoided in acute stages because of the risk of developing toxic megacolon with barium). On colonoscopy, areas of ulceration and submucosal thickening give the bowel a cobblestone appearance, with some skipped areas of normal bowel. In addition to the transmural inflammation, there are granulomas, abscesses, fissures, and fistula formation.

Symptoms include fever, weight loss, abdominal pain (usually the right lower quadrant), diarrhea (rarely associated with blood), and growth retardation in children. In children, Crohn disease is more common than ulcerative colitis. Complications include intestinal obstruction; toxic megacolon, which is usually more common in ulcerative colitis; malabsorption, particularly associated with fat-soluble vitamins and especially vitamin B_{12}; intestinal perforation; fistula formation; and development of gall and kidney stones. There is also a significant (5×) increase in the risk of developing colon cancer. Other areas may be affected, including the following:

- Joints: arthritis, ankylosing spondylitis
- Skin: erythema nodosum, aphthous ulcers, pyoderma gangrenosum
- Eyes: episcleritis, iritis, uveitis
- Liver: fatty liver, pericholangitis

Additional Reading: Crohn's disease: diagnosis and management.*Am Fam Physician*. 2018;98(11):661-669.

7. You are seeing a 37-year-old White man with complaints of diarrhea for the past 2-3 weeks. He denies blood in the stool, fever, and has no weight loss and no recent travel. Appropriate management at this time includes which one of the following?

A) Check stool cultures
B) Colonoscopy
C) Observation
D) Stool fat studies

The answer is C: Chronic diarrhea is a common and sometimes difficult problem encountered by physicians and patients. The condition is defined as diarrhea that continues for >4 weeks. The problem occurs in 1% to 5% of the population. Patients often present late in their course, after other symptoms such as weight loss, rectal bleeding, and abdominal pain have developed.

Diarrhea results from incomplete absorption of water from the bowel lumen because of a reduced rate of water absorption or osmotically induced luminal retention of water. Even mild changes in absorption can cause loose stools. It is usually impractical to test for the many causes of chronic diarrhea. Instead, a useful approach is to first categorize the type of diarrhea before testing and treating to limit the diagnostic possibilities. Chronic diarrhea can be categorized as watery, fatty (malabsorption), or inflammatory (bloody).

- Watery diarrhea may be subdivided into three causes:
- Secretory: Reduced water absorption in the colon due to bowel dysfunction.
- Osmotic: Water retention in the colon due to poorly absorbed substances (eg, lactose, mannitol).
- Functional: Hypermotility with smaller volumes and improvement at night and with fasting; consistent with irritable bowel syndrome.

Secretory diarrhea can be distinguished from osmotic and functional diarrhea by virtue of higher stool volumes (greater than 1 L/d) that continue despite fasting and occur at night. The fecal osmotic gap can also help distinguish secretory (<50 mOsm/kg) from osmotic diarrhea (>125 mOsm/kg). Persons with functional disorders have smaller stool volumes (less than 350 mL/d) and no diarrhea at night. Once the diarrhea is categorized, further testing becomes more specific.

- Fatty diarrhea: often with bloating and steatorrhea. From malabsorption or maldigestion as in celiac disease or sprue, with small intestine malabsorption provoked by gluten (wheat) ingestion in affected individuals.
- Inflammatory: Inflammatory bowel disease manifests as ulcerative colitis or Crohn disease.

Additional Reading: Chronic diarrhea in adults: evaluation and differential diagnosis. *Am Fam Physician*. 2020;101(8):472-480.

8. A 26-year-old mailman presents to your office with complaints of diarrhea. He states that he has had loose stools for the past week. You obtain a stool sample for fecal leukocytes and that the laboratory report indicates the presence of polymorphonuclear fecal leukocytes in his sample. This finding most likely supports which one of the following diagnoses?

A) A bacterial infection
B) A fungal infection
C) A parasitic infection
D) A viral etiology
E) Laxative abuse

The answer is A: Acute diarrhea is defined as stools occurring with increased frequency or decreased consistency. There are many different organisms. Bacterial agents include *E coli*, *Salmonella*, *Shigella*, *Campylobacter*, *Clostridium*, *Yersinia*, and *Vibrio cholerae*. Viral agents include rotavirus, enterovirus, and Norwalk agent. Parasitic infections include *G lamblia*, *Entamoeba histolytica*, *Cryptosporidium*, and *Strongyloides*. Fungal agents include *Candida*, *Histoplasma*, and *Actinomyces*.

Diagnosis is accomplished with stool culture and sensitivity studies; however, the presence of polymorphonuclear cells supports a bacterial cause. In most cases of acute diarrhea, the use of antibiotics is unnecessary; however, the empiric use of antibiotics, including trimethoprim-sulfamethoxazole, ciprofloxacin, or erythromycin, may be appropriate (although controversial) in severe cases in which stool cultures are pending, especially for those at risk of transmitting the offending organism to others.

Additional Reading: Acute diarrhea in adults. *Am Fam Physician*. 2022;106(1):72-80.

9. Which one of the following tests is recommended to be used to screen when celiac sprue is suspected?

A) Immunoglobulin A (IgA) and Immunoglobulin G (IgG) antigliadin antibodies
B) IgA tissue transglutaminase (tTG) antibodies
C) Shilling test
D) The scotch tape test
E) Withdrawal of lactose from the diet to monitor for improvement of symptoms

The answer is B: Celiac sprue is an inherited disorder that is characterized by intolerance to gluten, a cereal-type protein found in wheat, rye, oats, and barley. Symptoms in infancy include colic, failure to thrive, and, in severe cases, iron-deficiency anemia with the development of edema. In adults, symptoms include abdominal bloating and discomfort, with diarrhea, anemia, weight loss, arthralgias, and edema. Steatorrhea is usually present.

Laboratory findings usually include iron-deficiency anemia (in children), folate-deficiency anemia (in adults), low protein levels, and electrolyte abnormalities, and coagulation studies may be abnormal.

Celiac disease can be difficult to diagnose and may be confused with irritable bowel syndrome, inflammatory bowel disease, diverticulitis, intestinal infections, iron-deficiency anemia caused by menstrual blood loss, and chronic fatigue syndrome. IgA tTG antibodies (tTG) and IgA endomysial antibodies (EMAs) are appropriate first-line serologic tests to rule in celiac disease.

The tTG test uses a less costly enzyme-linked immunosorbent assay; therefore, it is the recommended single serologic test for celiac disease screening in the primary care setting. However, a minority of patients with celiac disease have IgA deficiency. Therefore, if the serum IgA tTG result is negative but clinical suspicion for the disease is high, a serum total IgA level may be considered. Antigliadin IgA and IgG antibodies are elevated in >90% of patients; however, they are nonspecific and no longer recommended to test for celiac disease.

A positive IgA tTG result should prompt small bowel biopsy to confirm the diagnosis. A jejunum biopsy would show a flat mucosa with a loss of intestinal villi. Before being tested, one should continue to eat a diet that includes foods with gluten, such as breads and pastas. If a person stops eating foods with gluten before being tested, the results may be negative for celiac disease even if the disease is present.

The Schilling test is used to diagnose pernicious anemia in patients with vitamin B_{12} deficiency, and the Scotch tape test is used in the diagnosis of pin worms. Withdrawal of lactose from the diet to monitor for improvement of symptoms can be utilized when assessing patients for lactose deficiency.

Additional Reading: Celiac disease: common questions and answers. *Am Fam Physician*. 2022;106(1):36-43.

11. Which one of the following signs and symptoms are associated with Sjögren syndrome?

A) Chronic diarrhea and a peripheral neuropathy
B) Chronic diarrhea with polycythemia
C) Glossitis, iritis, and hyperextensible joints
D) Hepatomegaly, chronic rhinitis, and palmar erythema
E) Parotid gland enlargement, xerostomia, and keratoconjunctivitis

The answer is E: Sjögren syndrome is a rare chronic inflammatory disorder that leads to dry mouth, dry eyes (keratoconjunctivitis sicca), dryness of other mucous membranes, and joint pain. Women are more commonly affected. The disease is often found in conjunction with autoimmune disorders such as scleroderma, rheumatoid arthritis, and lupus. The cause is unknown, but there has been a genetic link with the HLA-DR3 focus. Signs include keratoconjunctivitis, parotid gland enlargement, xerostomia, and loss of taste and smell. Other complications include alopecia, increased risk of pulmonary infections, pancreatitis, pericarditis, sensory neuropathies, interstitial nephritis, and renal tubular acidosis.

Laboratory findings include positive rheumatoid factor (seen in 70% of affected patients), elevated erythrocyte sedimentation rate (70% of affected patients), anemia (33% of affected patients), and leukopenia and eosinophilia (25% of affected patients). Diagnosis is accomplished with the Schirmer test, which measures the quantity of tears secreted in 5 minutes in response to irritation from a filter paper strip placed under each lower eyelid.

Many patients affected with Sjögren syndrome are at increased risk for lymphoma and Waldenström macroglobulinemia. Treatment is aimed at control of symptoms. In some cases, steroids and immunosuppressants may be used.

Additional Reading: Sjögren syndrome. In: Domino F, ed. *The 5-Minute Clinical Consult*. Wolters Kluwer; 2022.

12. A 63-year-old White female smoker presents for follow-up care after recovering from a bout of acute diverticulitis. She is wondering what she can do to avoid having a recurrence. You advise her that any of the following have been found to be helpful in preventing recurrent diverticulitis, except which one?

A) Exercise regularly.
B) Increase her daily dietary fiber intake.
C) Avoid eating nuts, corn, and popcorn.
D) Stop smoking.
E) Take *Lactobacillus casei* daily.

The answer is C: Interventions to prevent recurrences of diverticulitis include increased intake of dietary fiber, exercise, and weight loss for obese patients. Counseling for smoking cessation is recommended because smoking is associated with an increased incidence of complicated diverticulitis and less favorable outcomes (eg, surgery at a younger age and higher risk of recurrence).

Evidence from a prospective cohort study of more than 47,000 men found no evidence that avoiding nuts, corn, or popcorn decreased the risk of diverticulosis or diverticulitis. However, a prospective study found that mesalamine and *L casei* are effective in preventing recurrence. A meta-analysis of four randomized controlled trials with 1660 patients who had experienced at least one episode of diverticulitis found that rifaximin (Xifaxan) plus fiber provided 1 year of complete relief and fewer complications compared with fiber alone.

Additional Reading: Diverticular disease: rapid evidence review. *Am Fam Physician*. 2022;106(2):150-156.

13. A 21-year-old college student has come in after a 3-week trip to Central America. She has developed significant diarrhea, with abdominal pain and cramping—she also thinks that she saw some blood in her stool this morning. You decide to prescribe an antibiotic. The most effective drug for the treatment of traveler's diarrhea is which one of the following medications?

A) Metronidazole
B) Doxycycline
C) Azithromycin
D) Tetracycline
E) Trimethoprim-sulfamethoxazole

The answer is C: Travel to the third-world countries can be complicated by traveler's diarrhea. The incidence ranges from 4% to >50%. The most common pathogens are enteropathogens (eg, *E coli*) in approximately 80% of cases; occasionally, viruses such as the Norwalk agent or rotavirus are causative. Traveler's diarrhea usually is a self-limited disorder and often resolves without specific treatment; however, oral rehydration is often beneficial to replace lost fluids and electrolytes. Clear liquids are routinely recommended for adults.

Travelers who develop three or more loose stools in an 8-hour period—especially if associated with nausea, vomiting, abdominal cramps, fever, or blood in stools—may benefit from antimicrobial therapy. Antibiotics are usually given for 3 to 5 days. However, there are concerns about travelers who take antibiotics acquiring resistant organisms such as extended-spectrum β-lactamase–producing organisms or *Clostridioides difficile* infection as a result.

As empiric therapy, first-line antibiotics have traditionally been the fluoroquinolones, such as ciprofloxacin or levofloxacin. Increasing microbial resistance may limit their usefulness in many destinations. In addition, the use of fluoroquinolones has been associated with tendinopathies and the development of *C difficile* infection. The U.S. Food and Drug Administration (FDA) warns that the potentially serious side effects of fluoroquinolones may outweigh their benefit in treating uncomplicated respiratory and urinary tract infections; however, because of the short duration of therapy for traveler's diarrhea, these side effects are not believed to be a significant risk.

A potential alternative to fluoroquinolones is azithromycin, although enteropathogens with decreased azithromycin susceptibility have been documented in several countries. A new therapeutic option is rifamycin SV, which was approved by the FDA in November

2018 to treat traveler's diarrhea caused by noninvasive strains of *E coli* in adults.

Bismuth subsalicylate also may be used as treatment: 1 fluid ounce or two 262-mg tablets every 30 minutes for up to 8 doses in a 24-hour period, which can be repeated on a second day. If diarrhea persists despite therapy, travelers should be evaluated and treated for possible parasitic infection.

The traveler should also take precautions by eating only freshly prepared foods that are adequately cooked, eating freshly peeled fruits, drinking only boiled or bottled water, and avoiding tap water and ice made from tap water (even in alcoholic drinks).

Additional Reading: *Travelers' Diarrhea.* Center for Disease Control and Prevention. https://wwwnc.cdc.gov/travel/yellowbook/2020/preparing-international-travelers/travelers-diarrhea

14. Gilbert disease is associated with which one of the following?

A) An increased risk for liver cancer
B) Intravascular hemolysis
C) Mild elevations of unconjugated bilirubin
D) Overproduction of glucuronyl transferase

The answer is C: Gilbert disease is a persistent, lifelong condition that involves the deficiency of glucuronyl transferase. It affects as much as 5% of the population. There may be a familial component. Patients exhibit a persistent elevation in indirect (unconjugated) bilirubin. Stressful states and fasting may increase bilirubin levels. Patients do not exhibit symptoms, and there is no evidence of hemolysis. Gilbert syndrome can be distinguished from hepatitis by normal liver function tests, absence of urinary bile, and predominantly unconjugated bilirubin fractionation. Hemolysis is differentiated by the absence of anemia or reticulocytosis. Liver histology is normal, but biopsy is not needed for the diagnosis. No treatment is required, and no untoward effects are noted. Patients should be reassured that this is a benign condition and they do not have a liver disease.

Additional Reading: Gilbert disease. In: Domino F, ed. *The 5-Minute Clinical Consult*. Wolters Kluwer; 2017.

15. A 55-year-old Black male patient present to the emergency department with severe abdominal pain, which has been radiating to his back, along with persistent vomiting over the previous few hours. Other than a history of hypertriglyceridemia (512 mg/dL), he has been healthy. Acute laboratory test results are obtained and include the following abnormalities:

- White blood cell (WBC) count: 20,000
- Glucose: 295 mg/dL
- Aspartate aminotransferase (AST): 333 IU/L
- Lactate dehydrogenase: 375 IU/L

The most likely diagnosis to explain his presentation is which one of the following conditions?

A) Acute cholecystitis
B) Acute pancreatitis
C) Diabetic ketoacidosis
D) Hepatitis
E) Ruptured abdominal viscus

The answer is B: Acute pancreatitis is caused by biliary tract disease, alcoholism, hypertriglyceridemia, hypercalcemia, hyperparathyroidism, trauma, medications (eg, furosemide, valproic acid, and sulfasalazine), infections, and structural abnormalities of the biliary tract. Symptoms include constant, boring, abdominal pain that radiates to the back; nausea; and repeated vomiting with a low-grade fever. Physical examination shows a distended rigid abdomen with positive peritoneal signs, tachycardia, tachypnea, and signs of dehydration and shock.

Laboratory tests show an elevation in serum lipase (more sensitive) and amylase, elevated WBC count (12,000-20,000 per mm^3), elevated liver function tests, increased bilirubin, hyperglycemia, and hypocalcemia. Chest radiographs may show pleural effusions. Abdominal films may show the presence of a sentinel loop (ileus of the transverse colon). Ultrasonography or computed tomographic (CT) examination may show evidence of gallstones, dilation of the common bile duct, or edema of the pancreas. Pancreatitis associated with hemorrhage or necrosis of the pancreas has a mortality rate that approaches 50%. Hemorrhage is suspected if there is a grayish-blue discoloration of the back or flanks of the patient's body (Grey Turner sign) or affecting the periumbilical area (Cullen sign).

Treatment involves bowel rest with nasogastric suction and fluid resuscitation with correction of electrolyte disturbances. Various scoring systems have been developed to predict outcome at the time of admission. The Atlanta criteria use early prognostic signs, organ failure, and local complications to define disease severity. Early prognostic signs include a Ranson score of 3 or greater, or an APACHE II score of 8 or greater.

Newer risk scores include the Modified Glasgow (Imrie) prediction score, the bedside index of severity in pancreatitis, the BALI score, and the CT severity index. In a comparison of nine clinical and radiologic prognostic tools, none was demonstrated to be superior to the others by a statistically significant level.

An advantage of the BALI score is simplicity because it evaluates only four variables: blood urea nitrogen level, age, lactate dehydrogenase level, and interleukin 6 (IL-6) level. Measurements are taken at admission and can be repeated throughout the first 48 hours of hospitalization. A score of 3 is associated with a mortality rate ≥25%, and a score of 4 is associated with a mortality rate ≥50%. Given the ease of use of the BALI score as a prognostic tool, it should be considered if IL-6 levels are easily obtained.

Additional Reading: Acute pancreatitis: rapid evidence review. *Am Fam Physician*. 2022;106(1):44-50.

16. You are seeing a 27-year-old Hispanic man who has been diagnosed with ulcerative colitis. True statements regarding this condition include all, except which one of the following?

A) There is transmural involvement of the bowel wall.
B) The condition appears as a continuous area of involvement on colonoscopy.
C) There is a greater risk of developing intestinal cancer compared to Crohn disease.
D) The area of involvement is localized to the colon and rectosigmoid area.
E) Oral 5-aminosalicylic acid (5-ASA) compounds are effective in the treatment of ulcerative colitis.

The answer is A: Ulcerative colitis is characterized by inflammation of the bowel that is limited to the mucosal surface and submucosa of the bowel wall (ie, it is not transmural like Crohn disease). The area of involvement is localized to the colon and rectosigmoid area in a continuous fashion; this is unlike Crohn disease, which shows skipped areas of involvement. Symptoms include bloody diarrhea, abdominal pain, fever, and tenesmus.

Complications include intestinal perforation, development of toxic megacolon, and development of cancer (which is more commonly seen in patients with ulcerative colitis than in those with Crohn disease). Extracolonic involvement affects the skin, eyes, joints, and liver; however, the kidneys are not involved (as they are in Crohn disease).

Diagnosis is accomplished in the same manner as in Crohn disease (ie, colonoscopy or flexible sigmoidoscopy with biopsy or with x-ray contrast studies). Treatment of ulcerative colitis is similar to that for Crohn disease; however, the oral forms of 5-ASA (eg, sulfasalazine, olsalazine, and mesalamine) are more effective in controlling recurrences and the severity of outbreaks in ulcerative colitis. Close follow-up is necessary for ulcerative colitis and Crohn disease because of the increased risk of developing bowel cancer.

Additional Reading: Ulcerative colitis. In: Domino F, ed. *The 5-Minute Clinical Consult.* Wolters Kluwer; 2022.

17. The use of proton pump inhibitors has been associated with a deficiency in which one of the following vitamins?

A) Folate
B) Vitamin B_{12}
C) Vitamin C
D) Vitamin D

The answer is B: Vitamin B_{12} (cobalamin) deficiency is a common cause of macrocytic anemia and has been implicated in a host of neuropsychiatric conditions. The widespread use of gastric acid–blocking agents, which can lead to decreased vitamin B_{12} levels, may contribute to the development of vitamin B_{12} deficiency. Given the widespread use of these agents and the aging of the US population, the actual prevalence of vitamin B_{12} deficiency may be even higher than what statistics indicate.

Vitamin B_{12} deficiency is associated with hematologic, neurologic, and psychiatric symptoms. Neurologic manifestations from vitamin B_{12} deficiency include paresthesias, peripheral neuropathy, and demyelination of the corticospinal tract and dorsal columns (subacute combined systems disease). Vitamin B_{12} deficiency also has been linked to psychiatric disorders, including impaired memory, irritability, depression, dementia, and, rarely, psychosis.

Dietary sources of vitamin B_{12} are primarily meats and dairy products. In a typical Western diet, a person obtains approximately 5 to 15 μg of vitamin B_{12} daily, which is far greater than the recommended daily allowance of 2 μg. Normally, individuals maintain a large vitamin B_{12} reserve, which can last 2 to 5 years even in the presence of severe malabsorption. However, nutritional deficiency can occur in specific populations. Elderly patients and chronic alcoholics are at especially high risk. The dietary restrictions of strict vegans make them another, less common at-risk population. The role of B_{12} deficiency in hyperhomocysteinemia and the promotion of atherosclerosis are under investigation.

Diagnosis of vitamin B_{12} deficiency is based on measurement of serum vitamin B_{12} levels; however, about half of patients with subclinical disease have normal B_{12} levels. A more sensitive method of screening for vitamin B_{12} deficiency is measurement of serum methylmalonic acid and homocysteine levels, which are increased early in vitamin B_{12} deficiency. The use of the Schilling test for detection of pernicious anemia has been replaced for the most part by serologic testing for parietal cell and intrinsic factor antibodies.

Contrary to prevailing medical practice, supplementation with oral vitamin B_{12} is a safe and effective treatment for the B_{12} deficiency state compared to intramuscular injection. Even when intrinsic factor is not present to aid in the absorption of vitamin B_{12} (pernicious anemia) or in other diseases that affect the usual absorption sites in the terminal ileum, oral therapy remains effective.

Additional Reading: Common questions about the management of gastroesophageal reflux disease. *Am Fam Physician.* 2015;91(10):692-697.

18. You are seeing a 43-year-old nurse, who has recently undergone an endoscopy for severe dyspepsia, with a resultant diagnosis of an *H pylori* infection. Which one of the following is an acceptable treatment for this condition?

A) Bismuth, metronidazole, tetracycline, and omeprazole
B) Docusate, tetracycline, and metronidazole
C) Omeprazole, clindamycin, and sucralfate
D) Ranitidine, metronidazole, and ampicillin
E) Trimethoprim-sulfamethoxazole, sucralfate, and metronidazole

The answer is A: *H pylori* is a bacterium found in the stomach that is present in >80% of patients with duodenal ulcers and up to 60% of those with gastric ulcers. The incidence appears to increase with increasing age. Most *H pylori* colonization is asymptomatic. Test sensitivity is reduced if the patient is taking proton pump inhibitor (PPIs), bismuth, or antibiotics.

Tests include urea breath testing. The patient ingests a urea solution with a carbon isotope and then breathes into a container; in the presence of *H pylori*, urease hydrolyzes the urea to release labeled CO_2, which can be detected by a mass spectrometer. A stool antigen enzyme immunoassay is reliable in confirming successful treatment but should not be used to test for eradication of *H pylori* until at least 4 weeks after completion of therapy. Serology antibody tests for *H pylori* are useful in ruling out the diagnosis, but they lack specificity and are not reliable (because of persisting antibodies) for documenting eradication. The gold standard for diagnosis is biopsy and histologic examination.

The goals of treatment are to eradicate the microorganism and to prevent complications. Triple-therapy regimens are omeprazole, amoxicillin, and clarithromycin (OAC) for 10 days; bismuth subsalicylate, metronidazole, and tetracycline (BMT) for 14 days; and lansoprazole, amoxicillin, and clarithromycin (LAC), which has been approved for either 10 days or 14 days of treatment. Quadruple therapy (BMT plus omeprazole) appears to provide better eradication with similar safety and tolerability to triple-therapy regimens.

Patients should be tested for successful eradication of *H pylori* and those still infected after treatment with two different regimens should receive salvage therapy with a different regimen, such as a PPI, amoxicillin, and levofloxacin (Levaquin and others), if needed.

Additional Reading: *H. pylori* infection: ACG updates treatment recommendations. *Am Fam Physician.* 2018;97(2):135-137.

19. A 30-year-old man presents a week after he had been given a tetanus vaccine booster. He has been feeling OK but has developed a sterile abscess at the site of the injection. You have seen him in the past with recurrent oral and genital ulcers and frequent complaints of joint aches and pains. The most likely diagnosis to explain this presentation is which one of the following?

A) Behçet disease
B) Gonorrhea
C) Lyme disease
D) Systemic herpes
E) Syphilis

The answer is A: Named after a famous Turkish dermatologist, Behçet syndrome is an inflammatory disorder that may involve ocular, genital, articular, mucocutaneous, vascular, and central nervous system (CNS) structures. Symptoms usually develop when patients are in their 30s. Men are more severely affected than women. Symptoms include episodic and recurrent oral and genital aphthous-type ulcers, uveitis, arthritis (usually affecting the knees and ankles), skin lesions, thrombophlebitis, and vasculitis. Signs include cranial nerve palsies, seizures, mental disturbances, and spinal cord lesions.

The disease is usually chronic and is characterized by remissions and exacerbations. The syndrome is usually benign; however, severe ocular involvement can lead to blindness. Steroids and immunosuppressive medications (interferon, azathioprine, cyclosporine) have been used for treatment, especially in cases of severe uveitis and CNS involvement. Other medications used in treatment include thalidomide, chlorambucil, and colchicine. The disease is more commonly seen in Japan and Korea, as well as the eastern Mediterranean countries. Sterile abscesses or pustules at the site of an injection are hallmark findings for the disease.

Additional Reading: Behcet syndrome. In: Domino F, ed. *The 5-Minute Clinical Consult*. Wolters Kluwer; 2022.

20. You are seeing a 33-year-old patient who was told that his cousin has recently been diagnosed with Peutz-Jeghers syndrome. Which one of the following statements is true about this condition?

A) It is inherited as a sex-linked condition.
B) Patients have multiple polyps in the stomach and small and large intestines that commonly undergo malignant change.
C) Patients usually have hyperpigmentation around the oral cavity lips, soles of the feet, and dorsum of the hands.
D) The condition is associated with inflammatory bowel disease.
E) The condition is identified by elevation in carcinoembryonic antigen levels.

The answer is C: Peutz-Jeghers syndrome is a familial autosomal dominant condition that involves the development of multiple, benign, hamartomatous polyps in the stomach and in the small and large intestines. Malignant change has occurred but is rare. Those affected also have melanin-associated brownish-black hyperpigmentation around the oral cavity, lips, soles of the feet, and dorsum of the hands. The condition usually causes no problems except in severe cases in which abdominal pain, intestinal obstruction, or bleeding can occur. In these severe cases, surgery may be considered.

Additional Reading: *Peutz–Jeghers Syndrome*. GeneReviews. www.ncbi.nlm.nih.gov/books/NBK1266

21. A 32-year-old woman reports frequent bouts of constipation alternating with diarrhea. She frequently experiences abdominal discomfort, which is relieved with bowel movements. Stress tends to aggravate her symptoms. The most appropriate treatment includes which one of the following?

A) Mesalamine enemas
B) Metoclopramide
C) Peppermint oil
D) Steroid enemas
E) None of the above

The answer is C: Irritable bowel syndrome is defined as abdominal discomfort or pain associated with altered bowel habits for at least 3 d/mo in the previous 3 months, with the absence of organic disease. Cramping abdominal pain is the most common symptom along with diarrhea, constipation, or alternating diarrhea and constipation. The goals of treatment are symptom relief and improved quality of life.

Exercise, antibiotics, antispasmodics, peppermint oil, and probiotics appear to improve symptoms. Over-the-counter laxatives and antidiarrheals may improve stool frequency but not pain. Treatment with antidepressants and psychological therapies are also effective for improving symptoms compared with usual care. Lubiprostone is effective for the treatment of constipation-predominant irritable bowel syndrome.

Additional Reading: Irritable bowel syndrome: questions and answers for effective care. *Am Fam Physician*. 2021;103(12):727-736.

22. You are seeing a 39-year-old lawyer who has had long-standing problems with heartburn. You had sent him for an endoscopy and were told that he had some esophagitis and a biopsy was done. He is in for a follow-up of the biopsy result, which was consistent with Barrett esophagus. This condition is associated with which one of the following?

A) Adenocarcinoma of the esophagus
B) Overuse of proton pump inhibitors (PPIs)
C) Tracheoesophageal fistula
D) Transformation of esophageal columnar epithelium to squamous epithelium
E) Trauma from prior esophagogastroduodenoscopy

The answer is A: Barrett esophagus is the result of chronic gastroesophageal reflux. The condition causes metaplasia and transformation of squamous to columnar epithelium in the areas affected. Patients usually report symptoms of pyrosis (heartburn, a burning sensation in the upper abdomen), and dysphagia if strictures develop. Men are more commonly affected than women. The diagnosis is made with esophagoscopy and biopsy of suspected areas.

Treatment is accomplished with H_2 blockers and PPIs. PPIs strongly inhibit gastric acid secretion. They act by irreversibly inhibiting the H^+-K^+ adenosine triphosphatase pump of the parietal cell. By blocking the final common pathway of gastric acid secretion, the PPIs provide a greater degree and duration of gastric acid suppression compared with H_2 receptor blockers. Long-term use of PPIs in humans has not been associated with an increased risk of gastric carcinoma, although this was initially a concern. Prolonged use of the drugs has been associated with gastric atrophy; however, atrophy is more likely to be a problem in patients infected with *H pylori*.

PPIs are fairly well tolerated. The most common side effects are nausea, diarrhea, constipation, headache, and rash. Occasionally, severe cases of Barrett esophagitis are treated with surgery.

Because of a 10% increased risk for the development of adenocarcinoma in the affected areas, follow-up with endoscopy every 3 to 5 years is indicated, although screening endoscopy time frames are controversial. Treatment of gastroesophageal reflux disease associated with Barrett esophagus has not been shown to eliminate the metaplasia of that condition or the risk of malignancy. Consequently, patients with Barrett esophagus require periodic endoscopic biopsy to assess esophageal tissue for malignant changes.

Additional Reading: Common questions about barrett esophagus. *Am Fam Physician*. 2014;89(2):92-98.

23. You are seeing an intravenous drug abuser, who has developed hepatitis. You are concerned that he has a hepatitis B virus (HBV) infection. Which one of the following tests is useful to detect an acute HBV infection?

A) Hepatitis B e antigen
B) Hepatitis B surface antigen
C) Hepatitis B surface antibody
D) Hepatitis B immunoglobulin (IgG) core antibody
E) Hepatitis B antibody to the delta agent

The answer is B: The following are specific tests used when assessing a patient infected with HBV:

Hepatitis B surface antigen. This test detects the surface antigen of the HBV. It is usually detected 1 to 4 months after exposure to the virus. Its presence represents infection with the virus. In approximately 10% of cases, this test remains positive and no antibodies are formed. This state denotes the chronic carrier state.

Hepatitis B antibody. This test detects the presence of antibodies to the hepatitis B surface antigens. It usually occurs 5 months after exposure to the virus and persists for life. Its presence represents past infection and relative immunity to hepatitis B. It can also be used to check for antibodies after immunization for the HBV.

Hepatitis B core antibody immunoglobulin M and IgG. Anti-hepatitis B core antibody IgM is useful when trying to determine infection with the virus during the "window period" (ie, the time between the disappearance of the surface antigen and the development of the antibody). Its presence indicates a current infection with hepatitis B. Anti-hepatitis B core antibody IgG indicates a previous hepatitis B infection, and its presence remains indefinitely.

Hepatitis B e antigen. The presence of the e antigen indicates that the blood is highly infectious. It is associated with more severe cases and the development of the chronic carrier state. Its persistence for longer than 8 weeks indicates that a chronic carrier state has developed. In 90% of cases, hepatitis B e antigen-positive mothers infect their fetuses.

Hepatitis B antibody to the delta agent. Conversion from the hepatitis B e antigen to the anti-hepatitis B e indicates a lower infectivity rate and improvement in the patient's liver function status. It usually reflects a benign outcome.

Additional Reading: Hepatitis B: screening, prevention, diagnosis, and treatment. *Am Fam Physician*. 2019;99(5):314-323.

24. A 37-year-old painter is in for a recheck of his blood pressure (BP). He has been diagnosed with a chronic hepatitis C virus (HCV) infection. Overall, he is doing well and his BP is normal at today's visit. He has several questions about his liver given his HCV infection, and you advise him of several recommendations, except which one of the following?

A) Ibuprofen should be avoided.
B) Low-dose acetaminophen is useful for pain.
C) Milk thistle can help maintain lever health.
D) Alcohol intake can increase the risk of cirrhosis.
E) Vaccination for hepatitis A and B are not recommended.

The answer is E: HCV infection is the most frequent cause of chronic liver disease and the most common reason for liver transplantation. Chronic liver disease is the tenth leading cause of death in the United States. Preventive care can significantly reduce the progression of liver disease. Because alcohol in the setting of hepatitis C can increase the development of cirrhosis, patients with HCV infection should abstain from alcohol use. Because associated infections with hepatitis A or B virus can lead to liver failure, vaccination of both is recommended.

Medications that are potentially hepatotoxic should be avoided or used with caution in patients with chronic liver disease. In general, nonsteroidal anti-inflammatory drugs should be avoided; acetaminophen in a dosage below 2 g/d is a safer alternative. Many herbal remedies are potentially hepatotoxic and should also be avoided. Milk thistle can be used safely in patients who have chronic liver disease and may be beneficial. Weight reduction and exercise can improve liver function in patients with fatty infiltration of the liver.

Additional Reading: Hepatitis C: diagnosis and management. *Am Fam Physician*. 2021;104(6):626-635.

25. A 38-year-old describes severe rectal pain associated with pallor, diaphoresis, and tachycardia that lasts for only a few minutes. The pains occur mostly at night and are described as spasms. The most likely diagnosis is which one of the following?

A) Irritable bowel syndrome
B) Obstipation
C) Proctalgia fugax
D) Thrombosed hemorrhoids
E) Ulcerative colitis

The answer is C: Proctalgia fugax is a unique anal pain. Patients with proctalgia fugax experience severe episodes of spasmlike pain that often occur at night. Proctalgia fugax may only occur once a year or may be sporadic in waves of three or four times per week. Each episode lasts only minutes, but the pain is severe and may be accompanied by sweating, pallor, and tachycardia. Patients experience urgency to defecate yet pass no stool.

No specific etiology has been found, but proctalgia fugax may be associated with spastic contractions of the rectum or the muscular pelvic floor in irritable bowel syndrome. Other unproven associations are food allergies, especially to artificial sweeteners or caffeine.

Reassurance that the condition is benign may be helpful, but little can be done to treat proctalgia fugax. Medications are not helpful because the episode is likely to be over before the drugs become active. Sitting in a tub of hot water or, alternatively, applying ice may provide symptomatic relief. A low dose of diazepam at bedtime may be beneficial in cases of frequent and disabling proctalgia fugax.

Additional Reading: Benign anorectal conditions: evaluation and management. *Am Fam Physician*. 2020;101(1):24-33.

26. A 53-year-old waitress presents with a concern over a recent diagnosis of hepatitis C virus (HCV) infection. She is currently feeling well, and the illness was picked up on routine screening. Which one of the following statements regarding HCV infection is false?

A) Most patients are asymptomatic with the disease.
B) The course of the disease is quite variable.
C) Most patients develop chronic hepatitis.
D) The disease can be transferred through sexual contact.
E) Immune globulin is not effective for postexposure prophylaxis.

The answer is C: HCV is the most common chronic blood-borne infection in the United States. Identified in 1988 through molecular biologic techniques, HCV is an enveloped RNA virus that is classified as a separate genus in the Flaviviridae family. HCV is most efficiently transmitted through large or repeated percutaneous exposures to blood, such as transfusions or transplants from infected donors (although the blood supply has been screened for HCV since 1992), inadvertent contamination of supplies shared among patients undergoing chronic hemodialysis, or sharing of equipment among injection drug users. Transmission of HCV may also occur through high-risk (particularly anal) sex, perinatal exposure, percutaneous exposures in the health care setting, or exposure to the blood of an infected household contact.

There is no anti-HCV vaccine, and immune globulin does not prevent infection. There is no means to prevent mother to child transmission (estimated to occur 5% of the time), and breastfeeding is allowed for mothers with chronic HCV. The incubation period for newly acquired (acute) HCV infection ranges from 2 weeks to 6 months, averaging 6 to 7 weeks. The course of acute HCV is variable, and the majority are asymptomatic, 20% to 30% have jaundice, and 10% to 20% have nonspecific symptoms such as loss of appetite, fatigue, and abdominal pain; alanine aminotransferase (ALT) elevations are typically <800 IU/L and rarely exceed 1000 IU/L.

Most patients (80%) develop chronic HCV infection, with a typical, fluctuation in ALT between normal and 300 IU/L. No clinical features of the acute disease or risk factors for infection, including a history of percutaneous exposures, have been found to be predictive of chronicity. Because viral replication can be detected as early as 1 to 2 weeks after exposure, acute HCV is best diagnosed with an HCV RNA polymerase chain reaction assay. Emergence of the anti-HCV antibody is expected in 80% of patients by 3 months and 97% by 6 months and is the recommended test to screen for chronic HCV, which is currently recommended by the U.S. Preventive Services Task Force for all patients born between 1945 and 1965, as well as for those with risk factors for infection.

The persistence of HCV viremia beyond 6 months defines chronic infection, whereas clearance of detectable virus indicates either self-eradication or treatment success when measured 12 weeks after the end of treatment.

Additional Reading: Hepatitis C: diagnosis and management. *Am Fam Physician.* 2021;104(6):626-635.

27. A 41-year-old accountant presents with a flare of his eczema. He additionally reports that he has been taking omeprazole (Prilosec) over the counter because he has been having worsening of his heartburn the past couple of months. He finds that it helps but asks about any long-term side effects from taking this regularly. You tell him that evidence has shown that continuing to take this medication has been associated with all of the following, except which one?

A) *C difficile* colitis
B) Hypocalcemia
C) Lung cancer
D) Vitamin B_{12} deficiency

The answer is C: Proton pump inhibitors (PPIs) such as omeprazole (Prilosec) effectively inhibit acid production in the stomach. This reduces symptoms of acid-mediated gastritis, peptic ulcer disease, and gastroesophageal reflux. However, this reduction in stomach acidity can cause unintended consequences involving processes that are physiologically dependent on low pH in the gastrointestinal (GI) tract. Theoretical risks include decreased levels of vitamin B_{12}, iron, and magnesium, along with loss of bone density; associated increases in infections—particularly GI tract infections and pneumonia; and an increased risk for GI neoplasm. Another concern is interference with the absorption of other medications, particularly those that rely on an acidic environment.

The evidence is conflicting on these risks, but it seems that long-term use of PPIs is associated with an increased risk for pneumonia and GI tract infections, primarily *C difficile* colitis. PPIs may also decrease bone density in subsets of patients. These risks need to be weighed against the benefits that these medicines provide before prescribing them on a long-term basis.

Additional Reading: Common questions about the management of gastroesophageal reflux disease. *Am Fam Physician.* 2015;91(10):692-697.

28. A 33-year-old mailman comes to the office with complaints of loose watery stools for the past week. He reports that he has not been out of the country and has not eaten anything different than his wife and she has not been ill. Which of the following statements concerning diarrhea in the United States is true?

A) Antimicrobial resistance is not a concern when treating diarrhea.
B) Eradication of the causative agent is the goal of treatment.
C) Pathogens are not identifiable in more than 50% of cases of diarrhea.
D) Traveler's diarrhea is usually caused by a virus.

The answer is C: *Diarrhea* is defined as watery or liquid stools, usually with increases in daily frequency and in total stool weight (>200 g/d). The pathogens that commonly cause sporadic diarrhea in adults in the United States and other developed countries are *Campylobacter*, *Salmonella*, and *Shigella* species; *E coli*; *Yersinia* species; protozoa; and viruses. However, pathogens are not identifiable in more than one half of cases.

Traveler's diarrhea is caused by bacteria in approximately 80% of patients. Common pathogens are enterogenic *E coli*, *Salmonella*, *Shigella*, *Campylobacter*, *Vibrio*, *Yersinia*, and *Aeromonas* species. Death from diarrhea is rare, but infants, elderly patients, and those in long-term care facilities are at a greater risk. The goals of treatment include reducing the infectious period, length of illness, risk of transmission to others, risk of dehydration, and rates of severe illness.

Antimotility and antisecretory agents (bismuth subsalicylate reduces duration of diarrhea compared with placebo, but less effective than loperamide) are likely to be beneficial in the treatments of acute diarrhea in adults.

Empiric treatment of traveler's diarrhea shortened the length of illness, although it was occasionally associated with prolonged presence of the causative pathogen in the stool and the development of resistant strains. Empiric treatment of community-acquired diarrhea with ciprofloxacin shortened the length of illness by 1 to 2 days. Development of resistant strains occurred with the use of some antibiotics but not with others. Adverse effects were similar to those noted for traveler's diarrhea. One must balance the trade-off between the benefits and harms of using empiric antibiotics for mild to moderate diarrhea. However, in treating traveler's diarrhea in adults, the empiric use of antibiotics is likely to be beneficial.

Additional Reading: Acute diarrhea in adults. *Am Fam Physician.* 2022;106(1):72-80.

29. You are seeing a 63-year-old White woman who was diagnosed with diverticulosis on her screening colonoscopy a year ago and now presents with complaints of left lower quadrant pain, a low-grade fever, and difficulty moving her bowels. You diagnose her with acute diverticulitis. Which one of the following regimens is the most appropriate treatment for this situation?

A) Admit for intravenous fluids and antibiotics.
B) Advise clear liquid diet and to call back if unimproved.
C) Advise clear liquid diet and start metronidazole.
D) Advise clear liquid diet and start metronidazole with ciprofloxacin.

The answer is D: The treatment of diverticulitis depends on whether the patient has uncomplicated disease or complicated disease. Acute uncomplicated diverticulitis is successfully treated in most patients with conservative outpatient management. Although the elderly, immunocompromised patients, or those with comorbid conditions such as diabetes and renal failure are at risk for treatment failure.

Patients with mild diverticulitis can be treated with a clear liquid diet and 7 to 10 days of oral broad-spectrum antimicrobial therapy, which covers anaerobic microorganisms (eg, *Bacteroides fragilis* and Clostridia) and aerobic microorganisms (eg, *E coli*, *Klebsiella*, and *Proteus*). Single and multiple antibiotic regimens are equally effective as long as both groups of organisms are covered.

A typical oral antibiotic regimen is a combination of ciprofloxacin (or trimethoprim-sulfamethoxazole) and metronidazole. Moxifloxacin is appropriate monotherapy for outpatient treatment of uncomplicated diverticulitis. Amoxicillin/clavulanic acid monotherapy is acceptable as well. Improvement is expected in 48 to 72 hours, and patients should be instructed to advance the diet slowly at that time. Those who fail outpatient therapy (ie, persistent or increasing fever, pain, or leukocytosis after 2-3 days) need inpatient treatment.

Hospitalization is also required for those with more severe diverticulitis, particularly if demonstrating systemic signs of infection or peritonitis. Additionally, those who cannot tolerate oral antibiotics, who are immunocompromised, or who have comorbidities may also require hospitalization.

Additional Reading: Acute colonic diverticulitis: medical management. In: *UpToDate*. 2022.

30. You are seeing a 51-year-old White man and have suggested a colonoscopy to screen for colorectal cancer (CRC). He is in agreement with screening but wonders about his options. Which one of the following represents an optimal screening strategy for CRC?

A) Colonoscopy every 5 years
B) Computed tomographic (CT) colonography every 10 years
C) High-sensitivity fecal occult blood test (FOBT) every 2 years
D) Sigmoidoscopy every 5 years with high-sensitivity FOBT every 3 years
E) Sigmoidoscopy every 5 years

The answer is D: The U.S. Preventive Services Task Force (USPSTF) recommends screening for CRC in adults 50 to 75 years of age using colonoscopy, sigmoidoscopy, or high-sensitivity FOBT. Studies show that the optimal intervals for these tests are colonoscopy every 10 years, high-sensitivity FOBT annually, and sigmoidoscopy every 5 years combined with high-sensitivity FOBT every 3 years. Sigmoidoscopy every 5 years without high-sensitivity FOBT is significantly less effective in detecting CRC than are other screening tests. The USPSTF concluded that there is insufficient evidence to determine the net benefit of CT colonography and fecal DNA testing.

Additional Reading: *Colorectal Cancer: Screening*. www.uspreventiveservicestaskforce.org/Page/Document/UpdateSummaryFinal/colorectal-cancer-screening2?ds=1&s=colon_cancer_screening.

31. Which one of the following statements is correct concerning hepatitis C virus (HCV)?

A) There is no risk to infants if the mother is infected with HCV.
B) There is no risk associated with sexual intercourse with an individual with hepatitis C.
C) Cesarean section should be performed on mothers who test positive for hepatitis C to prevent transmission to the newborn.
D) Hepatitis C can spread by contaminated water supplies.
E) Hepatitis C does not appear to be transmitted in breast milk.

The answer is E: In an effort to reduce the risk of transmission to others, HCV-positive patients should be advised not to donate blood, organs, tissue, or semen; not to share toothbrushes, dental appliances, razors, or other personal care articles that might have blood on them; and to cover cuts and sores on the skin to keep from spreading infectious blood or secretions. HCV-positive patients with one long-term, steady sex partner do not need to change their sexual practices. They should, however, discuss the risk (which is low but not absent) with their partner. If they want to lower the small chance of spreading HCV to their partner, they may decide to use barrier precautions such as latex condoms. HCV-positive women do not need to avoid pregnancy or breast-feeding.

Potential, expectant, and new parents should be advised that about 5 of every 100 infants born to HCV-infected women become infected. This infection occurs at the time of birth, and no treatment has been shown to prevent the transmission. There is no evidence that the method of delivery is related to transmission; therefore, the need for cesarean section versus vaginal delivery should not be determined on the basis of HCV infection status.

Limited data on breastfeeding indicate that it does not transmit HCV, although it may be prudent for HCV-positive mothers to abstain from breastfeeding if their nipples are cracked or bleeding. Infants born to HCV-positive women should be tested for HCV infection and, if positive, evaluated for the presence or development of chronic liver disease.

HCV is not spread by sneezing, hugging, coughing, food or water, sharing eating utensils or drinking glasses, or casual contact. Persons should not be excluded from work, school, play, child care, or other settings on the basis of HCV infection status.

Additional Reading: Hepatitis C: diagnosis and management. *Am Fam Physician*. 2021;104(6):626-635.

32. Which one of the following statements is correct concerning chronic hepatitis C virus (HCV) infection?

A) Alanine aminotransferase (ALT) levels are typically twice normal in individuals with a chronic HCV infection.
B) HCV genotyping is not necessary to guide treatment.
C) Patients with chronic infections are treated if there are elevated ALT levels, along with hepatic fibrosis (Metavir score ≥2).
D) The risk of developing hepatocellular carcinoma is rare.
E) The risk associated of developing a chronic HCV infection is highest among IV drug users.

The answer is C: Most patients, who develop a chronic HCV infection, will have chronic fluctuations in their ALT levels ranging from normal to 300 IU/L. No clinical features of the acute disease or risk factors for infection (eg, history of intravenous drug abuse) have been found to be predictive of chronicity. Because viral replication can be detected as early as 1 to 2 weeks after exposure, acute HCV is best diagnosed with an HCV RNA polymerase chain reaction assay. Emergence of the anti-HCV antibody is expected in 80% of patients by 3 months and 97% by 6 months and is the recommended test to screen for chronic HCV, which is currently recommended by the U.S. Preventive Services Task Force for all patients born between 1945 and 1965, as well as for those with risk factors for infection.

Complications of chronic HCV infection include hepatocellular carcinoma, with an annual incidence of about 4% and decompensated cirrhosis (4%). One study reported an annual mortality rate of 4% in a cohort of patients with chronic HCV, with hepatocellular carcinoma as the main cause of death in 44% of patients. It is recommended that patients with HCV-related cirrhosis be followed with hepatic ultrasonography and α-fetoprotein measurement every 6 to 12 months for hepatocellular carcinoma. Additionally, those with cirrhosis or advanced fibrosis should be screened for varices using upper endoscopy every 1 to 2 years.

The persistence of HCV viremia beyond 6 months defines chronic infection, whereas clearance of detectable virus indicates either self-eradication or treatment success when measured 12 weeks after the end of treatment. Candidates for treatment are 18 years or older, are able to adhere to the treatment schedule, and have elevated serum ALT levels, along with hepatic fibrosis (Metavir score ≥2).

Assessing the degree of liver fibrosis and cirrhosis is used in patients with confirmed HCV infection to determine treatment. Although several noninvasive tests are currently available to estimate liver disease stage (such as FibroSure, Hepascore, ultrasound elastography, and others), a liver biopsy remains the gold standard to stage liver disease. The Metavir scoring system is used to grade fibrosis, and treatment should be considered in patients with substantial fibrosis (score of 2 points or greater). The Metavir score is as below:

Fibrosis	Points
None	0
Minimal scarring	1
Positive scarring with extension beyond area containing blood vessels	2
Bridging fibrosis with connection to other areas of fibrosis	3
Cirrhosis or advanced liver scarring	4

Treatment protocols can be complex and are evolving. Once a decision is made to treat an individual for chronic HCV, based on elevated transaminases and degree of fibrosis, the drug regimen is guided by the underlying HCV genotype (1a, 1b, 2, 3, 4, 5, 6). The classes of medication include the following:

- Ribavirin (Rebetol) inhibits viral RNA polymerase, thereby inhibiting protein synthesis.
- Pegylated interferon (peg
- interferon alfa-2a [Pegasys]; peginterferon alfa-2b [PEG-Intron]) inhibits viral replication by antiviral, antiproliferative, and immunomodulatory effects.
- Sofosbuvir (Sovaldi) is an NS5B inhibitor; which prevents HCV viral assembly and RNA polymerase, thus inhibiting viral replication.
- Harvoni (ledipasvir and sofosbuvir combination) is taken once daily to treat chronic HCV genotype 1 infection. Ledipasvir is an NS5A inhibitor that acts in combination with sofosbuvir to interfere with viral replication.
- Viekira Pak (ombitasvir [NS5A inhibitor], paritaprevir [NS3/4A inhibitor], and ritonavir [HIV-1 protease inhibitor]) tablets copackaged with dasabuvir tablets (NS5B inhibitor) is used to treat adults with chronic HCV genotype 1 infection. These drugs work together to inhibit the growth of HCV and may be used with or without ribavirin.

Additional Reading: Hepatitis C: diagnosis and management. *Am Fam Physician*. 2021;104(6):626-635.

33. You have obtained a hepatitis B virus (HBV) serology panel on a patient who has a history of intravenous drug use. The results are reported as following:

Hepatitis B surface antigen (HBsAg)	Negative
Hepatitis B surface core antibody (anti-HBc)	Positive
Hepatitis B surface antigen (anti-HBs)	Positive

Which one of the following statements is correct concerning these results and the implications for this patient?

A) He is susceptible to HBV infection.
B) He is immune to HBV because of recovery from a natural infection.
C) He is immune because of a prior immunization.
D) He has chronic HBV infection.
E) The results are inconclusive in determining his HBV status.

The answer is B: HBV serology testing is useful to determine a patients' status. The tests include the following:

HBsAg: A protein on the surface of the HBV. The presence of HBsAg indicates that the person is infectious. The body normally produces antibodies to HBsAg as part of the normal immune response to infection. HBsAg is the antigen used to make hepatitis B vaccine.

Anti-HBs): The presence of anti-HBs is generally interpreted as indicating recovery and immunity from HBV infection or the result of successful vaccination.

Hepatitis B core antibody (anti-HBc): Appears at the onset of symptoms in acute infection and persists for life. The presence of anti-HBc indicates previous or ongoing HBV infection. The IgM antibody (IgM anti-HBc) indicates recent infection with HBV.

The following table is helpful in interpreting HBV testing:

Additional Reading: *Interpretation of Hepatitis B Serologic Test Results*. Center for Disease Control and Prevention. www.cdc.gov/hepatitis/hbv/pdfs/serologicchartv8.pdf

➔ Immunologic testing for determining hepatitis B status - whether acutely or chronically infected or immune can be confusing. Inconclusive results should be repeated in 6-12 weeks. The incubation period for hepatitis B ranges from 60-150 days.

Serology	Result	Interpretation
HBsAg	Negative	Susceptible to infection
Anti-HBc	Negative	
Anti-HBs	Negative	
HBsAg	Negative	Immune due to a natural infection
Anti-HBc	Positive	
Anti-HBs	Positive	
HBsAg	Negative	Immune due to HBV vaccination
Anti-HBc	Negative	
Anti-HBs	Positive	
HBsAg	Positive	Acutely infected with HBV
Anti-HBc	Positive	
Immunoglobulin M (IgM) anti-HBc	Positive	
Anti-HBs	Negative	
HBsAg	Positive	Chronically infected with HBV
Anti-HBc	Positive	
IgM anti-HBc	Negative	
Anti-HBs	Negative	
HBsAg	Negative	Interpretation unclear; four possibilities: 1. Resolved infection (most common) 2. False-positive anti-HBc, thus susceptible 3. "Low-level" chronic infection 4. Resolving acute infection
Anti-HBc	Positive	
Anti-HBs	Negative	

Section V. Endocrinology

Questions related to endocrinology account for about 5% of the American Board of Family Medicine certifying examination. Remember, as this examination is for family physicians, the focus is on the primary care management of these conditions. As you study for the examination, ensure that you have a good overview of the following endocrinology topics.

1. Type 2 Diabetes Mellitus (T2DM)
   - Know the recommended screening strategies and the diagnostic criteria (A1c greater than 6.5; two fasting levels greater than 125; one random glucose level greater than 200 or more plus symptoms; two random glucose levels greater than 200 in a 3-hour glucose tolerance test).
   - Appreciate the workup for a patient with newly diagnosed T2DM.
   - Appreciate the use of nonpharmacologic treatments (diet/exercise).
   - Appreciate the use of A1c targets based on the American Diabetes Association recommendations with when to be aggressive and when aggressive care can be clinically inappropriate.
   - Understand comorbid conditions and how/when to screen/treat.
   - Know the commonly accepted first- and second-line medications for T2DM, how they work, and the clinical benefits and adverse effects of each class.
   - Appreciate how to manage diabetes for a surgical patient.
2. Type 1 Diabetes Mellitus (T1DM)
   - Know the diagnostic criteria and epidemiology for T1DM.
   - Appreciate the diagnosis and treatment of diabetic ketoacidosis.
   - Know the types of insulin (eg, glargine [Lantus] insulin is long-acting; lispro insulin is quick-acting).
   - Know how best to dose insulin (eg, two-thirds of the insulin dose should be given in the morning with two-thirds being intermediate and one-third regular, and one-third of the total insulin dose should be given in the evening with two-thirds intermediate and one-third regular).
   - Appreciate noninsulin therapies for T1DM.
3. Thyroid dysfunction
   - Recommended screening strategies for thyroid dysfunction based on age, diverse populations, and comorbid conditions. (For example, amiodarone can increase the risk of both hyperthyroidism and hypothyroidism.)
   - Appreciate the workup for a patient with newly diagnosed hyperthyroidism. (For example, Graves disease is the most common cause of hyperthyroidism in the United States, an autoimmune-mediated stimulation of the thyroid gland.)
   - Appreciate the workup for a patient with newly diagnosed hypothyroidism. (For example, the most common cause of hypothyroidism is Hashimoto thyroiditis, a brief hyperthyroidism state that progresses to a hypothyroid state. This is a chronic autoimmune thyroiditis that leads to the destruction of the thyroid gland.)
   - Understand the use of thyroid serum markers in diagnosing and treating thyroid dysfunction (eg, thyroid-stimulating hormone, triiodothyronine, and thyroxine).
   - Understand the workup for a thyroid nodule (eg, initial procedure of choice should be ultrasonography).
   - Appreciate the secondary complications of thyroid dysfunction (eg, untreated hyperthyroidism causes atrial fibrillation, osteoporosis, and heat intolerance).
4. Osteoporosis
   - Know the risk factors and recommended screening strategies/testing based on age, sex, and comorbid conditions.
   - Appreciate the workup for a patient with early-onset osteoporosis.
   - Understand the use of serum markers and frequency of diagnostic bone mineral density testing.
   - Appreciate the use of nonprescription treatments (eg, exercise, smoking cessation, calcium, and vitamin D supplementation).
   - Understand indications for medication treatment and the use of fracture risk calculators.
5. Other endocrine conditions
   - Appreciate the basic classification and diagnosis for diabetes insipidus. (For example, central diabetes insipidus is polyuria, polydipsia as a result of deficient antidiuretic hormone [ADH]. Nephrogenic diabetes insipidus results from a lack of renal response to ADH.)
   - Appreciate the basics of hyperaldosteronism. (For example, Conn syndrome is primary hyperaldosteronism. Clinical signs include weakness from hypokalemia.)
   - Understand parathyroid hormone interpretation. (For example, hyperparathyroidism results in hypercalcemia and hypercalcuria and is associated with renal stones [calcium oxalate] "stone, bones, abdominal groans, and psychotic moans.")
   - Appreciate the basics of Addison disease. (For example, Addison disease presents with weakness, hypotension, and hyperpigmentation [of mouth, palmar creases, and pressure points] and is most often due to an autoimmune destruction of the adrenal gland.)
   - Appreciate the behavioral and medical approaches for obesity.
   - Appreciate the basics of Cushing disease.

Each of the following questions or incomplete statements is followed by suggested answers or completions. Select the ONE BEST ANSWER in each case.

1. A 57-year-old White man is being seen in follow-up to discuss therapy for his newly diagnosed type 2 diabetes mellitus (T2DM). All of the following choices are consistent with the 2022 American Diabetes Association (ADA) recommendations for initiating pharmacologic therapy in T2DM, except which one?

A) Metformin is the preferred initial pharmacologic agent.
B) Insulin therapy is an option for initial therapy.
C) A second agent should be added if not at target by 3 months on a maximum dose of noninsulin therapy.
D) If not started earlier, insulin should be delayed until other agents have been utilized for at least a year.

The answer is D: The ADA has issued several recommendations for the initial pharmacologic management of T2DM:

- Metformin, if not contraindicated, is the preferred initial pharmacologic agent.

- Consider initiating insulin (with or without other agents) for newly diagnosed diabetics who are markedly symptomatic and/or with significantly elevated glucose or A1c levels.
- If noninsulin monotherapy at maximum dose does not achieve the A1c target over 3 months, then add a second oral agent, a glucagonlike peptide-1 (GLP-1) receptor agonist, or basal insulin.
- A patient-centered approach should be used to guide the choice of agent, considering efficacy, cost, side effects, weight, comorbidities, and hypoglycemia risk.
- Insulin therapy should not be delayed in patients who are not achieving glycemic goals.

There are now various medications available to treat T2DM:

- Sulfonylureas (glipizide, glimepiride, and others) increase insulin secretion by closing potassium channels on the surface of pancreatic β cells. Hypoglycemia can occur with any insulin secretagogue, and sulfonylureas can cause weight gain.
- Biguanides (metformin) decrease hepatic glucose output and, to a lesser extent, sensitize peripheral tissues to insulin. Metformin has been shown to decrease progression from impaired glucose tolerance to T2DM and it is the only hypoglycemic agent shown to reduce mortality rates in patients with T2DM.
- Thiazolidinediones (rosiglitazone, pioglitazone) increase insulin sensitivity in peripheral tissues and also decrease glucose production by the liver. These agents are not associated with hypoglycemia when used as monotherapy.
- α-Glucosidase inhibitors (acarbose) act in the small intestine, inactivating the enzyme that breaks down complex carbohydrates, slowing absorption of glucose, and flattening the postprandial glycemic curve.
- GLP-1 receptor agonists or incretin mimetics (Byetta, Victoza, and others) are given as subcutaneous injections. They act by increasing insulin secretion, reduce glucose release from liver after meals, delay food emptying from stomach, and promote satiety. They have a lower risk of causing hypoglycemia.
- Dipeptidyl peptidase-4 inhibitors (Januvia and others) inhibit the degradation of the incretins, GLP-1, and glucose-dependent insulinotropic peptide, resulting in an increase in insulin secretion and a reduction in glucose release from liver after meals.
- Sodium-glucose cotransporter 2 (SGLT2) inhibitors (Invokana and others) facilitate glucose reabsorption in the kidney. SGLT2 inhibitors block reabsorption resulting in an increase in glucose excretion in the urine, lowering blood glucose levels.

Additional Reading: American diabetes association standards of medical care in diabetes. *Diabetes Care*. 2022;45(suppl 1):S97-S112.

2. You are treating a 67-year-old White woman for hypertension (HTN). She is concerned about developing osteoporosis because her mother died from a hip fracture. Which one of the following antihypertensive medications would provide protection from osteoporosis?

A) Enalapril
B) Hydrochlorothiazide
C) Losartan
D) Metoprolol
E) Verapamil

The answer is B: In healthy elderly adults, low-dose hydrochlorothiazide preserves bone mineral density at the hip and spine. Hydrochlorothiazide produces small positive benefits on cortical bone density, which sustain for at least the first 4 years of treatment. They provide a further option in the prevention of postmenopausal bone loss, especially for women with HTN or a history of kidney stones. None of the other listed medications provide this protection.

Additional Reading: The effect of treatment with a thiazide diuretic for 4 years on bone density in normal postmenopausal women. *Osteoporos Int*. 2007;18(4):479-486.

3. A 54-year-old Latinx woman presents with complaints of frequent sweating episodes, palpitations, nervousness, and sensitivity to heat. She notes that she has been losing weight yet has been eating more. Which one of the following conditions is the most likely reason for her symptoms?

A) Addison disease
B) Cushing disease
C) Hyperthyroidism
D) Hypothyroidism
E) Menopause

The answer is C: The manifestations of hyperthyroidism are numerous and include goiter; widened pulse pressure; tachycardia; warm, moist skin; tremor; atrial fibrillation; nervousness; frequent diaphoresis; sensitivity to heat; palpitations; exophthalmos; pretibial myxedema; increased appetite with weight loss; diarrhea; and insomnia. The hallmark findings of Graves disease include the triad of goiter, exophthalmos, and pretibial myxedema. Anemia, present with hypothyroidism, is not seen with hyperthyroidism.

Although menopausal symptoms would include hot flashes and night sweats, mood changes are also often seen, but slowed metabolism and weight gain are more likely than weight loss and there would be accompanying irregular periods.

Addison disease is characterized by a gradual onset of fatigability, weakness, anorexia, nausea and vomiting, weight loss, skin and mucous membrane pigmentation, hypotension, and in some cases hypoglycemia depending on the duration and degree of adrenal insufficiency. The manifestations vary from mild chronic fatigue to life-threatening shock associated with acute destruction of the glands. Asthenia is the major presenting symptom.

Cushing disease is not associated with sweats and palpitations; however, weight gain, especially truncal obesity, and "moon faces" are common. While depression and irritability can be seen, so can be menstrual irregularities.

Additional Reading: Overview of the clinical manifestations of hyperthyroidism in adults. In: *UpToDate*. 2022.

4. A patient presents with complaints of palpitations and a racing heart. She has recently been losing weight. On examination, she is sweaty and you detect a goiter. You are concerned that she is experiencing a thyroid storm. Which one of the following medications should be avoided in this condition?

A) Acetaminophen
B) Aspirin
C) Propranolol
D) Propylthiouracil
E) Supersaturated potassium iodide

The answer is B: Thyroid storm is a life-threatening condition seen in patients with hyperthyroidism. The condition is usually precipitated by stress, illness, or manipulation of the thyroid during surgery. Signs and symptoms include diaphoresis, tachycardia, palpitations, weight loss, diarrhea, fever, mental status changes, weakness, and shock.

Treatment should be provided immediately and includes propylthiouracil, supersaturated potassium iodide, and propranolol. Other measures involve fluid replacement and control of fever with acetaminophen and cooling blankets. Avoid aspirin because it may increase triiodothyronine (T3) and thyroxine (T4) by reducing protein binding. Steroids may also be given to help prevent the conversion of T3 and T4 peripherally. The definitive therapy after control of the thyroid storm involves ablation of the thyroid gland with iodine-131 or surgery. After treatment, many patients become hypothyroid and may require replacement therapy.

Additional Reading: Overview of the clinical manifestations of hyperthyroidism in adults. In: *UpToDate*. 2022.

5. Which one of the following statements about hyperglycemic hyperosmolar nonketotic coma is true?

A) It is usually associated with type 1 adult-onset diabetes mellitus.
B) It is usually associated with fluid overload.
C) It is usually associated with a decreased serum lactate level.
D) Treatment involves intravenous administration of glucose.
E) Treatment involves fluid administration.

The answer is E: Hyperosmolar nonketotic coma secondary to hyperglycemia usually occurs in patients with type 2 diabetes mellitus. The condition occurs when serum glucose is elevated, leading to osmotic diuresis and the development of dehydration without ketosis. In most cases, the condition affects elderly, mildly obese patients who fail to keep adequate fluid intake to make up for the osmotic diuresis. Complications include mental status changes with the development of coma, acute renal failure, thrombosis, shock, and lactic acidosis.

Diagnosis depends on the detection of plasma glucose >600 mg/dL, serum lactate >5 mmol, and a serum osmolality >320 mOsmol/kg. Sodium and potassium levels are usually normal; however, blood urea nitrogen and creatinine are markedly elevated.

Treatment consists of fluid replacement (usually approximately 10 L) with potassium supplementation and the cautious administration of insulin. Triggering conditions such as infection, myocardial infarction, or stroke should be ruled out. Unfortunately, the mortality rate for hyperglycemic hyperosmolar nonketotic coma approaches 50% if not treated immediately.

Additional Reading: Clinical features and diagnosis of diabetic ketoacidosis and hyperosmolar hyperglycemic state in adults. In: *UpToDate*. 2022.

6. Which one of the following test results would be detected in a patient with Graves disease?

A) Decreased thyroid-stimulating hormone (TSH)
B) Increased TSH
C) Decreased thyroxine (T4) levels
D) Decreased triiodothyronine (T3) levels
E) None of the above

The answer is A: Graves disease is the most common form of hyperthyroidism seen predominantly in women between 20 and 40 years of age. The condition, also known as *toxic diffuse goiter*, is characterized by a triad of symptoms, including goiter, exophthalmos, and pretibial edema. Patients affected may report palpitations, tachycardia, heat intolerance with excessive sweating, weight loss, emotional lability, weakness and fatigue, diarrhea, or menstrual irregularities.

Laboratory findings include a decreased TSH and positive thyroid-stimulating antibodies (which are thought to bind to the TSH receptors and stimulate the gland to hyperfunction). T4 levels are usually elevated, but in rare cases may be normal with increased T3 levels. Treatment involves the use of propylthiouracil or methimazole, inorganic iodine, propranolol (especially in thyroid storm), radioactive iodine (but not in pregnant patients), and surgery.

Additional Reading: Grave's disease. In: Domino F, ed. *The 5-Minute Clinical Consult*. Wolters Kluwer; 2022.

7. Acromegaly is associated with which one of the following factors?

A) Excessive cortisol secretion
B) Excessive gastrin secretion
C) Excessive growth hormone
D) Inadequate parathyroid hormone
E) Thyroid dysfunction

The answer is C: The condition of acromegaly is associated with an excessive amount of growth hormone, which in most cases is caused by a pituitary tumor. If there is excessive growth hormone secretion before closure of the epiphyses during childhood, then the condition of excessive skeletal growth is referred to as gigantism. When excessive growth hormone occurs in adulthood, it is usually between the third and fifth decades and is referred to as *acromegaly*.

Associated conditions include coarsening of facial features with increased hand, foot, jaw, and cranial size; macroglossia; wide spacing of the teeth; deep voice; excessive coarse hair growth; thickening of the skin; excessive sweating as a result of increased number of sweat glands; and neurologic symptoms, including headaches, peripheral neuropathies, muscle weakness, and arthralgias. Insulin resistance is common; diabetes occurs in 25% of patients. Coronary artery disease, cardiomyopathy with arrhythmias, left ventricular dysfunction, and hypertension occur in 30% of patients. Sleep apnea occurs in 60%. Acromegaly is also associated with an increased risk of colon polyps and colonic malignancy.

The diagnosis is made by detecting elevated levels of growth hormone after the administration of a 100-g glucose load. Because of the pulsatility of growth hormone secretion, a single random growth hormone level is not useful. Further diagnostic tests include magnetic resonance imaging and computed tomographic scanning.

Treatment is usually surgery; however, radiation is considered in some patients to treat pituitary tumors. Bromocriptine and a long-acting somatostatin analogue (eg, octreotide acetate) may also be used as adjuncts to surgery to help shrink the tumor.

Additional Reading: Acromegaly. In: Domino F, ed. *The 5-Minute Clinical Consult*. Wolters Kluwer; 2022.

8. A 58-year-old secretary presents with asthenia and hyperpigmented changes on her elbows and inner cheek. She also has noted her blood pressure (BP) is low and she is dizzy when she stands. She has recently lost 10 pounds and has some nausea but no vomiting. A recent workup included a positive test for coccidioidomycosis. Appropriate testing at this time would include which one of the following?

A) Adrenocorticotropic hormone (ACTH) stimulation test
B) Colonoscopy
C) CT scan of the abdomen
D) Esophagoduodenoscopy
E) Glucose tolerance test

The answer is A: Addison disease results from a progressive destruction of the adrenal glands, which must involve the majority of the glands before adrenal insufficiency appears. The adrenal is a frequent site for chronic granulomatous diseases, predominantly tuberculosis but also histoplasmosis, coccidioidomycosis, and cryptococcosis. Although infection with tuberculosis at one time was the most common cause of Addison disease, now the most frequent cause is idiopathic atrophy, related to an autoimmune mechanism.

Adrenocortical insufficiency caused by gradual adrenal destruction is characterized by a gradual onset of fatigability, weakness, anorexia, nausea and vomiting, weight loss, skin and mucous membrane pigmentation, hypotension, and in some cases hypoglycemia depending on the duration and degree of adrenal insufficiency. The manifestations vary from mild chronic fatigue to life-threatening shock associated with acute destruction of the glands. Asthenia is the major presenting symptom. Early in the course, it may be sporadic, occurring at times of stress. Late in the course, the patient is continuously fatigued. Hyperpigmentation can occur. It commonly appears as a diffuse brown, tan, or bronze darkening of parts such as the elbows or creases of the hand and pigmented areas such as the areolae around the nipples. Bluish-black patches may appear on the mucous membranes. Some patients develop dark freckles, and a persistent tan following sun exposure can occur.

Hypotension with orthostasis is frequent, and BP may be in the range of 80/50 mm Hg or less. Abnormalities of the gastrointestinal tract are often the presenting complaint. Symptoms include anorexia with weight loss to severe nausea, vomiting, diarrhea, and vague and sometimes severe abdominal pain. Patients may also exhibit personality changes, usually consisting of excessive irritability and restlessness. Axillary and pubic hair may be decreased in women because of the loss of adrenal androgens.

The diagnosis of adrenal insufficiency is made with the ACTH stimulation testing to assess adrenal reserve capacity for steroid production. The best screening test is the cortisol response 60 minutes after cosyntropin is given intramuscularly or intravenously. Cortisol levels should increase appropriately. If the response is abnormal, then primary and secondary adrenal insufficiency can be distinguished by measuring aldosterone levels from the same blood samples. In secondary, but not primary, adrenal insufficiency, the aldosterone level is normal. In primary adrenal insufficiency, plasma ACTH and associated peptides are elevated because of loss of the usual cortisol-hypothalamic-pituitary feedback loop, whereas in secondary adrenal insufficiency, plasma ACTH values are low or "inappropriately" normal.

Additional Reading: Addison disease. In: Domino F, ed. *The 5-Minute Clinical Consult*. Wolters Kluwer; 2022.

Addison disease results from a progressive destruction of the adrenal glands. Infection with tuberculosis was previously the most common cause of Addison disease; now, the most frequent cause is idiopathic autoimmune atrophy.

9. You are evaluating a 16-year-old who is on insulin for type 1 diabetes mellitus (T1DM), which he developed during puberty. He has been sick for the past 3 days and you are concerned that he has developed diabetic ketoacidosis (DKA). Which one of the following factors would not be associated with a DKA diagnosis?

A) Acidosis
B) Dehydration
C) Hyperglycemia
D) Hyperkalemia
E) Hyperosmolarity

The answer is D: DKA occurs in diabetics when a severe lack of insulin leads to a breakdown of free fatty acids, with the production of acetoacetic acid, β-hydroxybutyric acid, and acetone, resulting in severe acidosis. The condition usually occurs in patients with T1DM and is often seen as the initial presentation. Triggering factors include infection, trauma, poor compliance with insulin administration, MI, cerebrovascular accident, alcohol intoxication, or dehydration. DKA is characterized by the following conditions:

- Hyperglycemia
- Acidosis
- Dehydration (secondary to osmotic diuresis)
- Hyperosmolarity
- Hypokalemia

Symptoms include mental status changes, tachypnea, fruity breath (secondary to acetones), and nausea and vomiting with abdominal pain. In severe cases, coma may occur.

Treatment involves the administration of insulin to lower glucose levels, fluid rehydration (usually >5 L), and replacement of potassium and other electrolyte losses. If the condition is severe, cardiovascular collapse may occur. Close follow-up with frequent monitoring of serum pH, electrolytes, and urine output is necessary during treatment.

Further tests should be conducted to rule out infection as a precipitating cause. Unfortunately, the white blood cell (WBC) count is not a reliable indicator for the presence of infection in those with DKA because the stress of the illness often causes the WBC count to increase to 15,000 to 30,000 cells/μL.

Additional Reading: Clinical features and diagnosis of diabetic ketoacidosis and hyperosmolar hyperglycemic state in adults. In: *UpToDate*. 2022.

10. Which of the following laboratory results best supports the diagnosis of subclinical hypothyroidism?

A) Normal thyroxine (T4), low thyroid-stimulating hormone (TSH)
B) Normal T4, high TSH
C) NormaT4, normal TSH
D) Low T4, high TSH
E) Low T4, borderline low TSH

The answer is B: The following are laboratory findings associated with hypothyroid dysfunction:

Diagnosis	Laboratory Findings
Overt hypothyroidism	High TSH, low T4
Subclinical hypothyroidism	High TSH, normal T4
Hypothyroidism secondary to hypopituitarism	Normal/borderline low TSH, low T4
Subclinical hyperthyroidism	Low TSH, normal T4
Euthyroid	Normal TSH, normal T4

Additional Reading: Hypothyroidism: diagnosis and treatment. *Am Fam Physician*. 2021;103(10):605-613.

Treatment is indicated for subclinical hypothyroidism with a with TSH >10 mIU/L.

11. A 53-year-old schoolteacher is asking for a blood test because she is worried about diabetes. Her older brother was recently diagnosed with diabetes, and she states that it runs in her family. Which of the following is a diagnostic criterion for the presence of diabetes mellitus?

A) A fasting plasma glucose level of 140 mg/dL
B) A random plasma glucose level >200 mg/dL
C) An abnormal glucose tolerance test
D) A hemoglobin A1c (HgA1c) level of 6.5
E) All of the above

The answer is E: Data suggest that as many as 5.7 million persons in the United States have undiagnosed diabetes. The American Diabetes Association consensus guidelines for the diagnosis of diabetes are based on various blood glucose measurements:

- A fasting blood glucose level of 126 mg/dL (7.0 mmol/L) or greater on two separate occasions. A diagnosis of "impaired fasting glucose" is made with fasting glucose levels between 100 and 125 mg/dL (5.6-6.9 mmol/L).
- A random blood glucose level of 200 mg/dL (11.1 mmol/L) or greater if classic symptoms of diabetes (eg, polyuria, polydipsia, weight loss, blurred vision, and fatigue) are present. Random blood glucose values of 140 to 180 mg/dL have a fairly high specificity of 92% to 98%; therefore, patients with these values should undergo more definitive testing. A low sensitivity of 39% to 55% limits the use of random blood glucose testing to confirm a diabetes diagnosis, unless the level is >200 mg/dL.
- The 2-hour oral glucose tolerance test is considered a first-line diagnostic test. A fasting glucose is drawn, and then the patient is instructed to drink a liquid containing 75 g of glucose. Blood glucose measurements are then taken again in 30, 60, and 120 minutes (2 hours) after the patient has taken the glucose solution. Normal blood values for a 75 g oral glucose tolerance test in those who are not pregnant are as follows:
    - Fasting: 60 to 100 mg/dL
    - 1 hour: less than 200 mg/dL
    - 2 hours: less than 140 mg/dL

A 2-hour value between 140 and 200 mg/dL is called impaired glucose tolerance. A glucose level of 200 mg/dL or higher at any of the intervals is used to diagnose diabetes.

- The HgA1c measurement has also been endorsed by the ADA as a diagnostic and screening tool for diabetes. One advantage of using HgA1c measurement is the ease of testing because it does not require fasting. An A1c level of greater than 6.5% on two separate occasions is considered diagnostic of diabetes. Levels 5.5% to 6.5% are consistent with "prediabetes." A1c measurements for diagnosis of diabetes should be performed by a clinical laboratory because of the lack of standardization of point-of-care testing in an office testing. Limitations of A1c testing include low sensitivity, possible racial disparities, and interference by anemia and some medications.

Additional Reading: Diabetes mellitus: diagnosis and screening. *Am Fam Physician*. 2016;93(2):103-109.

12. You are seeing a patient who is on thyroid replacement therapy and have recently increased her levothyroxine to 75 mcg/d. Which one of the following test is best for assessing the adequacy of this replacement dosage?

A) Triiodothyronine level
B) Thyroxine level
C) Thyroid-stimulating hormone (TSH) level
D) Thyroid-releasing hormone level
E) None of the above

The answer is C: Patients diagnosed with hypothyroidism should receive replacement therapy with levothyroxine. These patients can be monitored for effective replacement by evaluating their serum TSH levels. A low-level TSH usually results from overreplacement, and adjustments should be made in the dose of medication; monitoring is repeated in 6 to 8 weeks. Underreplacement is represented by an increased TSH level and can be corrected by increasing the dose of thyroxine; monitoring is repeated in 6 to 8 weeks. Checking TSH levels earlier usually does not provide enough time for the levels to stabilize.

Additional Reading: Hypothyroidism, adult. In: Domino F, ed. *The 5-Minute Clinical Consult*. Wolters Kluwer; 2017.

13. A 57-year-old nonbinary patient with diabetes presents with a sore that they have noticed on the side of their right foot; although not painful, it has been slowly enlarging. Which one of the following is true about diabetic foot ulcers?

A) They rarely become infected.
B) They are typically polymicrobial.
C) They usually respond to topical antibiotics.
D) They should not be debrided because of the risk of bacteremia.

The answer is B: Foot ulcers in diabetic patients result from a diminished sensation associated with peripheral neuropathy and peripheral vascular disease (which is also usually present). Persistent pressure from ill-fitting shoes or skin cracking secondary to tinea pedis may predispose the patient's feet to infection. Infections associated with foot ulcers are usually caused by *Staphylococcus*, *Streptococcus*, anaerobes, and gram-negative organisms.

Aerobic and anaerobic cultures should be taken when signs of infection, such as purulence or inflammation, are present. Cultures are best taken from purulent drainage or curetted material from the ulcer base. Because all ulcers are contaminated, culture of noninfected wounds is generally not recommended. Polymicrobial infections predominate in severe diabetic foot infections and include various aerobic gram-positive cocci, gram-negative rods, and anaerobes.

Treatment involves debridement of nonvital and necrotic tissue, as well as oral or intravenous antibiotics. In severe cases, amputation may be necessary. Topical antibiotics are of little help and may delay healing. Osteomyelitis should always be considered in severe and persistent cases. Periodic examinations and treatment by a podiatrist are recommended. Diabetics who smoke should be encouraged to stop, and alcohol use should be discouraged.

Additional Reading: Diabetes-related foot infections: diagnosis and treatment. *Am Fam Physician*. 2021;104(4):386-394.

14. You have been treating a 27-year-old mother for postpartum depression, and one of her concerns is that she has become obese because she has not been able to lose her "pregnancy weight." She is 5′ 6″ tall and weighs 168 pounds. You calculate her body mass index (BMI) as 27.1 kg/m^2. What is considered the BMI threshold for obesity?

A) 25 kg/m^2
B) 27 kg/m^2
C) 30 kg/m^2
D) 35 kg/m^2
E) 40 kg/m^2

The answer is C: The BMI is an approximate measure of body fat and is used to define obesity. It is based on height and weight. The BMI is calculated by dividing the square of the body height in meters, by the body mass (weight in kilograms), expressed in units of kg/m^2. Obesity is defined as a BMI of 30 kg/m^2 or greater. A BMI between 19 and 25 is considered normal. If a patient's BMI is 25 to 29.9, that individual is considered to be overweight. A person is categorized as obese if his or her BMI is 30 or higher.

Additional Reading: Obesity. In: Domino F, ed. *The 5-Minute Clinical Consult*. Wolters Kluwer; 2022.

15. You have been caring for a 66-year-old White man for several years and have been successfully treating his hypertension and elevated cholesterol levels. This past year, he has complained of erectile dysfunction, for which you have prescribed sildenafil (Viagra). He returns today noting that his breasts seem to be swollen and his nipples have been "leaking." This scenario is most likely due to which one of the following conditions?

A) Adrenal adenoma
B) Breast cancer
C) Diabetes mellitus
D) Prolactinoma
E) Testicular cancer

The answer is D: Prolactinomas are the most common functioning, secreting pituitary tumors. Galactorrhea, oligomenorrhea, amenorrhea, and infertility are seen in women with prolactinomas, whereas men experience impotence, infertility, and, less commonly, gynecomastia or galactorrhea. Prolactin levels >300 μg/L usually indicate a pituitary adenoma.

Some medications, including oral contraceptives, phenothiazines, tricyclic antidepressants, antihypertensives (eg, α-methyldopa), and opioid-type medications, may increase prolactin levels. Other causes for hyperprolactinemia include nipple stimulation, pregnancy, stress, sexual intercourse, sleep, hypoglycemia, hypothyroidism, sarcoidosis, paraneoplastic syndromes (bronchogenic carcinoma and hypernephroma), and chronic renal failure.

Treatment is controversial. With small tumors, close observation may be instituted if the patient is asymptomatic. For larger tumors, bromocriptine (a dopamine agonist) is prescribed to lower the serum prolactin level. Surgery or radiotherapy may be necessary.

Additional Reading: Hyperprolactinemia. In: Domino F, ed. *The 5-Minute Clinical Consult*. Wolters Kluwer; 2022.

16. A 62-year-old woman presents complaining of joint pain, polyuria, polydipsia, and generalized fatigue. Her past medical history is remarkable for recurrent kidney stones, and she has also suffered from depression. You obtain a plain film of her hands, as she is complaining that those joints are worse lately. The x-rays show osteopenia and subperiosteal resorption on the phalanges. Which of the following blood tests may best help determine the cause of her symptoms?

A) Angiotensin-converting enzyme level
B) Antinuclear antibody test
C) Bone densitometry
D) Parathyroid hormone (PTH) level
E) ESR

The answer is D: Primary hyperparathyroidism is a disorder caused by excessive secretion of PTH. It is usually caused by an adenoma of the parathyroid (90% of cases); carcinoma is rare (3% of cases). Most patients are asymptomatic; however, some may present with kidney stones, joint or back pain, polyuria and polydipsia, constipation, and fatigue. The condition is more common in women and in patients older than 50 years. It also occurs in high frequency three or more decades after neck irradiation.

Findings include hypercalcemia (ionized), hypophosphatemia (hyperphosphatemia suggests secondary hyperparathyroidism), excessive bone loss leading to cystic bone lesions, and osteitis fibrosa cystica. Hyperparathyroidism is the most common cause of hypercalcemia in the general population. Radiographs may show subperiosteal resorption of the phalanges and osteopenia.

Treatment usually involves surgical exploration and removal of a parathyroid adenoma. For patients with mild, asymptomatic primary hyperparathyroidism, the recommendations for surgery are controversial.

Additional Reading: Hyperparathyroidism. In: Domino F, ed. *The 5-Minute Clinical Consult*. Wolters Kluwer; 2022.

17. You are seeing a middle-aged White woman with complaints of weakness and fatigue over the past couple of months. She has lost her appetite and having episodes of diarrhea. Her husband notes that she seems to have developed darkening skin around her gums, nipples, and vagina. You suspect Addison disease, which is associated with which one of the following?

A) Increased adrenocorticotropic hormone (ACTH) production
B) Decreased ACTH production
C) Increased urine 17-hydroxysteroids and 17-ketosteroids
D) Hypernatremia
E) Hypothalamic dysfunction

The answer is A: Addison disease (primary adrenal insufficiency) is a condition resulting from adrenocortical insufficiency. Secondary adrenal insufficiency is due to a lack of ACTH production from the pituitary gland. The primary disease results in electrolyte disturbances—hyponatremia, hyperkalemia, low bicarbonate, and elevated blood urea nitrogen. The plasma renin and ACTH are increased with primary adrenal insufficiency. Other laboratory findings include moderate neutropenia, lymphocytosis, eosinophilia, low plasma cortisol, decreased urine 17-hydroxysteroids, and decreased 17-ketosteroids. There is also a failure of plasma cortisol to increase after administration of corticotropin (ACTH).

Symptoms include weakness, fatigue, anorexia with nausea, vomiting, and diarrhea. Physical findings include hypoglycemia, sparse axillary hair, and increased pigmentation of the gingival mucosa, nipples, labia, and linea alba.

Treatment involves the replacement of glucocorticoids and mineralocorticoids. Symptoms of adrenal crisis include severe abdominal pain, generalized muscle weakness, hypotension, and shock. Severe cases may result in death.

Additional Reading: Addison disease. In: Domino F, ed. *The 5-Minute Clinical Consult*. Wolters Kluwer; 2022.

Addison disease (primary adrenal insufficiency) is a condition resulting from adrenocortical insufficiency. Patients often present with darkening skin around gums, nipples, and genitalia.

18. Type 1 diabetes mellitus (T1DM) is associated with which one of the following metabolic abnormalities?

A) Excessive growth hormone secretion
B) Hypersensitivity to glucose
C) Lack of insulin production by the pancreas
D) Overproduction of glucagon
E) Tissue resistance to insulin

The answer is C: T1DM tends to occur in individuals younger than 30 years. The cause is complete failure of the β islet cells in the pancreas to produce insulin. A genetic predisposition and perhaps a viral or autoimmune reaction that destroys the insulin-producing β cells are believed to be the cause. The incidence among schoolchildren is reported to be 1 in 500.

Symptoms include polydipsia, polyphagia, polyuria, dry mouth, nausea, vomiting and abdominal pain, weight loss, and fatigue. In severe cases, the patient may present in DKA with stupor, coma, dehydration, labored Kussmaul-type respirations, abdominal distension, and pain. The treatment is aggressive fluid and electrolyte replacement along with exogenous insulin administration.

Diabetic complications include retinopathy, nephropathy, macrovascular disease, and diabetic foot ulcers. Judicious control of glucose may help to prevent these complications. Typically, patients require 0.5 to 1.0 U/kg/d of insulin.

Additional Reading: Diabetes mellitus, type I. In: Domino F, ed. *The 5-Minute Clinical Consult*. Wolters Kluwer; 2022.

19. You are seeing a 55-year-old man with diabetes who has been recently started on insulin therapy. He is arguing with his wife over the best location to give his injections—he has been using his thigh and she insists that he should do the injections in his belly as her aunt who had diabetes used to do. Which one of the following statements is true regarding insulin injections?

A) Absorption from the buttock is rapid and can be used as a site just before eating.
B) Rotation of injections to different zones of the body can cause wide variations in serum glucose levels.
C) Injection in the arm often leads to exercise-induced hypoglycemia.
D) The thigh is the best site for reliable and predictable absorption.

The answer is B: The abdomen is the best site for insulin administration because the insulin is more reliably and predictably absorbed. Injection in exercised areas (eg, the thigh) may lead to development of exercise-induced hypoglycemia. However, insulin injection at the arm does not cause as much exercise-induced hypoglycemia and thus can be used as an alternative injection site. Absorption from the buttocks is the slowest and is a good site to use at bedtime to avoid nocturnal hypoglycemia. Rotation of injection sites can lead to erratic absorption of insulin with wide variations in serum glucose levels. Thus, injection sites should remain within the same zone (abdomen, arm, or buttock) but rotated at different sites within the zone to prevent lipohypertrophy.

Additional Reading: *Insulin Routines American Diabetes Association*. www.diabetes.org/living-with-diabetes/treatment-and-care/medication/insulin/insulin-routines.html

20. Based on the U.S. Preventive Sevices Task Force (USPSTF) recommendation for all women, without fracture risk factors, screening dual-energy x-ray absorptiometry (DEXA) scan should start at which age?

A) 50 years
B) 55 years
C) 60 years
D) 65 years
E) 70 years

The answer is D: The USPSTF guideline, based on a systematic review of the evidence, recommends screening DEXA in all women 65 years and older, as well as in women 60 to 64 years of age who have increased fracture risk. The USPSTF states that the evidence is insufficient to recommend for or against screening in postmenopausal women younger than 60 years.

Additional Reading: *Screening for Osteoporosis*. www.uspreventiveservicestaskforce.org/uspstf/uspsoste.htm

21. Primary hypothyroidism is associated with a deficiency of which one of the following?

A) Thyroxine (T4)
B) Thyroid-stimulating hormone (TSH)
C) Thyroid-releasing hormone
D) Thyroid-stimulating antibodies

The answer is A: There are basically two types of hypothyroidism:

- Primary hypothyroidism (most common form), which is a deficiency of T4 that is caused by thyroid gland disease.
- Secondary hypothyroidism, which is associated with a deficiency in TSH from the pituitary gland or deficient thyroid-releasing hormone by the hypothalamus.

Hypothyroidism is seen more commonly in patients older than 55 years and in women. The most common form occurs as a result of Hashimoto thyroiditis followed by posttherapeutic hypothyroidism, especially after radioactive iodine therapy or surgery for hyperthyroidism. Symptoms include fatigue, weakness, cold intolerance, constipation, hair loss, menorrhagia, carpal tunnel syndrome, dry skin, nonpitting edema (also referred to as *myxedema*) caused by deposition of mucopolysaccharides, weight gain, memory impairment, depression, hoarseness, delayed relaxation of reflexes, altered mental status, and bradycardia.

The thyroid hormones, triiodothyronine (T3) and its prohormone, T4, are produced by the thyroid gland in response to TSH production from the pituitary gland and are primarily responsible for regulation of metabolism. Most of the T3 and T4 circulate in the blood bound to protein, while a small percentage is free (not bound). Blood tests are available to measure total T4, free T4, total T3, or free T3. Total T4 can be affected by the amount of protein available in the blood to bind to the hormone. Free T4 is not affected by protein levels and is the active form of thyroxine. The free T4 test is thought by many to be a more accurate reflection of thyroid hormone function, and its use has replaced that of the total T4 test.

A low free T4 with a high TSH is seen in primary hypothyroidism, whereas a low free T4 with a low TSH is indicative of secondary or tertiary hypothyroidism.

Additional Reading: Hypothyroidism: diagnosis and treatment. *Am Fam Physician*. 2021;103(10):605-613.

22. A 48-year-old woman with type 1 diabetes mellitus receives a corticosteroid injection for osteoarthritis of her right knee. Which one of the following is true regarding monitoring of her blood glucose levels?

A) Glucose levels should be closely monitored for 48 hours.
B) Glucose levels should be closely monitored for 7 days.
C) Glucose levels should be closely monitored for 14 days.
D) No additional monitoring is necessary.

The answer is D: A single intra-articular steroid injection has little effect on glycemic control, whereas soft tissue or peritendinous steroid injections can affect blood glucose levels for several days after the injection. Type 1 diabetics should be advised to closely monitor their blood glucose levels for 2 weeks following such injections.

Additional Reading: Musculoskeletal injections: a review of the evidence. *Am Fam Physician*. 2008;78(8):971-976.

23. You have recently diagnosed an overweight 48-year-old White woman with type 2 diabetes mellitus and decide to start treatment with metformin. She asks about potential side effects. Which one of the following statements concerning the use of metformin is true?

A) Weight gain is common with its use.
B) The most common side effect is headache.
C) Patients using metformin must have periodic liver function tests.
D) The most serious side effect is lactic acidosis.

The answer is D: Metformin belongs to the *biguanide* class of hypoglycemic drugs and decreases hepatic glucose production by inhibiting gluconeogenesis and decreasing insulin resistance. Metformin decreases plasma triglycerides and low-density lipoprotein cholesterol, and increases high-density lipoprotein cholesterol. Hypoglycemia does not typically occur with metformin monotherapy, and, in contrast to other hypoglycemic agents, weight is not usually gained. The most common side effects are gastrointestinal irritation, abdominal cramps, and diarrhea. Patients with inflammatory bowel disease and peptic ulcer disease are not good candidates for metformin therapy.

The most severe side effect is lactic acidosis, which can be fatal; however, the increased risk for lactic acidosis associated with metformin is controversial. A 2006 Cochrane systematic review of more than 200 trials evaluated the incidence of lactic acidosis among patients prescribed metformin vs nonmetformin antidiabetes medications. Of 100,000 people, the incidence of lactic acidosis was 5.1 cases in the metformin group and 5.8 cases in the nonmetformin group. The authors concluded that metformin is not associated with an increased risk for lactic acidosis. However, metformin should be used cautiously in men with a serum creatinine greater than 1.5 mg/dL, or greater than 1.4 mg/dL in women, and avoided in patients receiving intravenous radiographic iodinated contrast media.

Additional Reading: Drugs for type 2 diabetes. *Med Lett Drugs Ther*. 2019;61(1584):169-178.

24. A 40-year-old woman who is otherwise healthy presents to your office complaining of a lump in her neck. On examination, you palpate a 2-cm nodule in the left lobe of her thyroid gland. Appropriate management at this time includes which one of the following?

A) Fine-needle aspiration
B) Radiation ablation
C) Surgical excision
D) Thyroid uptake scan
E) Ultrasonography of the thyroid

The answer is A: Most thyroid nodules found incidentally are benign; however, children and the elderly have a higher incidence of malignancy. Previous studies have found that the prevalence of thyroid carcinoma was about 5% in palpable and nonpalpable nodules. Thyroid ultrasonography should be performed in patients with known or suspected thyroid nodules, but single thyroid nodules should be evaluated with a fine-needle aspiration biopsy.

Ultrasonographically guided fine-needle aspiration biopsy of thyroid nodules should be performed if the diameter of the nodule is 1.0 cm or greater (as in this patient) or if the patient has a history of radiation to the head, neck, or upper chest or a family history of thyroid carcinoma. Suspicious ultrasonographic characteristics, particularly associated calcifications, suggest the presence of psammoma bodies, which are associated with papillary carcinoma, and should also undergo a biopsy procedure.

In the absence of these findings, follow-up for every 6 to 12 months is appropriate because most occult carcinomas are papillary and rarely aggressive. Serum thyroid-stimulating hormone level should be measured during the initial evaluation of a patient with a thyroid nodule. If it is low, radionuclide scintigraphy should be performed. Hyperfunctioning nodules do not require biopsy.

Additional Reading: Thyroid nodules: advances in evaluation and management. *Am Fam Physician*. 2020;102(5)298-304.

25. You have recently diagnosed a 67-year-old White woman with osteoporosis and she is asking about taking raloxifene (Evista). You inform her that this is a selective estrogen receptor modulator. This class of medications has various effects, including which one of the following effects?

A) Estrogenlike effects on the breast
B) Estrogenlike effects on endometrium
C) Reduced risk of invasive breast cancer
D) Reduced risk of thromboembolic events

The answer is C: Raloxifene (Evista) is a selective estrogen receptor modulator with estrogenlike effects on bone and antiestrogen effects on the uterus and breast. It can reduce the risk of invasive breast cancer. The most common adverse effects of raloxifene are hot flushes and leg cramps. This drug is also associated with an increased risk of thromboembolic events.

Raloxifene is approved by the U.S. Food and Drug Administration for both prevention and treatment of postmenopausal osteoporosis. Although it has been shown to reduce the risk of vertebral fractures, it has not been proven to reduce the risk of nonvertebral fractures. Because of its tissue selectivity, raloxifene may have fewer side effects than are typically observed with estrogen therapy. The beneficial estrogenic activities of raloxifene include a lowering of total and low-density lipoprotein cholesterol levels, and it should be considered for women at high risk for invasive breast cancer.

Additional Reading: Osteoporosis and osteopenia. In: Domino F, ed. *The 5-Minute Clinical Consult*. Wolters Kluwer; 2022.

26. You are seeing a 66-year-old patient with diabetes back in follow-up for an infected foot ulcer, which has been very slow to heal. You are concerned that he has developed osteomyelitis in the bone underlying the ulcer. The imaging procedure of choice for detecting osteomyelitis in diabetic foot ulcers is which one of the following?

A) Computed tomographic scan
B) Indium scan
C) Magnetic resonance imaging (MRI)
D) Plain films
E) Technetium bone scan

The answer is C: Diabetic foot infection is defined as soft tissue or bone infection below the malleoli and is the most frequent cause of nontraumatic lower extremity amputation. Diabetic foot infections are diagnosed clinically on the basis of the presence of at least two classic findings of inflammation or purulence. Most infections are polymicrobial. The most common pathogens are aerobic gram-positive cocci, mainly *Staphylococcus* species. Osteomyelitis is a serious complication of diabetic foot infection that increases the likelihood of surgical intervention.

Although plain films of the feet are often ordered initially, MRI is the imaging procedure of choice for osteomyelitis in diabetic foot ulcers. MRI can show abnormal bone marrow signal, soft tissue masses, and cortical destruction characteristic of osteomyelitis. Unlike plain films, MRI can detect these changes early (within days) in infection. MRI also provides the anatomic detail, necessary when surgical debridement is required.

Treatment is based on the extent and severity of the infection and comorbid conditions. Mild infections are treated with oral antibiotics, wound care, and pressure off-loading in the outpatient setting. Surgical debridement and drainage of deep tissue abscesses and infections should be performed in a timely manner.

Additional Reading: Diabetes-related foot infections: diagnosis and treatment. *Am Fam Physician.* 2021;104(4):386-394.

27. You are seeing a 52-year-old patient who has been struggling with her weight for many years. A friend was recently prescribed a medication to help with weight loss. The use of medication to assist with weight loss should be reserved for patients with which one of the following?

A) A body mass index (BMI) greater than 20 kg/m^2
B) A BMI greater than 25 kg/m^2
C) A BMI greater than 30 kg/m^2
D) Weight gain greater than 20% in the past year
E) A calculated fat percentage greater than 35% of ideal body weight

The answer is C: Obesity is epidemic in the United States and other industrialized nations. The BMI is used to define obesity. The BMI is calculated by dividing the square of the body height in meters, by the body mass (weight in kilograms), expressed in units of kg/m^2. Obesity is defined as a BMI of 30 kg/m^2 or greater.

There are three classes of severity:

Class I (BMI of 30.0-34.9 kg/m^2)
Class II (BMI of 35.0-39.9 kg/m^2)
Class III (BMI of 40.0 kg/m^2 or higher)

The age-adjusted prevalence rates of classes I, II, and III obesity in American adults are estimated to be 14.4%, 5.2%, and 2.9%, respectively. These estimates represent a substantial increase in the prevalence of all three obesity classes since the mid-1990s. Although behavior modification strategies are helpful for most obese patients, they do not guarantee long-term weight loss maintenance. Without ongoing management, most or all of the weight patients lose can be regained within 3 to 5 years. This limitation contributes to the active development of pharmacologic approaches to obesity. Current guidelines consider pharmacotherapy to be an adjunct to lifestyle modification programs and are targeted toward at-risk patients (patients with a BMI of 30 or greater or a BMI of 27 or greater combined with medical comorbidities such as hypertension or insulin resistance).

Additional Reading: Several drugs are effective for weight loss in obese or overweight adults; it is unclear whether they improve health outcomes. *Am Fam Physician.* 2022;106(1):99A-99B.

28. You are seeing a 63-year-old White man in follow-up after falling and breaking his left wrist—the x-rays showed osteopenia and you obtained a dual-energy x-ray absorptiometry (DEXA) scan that was consistent with osteoporosis. Which one of the following conditions is related to the development of osteoporosis in men?

A) Hypogonadism
B) Inguinal hernia
C) Prolactinoma
D) Prostate cancer
E) Renal stones

The answer is A: Men, like women, are at risk of developing osteoporosis that may lead to increased risk of fractures. Hypogonadism is an independent risk factor for osteoporosis. DEXA should be performed in men who are at increased risk of osteoporosis and who are candidates for drug therapy. Initial laboratory test results in men with osteoporosis should include a complete blood count, liver function testing, thyroid-stimulating hormone level, serum testosterone, creatinine, calcium, and 25-OH vitamin D levels. Twenty-four hour urine calcium and creatinine levels to identify hypercalciuria are indicated in men with osteoporosis that occurs before the age of 60 years or if initial diagnostic methods fail to determine a cause of low bone mass.

Bisphosphonates decrease the risk of vertebral fracture in men with osteoporosis. Teriparatide (Forteo) decreases the risk of vertebral fractures and can be used for treatment of severe osteoporosis. Men should have an adequate intake of calcium (1200 mg daily) along with vitamin D (800 IU daily) to prevent osteoporosis.

Additional Reading: Osteoporosis in men. *Am Fam Physician.* 2010;82(5):503-508.

29. A 33-year-old obese patient is asking for medication to help her lose weight. A friend has been purchasing orlistat (Alli) over the counter and is wondering if it would be a good option for her. You inform her that orlistat has several effects, except which one of the following?

A) It decreases the absorption of fat from the gastrointestinal (GI) tract.
B) It needs to be used as an adjunct to diet.
C) It is modestly effective in increasing weight loss.
D) It can cause flatulence with discharge and oily spotting.
E) It is safe for use during pregnancy.

The answer is E: Orlistat inhibits pancreatic and gastric lipase, resulting in less fat being absorbed from the GI tract. It is available over the counter (Alli), but also by prescription (Xenical). Used as an adjunct to diet, it is modestly effective in weight loss. As the mechanism of action results in fatty stools, patients suffer from flatulence with discharge, oily spotting, and fecal urgency, although those effects can be modulated by eating a low-fat diet. Fat-soluble vitamin supplementation is also recommended. Orlistat is contraindicated for use during pregnancy.

Various other medications are now U.S. Food and Drug Administration–approved for weight loss; these include the following:

- Phentermine/topiramate (Qsymia): Phentermine (a sympathomimetic amine) is used in combination with topiramate (an anticonvulsant drug) and is the most effective weight loss drug currently available to date. Additionally, a continuation study found that the combination was effective in maintaining weight loss over 2 years.
- Lorcaserin (Belviq) is a selective serotonin 2C agonist that suppresses appetite. It is modestly effective for weight loss and many regain about 25% of their initial weight loss in the second year. Patients who do not lose ≥5% of their baseline weight by 12 weeks should stop taking the medication.
- Bupropion/naltrexone (Contrave) is a combination of bupropion (an antidepressant and smoking cessation drug) with naltrexone (an opioid receptor antagonist). Bupropion is an appetite suppressant, whereas naltrexone potentiates that effect. A titration protocol is used; if weight loss of ≥5% is not achieved after 12 weeks on the maintenance dosage, the drug should gradually be discontinued.
- Liraglutide (Victoza) an injectable glucagonlike peptide-1 agonist used for the treatment of type 2 diabetes mellitus has also been approved for weight loss as Saxenda for use in nondiabetic individuals.

Because of the inherent difficulties in treating obesity, physicians should attempt to develop continuous care programs emphasizing lifestyle modifications such as enduring changes in dietary and activity habits. Patients using behavior modification strategies to make these changes are more likely to succeed in long-term weight maintenance. Weight loss related to drug treatment is modest (5%-10%) and occurs in the first 6 months. Medication appears to be more effective at maintaining weight loss.

Additional Reading: Diet, drugs, and surgery for weight loss. *Med Lett Drugs Ther*. 2015;57(1462):21-28.

30. A 45-year-old African American woman presents with complaints of weight gain. She has always been a little overweight but has gained 20 pounds in the past few months, primarily around her waist and stomach. She has felt fatigue, but denies any pain or other symptoms. On examination, she appears to be developing a "moon face," and her blood pressure is 146/94 mm Hg and pulse rate 72 bpm. She has a normal cardiac examination and no peripheral edema. You suspect Cushing disease and would expect to find all of the following symptoms, except which one?

A) Depression/emotional lability
B) Excessive thirst
C) Glucose intolerance
D) Menstrual irregularity
E) Truncal striae

The answer is C: Cushing syndrome describes a condition resulting from long-term exposure to excessive glucocorticoids. The exogenous intake of steroids is the primary cause of secondary Cushing syndrome. When Cushing syndrome is due to excessive secretion of adrenocorticotropic hormone (ACTH) by a pituitary tumor (usually an adenoma), it is known as Cushing disease. Cushing disease is responsible for most of the cases of endogenous Cushing syndrome, with the remainder due to ectopic ACTH-secreting tumors and primary adrenal neoplasms. Cushing disease occurs most frequently in women of reproductive age, but it can affect men and women of any age. In addition to the above common signs, physical findings include the following:

- Obesity (usually central)
- Facial plethora
- Moon face (facial adiposity)
- Thin skin
- Hypertension
- Hirsutism
- Proximal muscle weakness
- Purple striae on the skin
- Acne
- Easy bruisability

Additional Reading: Cushing disease and cushing syndrome. In: Domino F, ed. *The 5-Minute Clinical Consult*. Wolters Kluwer; 2022.

31. A 57-year-old man who is being treated for hypertension with hydrochlorothiazide and amlodipine (Norvasc) comes in for routine follow-up. His routine basic metabolic panel is normal except for a mildly elevated calcium level. On further questioning, he notes that he has had problems with kidney stones in the past. After stopping his hydrochlorothiazide, which one of the following evaluations would be most appropriate?

A) Obtaining a 24-hour urine for calcium and creatinine
B) Ordering a 25-OH vitamin D, magnesium, and phosphorous
C) Ordering a parathyroid hormone (PTH) level
D) Ordering a sestamibi scan
E) Repeating a basic metabolic panel with ionized calcium

The answer is E: Isolated elevated calcium levels should be confirmed before pursuing further testing. After calcium elevation is confirmed, immediate treatment should be undertaken if hypercalcemia is severe. Otherwise, a history and physical examination would be appropriate, as well as 25-hydroxyvitamin D, magnesium, creatinine, and PTH levels. In patients with a normal or elevated PTH level, 24-hour urine calcium and creatinine levels can help to differentiate between primary hyperparathyroidism and familial hypocalciuric hypercalcemia. If the PTH level is low, 25-hydroxyvitamin D, 1,25-dihydroxyvitamin D, and PTH-related peptide levels should be checked to evaluate possible causes of hypercalcemia independent of the parathyroid. Sestamibi scan is indicated only after confirmation of hyperparathyroidism and typically in anticipation of surgical treatment.

Additional Reading: Parathyroid disorders. *Am Fam Physician*. 2013;88(4):249-257.

32. You are caring for a 20-year-old transgender woman in your primary care practice. She been taking estradiol 6 mg by mouth daily for gender-affirming hormone treatment but would like to start spironolactone today for better breast development. She has a past medical history of well-controlled asthma and has no surgical history. She is currently in college and denies any smoking/vaping, alcohol use or illicit drug use. Her last creatinine level was 0.7. Side effects of this new medication include all of the following except:

A) Hypotension
B) Hypokalemia
C) Gastrointestinal upset
D) Increased Urinary output

The answer is B: Antiandrogens reduce endogenous testosterone levels, allowing the full effect of estrogen therapy. The antiandrogen of choice in the United States is usually spironolactone (Aldactone), a potassium-sparing diuretic that directly inhibits testosterone secretion and inhibits androgen binding to the androgen receptor. Side effects of spironolactone include gastrointestinal upset, hyperkalemia, increased urinary output, and hypotension. It is contraindicated in patients with renal insufficiency or with serum potassium levels greater than 5.5 mEq/L. Spironolactone should not be given with digoxin, angiotensin-converting enzyme inhibitors, other potassium-sparing diuretics, and angiotensin receptor blockers.

Additional Reading: *Guidelines for the Primary and Gender-Affirming Care of Transgender and Gender Nonbinary People.* https://transcare.ucsf.edu/sites/transcare.ucsf.edu/files/Transgender-PGACG-6-17-16.pdf

33. Which of the following physiological changes due to testosterone therapy is reversible in gender-affirming hormone therapy for female-to-male (FTM) trans patients?

A) Clitoromegaly
B) Increased libido
C) Deepened voice
D) Male pattern hair loss

The answer is B: Within 1 year of testosterone therapy, the voice usually deepens, clitoromegaly occurs, and male pattern hair loss may be apparent. These changes in voice range, hair follicles, and clitoral size are permanent. Other effects, such as increased muscle mass, acne, increased libido and energy level, and amenorrhea, are reversible if testosterone is discontinued. FTM individuals report a better quality of life after receiving male hormones regardless of the duration of treatment.

Additional Reading: *Guidelines for the Primary and Gender-Affirming Care of Transgender and Gender Nonbinary People.* https://transcare.ucsf.edu/sites/transcare.ucsf.edu/files/Transgender-PGACG-6-17-16.pdf

Section VI. Integumentary System

This section covers topic related to the integumentary system, an organ system consisting of the skin, hair, nails, and associated exocrine glands, which protects the body from various environmental insults such as dehydration or abrasion. Interestingly the skin is the largest organ in the body, even though it is less than a centimeter thick. The following questions relate to this important system, which accounts for frequent family medicine encounters and for about 5% of the American Board of Family Medicine certifying examination. Additional topics are covered in Chapter 2, Care of Children and Adolescents. As you study for the examination, ensure that you have a good overview of the following topics:

1. Skin cancers
   - Understand the risk factors and the prevention of skin cancers (basal cell, squamous cell, melanoma).
   - Know the basic characteristics of basal cell carcinomas (eg, the most common form of skin cancer occurring in head, face, nose, ears, neck, trunk, and extremities).
   - Know the basic characteristics of squamous cell carcinomas (eg, actinic keratosis precursor, second-most common, not just sun-exposed areas).
   - Know the basic treatment for nonmelanotic skin cancers (eg, cryotherapy and surgical excision).
   - Know the basic characteristics of melanoma (eg, ABCD evaluation and malignant nature).
   - Understand the approach to dysplastic nevi.
   - Know the basic treatment for melanoma (eg, full thickness excisional biopsy with at least a 1-2 cm margin of normal tissue).
   - Appreciate the appropriate follow-up for a patient with a treated melanoma.
2. Common dermatologic conditions (eczema/psoriasis/rosacea/warts)
   - Know the basic characteristics of eczema and the atopic triad and the recommended nonpharmacologic and pharmacologic treatments for eczema.
   - Know the basic characteristics of psoriasis and the recommended nonpharmacologic and pharmacologic treatments for psoriasis.
   - Know the basic characteristics of rosacea and the recommended nonpharmacologic and pharmacologic treatments for rosacea (eg, avoiding triggers such as sun, spicy food, hot beverages, and alcohol; topical metronidazole; and oral antibiotics).
   - Know the basics about genital warts and treatment options.
3. Acne
   - Know the basic characteristics of acne. (For example, acne is a chronic inflammatory disease of the sebaceous follicle; primary lesion is comedone, noninflammatory lesions are open (blackhead) and closed comedones (whitehead); inflammatory lesions are papules, pustules, nodules, and cysts.)
   - Understand the basic pathophysiology of acne and the influence of endogenous and exogenous hormones (eg, effects of puberty and oral contraceptives).
   - Appreciate recommended nonpharmacologic treatments for acne.
   - Know the recommended first-line medications for acne. (For example, the fact medications begin with topical then oral antibiotics; what to use first for comedone acne—topical retinoids vs oral antibiotics.)
   - Understand the indications and risk factors for oral retinoids. (For example, isotretinoin [Accutane] is a teratogen and contraindicated for anyone at risk for pregnancy; side effects include erythema, irritation, and photosensitivity.)
4. Alopecia/hirsutism
   - Know the basic categories of alopecia and appropriate workup.
   - Understand the recommended treatments for alopecia.
   - Know the basic characteristics of hirsutism and workup.
   - Appreciate the recommended treatments for hirsutism.

Each of the following questions or incomplete statements is followed by suggested answers or completions. Select the ONE BEST ANSWER in each case.

1. A 27-year-old woman was concerned over warts on her vagina and is asking about treatment options. Which one of the following is true regarding the treatment of genital warts?

A) An alternative method is required if a single treatment fails to eradicate the wart.
B) Genital warts rarely spontaneously resolve.
C) Human papillomavirus (HPV) DNA does not remain in tissue after treatment.
D) The choice of treatment is based on cost, convenience, and adverse effects.

The answer is D: Genital warts can resolve spontaneously, remain the same, or increase in size. Although the primary treatment goal is to remove symptomatic warts, there is evidence that treatment may also reduce the persistence of HPV DNA in genital tissue and therefore may reduce the incidence of cervical cancer.

Treatment methods can be chemical or ablative. The choice of therapy is based on the number, size, site, and morphology of lesions, as well as patient preference, treatment cost, convenience, adverse effects, and physician experience. Assuming that the diagnosis is certain, switching to a different treatment modality is indicated if there has been no response after three treatment cycles with the initial treatment choice. Routine follow-up for 2 to 3 months is advised to monitor response to therapy and evaluate for recurrence.

Additional Reading: Management of external genital warts. *Am Fam Physician.* 2014;90(5):312-318.

2. You are performing a preemployment physical examination on a young lifeguard, and she is asking about how best to avoid sunburns. Which one of the following is true regarding sun exposure?

A) Patients allergic to thiazide diuretics may react adversely to *para*-aminobenzoic acid (PABA).
B) Repeated use of sunscreens can increase the risk of sun cancer.
C) Sunscreens with a sun protection factor of 10 provide adequate protection.
D) Steroids should be avoided in patients with sunburns because of their immunosuppressant properties.
E) The most dangerous solar rays are the ultraviolet A (UVA) type.

The answer is A: Sunburn (usually a first-degree burn) appears within the first few hours of exposure after a period of diminished sun exposure, such as being outdoors in the early summer. In most cases, sunburn is prevented with sun avoidance and the routine use of sunscreens. Sunburn can be treated with cold-water compresses and emollients, but steroids can be used for severe burns.

Ultraviolet light is divided into two types of rays: UVA (320-400 nm) and ultraviolet B (UVB; 280-320 nm). Although both types are associated with the development of skin cancer, the shorter UVB rays are more dangerous than UVA.

Sunscreens of at least sun protection factor of 15 and preferably sun protection factor of 30 should be used when persons are exposed to the sun. PABA, which is used in many sunscreens, is effective for preventing sunburns; however, those with allergies to thiazides, benzocaine, or sulfonamides may react adversely to PABA.

Additional Reading: Sunscreens revisited. *Med Lett Drugs Ther.* 2011;53(1359):17-18.

The U.S. Preventive Forces Task Force recommends (grade B recommendation) counseling for children, adolescents, and young adults aged 10 to 24 years who have fair skin about minimizing their exposure to ultraviolet radiation to reduce risk for skin cancer.

3. A young man is complaining of cold symptoms and wheezing. You listen to his lungs and observe several abnormal moles on his back. You suspect that he has dysplastic nevi syndrome. Which one of the following factors is associated with this syndrome?

A) The syndrome is characterized by scattered (<20) benign moles appearing on the torso, arms, and legs.
B) The syndrome is not genetically transmitted.
C) The syndrome is associated with an increased risk for the development of melanoma.
D) The number of dysplastic nevi does not increase after the first year of life.

The answer is C: Patients with dysplastic nevi syndrome are affected with numerous (>50) irregular, large moles. These moles are abnormal in appearance and show variegation of color. The moles more commonly occur on covered areas such as the breast, buttocks, and scalp. Unlike common moles, dysplastic nevi continue to appear as the patient ages.

The syndrome is a condition that is inherited as an autosomal dominant disease. Usually more than two family members are affected; however, sporadic cases do occur. Patients should be counseled to avoid sun exposure and are at increased risk for the development of melanoma; thus any suspicious lesion or change in nevi should be biopsied. Episodic digital photography of lesions can help determine if there are any changes seen over time.

Additional Reading: Atypical moles: diagnosis and management. *Am Fam Physician.* 2015;91(11):762-767.

4. An 11-year-old is brought into the office by his mother as he has an itchy rash over his arms and legs that started the night before. He thinks it is poison ivy as he was playing in the woods the past couple of days. She has been giving him diphenhydramine (Benadryl), which has helped a little, but he is scratching more. On examination, he appears healthy and the rash is confined to his arms and legs; you agree that this is *Rhus* dermatitis, which is associated with which one of the following?

A) A vesicular eruption in a dermatomal distribution
B) Fever and lymphadenopathy
C) An intensely pruritic, vesicular rash
D) Community outbreaks
E) Honey-colored weeping, crusty lesions

The answer is C: *Rhus* dermatitis is a contact dermatitis caused by cutaneous exposure to urushiol from species of *Toxicodendron* (*Rhus*), such as poison ivy, oak, or sumac. The vesicular rash can be intensely pruritic. When there is exposure to the plant within 24 to 48 hours, the extremities are often affected as they have come in contact with the urushiol. The condition is a result of a delayed hypersensitivity reaction that may take several days to appear.

Thorough washing with soap and water, preferably within 10 minutes of exposure, may prevent dermatitis. All contaminated clothes should be removed as soon as possible and cleaned. Frequent baths using colloidal oatmeal also relieve symptoms. Treatment of mild to moderate rash includes application of cold compresses or diluted aluminum acetate solution such as Burow solution or calamine lotion. The use of topical antihistamines and anesthetics should be avoided because of the possibility of increased sensitization.

Early application of topical steroid creams is useful to limit erythema and pruritus. However, occlusive dressings should be avoided on moist lesions. Refractory dermatitis can be treated with oral corticosteroids such as prednisone, with an initial dosage of 1 mg/kg per day, slowly tapering the dosage over 2 to 3 weeks. Shorter courses of steroids may be followed by rebound exacerbations after therapy is discontinued. Oral antihistamines may help reduce pruritus and provide sedation, when needed.

Herpes zoster may have a similar appearance but is in a dermatomal distribution and tends to be painful, not pruritic. *Staphylococcus* infection (impetigo) will have crusting and weeping and maybe itchy, and is usually painful, rather than itchy. Atopic dermatitis can be pruritic, but the skin is usually normal initially, and patients present with scaly excoriations from scratching.

Additional Reading: Diagnosis and management of contact dermatitis. *Am Fam Physician.* 2010;82(3):249-255.

5. Café au lait spots are associated with which one of the following disorders?

A) Addison disease
B) Dysplastic nevus syndrome
C) Neurofibromatosis
D) Peutz-Jeghers syndrome

The answer is C: The following are skin abnormalities noted in patients affected with the following disease processes:

Condition	Skin Findings
Neurofibromatosis (von Recklinghausen disease)	Café au lait spots
Peutz-Jeghers syndrome	Hyperpigmentation around the oral cavity and hamartomas of the intestine
Dysplastic nevus syndrome	Multiple pigmented nevi
Hypoadrenocorticism (Addison disease)	Hyperpigmentation of the gingiva, areola of the nipples, labia, and linea alba of the abdomen

Additional Reading: Neurofibromatosis type 1. In: Domino F, ed. *The 5-Minute Clinical Consult.* Lippincott Williams and Wilkins; 2022.

6. A 47-year-old waitress comes in with a concern about a dark mole on her leg. After you examine her skin, you reassure her that the mole is benign and that there are no worrisome characteristics seen. All of the following are considered worrisome characteristics for a melanoma, except which one?

A) Asymmetric border
B) Bleeding
C) Color change
D) Diameter less than 5 mm
E) Variegation of color

The answer is D: Skin lesions that represent concern for a melanoma usually possess certain characteristics, including:

A = Asymmetric and irregular borders
B = Bleeding or ulceration; persistent itching or tenderness
C = Color change or variegation of color
D = Diameter >6 mm

If any of these criteria are met, the lesion should be biopsied and sent for pathologic examination. Many often add an "E" for elevation as a fifth characteristic because nodular melanoma can increase up over time. Large, raised, and pigmented congenital lesions should also be biopsied. Patients who have a history of dysplastic nevi syndrome are at increased risk for the development of melanoma, particularly if a family member has been affected.

Additional Reading: Screening for skin cancer. *Am Fam Physician.* 2010;81(12):1435-1436.

7. Several drugs are known to cause a lupus like syndrome; in assessing a patient for lupus, which one of the following is a distinguishing feature between drug-induced and idiopathic systemic lupus erythematosus (SLE)?

A) In drug-induced lupus, there is an absence of antibodies to double-stranded DNA.
B) In drug-induced lupus, there are increased levels of complement.
C) In idiopathic SLE, a butterfly facial rash is seen.
D) Renal and central nervous system (CNS) involvement are common with drug-induced SLE.
E) There are no differences seen between the two conditions.

The answer is A: Two drugs known to cause a lupus like syndrome are procainamide and hydralazine. Most patients with drug-induced lupus do not have antibodies to double-stranded DNA, and they rarely have depressed levels of complement, which can distinguish drug-induced lupus from idiopathic SLE. Other laboratory abnormalities seen with drug-induced lupus include anemia, thrombocytopenia, and leukopenia. Additional findings often include a positive rheumatoid factor, false-positive Venereal Disease Research Laboratory result, and positive direct Coombs test.

In most cases, the symptoms resolve once the medication is discontinued; however, steroid administration may be needed in severe cases. Most symptoms are completely resolved in 6 months, but ANA test results may remain positive for years. Most affected patients complain of arthralgias, myalgias, fever, and pleuritic chest pain. Renal involvement and CNS involvement are rare with drug-induced lupus. Other medications associated with drug-induced lupus include chlorpromazine, methyldopa, and isoniazid.

Additional Reading: Systemic lupus erythematosus: primary care approach to diagnosis and management. *Am Fam Physician.* 2016;94(4):284-294.

8. A 42-year-old woman presents with a painful rash on her ear for the past several days and comes in now complaining of ringing in her ears. She has been healthy and takes no medications. You suspect Ramsay Hunt syndrome, which is associated with which one of the following characteristics?

A) Autoimmune destruction of auditory nuclei in the thalamus
B) Herpes zoster infection affecting the geniculate ganglion of the facial nerve
C) Spinothalamic disruption with loss of motor function in the upper face
D) Spontaneous progressive demyelination of motor neurons

The answer is B: Ramsay Hunt syndrome is a disorder caused by the herpes zoster virus that affects the geniculate ganglion of the facial nerve. The clinical manifestation includes unilateral peripheral facial palsy, with or without tinnitus, vertigo, or deafness. The syndrome can be distinguished from Bell palsy by the development of vesicular herpetic lesions that affect the pharynx, external auditory canal, and, occasionally, the eighth cranial nerve. Patients report painful lesions and lose their sense of taste associated with the anterior two-thirds of the tongue.

Additional Reading: Facial palsy in a 38-year-old man. *Am Fam Physician.* 2013;88(11):771-772.

9. A 31-year-old White man presents with recurrent cold sores on his lower lip. They seem to reoccur every spring when he spends more time outside and he is asking for you to prescribe treatment. You diagnose his condition as a herpes simplex virus (HSV) infection. Which one of the following statements about his condition is true?

A) Multinucleated giant cells are seen with Tzanck smears.
B) Recurrent outbreaks are usually more severe than an initial outbreak.
C) HSV type I is most commonly associated with genital infections.
D) Topical acyclovir is used for prophylaxis.
E) The rash usually consists of pustules, papules, and macules.

The answer is E: Herpes simplex virus infections are divided into type 1, which usually affects the oral mucosa, and type 2, which usually affects the genitals. The virus invades the nervous tissue and remains dormant in the skin or nerve ganglia.

Symptoms include recurrent, clear vesicles that usually occur in clusters and are extremely painful; fever; arthralgias; and adenopathy. Initial attacks are usually more severe and longer in duration than repeated attacks. Before the appearance of the vesicles, the patient may report paresthesias or tingling at the site of the outbreak. Transmission occurs by direct contact and is usually sexually transmitted, particularly for type 2. Repeated attacks are usually precipitated by excessive sunlight exposure, menstruation, stress, and febrile illnesses.

Laboratory tests include positive Tzanck smears (with the presence of multinucleated giant cells), cultures (gold standard for diagnosis), and rapid immunofluorescent antibody tests. The treatment of choice involves the use of topical and oral antiviral medication (acyclovir, valacyclovir, and famciclovir). Oral administration is more effective and should be begun at the initial onset of clinical symptoms. For severe cases, intravenous acyclovir may be used. In some cases, daily prophylactic oral therapy may be necessary.

Additional Reading: Nongenital herpes simplex virus. *Am Fam Physician*. 2010;82(9):1075-1082.

10. A 51-year-old male patient presents to your office with a violaceous skin lesion. He is human immunodeficiency virus (HIV)-positive and has been feeling relatively well over the past year, until he developed this rash. On examination you detect generalized lymphadenopathy, and microscopic examination of a skin punch biopsy shows spindle cells mixed with vascular tissue. The most likely diagnosis for this finding is which one of the following conditions?

A) Cherry hemangioma
B) Cryptococcal granuloma
C) Kaposi sarcoma
D) Malignant melanoma
E) Tina corpora

The answer is C: Kaposi sarcoma is a malignant skin lesion that was once rare but is now seen more commonly in acquired immunodeficiency syndrome (AIDS) patients, primarily among men who have sex with men, and remains the most frequent tumor associated with HIV infection. The lesion is characterized histologically by spindle cells mixed with vascular tissue. Before the detection of AIDS, the disease was predominantly found in Eastern Europe, Italy, and equatorial Africa and affected mostly Italian or Jewish men.

Symptoms include pink, violaceous, or red papules or plaques that affect any body surface and become widely disseminated with time and give rise to generalized lymphadenopathy. Serious cases can progress to visceral involvement.

Treatment is individualized on the basis of the extent and location of lesions, symptoms, comorbid factors, and patient preference. Up to 60% of cases will resolve within up to 1 to 2 years of effective antiretroviral therapy. Direct treatments include excision, cryotherapy, laser ablation, intralesional chemotherapy, external beam radiation, α-interferon, liposomal doxorubicin, or paclitaxel.

Additional Reading: Kaposi sarcoma. In: Domino F, ed. *The 5-Minute Clinical Consult*. Wolters Kluwer; 2022.

The U.S. Preventive Forces Task Force recommends (grade A recommendation) that clinicians screen for HIV infection in adolescents and adults aged 15 to 65 years. Younger adolescents and older adults who are at increased risk should also be screened.

11. A 16-year-old high school student presents with his mother as he seems to have developed an allergy to cold water. She reports that they recently installed a swimming pool and he gets itchy hives when swimming in the cold water. You diagnose him with cold-induced urticaria. Treatment options for this condition include all of the following, except which one?

A) Cimetidine
B) Cyproheptadine
C) Diphenhydramine
D) Hydroxyzine
E) Verapamil

The answer is E: This student is suffering from cold-induced urticaria. Urticaria is defined as an erythematous, pruritic rash that is often raised and occurs as discrete wheals and hives. The condition affects approximately 20% of the population. The rash involves the superficial layers of the skin. The center of the wheal is usually pale, and the rash blanches with pressure. Involvement of the deeper layers is referred to as angioedema.

The causes include allergen exposure; heat, cold, or sunlight exposure; and trauma. In many cases, a cause is never detected. The response is thought to be mediated by an immunoglobulin E antibody. Those affected by cold may have cryoglobulins or cryofibrinogen, which become activated. In extreme cases, bronchoconstriction and anaphylaxis can occur. Unfortunately, an underlying cause is identified in only approximately 20% of cases.

Treatment involves avoiding factors that trigger the response. Other treatment involves the use of antihistamine (H1) medications and histamine blockers (H2) such as cimetidine. Doxepin may also be beneficial. The drug of choice for cold-induced urticaria is cyproheptadine. Other causes of urticaria include medication use, malignancy, endocrinopathies, autoimmune diseases, insect bites, and infestations; psychogenic causes should also be investigated in complicated or persistent cases. Severe cases may require systemic steroids or the use of danazol.

Verapamil is useful for treating Raynaud phenomenon, which is also cold-induced.

Additional Reading: Urticaria. In: Domino F, ed. *The 5-Minute Clinical Consult*. Wolters Kluwer; 2022.

12. A 21-year-old surfer presents with complaints of an intensely itchy rash that has formed on the sole of his foot and is slowly spreading. On examination you observe a serpiginous-type of lesion with bullae forming at the affected site. Which one of the following is the most likely diagnosis?

A) Ascariasis
B) Bathing suit dermatitis
C) Cutaneous larva migrans
D) Leishmaniasis
E) Tinea pedis

The answer is C: Cutaneous larva migrans, also known as the "creeping eruption," is a common, self-limited, parasitic infection seen in patients who live in warm climates or have recently traveled to tropical regions, particularly if they have been to beaches and shady areas. The most common infective agent is a dog and cat hookworm, *Ancylostoma caninum* and *Ancylostoma braziliense*, respectively. Familial outbreaks of cutaneous larva migrans have been noted where the infection began with the household pet. When the animal defecates, the hookworms are shed and the larvae are picked up by humans through breaks in the skin, hair follicles, and even through intact skin.

The areas most often affected include the feet, hands, buttocks, thighs, and chest. The eruption begins as a pruritic lesion at the site of entry and progresses within a few hours into an inflamed papular or papulovesicular eruption. Serpiginous tracks left by the larvae's migration may also be seen. The eruption may spread up to 1 to 2 cm/d. Severe pruritus, vesicular and bullous lesions, local swelling, erosions, and folliculitis may be seen.

Biopsy is generally not useful, and blood tests rarely show eosinophilia or elevated immunoglobulin E levels. Destructive therapies, such as cryotherapy, are often ineffective. Isolated cutaneous cases are treated with topical thiabendazole, especially when applied ahead of the advancing lesions. Because of the risk of systemic infection and the ease of oral treatment, some recommend routine systemic treatment with oral thiabendazole, albendazole, or ivermectin. Although thiabendazole has significant side effects that include nausea, vomiting, diarrhea, and dizziness, albendazole and ivermectin are reliable and have fewer adverse effects. Ivermectin may be given as a single dose with no known toxic side effects.

Most people infected with ascariasis are asymptomatic; those with more severe infections can have various symptoms, depending on which part of the body is affected. After an individual ingests microscopic ascariasis eggs, they hatch in the small intestine and the larvae migrate through the bloodstream or lymphatic system into the lungs. Patients can have various gastrointestinal or pulmonary symptoms.

Additional Reading: Acute pruritic rash on the foot. *Am Fam Physician.* 2010;81(2):203-204.

13. You are examining a rash on the skin of a previously healthy 21-year-old White man. He had a mild cold a week ago, but otherwise has felt well. On examination his vital signs are normal and he appears healthy. The rash is characterized by numerous small, slightly scaly, oval-shaped lesions. The presentation is most consistent with which one of the following conditions?

A) Guttate psoriasis
B) Plaque psoriasis
C) Pityriasis alba
D) Pityriasis rosea
E) Scarlet fever

The answer is A: The condition of guttate psoriasis is characterized by numerous small, oval (teardrop-shaped) lesions that develop after an acute upper respiratory tract infection. These lesions are often not as scaly or as erythematous as the classic lesions of plaque-type psoriasis, which are usually located on extensor surfaces. Usually, guttate psoriasis must be differentiated from pityriasis rosea, another condition characterized by the sudden outbreak of red scaly lesions, which also often follows a mild upper respiratory tract infection.

Compared with pityriasis rosea, psoriatic lesions are thicker and scalier, and the lesions are not usually distributed along skin creases. In pityriasis rosea, oval patches generally spread across the torso, following the rib lines in a classic "Christmas-tree" distribution. Typically, it begins with a single "herald patch" lesion, followed in a week or so by a generalized body rash lasting up to 12 weeks.

Pityriasis alba is a chronic skin disorder that affects preadolescent children. This rash is characterized by hypopigmented patches of skin typically on the face, although the neck, upper chest, and arms are sometimes involved. Sometimes the rash is covered by very fine scales; the cause is unknown.

Scarlet fever can occur as a result of a group A streptococcal infection, typically in children between 5 and 15 years of age. The signs include a sore throat, fever, and a characteristic red rash that feels like sandpaper.

Additional Reading: Psoriasis. *Am Fam Physician.* 2013;87(9): 626-633.

14. A sexually active 23-year-old woman presents with several external genital warts on her vagina. In treating this patient, which one of the following is necessary to adequately address these lesions?

A) Apply acetowhite stain to the labia to identify the affected lesions
B) Biopsy a visible lesion
C) Obtain viral typing of the lesions
D) Remove visible warts

The answer is D: Genital warts caused by human papilloma virus infection are frequently seen in primary care. Evidence-based treatment recommendations are limited. Biopsy, viral typing, acetowhite staining, and other diagnostic measures are not routinely required. The goal of treatment is removal of visible warts; some evidence exists that treatment reduces infectivity, but there is no evidence that treatment reduces the incidence of cervical and genital cancer.

The choice of therapy is based on the number, size, site, and appearance of lesions, as well as patient preferences, cost, convenience, adverse effects, and clinician preference. Patient-applied therapies include imiquimod cream (Zyclara, Aldara), podofilox (*Condylox*), and sinecatechins ointment (Veregen). Trichloroacetic acid, cryotherapy, and surgical excision are used in the office.

Additional Reading: Management of external genital warts. *Am Fam Physician.* 2014;90(5):312-318.

15. A 32-year-old man presents to your office. Approximately 5 days ago, he was cleaning out an old trunk in his attic. That day, he noticed a red lesion with a clear center on his arm. Since then the center of the lesion has broken open with a craterlike scabbed appearance. The most likely diagnosis for this presentation is which one of the following?

A) Black widow spider bite
B) Brown recluse spider bite
C) Lyme disease
D) Psittacosis
E) Scorpion sting

The answer is B: The brown recluse spider (violin spider) may be identified by a dark, violin-shaped design on its back. These spiders are usually found in dark areas, woodpiles, attics, and other undisturbed locations. The bite is initially mild (burning at site) and goes unnoticed, although some localized pain develops within 30 to 60 minutes. Within 1 to 4 hours, an erythematous, pruritic area with an ischemic pale center develops, giving the appearance of a bull's-eye target lesion. The central zone may progress to form a pustule that eventually fills with blood and ruptures; within 3 to 4 days, a craterlike lesion with necrosis develops. Large tissue defects may occur and include muscle. Healing usually requires extended periods; if large areas are involved, skin grafting may be necessary in some cases.

Symptoms include headache, nausea and vomiting, low-grade fever, chills and sweats, generalized pruritus, malaise, arthralgias, severe pain (late in the course), and rash. Rare fatalities (none in the United States) have been reported with complications such as massive intravascular hemolysis with hemoglobinuria, renal failure, and disseminated intravascular coagulopathy.

Treatment with dapsone has been recommended. Because dapsone can cause agranulocytosis and hemolytic anemia, which may be exaggerated in patients with glucose-6-phosphate dehydrogenase (G6PD) deficiency, a G6PD test and complete blood count should be done before starting therapy. Systemic corticosteroids have shown no consistent or reliable benefit. Surgical debridement should be delayed until the area of necrosis is fully demarcated. Incision and suction is not recommended. Most bites require only local treatment. Ice therapy to the site may help reduce pain.

The black widow spider produces a protein venom that affects the nervous system. Reactions vary from minimal discomfort to severe reactions. The first symptom is acute pain at the site of the bite, followed by localized or generalized severe muscle cramps, abdominal pain, weakness, and tremor. In severe cases, nausea, vomiting, faintness, dizziness, chest pain, and respiratory difficulties may follow. The black widow spider is shiny black with a red hourglass-shaped mark on its abdomen.

Lyme disease is caused by a tick bite; the causative agent is the spirochete, *Borrelia burgdorferi*; and the classic skin finding is erythema migrans.

Psittacosis (parrot fever, ornithosis) is a zoonotic infectious disease caused by the *Chlamydophila psittaci* bacterium and contracted from infected parrots. Often asymptomatic, it can cause pneumonia.

Scorpions belong to the same class as spiders, mites, and ticks; scorpions have a stinger at the end of their tail, which transmits a toxin at the last tail segment. Most scorpion stings in the United States cause only minor pain and warmth at the sting site, although elsewhere the venom can cause severe allergic, neurotic, or necrotic reactions, and rarely, death. Contact with scorpions is generally accidental and they are nocturnal, so that stings occur most often at night.

Additional Reading: Arthropod bites and stings. *Am Fam Physician*. 2022;106(2):137-147.

16. A 62-year-old alcoholic man, currently being treated for gastritis, presents to the office complaining that his breasts seem to be swollen and have become painful over the past couple of months. The most likely explanation for this scenario is which one of the following?

A) Breast cancer
B) Milk alkali syndrome
C) Omeprazole use
D) Prolactinoma
E) Trauma

The answer is C: Gynecomastia is a condition characterized by enlargement of the breasts in men. It occurs when there is hypertrophy of breast tissue beneath the areola. In young adolescents, it is a natural response to the body's hormones. During this time, the breast may be tender. Patients and their parents should be reassured this is a natural response and will eventually resolve (usually within 3 years).

Gynecomastia in older men can result from medication use (eg, omeprazole and cimetidine, isoniazid, digitalis, phenothiazine, and testosterone), substance abuse (eg, alcohol and illegal drugs, including marijuana and heroin), endocrine disorders (eg, hypogonadism and hyperthyroidism), Klinefelter syndrome, liver disease, and neoplasm.

The workup of gynecomastia should include a chest radiograph; beta unit of β-human chorionic gonadotropin determination; luteinizing hormone, follicle-stimulating hormone, estrogen, and testosterone levels; liver and thyroid function tests. Typically, the estrogen-testosterone ratio is high. If the human chorionic gonadotropin is elevated, then a testicular ultrasonography should be performed to look for testicular tumor. Additionally, if the testes are small, a karyotype should be obtained to look for Klinefelter syndrome. Other testing may be necessary, if indicated.

Treatment involves stopping any offending medications and correcting the underlying abnormality. If the condition does not resolve, suppressive medication or surgery may be indicated.

Additional Reading: Gynecomastia. *Am Fam Physician*. 2012;85(7):716-722.

17. A 50-year-old White man, who is not feeling well, presents to your office. He has been having fever and night sweats, with myalgias over the past couple of months. He comes in because he has developed tender bumps on his lower legs and one bump seems to be breaking down. On examination you note tender nodules varying in size from 1 to 2 cm on his lower legs and ankles, with one that has superficial ulcer and others that appear to be older healing lesions that have a bluish hue to the surrounding skin. His presentation is most likely due to which of the following conditions?

A) Dermatomyositis
B) Giant cell arteritis
C) Polyarteritis nodosa (PAN)
D) Polymyositis
E) Pyoderma gangrenosum

The answer is C: PAN is a condition characterized by inflammation and necrosis of the muscular tissue supplied by small- and medium-size arteries. Dermatologic symptoms are common in PAN, and about 40% of patients present with skin lesions, including rash, purpura, gangrene, nodules, cutaneous infarcts, livedo reticularis, and Raynaud phenomenon. Skin involvement, which can be painful, occurs most frequently on the legs, with tender nodules 0.5 to 2 cm on the foot, ankle, and lower legs. The lesions turn bluish as they heal and can reoccur at the same site. Thirty percent of lesions will have weeping ulcers secondary to ischemia from the vasculitis.

Livedo reticularis is thought to be due to spasms of the blood vessels or a problem of the blood flow near the skin surface. It makes the skin look mottled in a net like pattern with clear borders. The condition most often shows up on the legs. Sometimes livedo reticularis is simply the result of being chilled.

Polyarteritis nodosa symptoms include fever, abdominal pain, peripheral neuropathy, headaches, seizures, weakness, and weight loss. Those with renal involvement may show hypertension, edema, azotemia, and oliguria. Other symptoms include angina, nausea, vomiting, diarrhea, myalgias, and arthralgias.

Laboratory studies show leukocytosis, proteinuria, microscopic hematuria, thrombocytosis, and an elevated erythrocyte sedimentation rate (ESR). Diagnosis is usually made with a biopsy of affected tissue, which shows necrotizing arteritis. The cause is unknown but may be associated with an autoimmune response, medication (eg, sulfonamides, iodide, thiazides, bismuth, and penicillins), or from infections. Involvement of the renal and visceral arteries is characteristic, but pulmonary arteries are usually spared. Affected individuals are usually between 40 and 50 years of age; men are more commonly affected.

Treatment involves avoidance of the offending agent and often long-term, high-dose steroid therapy and cyclophosphamide for severe cases and steroids alone for milder cases. The disease can be fatal if untreated.

Polymyositis is an idiopathic inflammatory myopathy with symmetrical, proximal muscle weakness. Histopathology demonstrates endomysial mononuclear inflammatory infiltrate and muscle fiber necrosis. Dermatomyositis is clinically similar to polymyositis, an idiopathic, inflammatory myopathy associated with characteristic skin findings that include a violet or dusky red rash seen on the face and eyelids and on skin around the nails, knuckles, elbows, knees, chest, and back. The rash can be patchy with bluish-purple discolorations and is often the first sign of dermatomyositis.

Giant cell arteritis, also known as temporal arteritis, is a vasculitis of the large and medium arteries of the head and neck. Giant cell arteritis typically presents with a headache and nonspecific systemic symptoms. The temporal artery is tender to palpations, and a high ESR is detected. The diagnosis is confirmed by patchy inflammation of arterial walls, characterized by the infiltration of mononuclear cells and the presence of giant cells from a temporal artery biopsy.

Pyoderma gangrenosum causes deep leg ulcers, with necrotic tissue, and can lead to chronic wounds. Ulcers initially present as small papules and progress to larger ulcers, causing pain and scarring.

Additional Reading: Systemic vasculitis. *Am Fam Physician.* 2011;83(5):556-565.

PAN is a condition characterized by inflammation and necrosis of the muscular tissue supplied by small- and medium-size arteries. Skin involvement occurs most frequently on the legs, with tender nodules 0.5 to 2 cm on the foot, ankle, and lower legs. The lesions turn bluish as they heal and can reoccur at the same site.

18. A 47-year-old mechanic comes in complaining of a sore on his lower left leg. He has had the lesion for a few weeks, and it is enlarging and getting worse. It started as a painful pimple after he bumped his leg on a car lift and has slowly enlarged, and the surrounding skin is breaking down. You are concerned that he has pyoderma gangrenosum and decide to treat him with which one of the following?

A) Infliximab
B) Oral antibiotics
C) Oral steroids
D) Methotrexate
E) Topical antibiotics

The answer is C: Pyoderma gangrenosum is a rapidly evolving and severely debilitating skin disease that is characterized by a painful hemorrhagic pustule that breaks down to form a chronic ulcer. The ulcer is associated with pus production, and there is usually a dusky red or purple halo around the ulcer. The cause of the lesions is unknown, but they tend to form at the sites of trauma (most commonly the legs), in middle-aged adults. The borders of the lesions are usually irregular, and the lesions are boggy and usually quite painful. Although as many as 50% of cases have no associated underlying abnormality, other diseases associated with pyoderma gangrenosum include Crohn disease, ulcerative colitis, leukemia, paraproteinemia, multiple myeloma, rheumatoid arthritis, hepatitis, and Behçet disease.

The diagnosis of pyoderma gangrenosum is usually made by the history and clinical findings. Laboratory tests show elevated erythrocyte sedimentation rate and leukocytosis. Treatment involves correction of the underlying disease and the use of high-dose oral steroids or intravenous pulse steroid therapy as first-choice therapy or systemic cyclosporine as an alternative with patients with certain medical conditions like renal insufficiency, hypertension, type 2 diabetes mellitus, and obesity.

Additional Reading: Pyoderma gangrenosum: treatment and prognosis. In: *UpToDate*. 2022.

19. A young woman is in for a routine gynecologic examination and is asking about how often she should do a self-breast examination for breast cancer screening. Which one of the following is true regarding breast self-examination (BSE) for breast cancer screening?

A) Teaching BSE reduces breast cancer mortality.
B) Teaching BSE should start as early as 16 years of age.
C) The goal of the BSE is to detect breast cancer.
D) The U.S. Preventive Services Task Force (USPSTF) recommends against teaching BSE.

The answer is D: Teaching BSE does not reduce breast cancer mortality and may increase false-positive rates. Two large randomized international trials did not demonstrate a mortality benefit from teaching BSE. A review of eight other studies did not show a benefit from BSE in the rate of breast cancer diagnosis, tumor stage, or the rate of breast cancer. Thus, the USPSTF recommends against teaching BSE.

However, given the number of times that women find lumps that lead to a breast cancer diagnosis, it warrants educating patients to recognize and report changes in their breasts. Thus, although there are no studies to support breast self-awareness, some organizations recommend encouraging women 20 years and older to recognize the normal feel of their breasts (rather than teaching formal BSE) and to report any changes to their physician.

Additional Reading: *Breast Cancer: Screening*. USPSTF; 2016. www.uspreventiveservicestaskforce.org/Page/Document/UpdateSummaryFinal/breast-cancer-screening

The USPSTF recommends (grade B recommendation) that primary care providers screen women who have family members with breast, ovarian, tubal, or peritoneal cancer with one of several screening tools designed to identify a family history that may be associated with an increased risk for potentially harmful mutations in breast cancer susceptibility genes (BRCA1 or BRCA2). Women with positive screening results should receive genetic counseling and, if indicated after counseling, BRCA testing.

20. A 16-year-old surfer presents with an erythematous, maculopapular rash that was noted in the area of his bathing suit. Initial treatment includes which one of the following?

A) Application of ice packs
B) Application of clotrimazole cream
C) Application of vinegar compresses
D) Application of zinc oxide ointment
E) Cryotherapy

The answer is C: Swimmers or surfers with seabather's eruption present with an urticarial maculopapular rash on areas of the body that were covered by the swimsuit. One study implicated larvae of the sea anemone *Edwardsiella lineata* as a causative agent. The rash may appear while the bather is in the water or up to 1.5 days later. The rash may last for 2 to 28 days; most reactions resolve within 1 to 2 weeks. Systemic symptoms include fever, nausea, vomiting, and headache and are more likely to affect children.

Initial treatment involves the topical application of heat or vinegar. Further treatment is symptomatic and may include topical corticosteroids, oral antihistamines, and oral steroids. Twice-daily application of thiabendazole (Mintezol) can be beneficial. The swimsuit should be cleaned thoroughly in hot water as well.

Additional Reading: Health issues for surfers. *Am Fam Physician*. 2005;71:2313-2317.

21. A 72-year-old retired professor presents with a painful rash that began yesterday and is developing on his forehead in the periorbital area. He is also complaining of myalgias and low-grade fevers. On examination, you note that the rash is vesicular on an erythematous base on the left side of his forehead and eye. Appropriate management for this patient would be which one of the following?

A) Antibiotics plus antiviral medications and follow-up for 3 to 5 days
B) Antiviral medication and follow-up for 3 to 5 days
C) Antiviral medication and ophthalmology referral
D) Hospitalization with IV antibiotics
E) Reassurance

The answer is C: The most common complication of herpes zoster is postherpetic neuralgia (ie, pain along cutaneous, dermatomal nerves persisting >30 days after the lesions have healed). The incidence of postherpetic neuralgia increases with age and is not commonly seen in patients younger than 60 years. Herpes zoster lesions can become secondarily infected with staphylococci or streptococci, and cellulitis may develop.

Herpes zoster involving the ophthalmic division of the trigeminal nerve can lead to ocular complications and visual loss. In these cases, immediate referral to an ophthalmologist is recommended. Other less common complications include motor paresis and encephalitis.

Additional Reading: Herpes zoster and postherpetic neuralgia: prevention and management. *Am Fam Physician*. 2011;83(12):1432-1437.

22. Osler-Weber-Rendu disease (OWRD) is a rare hereditary disorder that is associated with bleeding complications. All of the following statements about OWRD are true, except which one?

A) Laboratory studies show microcytic anemia.
B) OWRD is inherited as an autosomal dominant disorder.
C) OWRD is associated with telangiectasia lesions of the lips and gastrointestinal (GI) mucosa.
D) Patients can present with hemoptysis.
E) Treatment involves high-dose prednisone.

The answer is E: OWRD (also known as *hereditary hemorrhagic telangiectasia*) is a hereditary disorder that is associated with telangiectasia lesions on the face, lips, nasal and oral mucosa, and GI mucosa. The mode of transmission is autosomal dominant.

The condition can lead to significant GI hemorrhage or epistaxis. Some patients may have pulmonary arteriovenous malformations and may experience hemoptysis or dyspnea. Cerebral or spinal arteriovenous malformations may cause subarachnoid hemorrhage, seizures, or paraplegia.

Laboratory findings may demonstrate a microcytic anemia because of chronic blood loss and iron-deficiency anemia. Treatment is nonspecific and involves topical hemostatics and laser ablation of accessible lesions. In severe cases, blood transfusions may be necessary. Iron supplementation is also recommended.

Additional Reading: *Hereditary Hemorrhagic Telangiectasia*. GeneReviews; 1993. www.ncbi.nlm.nih.gov/books/NBK1351.

23. A 29-year-old truck driver presents with complaints of pain in his perirectal area for the past week. He has otherwise been healthy and has not been seen by a physician in 3 to 4 years. On examination, you note that he is rather hirsute and has an area of tenderness, redness, and induration just superior to the anus in the gluteal cleft. The area is warm and fluctuant but otherwise unremarkable. The most appropriate management at this time is which one of the following treatments?

A) Admit for intravenous antibiotics.
B) Incise and drain the area.
C) Recommend warm sitz baths.
D) Prescribe oral antibiotics and warm sitz baths.
E) Prescribe topical steroids, oral antibiotics, and warm sitz baths.

The answer is B: Pilonidal disease often affects young, white, hirsute men. The disease is related to acute abscesses or chronic draining sinuses that form in the sacrococcygeal region. These sinuses or pits may form a cavity often containing hair. The lesion is often painless unless it becomes infected. Treatment involves incision and drainage, and in most cases, antibiotics are not useful. Recalcitrant cases require marsupialization—a more involved procedure that involves incision and draining, removal of pus and hair, and sewing of the edges of the fibrous tract to the wound edges to make a pouch.

Additional Reading: Pilonidal disease. In: Domino F, ed. *The 5-Minute Clinical Consult*. Wolters Kluwer; 2022.

24. A 20-year-old college student presents with cold sores on her lower lip. She says that she gets these when she is stressed, and with final examinations next week she has a new outbreak. Which one of the following statements regarding orolabial herpes is false?

A) A recurrent infection is typically less severe but longer in duration.
B) Pain associated with lesions typically lasts 2 to 3 weeks.
C) Recurrent outbreaks are frequently triggered by exposure to ultraviolet (UV) sunlight.
D) The highest rate of infection occurs in preschool children.
E) Topical acyclovir is not particularly effective.

The answer is A: Orolabial herpes (gingivostomatitis) is the most prevalent form of mucocutaneous herpes infection. Overall, the highest rate of infection occurs during the preschool years. Female sex, history of sexually transmitted diseases, and multiple sexual partners have also been identified as risk factors for herpes simplex virus 1 (HSV-1) infection.

Primary herpetic gingivostomatitis usually affects children younger than 5 years. It typically takes the form of painful vesicles and ulcerative erosions on the tongue, palate, gingiva, buccal mucosa, and lips. Edema, halitosis, and drooling may be present, and tender submandibular or cervical lymphadenopathy is not uncommon. Hospitalization may be necessary when pain prevents eating or fluid intake. Systemic symptoms are often present, including fever

(38.4 °C-40 °C [101 °F-104 °F]), malaise, and myalgia. The pharyngitis and flulike symptoms are difficult to distinguish from mononucleosis in older patients.

The duration of the initial illness is 2 to 3 weeks, and oral shedding of the virus may continue for as long as 3 weeks. Recurrences typically occur two or three times per year, but the duration is shorter and the discomfort is less severe than that in primary infections. Recurrent lesions are often single and more localized, and the vesicles heal completely by 8 to 10 days. Pain diminishes quickly in 4 to 5 days. UV radiation predictably triggers recurrence of orolabial HSV-1, an effect that, for unknown reasons, is not fully suppressed by acyclovir. Pharmacologic intervention is therefore more difficult in patients with orolabial infection.

Topical medication for HSV-1 infection is generally not highly effective. In the treatment of primary orolabial herpes, oral acyclovir or valacyclovir can reduce the severity and duration of the outbreak. Standard analgesic therapy with acetaminophen or ibuprofen, careful monitoring of hydration status, and aggressive early rehydration therapy are usually sufficient to avoid hospitalization.

Although long-term suppression of orolabial herpes has not been addressed by clinical trials, episodic prophylaxis has been studied because of the predictable trigger effect of UV radiation. Short-term prophylactic therapy with acyclovir may be desirable in some patients who anticipate intense exposure to UV light (eg, skiers or those who work outdoors), although the clinical effect may vary. Early treatment of recurrent orolabial HSV-1 infection with high doses of antiviral medication has been found to markedly decrease the size and duration of lesions.

Additional Reading: Nongenital herpes simplex virus. *Am Fam Physician*. 2010;82(9):1075-1082.

25. A 67-year-old retired firefighter presents for follow-up of his hypertension, which is well controlled with a lisinopril/hydrochlorothiazide 20 mg/12.5 mg combination tablet. His blood pressure (BP) is well controlled (BP 132/68 mm Hg) and his pulse is regular at 74 bpm. He is feeling well but is concerned about a lesion that has developed on the back of his right hand over the past couple of months. The lesion on the dorsum of his hand is a dome-shaped lesion measuring 2 cm in diameter with an area of central necrosis and a protruding mass of keratin. Which one of the following is the most likely diagnosis?

A) Basal cell carcinoma
B) Dermatofibroma
C) Infected sebaceous cyst
D) Keratoacanthoma
E) Nodular malignant melanoma

The answer is D: Keratoacanthoma appears as a skin-colored or pink smooth lesion that becomes dome-shaped during a period of relatively rapid growth. Onset is rapid; usually the lesion reaches its full size within 1 to 2 months. Common sites include the face, dorsum of the hands, and forearms. When mature, it is volcano-shaped, with protruding masses of keratin.

Keratoacanthomas are not malignant and often regress spontaneously, but atypical lesions may actually be squamous cell carcinoma. Many dermatopathologists include keratoacanthoma in the spectrum of squamous cell carcinoma. Total excision is the preferred treatment for most solitary keratoacanthomas. For smaller lesions, electrodesiccation and curettage or blunt dissection is sufficient. Mohs surgery can be used in difficult areas, especially around the nose and ears.

Alternative therapies include oral isotretinoin, topical (Efudex) and intralesional (Adrucil) fluorouracil, intralesional methotrexate (Rheumatrex), and intralesional 5-interferon alfa-2a (Roferon-A). Radiotherapy is an option for patients with recurrence or larger lesions.

Basal cell carcinoma develops slowly and is seen as a nodule with an eroded center and a "rolled border." The center appears as if gnawed, hence the name "rodent ulcer."

Sebaceous cysts are subcutaneous and may erode through the skin surface. They possess a soft cheesy material, not scaly keratin.

Malignant melanoma is evaluated by the "ABCD" mnemonic. A stands for asymmetry, B is for an irregular border, C is for variations of color (from black to red, white, and blue hues), and D is for diameter greater than 1 cm.

Dermatofibromas are firm nodules, the overlying skin is slightly thickened, and they may be black, red, or brown-colored. Their diameter is generally about a centimeter and there can be multiple lesions. Dermatofibromas are benign focal proliferation of fibroblasts in the skin.

Additional Reading: Diagnosing common benign skin tumors. *Am Fam Physician*. 2015;92(7):601-607.

26. A 33-year-old White man with human immunodeficiency virus (HIV) infection presents for a follow-up visit. He complains of gum pain and his gums bleed when he brushes his teeth. On examination you note a bright erythematous line along the gingival margin and diagnose HIV gingivitis. This condition is associated with which one of the following?

A) Bacterial endocarditis
B) Dental caries
C) Infective glossitis
D) Loss of teeth
E) Necrotizing ulcerative gingivitis

The answer is E: HIV-infected patients can suffer from various periodontal diseases. Mild inflammation (HIV gingivitis) can progress to localized acute necrotizing ulcerative gingivitis, and periodontitis can progress to necrotizing stomatitis. Patients with HIV gingivitis present with a bright erythematous line along the gingival margin and complain of spontaneous bleeding. In acute necrotizing ulcerative gingivitis, the gingiva appears erythematous, with ulcerations of the papillae that become tender and bleed when teeth are brushed. Rapid bone and soft tissue loss and loosening teeth are characteristics of HIV periodontitis. Patients complain of "deep" pain, and the condition can rapidly progress to large areas of necrotizing stomatitis.

Patients with HIV gingivitis should be referred to an oral surgeon for debridement, scaling, and curettage of the involved areas. This treatment is followed by administration of metronidazole (Flagyl), irrigation with Povidone–iodine, and daily mouth rinsing with chlorhexidine gluconate (Peridex). Because it may potentiate peripheral neuropathy, metronidazole should not be given to patients taking didanosine (Videx) or zalcitabine (Hivid). In these patients, clindamycin or amoxicillin may be used.

Additional Reading: Complications of HIV infection: a systems-based approach. *Am Fam Physician*. 2011;83(4):395-406.

27. You are seeing a 27-year-old engineer who is concerned about his deformed toenails, which have slowly worsened over time. He has been healthy and keeps fit by working out at the neighborhood gym on a regular basis. On examination, the great toenail on his right foot is thickened and lifted above the nail bed, and he has similar changes on his other toenails, but they are not nearly as affected. You diagnose tinea unguium. Which one of the following statements regarding onychomycosis is true?

A) Ciclopirox (Penlac) is effective for the treatment of onychomycosis.
B) Fungi are responsible for 90% of nail dystrophies.
C) Griseofulvin and ketoconazole are the first-line oral medications for the treatment of onychomycosis.
D) Periodic testing of renal function is indicated with the use of antifungal medication.
E) *Trichophyton rubrum* is the most common infectious agent.

The answer is E: Onychomycosis is a fungal infection of the nail bed, matrix, or plate. Toenails are affected more often than fingernails. The infection is usually caused by *T rubrum*, which invades the nail bed and the underside of the nail plate beginning at the hyponychium and then migrating proximally through the underlying nail matrix. Fungi are responsible for only about a half of nail dystrophies; thus, the diagnosis of onychomycosis should be confirmed by potassium hydroxide preparation looking for fungi microscopically or by obtaining a fungal culture of the nail clippings. Psoriasis, lichen planus, contact dermatitis, trauma, nail-bed tumor, and yellow nail syndrome may be mistakenly diagnosed as onychomycosis.

Ciclopirox nail lacquer is U.S. Food and Drug Administration–approved for the treatment of mild to moderate onychomycosis caused by *T rubrum* without involvement of the lunula. Although safe and relatively inexpensive, ciclopirox therapy is less effective than treatment with triazole and allylamine antifungal oral medications. Terbinafine (Lamisil) and itraconazole (Sporanox) are considered first oral line, and fluconazole (Diflucan) is an alternative for those who cannot tolerate the first-line agents. Griseofulvin and ketoconazole are no longer considered appropriate treatment choices for the treatment of onychomycosis. Ketoconazole has a black-boxed warning given the association with liver failure.

Liver enzyme monitoring is recommended before continuous medication therapy is initiated and every 4 to 6 weeks during treatment with all antifungals.

Additional Reading: Antifungal drugs. *Treat Guidel Med Lett.* 2012;10(120):61.

Section VII. Nephrology

Questions related to nephrology account for only about 2% of the American Board of Family Medicine certifying examination. So do not fret if this is a weak area for you; however, as you study for the examination, ensure that you have a good overview of the following topics.

1. Acute and chronic renal failure
   - Understand the risk factors and how to diagnose and treat acute renal failure (eg, typical clinical setting and laboratory findings and leading causes).
   - Know the criteria and treatment for nephrotic syndrome.
   - Appreciate the leading causes of and the classification for chronic renal failure.
   - Know how to treat chronic renal failure (eg, role of angiotensin-converting enzyme and angiotensin receptor blockers, dietary advice, and erythropoietin indications).
2. Hematuria
   - Know the diagnostic approach for microscopic hematuria.
   - Know the workup for gross hematuria.
   - Know the risk factors for bladder cancer.
   - Know how glomerulonephritis is diagnosed and the treatments and prognosis for various types of glomerulonephritis.
   - Appreciate the risk factors for and the types of kidney stones.
   - Know the evidence-based workup for kidney stones and appreciate the treatment of renal colic (eg, which stones are likely to pass spontaneously).
   - Know what types of treatment are indicated to prevent recurrent renal stone formation for various types of stones.

Each of the following questions or incomplete statements is followed by suggested answers or completions. Select the ONE BEST ANSWER in each case.

1. Type II renal tubular acidosis is associated with which one of the following issues?

A) Hyperkalemia
B) A decreased ability to reabsorb bicarbonate by the proximal tubules
C) Urine pH that is normal when plasma bicarbonate levels are normal
D) Plasma bicarbonate levels that are easily restored with supplementation

The answer is C: Renal tubular acidosis is classified by type as outlined below. Types I and II are associated with chronic metabolic acidosis, mild volume loss, and hypokalemia. The hypokalemia may lead to muscle weakness, hyporeflexia, and paralysis. The ability of the proximal tubules to reabsorb bicarbonate is decreased so that urine pH is >7 (alkalotic) despite normal levels of plasma bicarbonate but may be <5.5 at low levels of plasma bicarbonate.

Type I (distal) is a disorder that affects adults and is considered a familial disorder in children. Sporadic cases may be primary (especially in women) or secondary (eg, an autoimmune disease such as Sjögren syndrome; medications, including amphotericin B or lithium therapy; kidney transplantation; nephrocalcinosis; renal medullary sponge kidney; and chronic renal obstruction). Familial cases may be autosomal dominant and are often associated with hypercalciuria. The urine pH is never <5.5.

Type II (proximal) is associated with several inherited diseases (eg, Fanconi syndrome, fructose intolerance, Wilson disease, and Lowe syndrome), multiple myeloma, vitamin D deficiency, and chronic hypocalcemia with secondary hyperparathyroidism. It may occur after renal transplant, exposure to heavy metals, and after treatment with certain medications, including acetazolamide, sulfonamides, tetracycline, and streptozocin. The ability of the proximal tubules to reabsorb bicarbonate is decreased so that urine pH is >7 at normal levels of plasma bicarbonate but may be <5.5 at low levels of plasma bicarbonate.

Type III is a combination of types I and II and is seldom seen.

Type IV is a condition associated with mild renal insufficiency in adults with diabetes mellitus, human immunodeficiency virus nephropathy, or interstitial renal damage (systemic lupus erythematosus, obstructive uropathy, sickle cell disease). It may also be produced by drugs that interfere with the renin-aldosterone system (eg, nonsteroidal anti-inflammatory drugs, angiotensin-converting enzyme inhibitors, potassium-sparing diuretics, trimethoprim). Aldosterone deficiency or unresponsiveness of the distal tubule to aldosterone results in type IV, with reduced potassium excretion, causing hyperkalemia, which reduces ammonia production and acid excretion by the kidney. Urine pH is usually normal.

Additional Reading: Overview of renal tubular acidosis. In: *UpToDate*. 2021.

2. You are treating a 23-year-old White man with Goodpasture syndrome who is complaining of mild hemoptysis. Which one of the following conditions would you also expect to find associated with this condition?

A) Angioedema
B) Glomerulonephritis
C) Hemorrhagic cystitis
D) Renal lithiasis
E) Urethritis

The answer is B: Goodpasture syndrome is a condition manifested by pulmonary hemorrhages and progressive glomerulonephritis. Circulating basement membrane antibodies are responsible for the renal and pulmonary abnormalities. Patients with Goodpasture syndrome are typically young men (5–40 years; male-female ratio of 6:1); however, there is a bimodal peak at approximately 60 years of age. Men and women are equally affected at older ages. Symptoms include severe hemoptysis, shortness of breath, and renal failure.

Laboratory findings include iron-deficiency anemia, hematuria, proteinuria, cellular and granular casts in the urine, and circulating antiglomerular antibodies. Chest radiographs show progressive, bilateral, fluffy infiltrates that may migrate and are asymmetrical. Renal biopsy may be necessary to make the diagnosis.

Treatment involves high-dose steroids, immunosuppression, and plasmapheresis, which may help preserve renal function. If significant injury to the kidneys occurs, then dialysis or transplant may be necessary. Untreated, Goodpasture syndrome can be fatal.

Additional Reading: Anti-GBM antibody (Goodpasture's) disease: pathogenesis, clinical manifestations and diagnosis. In: *UpToDate*. 2022.

3. A 20-year-old otherwise healthy woman presents with cloudy urine, burning on urination, and urinary frequency. The patient has no allergies. On examination, she is afebrile, with mild suprapubic pain to palpation but no costovertebral angle tenderness. Urinalysis is positive for nitrites and leukocyte esterase. Which one of the following is the most appropriate treatment at this time?

A) Admit for intravenous antibiotics.
B) Administer trimethoprim/sulfamethoxazole (TMP-SMX) on an outpatient basis for 7 days.
C) Administer nitrofurantoin on an outpatient basis for 5 days.
D) Advise the patient to increase fluid intake, especially with cranberry juice.
E) Arrange for an intravenous pyelogram.

The answer is C: Urinary tract infections are more common in sexually active women. Symptoms include dysuria, urinary frequency, enuresis, incontinence, suprapubic tenderness, flank pain, or costovertebral angle tenderness (which usually indicates pyelonephritis). Gram-negative bacteria that originate from the intestinal tract (ie, *E coli*, *Staphylococcus saprophyticus*, *Klebsiella*, *Enterobacter*, *Proteus*, and *Pseudomonas*) are usually the causative organisms. Diagnosis is accomplished by microscopic or dipstick evaluation of a clean-catch midstream urine sample. Urine culture confirms the diagnosis.

Treatment is oral (and in most cases sulfa-containing) antibiotics. With no complicating clinical factors, reasonable empiric treatment for presumed cystitis before organism identification is a 3-day regimen of any of the following: oral nitrofurantoin, fosfomycin, or TMP-SMX in regions where the uropathogen resistance is less than 20%.

Phenazopyridine hydrochloride may be necessary for 1 to 3 days if significant dysuria is present. Affected patients should also be encouraged to increase their fluid intake.

Additional Reading: Diagnosis and treatment of acute uncomplicated cystitis. *Am Fam Physician*. 2011;84(7):771-776.

4. A 52-year-old woman presents for follow-up with her wife after passing another kidney stone last month. He has passed several calcium oxalate kidney stones over the past few years and her wife returns for recommendations on her diet. The most appropriate advice would be to recommend which one of the following?

A) Increase her sodium intake.
B) Increase her dietary protein intake.
C) Restrict her calcium intake.
D) Restrict her intake of yellow vegetables.
E) Take potassium citrate supplements with her meals.

The answer is E: Calcium oxalate stones are the most common of all renal calculi. A low-sodium, restricted-protein diet with increased fluid intake reduces stone formation. A low-calcium diet has been shown to be ineffective. Oxalate restriction also reduces stone formation. Oxalate-containing foods include spinach, chocolate, tea, and nuts, but not yellow vegetables. Potassium citrate should be taken at mealtime to increase urinary pH and urinary citrate.

Additional Readings:
1. Medical management of common urinary calculi. *Am Fam Physician*. 2006;74(1):86-94.
2. Effect of potassium citrate on calcium phosphate stones in a model of hypercaliciuria. *J Am Soc Nephrol*. 2015;26(12):3001-3008. doi:10.1681/ASN.2014121223.

5. You are seeing a patient in the emergency department who has been involved in a motor vehicle accident. His urine dipstick is positive for hemoglobin, but no erythrocytes are seen on a reflex microscopic examination of the urinary sediment. Which one of the following is the most likely diagnosis in this situation?

A) Intravascular hemolysis
B) Splenic laceration
C) Myocardial contusion
D) Renal contusion
E) Rhabdomyolysis

The answer is E: A positive urine dipstick for hemoglobin results from free hemoglobin or myoglobin in the urine. When hemoglobin is released from erythrocytes, it is bound by haptoglobin, and once the haptoglobin becomes saturated, free hemoglobin spills into the urine.

Free hemoglobin appears in the urine when there is intravascular hemolysis, which can be seen with a transfusion reaction. However, myoglobinuria is associated with rhabdomyolysis and occurs when there is significant muscle injury with the release of myoglobin into the bloodstream.

Causes include electrical shock or massive muscle trauma as occurs with a motor vehicle accident, as seen in this case. Other causes may include toxin exposures, metabolic disorders, inflammatory conditions, and infection. Thus myoglobinuria causes a positive urine test for blood (hemoglobin) in the absence of urinary erythrocytes as seen in this situation.

Additional Reading: Clinical manifestations and diagnosis of rhabdomyolysis. In: Dashe. *UpToDate*. 2021.

6. A 31-year-old woman has had frequent urinary tract infections over the years and presents with recurrent dysuria. She has felt ill for the past couple of days and presents now with nausea and vomiting. On examination, she has a temperature of 103.2 °F and flank pain. The most appropriate treatment at this time would be which one of the following?

A) Hospitalize and administer intravenous fluids and antibiotics.
B) Advise oral rehydration and oral antibiotics for 10 to 14 days.
C) Obtain a surgical consultation for exploratory laparotomy.
D) Order extracorporeal shock wave lithotripsy.
E) Make NPO (nothing by mouth) with nasogastric suction.

The answer is A: Acute pyelonephritis is an infection of the upper urinary tract. It affects the kidneys' collecting system and renal parenchyma. The most common causative agent is *E coli*. Other causative agents include *Proteus*, *Pseudomonas*, *Enterobacter*, *Klebsiella*, *Staphylococcus*, and *Enterococcus*. Symptoms include lower abdominal pain, flank tenderness, fevers, chills, nausea, and vomiting as seen in this patient. Physical findings include tenderness of the costovertebral angle and the abdomen. Laboratory findings include elevated white blood cell (WBC) count, elevated erythrocyte sedimentation rate, pyuria, bacteriuria, hematuria, proteinuria, and possible WBC cast. Severe cases may cause bacteremia (20% of patients) and urosepsis.

Treatment includes antibiotics directed at gram-negative organisms. For empirical oral therapy, a fluoroquinolone is recommended. Should fluoroquinolone resistance exceed 10%, a single initial intravenous dose of a long-acting antibiotic such as ceftriaxone 1 g is recommended. Patients with mild to moderate symptoms can be managed as outpatients. Hospitalization is required if the patient has a high fever (as seen in this case), dehydration, or other complicating medical conditions (eg, pregnancy and diabetes).

For parenteral therapy, a fluoroquinolone, aminoglycoside ± ampicillin, or an extended-spectrum cephalosporin ± an aminoglycoside can be used. Duration of antibiotic therapy depends on clinical response but should be at least 10 to 14 days. Intravenous antibiotics should be continued until the patient is afebrile. Repeated cultures after treatment should be performed; if the patient has had repeated infections, further workup, including an intravenous pyelography or voiding cystourethrogram, may be necessary.

Additional Reading: Pyelonephritis. In: Domino F, ed. *The 5-Minute Clinical Consult*. Wolters Kluwer; 2022.

7. Which one of the following clinical findings is consistent with the syndrome of inappropriate antidiuretic hormone (SIADH)?

A) Hypernatremia
B) Hypertonic urine
C) Hypovolemia
D) Hyperosmolality
E) Increased glomerular filtration rate

The answer is B: SIADH is defined as less than maximally dilute urine in the presence of plasma hypo-osmolality and hyponatremia. The condition is associated with several disorders, including small cell carcinoma of the lung, Guillain-Barré syndrome, acute intermittent porphyria, other pulmonary disorders (eg, pneumonia and tuberculosis), and neurologic disorders (eg, meningitis, tumors, trauma, and stroke). It is seen as a side effect of many medications as well, including selective serotonin reuptake inhibitor antidepressants. In many cases, the condition may be idiopathic. The cause is the inappropriate release of antidiuretic hormone (ADH) with respect to the body's fluid osmolality. As the osmolality is low, the kidneys should be releasing fluid (diuresis), but ADH is being released, so that the kidneys instead retain fluid resulting in low plasma osmolality and low sodium. Findings include the following:

- Hyponatremia and hypo-osmolality of body fluids
- Normal glomerular filtration rate
- Urine hypertonicity (usually >300 mOsmol/kg) despite a subnormal plasma osmolality and serum sodium concentration
- Euvolemia or hypervolemia without the presence of edema
- Urinary sodium wasting that increases with salt loading

Symptoms include confusion, anorexia, lethargy, and muscle cramps. Treatment involves fluid restriction—often less than 1200 mL daily. More severe cases may require replacement of sodium and potassium deficits. Care should be taken not to replace deficits too quickly because of the risk of central pontine myelinolysis.

Additional Reading: Diagnosis and management of sodium disorders: hyponatremia and hypernatremia. *Am Fam Physician*. 2015;91(5):299-307.

8. A blood urea nitrogen (BUN)–serum creatinine ratio greater than 20 is associated with which one of the following conditions?

A) Dehydration
B) Renal stones
C) Bladder outlet obstruction
D) Hypercalcemia
E) Renal artery stenosis

The answer is A: Acute renal failure is divided into three categories:

Prerenal. This is due to inadequate renal perfusion. It can be caused by volume depletion (dehydration), cardiac or hepatic failure, and sepsis. Laboratory tests reveal a low urinary sodium (<20 mEq/L) and a high urine to plasma creatinine ratio (>20:1). The BUN to serum creatinine ratio is higher than 20.

Postrenal. This is usually caused by obstruction by renal calculi or bladder outlet obstruction (eg, prostate enlargement). Laboratory tests show a high urinary sodium (>40 mEq/L) and a low urine to plasma creatinine ratio (<20:1). The BUN–serum creatinine ratio is lower than 20.

Intrarenal. This was previously known as acute tubular necrosis. Causes include ischemia, hypertension (HTN), vasculitis, metabolic disorders (eg, hypercalcemia and hyperuricemia), toxins, x-ray dyes, myoglobinuria, and medications (eg, aminoglycosides, penicillins, and anesthetic agents). Laboratory tests show results similar to postrenal azotemia.

Prerenal and postrenal causes for acute renal failure are potentially reversible. If caught early, some forms of intrarenal azotemia (eg, drug effects, infections, and HTN) can be reversed.

Additional Reading: Acute kidney injury: a guide to diagnosis and management. *Am Fam Physician*. 2012;86(7):631-639.

Acute renal failure can be due to inadequate renal perfusion (prerenal disease), caused by volume depletion (dehydration), cardiac or hepatic failure, or sepsis. The blood urea nitrogen (BUN)–serum creatinine ratio is higher than 20a.

9. A 33-year-old White man presents for a visit after passing a 4-mm calcium oxalate stone. This was his first episode of nephrolithiasis, but he is worried and wants to know how he can prevent developing more kidney stones in the future, as this was a painful experience for him. You would advise which of the following?

A) Drink up to 2 L of water per day.
B) Increase his consumption of meats and grains.
C) Increase the level of fructose in his diet.
D) Restrict foods high in oxalate, such as spinach and rhubarb.

The answer is A: Recommendations to prevent recurrent nephrolithiasis include increasing fluid intake up to 2 L of water daily (larger amounts are not recommended because they may lead to electrolyte disturbances). Dietary changes depend on the composition of the passed stone. If no stone is available for analysis, a 24-hour urine collection is advised for calcium, phosphorus, magnesium, uric acid, and oxalate.

Approximately 60% of all stones are calcium oxalate. Uric acid stones account for up to 17% of stones and, like cystine stones, form in acidic urine. Alkalinization of the urine to a pH of 6.5 to 7.0 may reduce stone formation in patients with these types of stones. This includes a diet with plenty of fruits and vegetables, and limiting acid-producing foods such as meat, grains, dairy products, and legumes. Drinking mineral water, which is relatively alkaline with a pH of 7.0 to 7.5, is also recommended. Restriction of dietary oxalates has not been shown to be effective in reducing stone formation in most patients.

Acidification of the urine to a pH < 7.0 is recommended for patients with the less common calcium phosphate and struvite stones (magnesium ammonium phosphate). This can be accomplished by consumption of at least 16 oz of cranberry juice per day or by taking betaine, 650 mg three times daily.

Additional Reading: Treatment and prevention of kidney stones: an update. *Am Fam Physician*. 2011;84(11):1234-1242.

10. A 66-year-old woman presents for a follow-up visit a month after you had prescribed enalapril (Vasotec) to treat heart failure. She is feeling okay but feels that her ankles are swollen. Her serum creatinine level is 2.6 mg/dL (0.6-1.5) and potassium level is 5.8 mEq/L (N 3.4-4.8). Her baseline values were normal 2 months ago. Which one of the following is a side effect of angiotensin-converting enzyme (ACE) inhibitors and is the most likely cause of these changes in renal function?

A) Impaired autoregulation of glomerular blood flow
B) Interstitial nephritis
C) Microangiopathic arteriolar thrombosis
D) Proximal renal tubular toxicity
E) Rhabdomyolysis

The answer is A: Renal blood flow is autoregulated to sustain pressure within the glomerulus, by angiotensin II–related vasoconstriction. ACE inhibition impairs this renal autoregulatory function, resulting in a decreased glomerular filtration rate, and can cause acute renal injury. This is usually reversible if recognized and the offending medication is stopped.

Nonsteroidal anti-inflammatory drugs can exert a similar effect, but they can also cause glomerulonephritis and interstitial nephritis. Statins, haloperidol, and drugs of abuse (cocaine, heroin) can cause rhabdomyolysis with the release of myoglobin, which causes acute renal injury.

Microangiopathic arteriolar thrombosis is a rare mechanism of injury to the kidney and may be caused by clopidogrel, quinine, or certain chemotherapeutic agents.

Additional Reading: Drug-induced nephrotoxicity. *Am Fam Physician*. 2008;78(6):743-750.

11. A 22-year-old sexually active woman calls the office with complaints of dysuria that began last night. She is otherwise healthy and has no other symptoms. The best management of this situation would include which one of the following?

A) Continued observation with a return call if she develops a fever.
B) Obtain a midstream urinalysis followed by microscopic evaluation and treatment if positive.
C) Obtain a urine culture and prescribe an appropriate antibiotic, once sensitivities are determined.
D) Prescribe a course of empiric antibiotic for 5 days.

The answer is D: A urinary tract infection (UTI) is typically classified as "complicated" in pregnant women and in those with comorbidities (eg, diabetes mellitus, recent urinary tract instrumentation, chronic renal disease, urinary tract abnormalities, and immunosuppression). For these women, empiric therapy is recommended with a urine culture to confirm the diagnosis and to determine antibiotic sensitivities. Women with complicated UTIs require longer courses of broader-spectrum antibiotics. Women with uncomplicated UTIs can be treated empirically with a 5-day course of nitrofurantoin, a 3-day course of trimethoprim-sulfamethoxazole (Bactrim, Septra) if resistance to *E coli* is less than 20%, or Fosfomycin (Monurol) in a single-day course.

It is unclear whether age alone increases the risk of a complicated infection, and few studies have evaluated shorter antibiotic courses in older patients. Physicians should use their own judgment to decide if otherwise healthy women older than 65 years with uncomplicated infections can be treated for only 3 days or whether a longer course is indicated. Physicians should follow up with patients after 3 days by telephone or in person to ensure clinical improvement.

Additional Reading: Diagnosis and treatment of acute uncomplicated cystitis. *Am Fam Physician*. 2011;84(7):771-776.

12. A urine culture obtained from an asymptomatic patient grows more than 100,000 colony-forming units. For which one of the following patients is treatment indicated?

A) A 94-year-old nursing home resident
B) A 78-year-old scheduled for cataract surgery
C) A 72-year-old business executive
D) A 68-year-old with a history of breast cancer
E) A 28-year-old pregnant woman at 38 weeks' gestation

The answer is E: Asymptomatic bacteriuria is defined as the presence of >100,000 colony-forming units per mL of voided urine in persons with no symptoms of a urinary tract infection (UTI). The largest patient population at risk for asymptomatic bacteriuria is the elderly (particularly women). Up to 40% of elderly men and women may have bacteriuria without symptoms. Although early studies noted an association between bacteriuria and excess mortality, more recent studies have failed to demonstrate any such link. Aggressively screening elderly persons for asymptomatic bacteriuria and subsequent treatment of the infection has not been found to reduce infectious complications or mortality. Consequently, this approach is currently not recommended.

Three groups of patients with asymptomatic bacteriuria have been shown to benefit from treatment: (1) pregnant women, (2) patients with renal transplants, and (3) patients who are about to undergo genitourinary tract procedures. Between 2% and 10% of pregnancies are complicated by UTIs; if left untreated, 25% to 30% of these women develop pyelonephritis. Pregnancies that are complicated by pyelonephritis have been associated with low-birth-weight infants and prematurity. Thus, pregnant women should be screened for bacteriuria by urine culture at 12 to 16 weeks of gestation. The presence of 100,000 colony-forming units of bacteria per milliliter of urine is considered significant. Pregnant women with asymptomatic bacteriuria should be treated with a 3- to 7-day course of antibiotics, and the urine should subsequently be cultured to ensure cure and the avoidance of relapse.

Additional Reading: Asymptomatic bacteriuria. *Am Fam Physician*. 2020;102(2):99-104.

13. You are assessing a 33-year-old man with right flank pain. He has been having intermittent pain for the past couple of days and his urinalysis is positive for erythrocytes, but his leukocyte esterase and urinary nitrates are negative. You suspect that he has a ureteral obstruction secondary to renal lithiasis. Which one of the following is the best test to detect such a condition?

A) An intravenous pyelogram (IVP)
B) Abdominal magnetic resonance imaging (MRI)
C) Noncontrast helical computed tomographic (CT) scan
D) Plain abdominal radiographs
E) Abdominal ultrasonography

The answer is C: The most common cause of the sudden onset of flank pain in adults is acute urolithiasis. Identification of a stone in the ureter with resultant partial or complete ureteral obstruction confirms the suspected diagnosis. Noncontrast helical CT has the advantages of avoiding contrast exposure (required for the IVP), identifying radiolucent calculi, and evaluating nearby structures and requires a shorter time for examination than MRI. As a result, helical CT is a better test for assessing acute urolithiasis.

Abdominal ultrasonography has a high specificity in evaluating stones, but its sensitivity is lower than that of helical CT. Plain films are used to follow patients with known radiopaque (ie, calcium) stones.

Additional Reading: Kidney stones: diagnosis and acute management of suspected nephrolithiasis in adults. In: *UpToDate*. 2022.

14. You are following a 57-year-old diabetic, and a recent metabolic panel revealed a glomerular filtration rate (GFR) of 31 mL/min. This result is consistent with renal insufficiency and would be considered what stage of chronic renal failure?

A) Stage 1
B) Stage 2
C) Stage 3
D) Stage 4
E) Stage 5

The answer is C: In 2012, Kidney Disease: Improving Global Outcomes (KDIGO) classified chronic kidney disease in six categories by GFR estimation:

- G1: kidney damage with normal or increased GFR ≥90 mL/min/1.73 m^2
- G2: mild ↓ GFR 60 to 89 mL/min/1.73 m^2
- G3a: mild to moderate ↓ GFR 45 to 59 mL/min/1.73 m^2
- G3b: moderate to severe ↓ GFR 30 to 44 mL/min/1.73 m^2
- G4: severe ↓ GFR 15 to 29 mL/min/1.73 m^2
- G5: kidney failure: GFR <15 mL/min/1.73 m^2 or dialysis

Additional Reading: Chronic kidney disease. In: Domino F, ed. *The 5-Minute Clinical Consult*. Wolters Kluwer; 2022.

15. You are seeing a 36-year-old woman who presents with complaints of back pain and pink-tinged urine. You suspect a renal stone, but the ultrasonography demonstrates polycystic kidneys. True statements about polycystic kidney disease (PKD) include all of the following, except which one?

A) PKD can also be associated with liver cysts.
B) PKD is often an asymptomatic condition.
C) PKD usually results in renal failure in young children.
D) Autosomal dominant PKD (ADPKD) is one of the most common human genetic disorders.

The answer is C: PKD refers to genetic disorders that result in numerous renal cysts. Although kidneys usually are the most severely affected organs, cysts can develop in liver and elsewhere in the body, including cerebral and cardiac arteries. The disease is often asymptomatic but is related to several complications, including HTN and renal failure. PKD cysts can enlarge the kidney and replace much of the normal structure, resulting in CKD, which may progress to renal failure.

The two main types of PKD are ADPKD and autosomal recessive PKD. The diagnosis of ADPKD relies principally on imaging of the kidney with renal ultrasonography. Typical findings include large kidneys and extensive cysts scattered throughout both kidneys. In certain settings, genetic testing is required for a definitive diagnosis. ADPKD is one of the most common human genetic disorders. Mutations in one of two genes (*PKD1* and *PKD2*) have been identified in the majority of patients with ADPKD.

PKD does not cause signs or symptoms until cysts are half an inch or larger and is often not diagnosed until later in life. When present, the most common symptoms are flank pain and headaches. The pain can be temporary or persistent and mild or severe. Hematuria may also be a sign of ADPKD. Hypertension is present in about half of those with ADPKD. Renal failure, on average, develops before the age of 60 years.

Additional Reading: Polycystic kidney disease. In: Domino F, ed. *The 5-Minute Clinical Consult*. Wolters Kluwer; 2022.

16. You are seeing a 65-year-old Black man for follow-up. He had presented with hematuria and was diagnosed with renal cell carcinoma (RCC). You inform him that all of the following statements about RCC are true, except which one?

A) RCC is usually treated with chemotherapy followed by surgery to remove the affected kidney.
B) RCC often metastasizes.
C) RCC usually does not cause renal failure.
D) RCC is associated with paraneoplastic syndromes.

The answer is A: RCC accounts for 3% to 4% of all adult cancers and 2.3% of all cancer deaths, making it the seventh most common malignant tumor in men and ninth in women. It is more common in Black men. It is characterized by varied presentations, including paraneoplastic syndromes, vascular findings, and metastases to uncommon sites. About a third of patients will present with metastatic disease at the time of diagnosis. Early, aggressive surgical management provides the best opportunity for cure. Chemotherapy is optional and renal failure is unusual.

Additional Reading: Renal cell carcinoma. In: Domino F, ed. *The 5-Minute Clinical Consult*. Wolters Kluwer; 2022.

17. You are treating a 67-year-old man for hypertension, which has been resistant to your prescribed therapy. His examination is benign, but you are considering that he may have secondary hypertension (HTN) and consider renal artery stenosis (RAS) as the cause. All of the following statements about RAS are true, except which one?

A) RAS is the most common cause for secondary HTN.
B) RAS rarely affects both renal arteries.
C) RAS can lead to renal failure.
D) RAS is best diagnosed with a duplex renal ultrasonography.

The answer is D: Renal artery stenosis refers to the narrowing of one or both renal arteries. This results in decreased perfusion to the kidneys, which respond as if the patient has low blood pressure. Renin is released, which causes an increase in vascular resistance, causing systemic (secondary) HTN.

HTN in young children is usually secondary to some identifiable cause. Of those with secondary HTN, most have intrinsic renal disease (eg, renal scarring, dysplasia, and chronic nephritis). RAS accounts for about 10% of secondary HTN in children, and 5% of adults with HTN have RAS. It is the most common cause of secondary HTN in older adults (>65 years).

The preferred method of imaging for suspected RAS is controversial. Angiography is the diagnostic standard for detecting RAS, but it is invasive. Magnetic resonance imaging with gadolinium contrast or computed tomographic (CT) angiography is equally accurate in visualizing stenosis as an initial diagnostic test. If MRI and CT angiography are contraindicated, renal Doppler can be used; Doppler provides useful information regarding blood flow, but its accuracy is affected by body habitus and operator skill.

Additional Reading: Hypertension, secondary and resistant. In: Domino F, ed. *The 5-Minute Clinical Consult*. Wolters Kluwer; 2022.

18. You are seeing a 43-year-old White man in your office as he had a health screening at his work and was told that he had blood in his urine. He states that he has not noticed blood when he urinates and he feels well and denies any recent trauma. You review his urinalysis and note that he has 6 red blood cells (RBCs) per high power field (HPF) on the microscopic evaluation. What is the next step in addressing this patient's hematuria?

A) Reassurance as he has <10 RBCs/HPF.
B) Referral for cystoscopy.
C) Evaluate for UTI and other benign causes (eg, vigorous exercise).
D) Obtain urine cytology.

The answer is C: For many patients with microscopic hematuria, a specific cause is not found. However, a full evaluation is recommended as malignancies are detected in up to 5% of patients with microscopic hematuria and in up to 40% of patients with gross hematuria. The first step with a positive dipstick for blood is to perform a microscopic evaluation, and there is general consensus that ≥3 RBCs/HPF in two of three urine specimens signals microscopic hematuria. Thus reassurance is not appropriate for this patient. The first step is to evaluate for a UTI and other benign causes (eg, vigorous exercise) and, if found, to treat. Additionally, the urine should be evaluated to ensure that there are no signs of underlying renal disease (eg, casts and proteinuria). If no obvious causes are found, then renal imaging and referral for cystoscopy should be pursued.

Additional Reading: Assessment of asymptomatic microscopic hematuria in adults. *Am Fam Physician*. 2013;88(11):747-754.

> **Finding three or more RBCs/HPF in two of three urine specimens signals microscopic hematuria, which needs further investigation.**

19. A 44-year-old man presents to your office for follow-up of recurrent kidney stones. He states that he is eating a normal diet but avoids soft drinks. Which one of the following would help him to avoid a recurrence of his kidney stones?

A) Drinking two cans of cola-flavored soft drinks daily
B) Eating a high-protein diet
C) Taking a loop diuretic daily
D) Taking a thiazide diuretic daily

The answer is D: The first treatment for patients with recurrent nephrolithiasis is to recommend that they increase their daily fluid intake so as to urinate 2 L or more each day. Increasing fluid intake decreases the recurrence of stones by at least 50%. Reducing cola-based soft drink intake may help as they are acidified with phosphoric acid; however, fruit-flavored drinks, which are acidified with citric acid, do not appear to have the same effect. There is little evidence that other dietary changes help significantly. If increasing daily fluids is not practical or effective, prescribing thiazide diuretics, citrate, or allopurinol is recommended.

Additional Reading: Prevention of recurrent nephrolithiasis: dietary and pharmacologic options recommended by the ACP. *Am Fam Physician*. 2015;92(4):311.

20. A 67-year-old woman is admitted with congestive heart failure and stage 3 chronic kidney disease. Her serum potassium level is 6.9 mEq/L (N 3.6-5.0). Which one of the following is the best initial management to reduce her potassium level?

A) Intravenous calcium gluconate solution
B) Intravenous furosemide
C) Intravenous insulin and glucose
D) A rectal sodium polystyrene sulfonate (Kayexalate) retention enema
E) Hemodialysis

The answer is C: This patient has severe hyperkalemia and needs urgent treatment. Intravenous insulin followed by glucose will shift potassium intracellularly and is an effective treatment. Sodium polystyrene sulfonate is not recommended as an urgent treatment and would not be an initial treatment for severe hyperkalemia. Intravenous calcium gluconate solution does not lower serum potassium but is indicated to prevent arrhythmias in patients with hyperkalemia and electrocardiographic changes. Intravenous furosemide is not a treatment for hyperkalemia, although hypokalemia is a common side effect. Hemodialysis is a treatment for severe hyperkalemia but is not considered a first-line treatment.

Additional Reading: Potassium disorders: hypokalemia and hyperkalemia. *Am Fam Physician*. 2015;92(6):487-495.

21. A 50-year-old man with autosomal dominant polycystic kidney disease (ADPKD) sees you for a routine visit and to ask about a screening colonoscopy. His blood pressure is 154/94 mm Hg, pulse rate 84 beats per minute, and respiratory rate 17/min, and he has an oxygen saturation of 99%. You obtain a basic metabolic panel that reveals a glomerular filtration rate of 49 mL/min/1.73 m^2. Which one of the following medications is the preferred initial therapy for controlling his hypertension?

A) Amlodipine (Norvasc)
B) Furosemide
C) Lisinopril (Prinivil, Zestril)
D) Metoprolol
E) Spironolactone (Aldactone)

The answer is C: ADPKD is the most common genetic kidney disease and accounts for about 5% of end-stage kidney disease in the United States. Many patients are asymptomatic, but early symptoms can include flank pain, gross hematuria, or recurrent urinary tract infections. All ADPKD patients eventually develop a loss of renal function, and approximately 80% develop end-stage renal disease by age 70. The most common extrarenal manifestation of ADPKD is hypertension; thus, an angiotensin-converting enzyme inhibitor (ACEI; eg, lisinopril) is the recommended first-line therapy. Angiotensin receptor blockers are acceptable in patients who cannot tolerate ACEIs.

Additional Reading: Autosomal dominant polycystic kidney disease. *Am Fam Physician*. 2014;90(5):303-307.

Section VIII. Neurology

Questions related to neurology account for only about 2% of the American Board of Family Medicine certifying examination. Remember, as this examination is for family physicians, the focus is on the primary care management of these conditions. As you study for the examination, ensure that you have a good overview of the following neurologic topics:

1. Headache
   - Know the red flags when assessing a patient presenting with a headache and the indications for use of imaging (eg, worst headache of your life is the classical description for subarachnoid hemorrhage).
   - Understand the classification and diagnostic criteria for headaches (eg, muscle tension and cluster).
   - Know the classification and signs/symptoms for migraine headaches.
   - Appreciate the hormonal influences on headaches. (For example, menstrual migraine starts 2 days before menstruation and end when menses ends. Estrogen withdrawal is likely the trigger. Oral contraceptives are contraindicated in migraine with aura because of an increased risk of stroke.)
   - Understand the commonly accepted first-line treatments for headaches.
   - Understand the medications used for abortive versus preventive treatment for migraines.
2. Common neurologic conditions
   - Understand the classification for seizures (eg, complex partial seizure—consciousness is impaired with amnesia, confusion, and repetitive behaviors; absence [petit mal] seizures—brief in duration, "staring off into space").
   - Understand the approach to and workup for febrile seizures.
   - Know the basics of trigeminal neuralgia.
   - Know the approach to neuropathy.
   - Know the approach to insomnia.
   - Know the signs and symptoms and the workup for a transient ischemic attack (TIA).
   - Understand the commonly accepted first-line treatments for TIA.
   - Learn the initial treatment for acute stroke syndrome, including the appropriate use of thrombolytics.
   - Know the management for poststroke care.
3. Degenerative (and other) neurologic disorders
   - Understand the approach to tremor (eg, rest vs intention).
   - Know the criteria for and differential diagnosis for dementia (eg, Lewy body dementia and delirium).
   - Know the diagnostic criteria for Alzheimer disease.
   - Know the diagnostic criteria for Parkinson disease.
   - Know the diagnostic criteria for amyotrophic lateral sclerosis.
   - Know the diagnostic criteria for multiple sclerosis. (For example, diagnosis must be two attacks at least 1 month apart, and there must be more than one area damaged to the brain.)
   - Understand the use of medications for dementia (eg, anticholinesterase and antipsychotics).

Each of the following questions or incomplete statements is followed by suggested answers or completions. Select the ONE BEST ANSWER in each case.

1. Primary insomnia is usually associated with which one of the following conditions?

A) Restless legs syndrome (RLS)
B) Periodic limb movements
C) Obstructive sleep apnea
D) Circadian rhythm sleep disorders
E) None of the above

The answer is E: Insomnia is defined as inadequate or poor-quality sleep characterized by one or more of the following: difficulty falling asleep, difficulty maintaining sleep, waking up too early in the morning, or sleep that is not refreshing. Insomnia is often associated with daytime consequences such as fatigue, difficulty concentrating, and irritability. Periods of insomnia lasting between one night and a few weeks are defined as acute insomnia. Chronic insomnia refers to sleep difficulty occurring at least 3 nights/wk for 1 month or more. Primary insomnia occurs in the absence of any associated conditions, such as specific sleep disorders, including RLS, periodic limb movement disorder, sleep apnea, and circadian rhythm sleep disorders.

RLS is characterized by unpleasant sensations in the legs or feet, which are temporarily relieved by movement. Symptoms are worse in the evening, especially when a person is lying down and remaining still. The sensations cause difficulty falling asleep and are often accompanied by periodic limb movements.

Periodic limb movement disorder is characterized by bilateral repeated and rhythmic, small-amplitude jerking or twitching movements in the lower extremities and, less frequently, in the arms. These movements occur every 20 to 90 seconds and can lead to awakenings, which are usually not noticed by the patient. Often, the patient reports that sleep is not refreshing. In many cases, the bed partner is more likely to report the movement problem.

Obstructive sleep apnea is most commonly associated with snoring, daytime sleepiness, and obesity but occasionally presents with insomnia.

Circadian rhythm sleep disorders, including sleep-work insomnia, are characterized by an inability to sleep because of a disturbance between the circadian sleep rhythm and the desired or required sleep schedule.

When primary insomnia persists beyond one or two nights or becomes predictable, treatment should be considered. Pharmacologic treatment is usually effective, especially short-acting hypnotics. Sleep hygiene measures may also be useful. Chronic insomnia may be more difficult to treat. Because chronic insomnia is often multifactorial in etiology, a patient may need multiple treatment modalities, including medication and behavioral therapy. If an underlying medical or psychiatric condition is identified, this condition should be treated first.

Additional Reading: Primary insomnia in older persons. *Am Fam Physician*. 2013;87(4):280-281.

2. A secondary cause of restless legs syndrome (RLS) is which one of the following conditions?

A) Alcohol abuse
B) Bismuth overdose
C) Heavy metal intoxication
D) Iron deficiency
E) Vitamin B_{12} deficiency

The answer is D: RLS is a neurologic movement disorder that is often associated with a sleep disturbance. The diagnosis of RLS is based on the patient's (and/or sleep partners) history. Patients with RLS have an irresistible urge to move their legs, which is usually secondary to uncomfortable sensations that are worse during periods of inactivity and often interfere with sleep. It is estimated that between 2% and 15% of the population may experience symptoms of RLS. Primary RLS may have a genetic origin.

Causes of secondary RLS include iron deficiency, neurologic lesions, pregnancy, and uremia. Patients with iron deficiency may receive symptom relief by taking supplemental iron. A ferritin level of less than 50 ng/mL may cause or exacerbate RLS. Although levels above 10 to 20 ng/mL are reported as normal, supplemental iron may improve symptoms in individuals with levels less than 50 ng/mL. Iron is not beneficial in individuals with ferritin above this level.

Additional Reading: AASM updates treatment guidelines for restless legs syndrome and periodic limb movement disorder. *Am Fam Physician*. 2013;87(4):290-292.

3. A 67-year-old Black man with a history of hypertension and tobacco abuse presents to the emergency department (ED) with complaints of left-sided arm weakness and slurring of his words. You have diagnosed him with a stroke, and an emergent computed tomographic (CT) scan was negative for hemorrhage. He meets criteria to receive thrombolytic therapy with recombinant tissue plasminogen activator. This medication can be given up to __ after the onset of stroke symptoms?

A) 1 hour
B) 2 hours
C) 3 hours
D) 6 hours
E) 12 hours

The answer is C: Patients who arrive at the ED within 180 minutes of symptom onset should undergo evaluation to determine if they are candidates for thrombolytic therapy. Initial testing should include a complete blood count with platelet count, prothrombin time (International Normalized Ratio), partial thromboplastin time, and electrolyte and glucose levels. CT scanning of the head should be performed immediately to ensure that there is no evidence of brain hemorrhage or mass. Criteria for using tissue plasminogen activator include the following:

- Onset <3 hours
- Blood pressure < 185/110; glucose >50
- No seizure at onset
- No recent invasive surgery, no history of intracranial hemorrhage, or no stroke/serious head trauma in the past 3 months
- Not rapidly improving or only minor symptoms

Patients who do not meet these criteria should be given aspirin.

Additional Reading: Stroke. In: Domino F, ed. *The 5-Minute Clinical Consult*. Wolters Kluwer; 2022.

4. A recognized complication of obstructive sleep apnea is which one of the following conditions?

A) Congestive heart failure
B) Diabetes mellitus
C) Hyperlipidemia
D) Migraines
E) Restless legs syndrome

The answer is A: Obstructive sleep apnea occurs most often in moderately or severely obese persons. Men are affected more often than women (4% of men and 2% of women in middle age). Upper airway narrowing leads to obstruction during sleep. In severely obese persons, a combination of hypoxemia and hypercapnia may induce central apnea as well.

By definition, apneic periods last at least 10 seconds (some for 2 minutes). Repeated nocturnal obstruction may cause recurring cycles of sleep, obstructive choking, and arousal with gasping for air. Daytime drowsiness usually results from the repeated cycles. Similar but less-pronounced cycles occur in nonobese persons, possibly secondary to developmental or congenital abnormalities of the upper airway.

Complications of sleep apnea include cardiac abnormalities (eg, sinus arrhythmias, extreme bradycardia, atrial flutter, ventricular tachycardia, and heart failure), hypertension, excessive daytime sleepiness, morning headache, and slowed mentation. The mortality rate from stroke and myocardial infarctionss is significantly higher in persons with obstructive sleep apnea than in the general population.

Additional Reading: Sleep apnea, obstructive. In: Domino F, ed. *The 5-Minute Clinical Consult*. Wolters Kluwer; 2022.

5. A 23-year-old White woman with a generalized seizure disorder is brought into the emergency department in status epilepticus. Which one of the following drugs should be administered initially?

A) Lorazepam
B) Fosphenytoin
C) Pentobarbital
D) Phenytoin
E) Phenobarbital

The answer is A: Lorazepam should be administered intravenously over a minute to assess its effect. Diazepam or midazolam may be substituted if lorazepam is not available. If seizures continue at this point, additional doses of lorazepam should be infused and a second intravenous line placed to begin a concomitant phenytoin (or fosphenytoin) loading infusion. Even if seizures terminate after the initial lorazepam dose, therapy with phenytoin or fosphenytoin is generally indicated to prevent the recurrence of seizures.

Additional Reading: Convulus status epilepticus in adults: management. In: *UpToDate*. 2022.

Status epilepticus is best controlled with a benzodiazepine. Lorazepam should be administered intravenously. Diazepam or midazolam may be substituted if lorazepam is not available.

6. A mother presents with her young son concerned that he is at risk for familial periodic paralysis, as she was told that her husband's cousin had such a diagnosis. Which one of the following statements about familial periodic paralysis is true?

A) It is an autosomal recessive transmitted disorder.
B) It involves disturbances of potassium regulation.
C) It is associated with permanent muscle weakness.
D) It is aggravated by administration of acetazolamide.
E) It most commonly affects the elderly.

The answer is B: Familial periodic paralysis is an autosomal dominant transmitted disorder that is characterized by episodes of paralysis, loss of deep tendon reflexes, and failure of the muscles to respond to electrical stimulation. Onset is usually early in life; episodic weakness beginning after age 25 is almost never due to periodic paralysis. There is no alteration in mental status—patients remain alert during attacks. Muscle strength is normal between attacks. There are two basic types:

1. *Hypokalemic.* Attacks usually begin in adolescence. Symptoms occur the day after vigorous exercise. The symptoms are usually mild and may affect particular muscle groups (proximal muscles) or involve all extremities at once. Oropharyngeal and respiratory muscles are unaffected. The weakness usually lasts 24 to 48 hours. Meals high in carbohydrates and sodium may precipitate the attacks.
2. *Hyperkalemic.* Attacks usually occur earlier in childhood. They are shorter in duration, more frequent, and less severe. Attacks are usually associated with myotonia. Most patients are actually normokalemic during the attacks; however, the administration of potassium can precipitate the attack—thus the name. Diagnosis is made by the history, and serum potassium levels should be drawn during the attacks to determine the specific type of paralysis. Provocative testing with glucose and insulin can be used (in hypokalemic forms) with caution in those who have infrequent attacks. The treatment of choice for both types is acetazolamide. Potassium chloride may help abort hypokalemic attacks; calcium gluconate and furosemide may help abort hyperkalemic attacks.

Additional Reading: Hypokalemic periodic paralysis. In: *UpToDate*. 2020.

7. You are seeing a 19-year-old White woman who has been struggling with hiccups for the past week. She asks if there is a medication that she can take as she has tried several "home remedies"—even standing on her head while drinking a glass of sugar water without success. Which one of the following medications can help to treat her refractory hiccups?

A) Acetazolamide
B) Chlorpromazine
C) Chloral hydrate
D) Clonidine
E) Gabapentin

The answer is B: Hiccups are sudden, repeated, involuntary contractions of the diaphragm followed by abrupt closure of the glottis. They result from stimulation of the efferent and afferent nerves that innervate the diaphragm. Causes include excitement, alcohol consumption, and gastric distension caused by overeating. Low CO_2 levels tend to accentuate hiccups, and high levels tend to prevent them.

"Home remedies" include breathing into a paper bag, rapidly drinking a glass of water, swallowing dry bread, holding one's breath, or consuming crushed ice. In addition, gastric decompression may provide relief.

For refractive hiccups, chlorpromazine may be given orally or intravenously. Other medications include phenobarbital, scopolamine, metoclopramide, and narcotics. In severe cases, surgery to disrupt the phrenic nerve or to inject the phrenic nerve with a procaine solution may be performed.

Additional Reading: Hiccups. In: Domino F, ed. *The 5-Minute Clinical Consult*. Wolters Kluwer; 2022.

8. A 57-year-old teacher presents to your office complaining of headaches, which have been occurring almost daily for the past month. He describes the headache as being pronounced in the morning on awakening, associated with nausea and vomiting. The most likely diagnosis is which one of the following?

A) Brain tumor
B) Classic migraine headache
C) Cluster headache
D) Muscle tension headache
E) Sinus headache

The answer is A: There are several types of headache associated with specific clinical histories. The following are some common types and their distinguishing features:

- *Headaches associated with tumors.* Pain occurs daily, becomes more frequent and severe as time passes, and may be associated with focal neurologic deficits or visual disturbances. Patients may report pain more in the morning on awakening, nausea, vomiting, or the pain may be worse with bending over.
- *Migraine headaches.* These usually are pulsating and unilateral in location. They occur infrequently, are throbbing, and are associated with photophobia (in some cases an aura preceding the headache), nausea, and vomiting; sleep usually provides relief. They typically last 4 to 72 hours.
- *Cluster headaches.* More common in middle-aged men, these headaches are usually described as a unilateral, sharp (ie, "feels like an ice pick"), agonizing pain located in the orbital area, in many cases occurring 2 to 3 hours after the patient falls asleep; they are associated with tearing, nasal congestion, rhinorrhea, and autonomic symptoms on the same side as the headaches. Frequency of attacks ranges from 1 to 8 daily.
- *Muscle tension headaches.* These are associated with a bandlike tightness that encircles the scalp area, usually occurring on a daily basis and usually worse at the end of a workday.
- *Sinus headaches.* These are usually associated with facial pain or pressure in the sinus area from infection with associated purulent sinus drainage.

Additional Reading: Approach to acute headache in adults. *Am Fam Physician*. 2013;87(10):682-687.

9. A 61-year-old cashier presents to your office with complaints of slurring word and tingling in her right arm that lasted for about 10 minutes earlier in the day. She is feeling well now, but her husband insisted that she get it checked out. She has a history of elevated BP readings but has never taken any medication. She is overweight and leads a sedentary lifestyle. She used to smoke but quit when she turned 50, after smoking a pack per day since the age of 16 years. Her examination is benign, although her blood pressure (BP) is elevated at 148/96. Which one of the following actions is warranted at this time?

A) Admit to the hospital for a workup and observation.
B) Start an antihypertensive agent and see her back the next day.
C) Start aspirin and advise to call back if symptoms return.
D) Start warfarin and obtain an International Normalized Ratio the next day.

The answer is A: Transient ischemic attack (TIA) is considered a significant warning sign of impending stroke. It is crucial to recognize these events to prevent permanent disability or death in affected individuals. The 90-day risk of stroke after a TIA has been estimated to be approximately 10%, with one-half of strokes occurring within the first 2 days of the attack. The 90-day stroke risk is even higher when a TIA results from internal carotid artery disease.

The ABCD2 TIA Scoring System (age, BP, clinical features, duration, diabetes) can be used to determine risk, and if the score is >3, it is recommended that the patient be admitted and workup for a possible stroke. The scoring is as follows:

Sign/symptom	Points
Age ≥ 60 y	1
Systolic blood pressure ≥ 140 mm Hg or diastolic blood pressure ≥ 90 mm Hg	1
Unilateral weakness	2
Speech impairment without weakness	1
TIA duration ≥ 60 min	2
TIA duration 10-59 min	1
Diabetes mellitus	1
Consider admission total points	≥3

This patient's score is 5, so admission is warranted. An urgent computed tomographic scan or magnetic resonance imaging is performed within 24 hours to rule out an infarct, and a carotid ultrasonography is obtained for those >60 years of age. Risk factors (HTN, hyperlipidemia, diabetes) should be controlled. If indicated, smoking cessation and weight loss are also important.

In considering other actions, patients should be anticoagulated (eg, warfarin), if found to have atrial fibrillation, but started on an antiplatelet (eg, aspirin), if not. A carotid endarterectomy is recommended for critical stenosis.

Additional Reading: Transient ischemic attack: Part II. Risk factor modification and treatment. *Am Fam Physician.* 2012;86(6):527-532.

10. During which of the following stages of sleep does most dreaming occur?

A) Stage 1 non–rapid eye movement (REM) sleep
B) Stage 2 non-REM sleep
C) Stage 3 non-REM sleep
D) Stage 4 non-REM sleep
E) REM sleep

The answer is E: REM sleep is a phase of sleep characterized by random movement of the eyes, low muscle tone throughout the body, and the propensity of the sleeper to dream. There are two distinct states of sleep: REM sleep, which accounts for about 2 hours (25%) of the night's sleep, and non-REM sleep, which make up the remainder of sleep. Non-REM sleep is classified into four stages (1, 2, 3, and 4) based on electroencephalographic patterns. Sleep is a cyclical phenomenon with four to five REM periods nightly that always follow non-REM sleep and end each cycle.

The first period of REM sleep occurs approximately 1.5 to 2 hours after sleep has occurred and lasts approximately 10 minutes. A night's sleep cycles through the different stages and reenters REM stage three or four times for longer periods (15-45 minutes), usually in the past several hours of sleep. Non-REM sleep is characterized by slow waves on electroencephalography (EEG), with stage 4 being the deepest stage of sleep. REM sleep is characterized by low-voltage, fast activity on EEG. Most night terrors, sleep walking, and sleep talking occur during stage 4 sleep. In REM sleep, muscle tone is decreased, but depth of respiration is increased.

As patients become older, the length of REM sleep remains the same; however, there are significant decreases in stages 3 and 4 sleep and an increase in wakeful periods during the night. In addition, it takes elderly patients a longer period to fall asleep. Wakefulness is characterized by alpha wave activity on EEG.

Additional Reading: Management of common sleep disorders. *Am Fam Physician.* 2013;88(4):231-238.

11. Patients with Charcot-Marie-Tooth syndrome experience various signs and symptoms. Which one of the following statements about this syndrome is true?

A) Decreased sense of pain, temperature, and vibration
B) Foot drop
C) Hypertrophy of the distal leg muscles
D) Hyperreflexia

The answer is B: Charcot-Marie-Tooth syndrome (or peroneal muscular atrophy) is an autosomal dominant inherited disorder, affecting the peripheral nervous system. Manifestations include weakness and atrophy of the peroneal and distal leg muscles, which often result in a foot drop. The condition affects motor and sensory nerves. Other features include impaired sensation and absent or hypoactive deep tendon reflexes. There are two types:

Type 1: Usually occurs in middle childhood. Features include the development of a foot drop; decrease in pain, temperature, and vibratory sense; slow nerve conduction velocities; and loss of reflexes.

Type 2: Usually occurs later in life and is slower in its clinical course than type 1. Nerve conduction velocities are usually normal.

Patients with Charcot-Marie-Tooth syndrome typically present with abnormal high-stepped gait with frequent tripping or falling. Despite involvement with sensory nerves, complaints of limb pain and sensory disturbance are unusual. Treatment consists of braces to help prevent the associated foot drop. Surgery is reserved for those with severe foot deformities. Chemotherapeutic agents known to affect peripheral nerves should be used with great caution. Vincristine use should be avoided.

Additional Reading: *Charcot-Marie-Tooth Disease Fact Sheet.* National Institute of Neurological Disorders and Stroke; 2021. http://www.ninds.nih.gov/disorders/charcot_marie_tooth/detail_charcot_marie_tooth.htm

12. A 57-year-old previously healthy accountant sees you because of a tremor, which is most noticeable in his hands when he is holding something or writing. He has noticed that it seems better after having a beer or two at night. On examination, you note a very definite tremor when he unbuttons his shirt. His gait is normal and there is no resting tremor. Of the following, which medication would be the best choice for this patient?

A) Amantadine (Symmetrel)
B) Levodopa/carbidopa (Sinemet)
C) Lithium carbonate
D) Propranolol

The answer is D: Parkinson disease and essential tremors are the primary concerns in a person of this age who presents with a new tremor. A coarse, resting, pill-rolling tremor is a characteristic of Parkinson disease.

Essential tremor is the most common movement disorder. Its onset occurs anywhere between the second and sixth decades of life and its prevalence increases with age. The tremor is usually bilateral. The tremor is minimal or absent at rest. The tremor is slowly progressive over a period of years, and the specific pathophysiology of essential tremor remains unknown. Essential tremor occurs sporadically or can be inherited (in 50% of patients, inheritance is autosomal dominant). It most commonly affects the hands, but can also affect the head, voice, tongue, and legs. In many cases, essential tremor is alleviated by small amounts of alcohol, an effect not found in Parkinson disease.

β-Adrenergic blockers (eg, propranolol) have been the mainstay of treatment for essential tremors. Primidone has been effective in the treatment of essential tremor, and in head-to-head studies with propranolol, it has been shown to be superior after 1 year, although this is a barbiturate and should be used cautiously.

Levodopa in combination with carbidopa and amantadine is useful in the treatment of parkinsonian tremor but not essential tremor. Lithium is used as a mood stabilizer in treating bipolar disease.

Additional Reading: Tremor: sorting through the differential diagnosis. *Am Fam Physician*. 2018;97(3):180-186.

Essential tremor occurs anywhere between the second and sixth decades of life, and its prevalence increases with age. The tremor is usually bilateral and absent (or minimal) at rest.

13. A 42-year-old man presents with ataxia and his wife feels that his hearing has decreased as well. On examination, you detect multiple pigmented skin lesions. Interestingly, he notes that other members of his family are similarly affected. The most likely diagnosis is which one of the following conditions?

A) Hemochromatosis
B) Malignant melanoma
C) Measles
D) Neurofibromatosis
E) Sturge-Weber syndrome

The answer is D: Neurofibromatosis type 1 (NF1) and 2 (NF2) are neurocutaneous syndromes (phakomatoses). Although they share a name, they are distinct and unrelated conditions with genes on different chromosomes. NF2 is a rare condition that causes bilateral vestibular schwannomas. As many as 33% of patients are asymptomatic. Symptomatic patients may have blindness, dizziness, ataxia, deafness secondary to acoustic neuromas, or other symptoms related to nerve compression from neuromas. The diagnosis of neurofibromatosis is supported by the detection of more than six pigmented lesions or one lesion larger than 1.5 cm.

Asymptomatic patients do not require further therapy; however, those who exhibit symptoms may require surgery or radiation to remove offending neuromas. Genetic counseling is recommended.

Hemochromatosis is also an inherited disorder, due to a mutation in the *HFE* gene, resulting in excess iron accumulation in organs, most commonly the liver, adrenals, heart, skin, gonads, joints, and the pancreas, disrupting function. Patients can present with cirrhosis, polyarthropathy, adrenal insufficiency, heart failure, or diabetes.

Sturge-Weber syndrome is also one of the phakomatoses, with neurologic and skin findings. Symptoms include port-wine stains of the face, glaucoma, seizures, mental retardation, and cerebral malformations and tumors.

Additional Reading: Neurofibromatosis type 2. In: Domino F, ed. *The 5-Minute Clinical Consult*. Wolters Kluwer; 2022.

14. Your office is offering the annual flu vaccine and coronavirus disease 2019 booster, and one of your patients is concerned about developing Guillain-Barré syndrome from the immunizations. You inform her that the risk of developing Guillain-Barré syndrome is rare. This syndrome is most closely associated with which one of the following findings?

A) Descending asymmetric paralysis
B) Low levels of protein in the cerebrospinal fluid (CSF)
C) Normal electromyographic (EMG) findings
D) Symptoms that usually begin in the lower extremities

The answer is D: The cause of Guillain-Barré syndrome is not known but believed to be associated with an immunologic response. The disorder usually appears days or weeks after a respiratory or gastrointestinal tract infection and rarely following recent surgery or an immunization.

The syndrome is a demyelinating polyradiculopathy that usually presents with symmetrical weakness of the proximal muscles. Paresthesias of the toes and fingers may also occur. The symptoms usually begin in the lower extremity and may progress to involve the arms and face (ascending symmetric paralysis).

In severe cases, the respiratory muscles may be affected, and the patient may require mechanical ventilation. Other symptoms include tachycardia, hypotension, hypertension, diaphoresis, hyporeflexia, and loss of sphincter control.

Laboratory findings include elevated protein levels and minimal lymphocytic pleocytosis in CSF samples, altered EMG findings, and evidence of demyelination on nerve biopsies. Treatment involving the use of plasmapheresis and intravenous Ig has been shown to be beneficial, particularly early in the course of the disease (ie, within the first few days). Steroids have not been shown to be beneficial and may actually worsen the outcome. Most cases resolve spontaneously, but recovery may take months. Mortality is approximately 10%. Up to 20% of patients may be left with persisting deficits. Approximately 3% may develop relapses, sometimes years later.

Additional Reading: Guillain-Barre syndrome. *Am Fam Physician*. 2013;87(3):191-197.

15. You are seeing a 53-year-old White woman who has been plagued by restless legs syndrome (RLS) and she is asking you to prescribe medication to help. Which one of the following medications is effective for RLS?

A) Cobalamin
B) Diltiazem
C) Ropinirole
D) Haloperidol
E) Phenytoin

The answer is C: RLS is a relatively common problem seen by family physicians. The condition is characterized by repeated movements and paresthesias of the lower extremities (occasionally the arms). Patients may describe a tingling irritation or a drawing or crawling sensation that prevents the onset of sleep or may disturb sleep. The symptoms are often relieved by movement.

Laboratory and neurologic tests are usually normal, although associated conditions include iron deficiency, diabetes, uremia, pregnancy, rheumatoid arthritis, and vitamin B_{12} deficiency.

Treatment includes the use of levodopa/carbidopa (Sinemet), ropinirole (Requip), pramipexole (Mirapex), pergolide (Permax), gabapentin (Neurontin), carbamazepine (Carbatrol), and other antiepileptics, opiates, and benzodiazepines.

Additional Reading: AASM updates treatment guidelines for restless legs syndrome and periodic limb movement disorder. *Am Fam Physician*. 2013;87(4):290-292.

16. A 72-year-old woman presents to the emergency department with the acute onset of right-sided hemiplegia. She has a history of hypertension and has been treated with amlodipine. She is conscious but confused and agitated, and an emergent head computed tomographic scan is negative for cerebral hemorrhage. She has no cardiac findings, although her blood pressure (BP) is elevated at 210/110 mm Hg. Appropriate management at this time to address her elevated BP would be which one of the following?

A) Administer an additional dose of her amlodipine
B) Administer intravenous labetalol
C) Administer oral clonidine
D) Administer sublingual nifedipine
E) Observation

The answer is B: BP increase following an ischemic stroke is a response, not a cause of arterial occlusion in an effort to maintain cerebral perfusion and perfuse the penumbra (the ischemic area surrounding the infarct). Guidelines recommend lowering the BP only if the SBP is >220 or diastolic is >120 mm Hg. An additional consideration is if the patient is a candidate to receive tissue plasminogen activator thrombolysis (BP needs to be <185/110 mm Hg). The recommended approach is to administer labetalol (10 mg intravenously every 10 minute). The goal is to reduce BP by 15% to 25% in the first day, with continued BP control.

Aggressive treatment of hypertension in ischemic strokes worsens function by reducing perfusion pressure. The 2009 CHHIPS trial (Controlling Hypertension and Hypotension Immediately Post Stroke) showed that a drop in either systolic or diastolic BP > 20 points was associated with higher rates of mortality, and that the administration of antihypertensive medications to patients with systolic BP > 180 was also associated with an increased risk of death.

The maximal dose of labetalol is 300 mg. Alternative treatments include 1 to 2 inches of transdermal nitropaste or nicardipine infusion at 5 mg/h, titrated up to a maximum dose of 15 mg/h.

Additional Reading: Stroke. In: Domino F, ed. *The 5-Minute Clinical Consult*. Wolters Kluwer; 2022.

17. A 43-year-old White woman presents with a migraine headache. She reports that her headaches are like a band around her head and she is wondering if she should use sumatriptan to treat her headaches. You indicate that you are not sure that sumatriptan is the best treatment for her headache. Which one of the following best describes symptoms associated with a common migraine headache?

A) An aura preceding the onset of the headache
B) Recurrent headaches lasting less than 4 hours
C) Unilateral, throbbing headache
D) Bilateral, bandlike headache
E) Rhinitis with facial pain

The answer is C: There are basically two types of migraine headaches: those with an aura (classic migraine) and those without an aura (common migraine). A classic migraine is characterized by recurrent attacks of a moderate to severe unilateral, throbbing headache that is usually preceded by visual prodrome, which may include scotomata, zigzag lines, or other visual distortions. Patients also report nausea, vomiting, photophobia, mood swings, food cravings, and a heightened perception of smell. The unilateral "throbbing" headache may become generalized and usually lasts 4 to 72 hours.

Migraines usually begin at 10 to 40 years of age and are more common in women. Patients usually report a positive family history. The pathophysiology is not fully understood. Whether vasodilation or vasoconstriction is a cause or an effect of the migraine is unclear.

Triptans such as sumatriptan that activate serotonin receptors (5-hydroxytryptamine) block neurogenic inflammation and can abort migraine pain in approximately 70% of patients. This patient's symptoms are more consistent with a muscle tension headache, and sumatriptan is not indicated.

Migraine attacks may be triggered by emotional or physical stress, lack of sleep, specific foods (eg, chocolate and cheese), alcohol, oral contraceptives, or menstruation. Migraines usually disappear during pregnancy. Most patients experience a decrease in the number and intensity of headaches as they age. Common migraines are identical to classic migraines except that the patient does not have an aura, and the headache may last longer.

Additional Reading: Treatment of acute migraine headache. *Am Fam Physician*. 2011;83(3):271-280.

18. A 76-year-old woman presents to your office complaining of a headache that she has had off and on for the past couple of weeks. She describes the headache as affecting the right side of her head, and she has tenderness over the right temple area. She also complains of some blurry vision as well. You obtain some laboratory results and she has a mild anemia, with an erythrocyte sedimentation rate (ESR) of 110 mm/h. The most appropriate management at this time would be which one of the following?

A) A computed tomographic scan of the head
B) Administration of high-dose steroids
C) Administration of a nonsteroidal anti-inflammatory drug
D) A magnetic resonance imaging of the head
E) A referral to an ophthalmologist

The answer is B: This patient's presentation is suspicious for temporal arteritis, an inflammatory disease that predominantly affects the temporal and occipital arteries, although other arteries of the aortic arch may be involved. Systemic symptoms include low-grade fever, malaise, weakness, anorexia, weight loss, painful joints, headaches in the temporal distribution, and visual disturbances.

Most cases occur in patients older than 50 years, and women are more commonly affected than men. Although the cause is unknown, it is believed to be autoimmune in origin. Granulomatous inflammatory lesions involving the arteries are seen.

The diagnosis is made by the clinical history and an elevated ESR (usually greater than 100 mm/h). Leukocytosis and mild normochromic normocytic anemia are also usually seen. A biopsy of the temporal artery showing inflammation provides the definitive diagnosis.

If left untreated, the most serious complication of temporal arteritis is blindness. If temporal arteritis is suspected, high doses of corticosteroids (60 mg daily) should be initiated immediately. Monitoring the patient's ESR can determine dose reduction of steroid therapy. Significant improvement is usually seen within 4 weeks of therapy. Extended therapy (up to 2 years) may be necessary to control the disease.

Polymyalgia rheumatica (PMR) occurs in 40% to 60% of patients with temporal arteritis. PMR is a generalized inflammatory disorder that tends to affect middle-aged and elderly patients (usually older than 50 years). Onset of symptoms is usually rapid and includes fever, generalized fatigue, weight loss, and pain and stiffness associated with the shoulder girdle that may extend to involve other areas, including the pelvis.

Corticosteroids are also used to treat PMR, but in smaller doses (5-20 mg/d of prednisone) than required for temporal arteritis. The diagnosis of PMR is usually based on clinical findings supported by laboratory tests; however, temporal arteritis is usually confirmed with a temporal artery biopsy. Treatment usually requires months of a slow, gradual taper of steroids while following the ESR. In some cases, medication may be needed for extended periods (up to 1 year); relapses requiring extended courses are not unusual.

Additional Reading: Arteritis, temporal. In: Domino F, ed. *The 5-Minute Clinical Consult*. Wolters Kluwer; 2022.

19. A 37-year-old man presents urgently with his husband, as he awoke with a right-sided facial droop, and they are concerned that he has had a stroke. He is otherwise healthy and on no medication. You suspect Bell palsy. In making your diagnosis you consider that the distinguishing feature of Bell palsy versus a more worrisome central nervous system (CNS) lesion (eg, stroke and tumor) is to find which one of the following?

A) Involvement of the forehead muscles
B) Inability to close the affected eye
C) Lack of involvement below the eyes
D) Slurred speech

The answer is A: The distinguishing feature between Bell palsy and more worrisome CNS lesions is that Bell palsy involves the entire face (including muscles of the forehead), whereas CNS lesions tend to affect the face below the eyes and other areas including the arms and legs.

Bell palsy is characterized by a sudden onset of unilateral facial paralysis. It is thought to be the result of an infection (usually viral) affecting the facial nerve, which involves compression of the nerve within the temporal bone. Symptoms usually develop as pain behind the ear preceding the facial paralysis. In some cases, the patient cannot close the affected eye because of widening of the palpebral fissures.

In 80% to 90% of cases, the physical findings resolve completely within weeks to months after onset; however, in some isolated cases, permanent deficits may occur. Treatment involves the use of steroids, but they are somewhat controversial and are of questionable proven benefit. If the patient has difficulty closing the affected eye, it should be patched for protection against excessive drying.

Additional Reading: Bell palsy. In: Domino F, ed. *The 5-Minute Clinical Consult*. Wolters Kluwer; 2022.

20. A 33-year-old nurse presents to your office complaining of sensations of numbness, weakness, and difficulty with coordination and her gait. Her symptoms are worse after a hot shower. You referred her to a neurologist who performed a spinal tap, and she is calling your office to discuss the results. Her cerebral spinal fluid shows oligoclonal immunoglobulin G (IgG) bands. The most likely diagnosis to explain this presentation includes which one of the following?

A) Amyotrophic lateral sclerosis (ALS)
B) Huntington disease
C) Multiple sclerosis
D) Neurofibromatosis
E) Parkinson disease

The answer is C: Multiple sclerosis is a slowly demyelinating disease that affects the central nervous system (CNS). It is typically characterized by remissions and exacerbations that are separated in time and involve different areas of the CNS; some patients suffer from a more progressive course. The cause is unknown but may be related to a combination of genetic factors and perhaps infection with a slow or latent virus. Women are affected more than men (2:1), and there appears to be a geographic predominance, with those in the northern United States affected more than those in the southern United States. The onset is usually between 20 and 40 years of age, and the geographic factor is present even if the individual relocates to a tropical climate (as long as they spent their first 15 years in the north).

The pathology involves multiple plaques of demyelination that are found throughout the CNS. Symptoms include paresthesias, including Lhermitte symptom (sensation of a momentary electric current or shock when the neck is flexed), weakness, loss of coordination, or visual disturbances (monocular visual loss), initially followed by emotional lability, gait disturbances, and spasticity in more severe cases.

Signs include optic neuritis, speech difficulties, cranial nerve palsies, increased deep tendon reflexes, nystagmus, tremor, urinary incontinence, and impotence. Symptoms increase with exposure to heat. Diagnosis is usually made by the history, appearance of oligoclonal bands of IgG in the cerebrospinal fluid, and magnetic resonance imaging scans showing plaques of demyelination in the paraventricular white matter. Evoked potential nerve tests may also be abnormal.

Treatment is usually supportive; however, steroids and immunosuppressive drugs have been used, including interferon β-1b (Betaseron) and interferon β-1a (Avonex). Glatiramer acetate (Copaxone) is interferon-type medications used in the relapsing-remitting forms.

ALS, also called Lou Gehrig disease, after the baseball player who died from it, is a progressive nervous system disease that results in the loss of muscle control. It often begins with muscle twitching and weakness in a limb, or slurred speech. Eventually, ALS affects control of the muscles needed to move, speak, eat, and breathe, resulting in death.

Huntington disease, named for Dr. Huntington who first described it in the late 1800s, is a progressive brain disorder caused by a single defective gene on chromosome 4 that codes for huntingtin protein. The disease presents with abnormal involuntary uncontrolled movement of the arms, legs, head, face and upper body along with mood changes and cognitive decline. Symptoms develop in middle aged adults.

Neurofibromatoses are a group of genetic disorders that cause tumors to form anywhere in the nervous system, including the brain, spinal cord and peripheral nerves. Symptoms depend on the location of the tumors and can include hearing loss, intellectual disability, loss of vision, and pain.

Parkinson disease is a progressive decline in motor function due to the loss of dopaminergic nerve cells in the basal ganglia. Classic symptoms include slowed movements, tremors, and balance problems.

Additional Reading: Multiple sclerosis. In: Domino F, ed. *The 5-Minute Clinical Consult*. Wolters Kluwer; 2022.

21. You are seeing an adolescent boy with his mother, who is concerned over a recent diagnosis of Tourette syndrome and she is anxious about associated problems that he may have as he grows up. She is particularly worried that he might develop seizures as he gets older because his cousin suffers from epilepsy. You advise her that which one of the following conditions is usually associated with this syndrome?

A) Attention-deficit disorder
B) Cardiac arrhythmias
C) Hypertension
D) Hypothyroidism
E) Partial or complex seizures

The answer is A: Tourette syndrome is a neurologic disorder characterized by repetitive, stereotyped, involuntary movements, and vocalizations called tics. The disorder is named for Dr Georges Gilles de la Tourette, a French neurologist who first described the condition in 1885. Tics are noticed in childhood, with the average onset between the ages of 3 and 9 years, and men are affected about three to four times more often than women. Most people with Tourette syndrome experience symptoms in their early teens, with improvement occurring in the late teens and continuing into adulthood. The condition is often associated with psychiatric comorbidities, mainly attention-deficit/hyperactivity disorder and obsessive-compulsive disorder. The other conditions listed are not associated with Tourette syndrome.

Additional Reading: Tourette's syndrome. *Am Fam Physician*. 2008;77(5):651-658; 782-783.

22. A 49-year-old accountant presents for follow-up of her trigeminal neuralgia and she is asking about treatment options as she noted that her bouts of pain have been increasing in severity and frequency over the past couple of months and the Tylenol that she has been using seems ineffective. The drug of choice for the treatment of trigeminal neuralgia is which one of the following?

A) Carbamazepine
B) Naproxen
C) Phenobarbital
D) Prednisone
E) Valproic acid

The answer is A: Trigeminal neuralgia is a disorder that involves the nucleus of the trigeminal nerve. This disorder is characterized by severe, unilateral, sharp, lancing type of pain that occurs in the distribution of the trigeminal nerve. Most patients are of middle age or elderly. The symptoms usually occur in recurrent bouts and can be incapacitating. Women tend to be more frequently affected than men.

Precipitating factors include touching the affected area and movement of the face (as with eating, talking, and brushing one's teeth), shaving, or feeling a cool breeze on the face. Patients afflicted with trigeminal neuralgia show no physical signs. If deficits are noted during neurologic examination, then alternative diagnosis, including masses impinging on the trigeminal nerve, demyelinating processes, or vascular malformation, should be considered.

In most cases, the momentary bouts of pain become more and more frequent, and remissions become shorter and shorter. A dull ache that is persistent between the episodes of severe stabbing pain may develop. Remissions may occur and last for weeks or even months.

The treatment of choice is carbamazepine, which requires monitoring of serial blood counts and liver function tests. Alternative medications include phenytoin and baclofen. Other treatments include injecting glycerol into the offending nerve, surgery to decompress nerve fibers from blood vessels and bony structures, and radiofrequency rhizotomy if medical therapy fails.

Additional Reading: Trigeminal neuralgia. *Am Fam Physician*. 2016;94(2):133-135.

The drug of choice for the treatment of trigeminal neuralgia is carbamazepine.

23. A 24-year-old presents to your office with complaints of severe premenstrual syndrome (PMS) symptoms. On review of the symptoms, she also reports numbness in both of her feet. The most likely cause for her symptoms related to her feet is which one of the following?

A) Excessive nonsteroidal anti-inflammatory drug use
B) Excessive vitamin B_6 intake
C) Folate deficiency
D) Iron-deficiency anemia

The answer is B: Supplementation with 50 to 100 mg of vitamin B_6 per day may improve PMS symptoms; however, some women will take larger daily doses. The recommended dietary allowance is about 2 mg/d. High intake has been associated with toxicity, including neuropathy. An intake of 200 mg/d may cause reversible damage, and an intake of 2000 mg/d or greater is associated with peripheral neuropathy. In some European countries, the quantity of vitamin B_6 that may be purchased or prescribed has been restricted to reduce the risk of toxicity from excessive use.

Selective serotonin reuptake inhibitors have been shown to be effective in relieving PMS symptoms; however, paroxetine (Paxil) should be avoided because of its increased risk for congenital abnormalities when taken in the first trimester of pregnancy.

Additional Reading: Premenstrual syndrome and premenstrual dysphoric disorder. *Am Fam Physician*. 2016;94(3):236-240.

24. A 55-year-old man with a medical history of diabetes mellitus, hypertension, and dyslipidemia presented to the emergency department with several hours of left-sided arm weakness. A magnetic resonance image of his brain was consistent with an acute ischemic stroke in the middle cerebral territory. Which of the following is the best medical management for this patient?

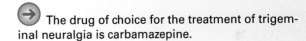

A) Aspirin
B) Heparin
C) Ibuprofen
D) Clopidogrel
E) Warfarin

The answer is A: Aspirin (160-300 mg) initiated within 48 hours of symptom onset results in a net decrease in morbidity and mortality caused by acute ischemic stroke regardless of the availability of computed tomographic scanning. Aspirin should not be used in patients receiving thrombolytic therapy, but that does not apply in this instance, as thrombolytic therapy must be started with 3 hours of symptom onset.

Ibuprofen (Motrin) may decrease aspirin's effectiveness in acute ischemic stroke. A Cochrane systematic review summarizing 15 trials (n = 16,558) comparing anticoagulants (unfractionated heparin or low-molecular-weight heparin) versus aspirin in acute ischemic stroke was published. No significant difference was found in rates of death or dependency, recurrent stroke, neurologic deterioration, or deep vein thrombosis/pulmonary embolism. However, anticoagulants were associated with higher rates of symptomatic intracranial hemorrhage, major extracranial hemorrhage, and all-cause mortality.

Two trials have evaluated the use of clopidogrel (Plavix) for secondary stroke prevention. One trial compared clopidogrel with aspirin alone and the other with a combination of aspirin and dipyridamole. Results from both trials found that rates of primary outcomes were similar between treatment groups. Adverse effects of clopidogrel include diarrhea and rash, although gastrointestinal symptoms and hemorrhage are less common than in persons taking aspirin. Proton pump inhibitors have been shown to reduce the effectiveness of clopidogrel and may also increase the risk of major cardiovascular events when taken with clopidogrel.

Compared with clopidogrel alone, the combination of clopidogrel and aspirin for prevention of vascular effects in persons with a recent transient ischemic attack or ischemic stroke was not found to have a significant benefit. There was a significantly increased risk of major hemorrhage in persons taking combination therapy compared with in those taking clopidogrel alone. When compared with aspirin alone, the combination of clopidogrel and aspirin did not have a statistically significant benefit but did increase the risk of bleeding in patients who had previously had a stroke.

Additional Reading: Antiplatelet agents for preventing early recurrence of ischemic stroke or TIA. *Am Fam Physician*. 2021;103(5):Online.

25. A 41-year-old woman presents with complaining of recurring headaches. They are typically unilateral, have a pulsatile quality, and are associated with nausea, and occasionally she experiences photophobia as well. The patient describes the headaches as intense, usually requiring her to limit her activities and can last for 1 to 2 days. She has tried several over-the-counter migraine medications that help a little, but asks you to prescribe something "stronger." All of the following would be recommended choices to use as first-line abortive therapy, except which one?

A) Acetaminophen/aspirin/caffeine compounds
B) Butalbital/aspirin/caffeine (Fiorinal)
C) Naprosyn
D) Sumatriptan (Imitrex)

The answer is B: Several different medications are recommended as first-line abortive therapies to treat acute migraine. But there are only a few trials directly comparing different medication classes and no definitive algorithms about which class works best. Nonsteroidal anti-inflammatory drugs and acetaminophen/aspirin/caffeine compounds are recommended as first-line therapies and can be obtained over the counter. Triptans are effective and safe for treatment of acute migraine and are recommended as first-line therapy but require a prescription. Opiates and barbiturates are not recommended because of their potential for abuse. Acetaminophen and oral corticosteroids alone are not effective.

Additional Reading: Treatment of acute migraine headache. *Am Fam Physician*. 2011;83(3):271-280.

26. Which one of the following is not a risk factor for stroke?

A) Alcohol consumption
B) Diabetes mellitus
C) Dyslipidemia
D) Hypertension (HTN)
E) Sickle cell disease

The answer is A: Stroke is a vascular phenomenon and the classic atherosclerotic risk factors are associated with stroke. These include diabetes, dyslipidemia, HTN, obesity, and sedentary lifestyles along with tobacco abuse. Unfortunately, children with sickle cell disease are also at increased risk.

Interestingly, studies have suggested that one alcoholic drink a day may lower a person's risk for stroke, and recommendations are for moderate alcohol consumption range from one to two drinks per day. Despite this potential benefit, patients should not be counseled to drink alcohol, and heavier drinking (more than three drinks per day) may actually increase the risk of stroke.

Blood pressure (BP) control after a transient ischemic attack (TIA) is associated with a 30% to 40% relative risk reduction, with larger BP decreases conferring a greater decrease in stroke risk.

Current smoking has been shown to increase BP, augment atherosclerosis, and increase the risk of stroke two- to fourfold compared with not smoking. There is a dose-response relationship between smoking and cerebral ischemia, with the heaviest smokers at the highest risk.

More than one in four persons will become clinically obese, and increased waist to hip ratio increases the risk of stroke. Regular physical activity has been shown to reduce the risk of TIA and stroke. High-intensity activity leads to a relative risk reduction of 64%, compared with inactivity.

Diets rich in fruits and vegetables, such as the Mediterranean diet, can help control body weight and have been shown to reduce the risk of stroke and myocardial infarction by at least 60%. The American Heart Association/American Stroke Association recommends weight reduction, at least 30 minutes of moderate to intensity physical activity daily, and a diet low in sodium and high in fruits, vegetables, and low-fat dairy products, such as the DASH diet.

Diabetes is a well-established risk factor for cardiovascular disease and confers a hazard ratio of 2.27 for ischemic stroke. Patients with newly diagnosed diabetes have double the rate of stroke compared with the general population, making early intervention and risk factor modification imperative. In most patients who have had a TIA, the A1c target is less than 7% as A1c reduction to targets of less than 6% has not been shown to decrease cardiovascular deaths or all-cause mortality.

Dyslipidemia has also been shown to be a significant risk factor for ischemic stroke. A large prospective cohort study showed a strong association between serum cholesterol levels and cerebral ischemia, with risk increasing proportionally to serum levels. In addition, a large meta-analysis studying the effect of statins on stroke reduction showed that the larger the reduction in low-density lipoprotein cholesterol levels, the greater the reduction in stroke risk.

Additional Reading: Transient ischemic attack: Part II. Risk factor modification and treatment. *Am Fam Physician*. 2012;86(6):527-532.

27. A 25-year-old White woman presents complaining of numbness in her toes; she is concerned because her uncle died of amyotrophic lateral sclerosis (ALS) and she was told that it runs in families. Which one of the following statements about ALS is true?

A) Dementia is a common late finding.
B) It is associated with destruction of motor neurons.
C) It is associated with destruction of sensory function.
D) It often improves with the administration of high-dose intravenous steroids.
E) The onset of symptoms is usually before 20 years of age.

The answer is B: ALS, also known as Lou Gehrig disease, is a progressive motor neuron disease that affects the corticospinal tracts. Onset of the disease is usually after 40 years of age, and the disease is more common in men. Approximately 5% to 10% of cases are familial and are associated with an autosomal dominant mode of transmission.

The hands are usually affected first with cramps, followed by weakness. Other manifestations include atrophy, muscle fasciculation, spasticity, and increased reflex response. There is usually a combination of upper and lower motor neuron signs. Dysarthria and dysphagia may occur; however, extraocular muscles, sensory function, sexual function, and urinary continence are usually not affected. Dementia is usually not present, although later in the illness, inappropriate, involuntary, and uncontrollable laughter or crying may occur (pseudobulbar palsy).

Diagnosis is usually made with electromyographic findings that correlate with the clinical presentation. Unfortunately, there is no treatment other than supportive care. Baclofen has been used to treat muscular spasticity and cramping. Death as a result of respiratory failure usually occurs within 5 years.

Additional Reading: Amyotrophic lateral sclerosis. In: Domino F, ed. *The 5-Minute Clinical Consult*. Wolters Kluwer; 2022.

28. You are seeing a 73-year-old White woman who has been taking large dose of antioxidants, including vitamin A as she is concerned about developing cancer as she gets older. You inform her that antioxidants are best consumed as fruits and vegetables, and that large dose of supplements can actually cause harm. Toxicity associated with excess vitamin A intake has been associated with which one of the following?

A) Increased intracranial pressure and vomiting
B) Night blindness
C) Peripheral neuropathy
D) Pulmonary fibrosis
E) Renal stones

The answer is A: Excessive ingestion of vitamin A may cause acute or chronic toxicity. Acute toxicity especially in children may result from taking large doses (>300,000 IU). The condition is associated with increased intracranial pressure and vomiting, which may lead to death. After discontinuation, recovery is usually spontaneous, with no residual damage.

Infants who are given 20,000 to 60,000 IU/d of water-soluble vitamin A may show evidence of toxicity within a few weeks. Birth defects have been reported in the children of women receiving isotretinoin (a vitamin A derivate) for skin conditions during pregnancy.

Megavitamin tablets containing vitamin A have occasionally induced acute toxicity when taken long term. Chronic toxicity usually affects older children and adults after taking daily doses of >100,000 IU for an extended course over several months.

Additional Reading: Overview of vitamin A. In: *UpToDate*; 2022.

29. A 62-year-old woman with long-standing type 2 diabetes presents with concern over weakness of her lower left leg and discomfort in her anterior thigh for the past week. Her knee has given out on a couple of occasions as well, although she has caught herself to avoid a fall and she has no recent injury. On examination, you find decreased sensation to pinprick and light touch over the left anterior thigh and reduced strength on hip flexion and knee extension. The straight leg raising test is normal. Which of the following is the most likely cause of this condition?

A) Diabetic polyneuropathy
B) Femoral neuropathy
C) Iliofemoral atherosclerosis
D) Meralgia paresthetica
E) Spinal stenosis

The answer is B: Femoral neuropathy can be a mononeuropathy or affect both limbs and is commonly seen with diabetes mellitus, although it has been found to be secondary to several conditions that are common in diabetics and not specifically to the diabetes.

Diabetic polyneuropathy is characterized by symmetric and distal limb sensory and motor deficits.

Iliofemoral atherosclerosis, a relatively common complication of diabetes mellitus, may produce intermittent claudication involving one or both calf muscles but would not produce the motor weakness noted in this patient.

Meralgia paresthetica, or lateral femoral cutaneous neuropathy, may be secondary to diabetes mellitus, but is manifested by numbness and paresthesia over the anterolateral thigh with no motor dysfunction.

Spinal stenosis causes pain in the legs, but is not associated with the neurologic signs seen in this patient, nor is it associated with knee problems.

Additional Reading: Evaluation and prevention of diabetic neuropathy. *Am Fam Physician*. 2005;71(11):2123-2128.

Diabetic polyneuropathy is characterized by symmetric and distal limb sensory and motor deficits.

30. You are caring for a 36-year-old man with severe alcohol use disorder who has been admitted with increasing confusion and you are concerned that he has developed Wernicke-Korsakoff syndrome. Which one of the following treatments should administered when a patient is suspected of having this syndrome?

A) Administration of intravenous (IV) glucose followed by thiamine
B) Administration of folic acid followed by IV dextrose
C) Administration of haloperidol intramuscularly
D) Administration of thiamine followed by IV dextrose
E) Administration of IV lactated Ringer's solution with naloxone

The answer is D: Wernicke-Korsakoff syndrome refers to the coexistence of Wernicke encephalopathy and Korsakoff psychosis. Wernicke encephalopathy is characterized by gait ataxia, mental confusion, nystagmus, vomiting, fever, and ophthalmoplegia. The disease is primarily seen in alcoholics but can also occur in hyperemesis gravidarum or the use of vitamin-free nutrition (eg, fad diets). The cause is thiamine deficiency (also known as *beriberi*).

Wernicke encephalopathy is a medical emergency and requires prompt attention; otherwise, permanent brain damage or even death may occur. If Wernicke encephalopathy is suspected, thiamine should always be administered before dextrose. Administration of glucose solution before thiamine administration may exhaust a patient's reserve of B vitamins and worsen his or her condition.

Korsakoff psychosis is also related to thiamine deficiency and may follow Wernicke disease. Symptoms include retrograde amnesia, impaired learning ability, and confabulation. Treatment also involves the administration of thiamine.

Additional Reading: Evaluation of suspected dementia. *Am Fam Physician*. 2011;84(8):895-902.

31. You are caring for an older woman who had recovered from polio in her right leg in her childhood. She has been developing some numbness in that leg over the past few weeks and is concerned that the polio has come back. True statements about postpolio syndrome include all of the following, except which one?

A) The syndrome represents a recurrence of the polio infection.
B) Symptoms typically occur 15 to 30 years after the initial infection.
C) The areas affected during the original infection are the same areas affected with the post-polio syndrome.
D) Treatment is supportive and involves rest.

The answer is A: Postpolio syndrome is a constellation of symptoms that affects patients previously infected with the poliovirus. The new symptoms are not due to reinfection of the poliovirus, but secondary to other conditions such as diabetes, disk herniation, or degenerative joint disease and/or aging.

Typically, symptoms occur 15 to 30 years after the initial infection and include progressive generalized weakness, muscle pain, cramps, fasciculations, and atrophy. Other findings include cold, cyanotic extremities that have adequate pulses, and diffuse joint pain. Typically, the areas that were affected during the original infection are the same areas affected with the postpolio syndrome. Treatment is supportive and involves rest.

Additional Reading: Post-polio syndrome. In: *UpToDate*. 2021.

32. A 73-year-old man presents to your office, as he has been having episodes over the past couple of months where his eyelid droops and he has been experiencing occasional double vision. He is worried about stroke, but you are considering myasthenia gravis as the diagnosis. Which one of the following statements about myasthenia gravis is true?

A) Symptoms are aggravated by the administration of edrophonium.
B) Symptoms rarely fluctuate and usually spare the facial nerves.
C) Symptoms usually involve problems with sensory function.
D) Symptoms also include dysarthria, dysphagia, and proximal muscle weakness of the limbs.

The answer is D: Myasthenia gravis is a disorder of the neuromuscular junction and is thought to be associated with an autoimmune attack on the postsynaptic acetylcholine receptor sites, which prevents neurosynaptic transmission. It may occur at any age and may be associated with thymic tumors, thyrotoxicosis, lupus, or rheumatoid arthritis. It appears to be linked to the HLA-DR3 genetic focus.

Episodic muscle weakness is a symptom that often fluctuates in intensity, particularly in muscles associated with the cranial nerves; this includes ptosis, diplopia, dysarthria, dysphagia, and proximal muscle weakness in the limbs. These symptoms improve when cholinesterase-inhibiting medications (eg, neostigmine) are administered. Sensory function and deep tendon reflexes are unaffected.

Diagnosis is usually confirmed by the edrophonium (Tensilon) test, which involves administration of an anticholinesterase medication. This test can help distinguish between a myasthenic and a cholinergic crisis. The patient is given 2 mg of edrophonium intravenously. If the patient's symptoms improve, the diagnosis of myasthenia gravis is confirmed. If symptoms become worse, a cholinergic crisis should be suspected. Because of the potential for respiratory arrest, atropine must be available as an antidote. Other findings that support the diagnosis of myasthenia gravis include the detection of acetylcholine receptor antibodies in the patient's serum and the detection of thymomas by chest computed tomographic scans.

Treatment is with the use of anticholinesterase medications (eg, pyridostigmine and neostigmine), thymectomy, corticosteroids, immunosuppressive agents, and plasmapheresis.

Additional Reading: Myasthenia gravis. In: Domino F, ed. *The 5-Minute Clinical Consult*. Wolters Kluwer; 2022.

33. A young man with acquired immunodeficiency syndrome (AIDS) has been admitted with increasing confusion and has been diagnosed with cryptococcal meningitis. The treatment of choice for this infection is which one of the following treatments?

A) Acyclovir
B) Amantadine
C) Amphotericin B and flucytosine
D) Metronidazole
E) Penicillin G

The answer is C: Cryptococcosis is an infection caused by the fungus *Cryptococcus neoformans* that usually involves the lungs, which spreads to the meninges and other organs. The disease is found worldwide and affects immune-deficient patients with lymphoma and AIDS or those chronically taking steroids.

Symptoms include headaches, blurred vision, and mental status changes. In addition, the patient usually reports a persistent cough, which reflects pulmonary involvement. The disease is acquired by respiratory transmission. Skin lesions and the development of osteomyelitis are infrequent; however, as many as 33% of patients with meningeal involvement also have renal involvement.

Laboratory tests show cerebrospinal fluid with an increased protein, a white cell count that is mostly lymphocytes, and a decreased glucose level with meningeal involvement. Culture of sputum, blood, urine, or other areas of involvement is diagnostic. The diagnosis is also supported with the evidence of budding yeast seen with India ink preparation.

The treatment of choice for cryptococcal meningitis is intravenous amphotericin B and oral flucytosine until lumbar cultures are clear, followed by lifelong prophylaxis with fluconazole. Amphotericin and itraconazole are alternatives. Nonprogressive pulmonary cryptococcosis may not require treatment in patients who are not immunocompromised.

Additional Reading: C. neoformans infection. In: Fungal Diseases. www.cdc.gov.

34. A 65-year-old woman whom you have cared for over the years presents to your office today with complaints of muscle cramping. She has also been feeling depressed and her skin has been very dry. Her medical history is remarkable for a long-standing seizure disorder that has been controlled with phenytoin (Dilantin). While taking her vital signs, she develops carpopedal spasms after application of the blood pressure (BP) cuff. The most likely diagnosis is which one of the following conditions?

A) Hypothyroidism
B) Hyperventilation with panic attacks
C) Hyperkalemia
D) Hypocalcemia
E) Hyponatremia

The answer is D: Hypocalcemia is defined as a decrease in total plasma calcium concentration <8.8 mg/dL in the presence of normal plasma protein concentration. Causes include hypoparathyroidism, vitamin D deficiency, renal tubular disease, magnesium depletion, acute pancreatitis, hypoproteinemia, septic shock, hyperphosphatemia, and drugs, including phenytoin, phenobarbital, and rifampin.

Most patients are asymptomatic. Symptoms, when present, include muscle cramps involving the legs and back, mental status changes, dry skin, depression, and psychosis. Papilledema may occasionally occur, and cataracts may develop after prolonged hypocalcemia. Severe hypocalcemia (<7 mg/dL) may cause tetany, laryngospasm, or generalized seizures.

With hypocalcemia giving rise to latent tetany, the patient may exhibit a positive Chvostek sign (involuntary twitching of the facial muscles caused by a light tapping of the facial nerve just anterior to the exterior auditory meatus) or a positive Trousseau sign (carpopedal spasm caused by reduction of the blood supply to the hand with a BP cuff inflated to 20 mm Hg above the SBP applied to the forearm after 3 minutes). Carpopedal spasms result in flexion of the hands at the wrists and of the fingers at the metacarpophalangeal joints and extension of the fingers at the phalangeal joints; the feet are dorsiflexed at the ankles and the toes are plantar-flexed.

Hypocalcemia can cause heart block and arrhythmias. Electrocardiographic changes show prolongation of the QTc and ST intervals. T-wave peaking or inversion can also occur.

Severe hypocalcemic tetany is treated initially with intravenous infusion of calcium salts (calcium gluconate). In chronic hypocalcemia, oral calcium and vitamin D supplements are usually sufficient. Treatment of hypocalcemia in patients with renal failure must be combined with dietary phosphate restriction and phosphate-binding agents such as calcium carbonate to prevent hyperphosphatemia and metastatic calcification.

Additional Reading: Clinical manifestations of hypocalcemia. In: *UpToDate*. 2022.

35. Shy-Drager syndrome is best characterized by which one of the following signs?

A) Autonomic dysfunction
B) Unilateral foot drop
C) Peripheral neuropathy
D) Proximal muscle weakness
E) Muscle atrophy

The answer is A: Shy-Drager syndrome (multiple system atrophy) affects multiple organ systems and causes neurologic damage, including autonomic dysfunction with cerebellar ataxia, parkinsonism, corticospinal, and corticobulbar tract dysfunction. Patients may experience orthostatic hypotension, impotence, urinary retention, fecal incontinence, decreased sweating, iris atrophy, and decreased tearing and salivation.

Treatment consists of intravascular volume expansion with the administration of fludrocortisone, application of constrictive garments to the lower extremities, and the administration of an α-adrenoreceptor stimulator midodrine. Bulbar dysfunction and laryngeal stridor can be fatal if not treated.

Additional Reading: *Multiple System Atrophy With Orthostatic Hypotension*. 2021. www.ninds.nih.gov/disorders/msa_orthostatic_hypotension/msa_orthostatic_hypotension.htm.

36. A young dairy farmer comes in with concern over mad cow disease (bovine spongiform encephalopathy [BSE]) because several of his cows have become ill and one has died. Mad cow disease has symptoms similar to which one of the following conditions?

A) Chronic fatigue syndrome
B) Creutzfeldt-Jakob disease
C) Lyme disease
D) Malaria
E) Syphilis

The answer is B: BSE presents as an encephalopathy, which progresses to an eventual death. BSE is transferred among cows through feed made from the rendered carcasses of cattle that contain a prion that has been linked to BSE. A prion is an infectious protein agent that can lead to diseases, similar to a viral infection. In the United Kingdom, a human illness called "new-variant Creutzfeldt-Jakob disease" gave rise to a theory that BSE can be transferred to humans who eat contaminated beef. Because of the potential risk of human transmission, the use of mammalian tissues such as meat, bone meal, meat by-products, and cooked bone marrow in feed for cattle and other ruminant animals has been banned in the United States.

Additional Reading: *BSE (Bovine Spongiform Encephalopathy, or Mad Cow Disease)*. Center for Disease Control and Prevention. http://www.cdc.gov/ncidod/dvrd/bse

37. A 62-year-old man presents with shaking of his left leg, which has been slowly increasing over the past few months. You are concerned that he is developing Parkinson disease. True statements about Parkinson disease include all of the following, except which one?

A) The tremor occurs at rest.
B) The classic presentation involves a pill-rolling tremor.
C) Rigidity and joint stiffness accompany the tremor.
D) Falls are frequent because of rapid movements.

The answer is D: Tremor is a symptom of many disorders, including Parkinson disease, essential tremor, orthostatic tremor, cerebellar disease, peripheral neuropathy, and alcohol withdrawal. Tremors may be classified as postural, rest, or action tremors. Symptomatic treatment is directed to the tremor type.

The tremor in Parkinson disease occurs at rest and is characterized by a frequency of 4 to 6 Hz and medium amplitude. It is not also classically referred to as a *pill-rolling* tremor of the hands but can also affect the head, trunk, jaw, and lips. Parkinson has been referred to as "shaky, slow, stiff, and stumbling," reflecting the cardinal motor symptoms of a resting tremor, bradykinesia (slow movements), rigidity, and postural instability with falls that tend to occur as the disease progresses.

Combination therapy with carbidopa and levodopa is commonly used for parkinsonian tremor, to replace the dopamine that is lacking in the substantia nigra.

Additional Reading: Differentiation and diagnosis of tremor. *Am Fam Physician*. 2011;83(6):697-702.

38. You are seeing a 57-year-old man who complains of difficulty with his gait and numbness and a loss of sensation in the soles of the feet. He had been treated for syphilis in his youth. His presentation is most consistent with which one of the following conditions?

A) Granuloma inguinale
B) Syphilitic polyneuropathy
C) Tabes dorsalis
D) Tuberculosis

The answer is C: Tabes dorsalis (syphilitic myelopathy) is due to a slow demyelination of the neural tracts in the dorsal columns of the spinal cord. These nerves help to maintain a person's sense of position (proprioception), vibration, and discriminative touch.

The main symptom is a periodic, insidious, progressive stabbing pain that affects the lower extremities. Over time, the patient may experience increasing difficulty with gait, particularly in poorly illuminated areas. Paresthesias and loss of sensation are commonly associated with the soles of the feet. Other findings include a thin appearance with sad- or depressed-appearing facies, Argyll Robertson pupils (react poorly to light but well to accommodation), positive Romberg sign, loss of reflexes in the lower extremities, bladder disturbances, and visible ataxia. Acute abdominal pain with vomiting (visceral crisis) can occur in 15% to 30%.

In tabes dorsalis, the rapid plasma reagin and Venereal Disease Research Laboratory tests may not be positive; however, the fluorescent treponemal antibody-absorption test is usually positive. Treatment involves the administration of a prolonged course of high-dose penicillin to treat syphilis. Pain medications along with chlorpromazine and carbamazepine may be helpful for the control of pain. Unfortunately, tabes dorsalis often progresses despite treatment.

Tabes dorsalis is also known as syphilitic myelopathy; the infection does not cause a polyneuropathy. Granuloma inguinale (also known as donovanosis) is characterized by ulcerative genital lesions caused by a *Klebsiella granulomatis* infection. It is treated with doxycycline. Tuberculosis primarily presents with respiratory symptoms, because of an infection caused by the bacterium *M tuberculosis*.

Additional Reading: *Syphilis Treatment and Care*. www.cdc.gov/std/syphilis/treatment.htm

39. Friedreich ataxia (FA) is a rare inherited disease that damages the nervous system. True statements about FA include all of the following, except which one?

A) It is inherited as an autosomal recessive trait.
B) It usually begins in early adulthood.
C) It leads to impaired muscle coordination (ataxia) that worsens over time.
D) Most individual dies due to dementia-related complication.

The answer is D: FA is inherited as an autosomal recessive a mutation of the *FXN* gene. Although rare, FA is the most common form of hereditary ataxia, affecting about 1 in every 50,000 people in the United States. FA usually begins in childhood and leads to impaired muscle coordination (ataxia) that worsens over time. The disorder is named after Nikolaus Friedreich, a German doctor who first described the condition in the 1860s.

In FA the spinal cord and peripheral nerves degenerate; the cerebellum is also affected, but to a lesser extent. Neuronal damage results in awkward, unsteady movements and impaired sensory functions. The disorder does not affect cognition.

Symptoms typically begin between the ages of 5 and 15 years, although they sometimes appear in adulthood and on rare occasions as late as 75 years of age. The first symptom to appear is usually gait ataxia or difficulty walking. The ataxia gradually worsens and slowly spreads to the arms and the trunk. There is often loss of sensation in the extremities, which may spread to other parts of the body. Dysarthria (slowness and slurring of speech) develops and can get progressively worse. Many individuals with later stages of FA develop hearing and vision loss.

The rate of progression varies from person to person. Generally, within 10 to 20 years after the appearance of the first symptoms, the person is confined to a wheelchair, and in later stages of the disease, individuals may become completely incapacitated.

Additional Reading: Friedreich ataxia. In: *UpToDate*. 2022.

Section IX. Hematology

Questions related to hematology account for about another 2% of the American Board of Family Medicine certifying examination. As you study for the examination, ensure that you have a good overview of the following topics:

1. Anemia
   - Appreciate the workup for microcytic anemia.
   - Understand the treatment of iron-deficiency anemia.
   - Appreciate the workup for macrocytic anemia.
   - Understand the treatment of pernicious anemia.
   - Know the diagnostic criteria for anemia of chronic disease.
   - Understand the appropriate use of Procrit.
2. Oncology topics
   - Appreciate an overview of lymphoma (eg, non-Hodgkin lymphoma is the most common type in the United States; Hodgkin lymphoma is associated with Reed-Sternberg cells and supraclavicular lymph nodes).
   - Appreciate an overview of leukemia (eg, in adults, chronic lymphocytic leukemia and acute myelogenous leukemia are the most common; acute lymphoblastic leukemia in children; Philadelphia chromosome is associated with chronic myelocytic leukemia).
   - Appreciate an overview of multiple myeloma (eg, disease of the elderly due to plasma cell malignancy; associated with Bence Jones protein in the urine; treatment includes bisphosphonates).

Each of the following questions or incomplete statements is followed by suggested answers or completions. Select the ONE BEST ANSWER in each case.

1. Patients with chronic renal disease have an associated anemic condition; this anemia is usually caused by insufficient levels of which one of the following substances?

A) Erythropoietin
B) Folate
C) Iron
D) Renin
E) Vitamin B_{12}

The answer is A: Serum recombinant erythropoietin is used to treat refractory anemia in patients with chronic renal disease. The synthetic drug replaces erythropoietin that is normally produced by the kidneys and lacking in renal disease, with the resultant anemic state. The drug does not appear to accelerate the preexisting renal disease. Hemoglobin goals should not exceed 11 g/dL (110 g/L) in patients receiving erythropoiesis-stimulating agents because of the risk of major cardiovascular events associated with higher levels. Iron supplementation must be given to achieve an adequate erythropoietin response.

Additional Reading: Update on the management of chronic kidney disease. *Am Fam Physician*. 2012;86(8):749-754.

2. A 37-year-old woman presents to your office with complaints of a speckled rash on her legs. On examination, you notice petechiae on her lower extremities and order a complete blood count. The platelet count is reported out as 10,000 cells/cm. All of the following signs can be seen with this degree of thrombocytopenia, except which one would be unlikely to be present?

A) Ecchymosis at the site of minor trauma
B) Epistaxis
C) Hemarthrosis
D) Oral mucosal bleeding
E) Vaginal bleeding

The answer is C: Thrombocytopenia is caused by decreased platelet production, splenic sequestration of platelets, increased platelet destruction or use, or dilution of platelets. Severe thrombocytopenia results in a characteristic pattern of bleeding: multiple petechiae in the skin, often most evident on the lower legs; scattered small ecchymoses at sites of minor trauma; mucosal bleeding (epistaxis, bleeding in the gastrointestinal [GI] and genitourinary tracts, vaginal bleeding); and excessive bleeding following surgical procedures. Heavy GI bleeding and bleeding into the central nervous system may be life-threatening.

However, thrombocytopenia does not cause massive bleeding into tissues, so that deep visceral hematomas and hemarthroses (bleeding into a joint) would not be present. This type of bleeding is characteristic of bleeding secondary to coagulation disorders such as hemophilia.

Medications associated with thrombocytopenia include heparin (up to 5%, even with very low doses), quinidine, quinine, sulfa preparations, oral antidiabetic drugs, gold salts, and rifampin.

Additional Reading: Thrombocytopenia. *Am Fam Physician*. 2012;85(6):612-622.

3. Iron-deficiency anemia is one of the most common anemias seen in the family physician's office. This type of anemia is associated with which one of the following findings?

A) Elevated serum iron levels
B) Hyperchromic, macrocytic morphology
C) Increased serum ferritin levels
D) Increased total iron-binding capacity (TIBC) levels
E) Normal bone marrow biopsy results

The answer is D: Iron-deficiency anemia produces a hypochromic, microcytic anemia. Causes include excessive menstruation, gastrointestinal blood loss, inadequate iron consumption, malabsorption, pregnancy, or excessive growth in the absence of adequate iron consumption during infancy.

Symptoms may include generalized weakness and fatigue, facial pallor, glossitis, cheilosis, and angular stomatitis. In chronic, severe cases, patients may have pica (eg, craving for dirt, paint), pagophagia (craving for ice), or dysphagia associated with a postcricoid esophageal web. Physical examination may show skin pallor, dry brittle nails, and tachycardia with perhaps a flow murmur.

Laboratory evaluation will reveal microcytic, hypochromic morphology on the blood smear, and the red blood cell (RBC) indices become microcytic when the hematocrit falls below 32%. Laboratory tests will show a decreased hemoglobin and hematocrit, low serum iron concentration, low ferritin, and increased TIBC. Bone marrow aspiration shows diminished iron stores with small, pale RBCs.

Treatment is the administration of iron replacement for 6 to 12 months until iron stores are replenished. The addition of ascorbic acid enhances iron absorption without increasing gastric distress.

Additional Reading: Iron deficiency anemia: evaluation and management. *Am Fam Physician*. 2013;87(2):98-104.

4. A 65-year-old woman presents with complaints of a sore tongue and diarrhea. She has been losing weight and recently has been having tingling in her hands and feet. Her laboratory work reveals a macrocytic anemia. The most likely condition to account for her constellation of signs and symptoms is which one of the following?

A) Colon cancer
B) Iron-deficiency anemia
C) Multiple myeloma
D) Pernicious anemia
E) Thalassemia minor

The answer is D: Vitamin B_{12} (cobalamin) deficiency is associated with several different conditions, including pernicious anemia (lack of intrinsic factor required for vitamin B_{12} absorption), celiac sprue, Crohn disease, and previous gastrectomy. Causes for vitamin B_{12} deficiency include inadequate diet, inadequate absorption, inadequate use, increased requirement, and increased excretion.

Symptoms include anorexia, weight loss, paresthesias, ataxia, dementia, neuropsychiatric changes, and diarrhea. Signs include glossitis (a smooth and erythematous tongue with loss of the lingual papillae), tachycardia, abnormal reflexes, positive Romberg sign, and abnormal positional and vibratory sensation.

Laboratory findings include a macrocytic anemia, diminished vitamin B_{12} levels, and low reticulocyte counts. Mild thrombocytopenia, leukopenia, elevated lactate dehydrogenase, and indirect bilirubin levels due to ineffective erythropoiesis are also seen.

Treatment consists of removing the underlying cause of vitamin B_{12} deficiency. Vitamin replacement therapy can be used. Iron deficiency, which coexists in up to one-third of patients, should be ruled out. The recommended daily allowance is 2 μg. Vitamin B_{12} is usually used slowly and, unless there is absence of the vitamin for months, there are sufficient stores to prevent deficiency. A strict vegetarian diet avoids the consumption of meat, dairy products, seafood, and poultry (including eggs). Unfortunately, vegetarians often lack adequate vitamin B_{12}; physicians should look for deficiencies in this population. Meat substitutes, enriched yeast, and soybean milk are alternative sources for vitamin B_{12}.

Iron-deficiency anemia and thalassemia minor would present with a microcytic anemia. Anemia is a common complication in patients with multiple myeloma but is usually normocytic.

Additional Reading: Update on vitamin B_{12} deficiency. *Am Fam Physician*. 2011;83(12):1425-1430.

5. Sickle cell anemia is an autosomal dominant inherited hemolytic anemia that predominantly affects African Americans, with approximately 8% of the African American population effected. Which one of the following statements about sickle cell anemia is true?

A) Hydroxyurea is contraindicated for patients with sickle cell anemia.
B) Individuals with sickle cell should avoid influenza vaccination.
C) Patients with sickle cell should receive pneumococcal vaccination.
D) The disease is a sex-linked, recessive, inherited disorder.
E) The condition is related to a defective β chain with sickling under conditions of low CO_2.

The answer is C: Sickle cell anemia has various signs and symptoms that are caused by the abnormal sickling shape of the RBCs, which occurs under low oxygen (pO_2) conditions. This defect occurs because of a mutation in the *Beta-hemoglobin* gene found on chromosome 11 (valine substituted for glutamic acid at the sixth position of the β chain). This abnormal hemoglobin is called hemoglobin S (HbS). The condition is manifested in a milder heterozygote form (referred to as sickle cell trait) and in the more severe homozygote form.

Signs and symptoms include anemia, jaundice, arthralgias, fever, painful aplastic crises that are characterized by severe abdominal and joint pain, poor-healing ulcers associated with the pretibial area, nausea, vomiting, hemiplegia, and cranial nerve palsies. Other manifestations include pulmonary and renal dysfunction, cardiomegaly, hepatosplenomegaly, cholelithiasis, and aseptic necrosis of the femoral heads. Heterozygous individuals are usually unaffected by these complications.

Laboratory findings include normocytic, normochromic anemia with a peripheral smear showing sickled red cells with Howell-Jolly bodies and target cells, leukocytosis with a left shift, thrombocytosis, elevated bilirubin levels, and elevated urinary and fecal urobilinogen. Erythrocyte sedimentation rates are usually normal. Diagnosis is usually made by hemoglobin electrophoresis demonstrating HbS chains. Heterozygous individuals usually show hemoglobin A and HbS chains.

Treatment is symptomatic and may include transfusions in severe cases, hydration, pain control, and possible corticosteroids. Hydroxyurea is also useful in the treatment of sickle cell anemia. Most crises are precipitated by infections, and treatment should provide coverage for these infections. Because of splenic dysfunction, those affected are at an increased risk for bacterial infections, particularly pneumococcal and *Salmonella* infections; therefore, they should receive the pneumococcal vaccine. Genetic counseling should also be instituted for those affected. Life spans may be shortened for those affected but have been increasing.

Additional Reading: Anemia, sickle cell. In: Domino F, ed. *The 5-Minute Clinical Consult*. Wolters Kluwer; 2022.

➔ **Sickle cell anemia has various and symptoms that are caused by the abnormal sickling shape of the red blood cells, which occurs under low blood oxygen conditions.**

6. A 46-year-old man presents for a follow-up visit for his diabetes and he has increasing complaints of joint pain. His neighbor had commented that he seemed nicely tanned this winter, yet he has not been in the sun. On examination, you also note a bronze discoloration of his skin and detect testicular atrophy. His laboratory test results show an A1c level of 7.2% and he has an elevated serum iron level of 500 μg/dL, serum ferritin of 2000 ng/mL, and a transferrin saturation of 80%. The most likely diagnosis that would account for this presentation is which one of the following?

A) Alcoholism
B) Gilbert disease
C) Hemochromatosis
D) Hepatitis C infection
E) Wilson disease

The answer is C: Hemochromatosis is a result of excessive iron deposition in the body (hemosiderosis) that leads to damage of bodily tissues. Primary hereditary hemochromatosis is an autosomal recessive trait. Persons who are homozygous for the *HFE* gene mutation C282Y comprise 90% of phenotypically affected persons. It is the most common form of hemochromatosis, affecting approximately 5 in 1000 persons. End-organ damage or clinical manifestations of hereditary hemochromatosis occur in approximately 10% of persons homozygous for C282Y. Complications include the following:

- Cirrhosis
- Diabetes mellitus
- Multiple joint pain
- Abdominal pain
- Chondrocalcinosis
- Bronze discoloration of the skin
- Cardiomyopathy that may result in congestive heart failure and cardiac arrhythmias
- Hepatomas
- Pituitary dysfunction leading to testicular atrophy and decreased sexual drive

The onset is usually in the fourth and fifth decades of life. The condition is rare before middle age. Diagnosis in women usually occurs after menopause because menstrual blood loss helps provide protection from iron overload. Laboratory findings show serum iron >300 mg/dL, serum ferritin >1000 ng/mL, and transferrin saturation >50%. Liver biopsy confirms the diagnosis when hepatic siderosis and cirrhosis are suspected.

Treatment involves phlebotomy (500 mL/wk), which removes 200 to 250 mg of excess iron from the body. The chelating agent deferoxamine is used in more severe cases; it acts by promoting urinary excretion of iron. Family members of those affected should be screened for hemochromatosis with human leukocyte antigen typing and iron studies.

Additional Reading: Hereditary hemochromatosis. *Am Fam Physician*. 2013;87(3):183-190.

7. Polycythemia vera is a rare condition that is seen more commonly in Jewish men older than 60 years. Which one of the following statements about this condition is true?

A) It is associated with an increased life span of the red blood cell (RBC).
B) It is associated with a neurodegenerative condition of the thalamus.
C) It is a chronic myeloproliferative disorder that is associated with increased levels of hemoglobin concentration and RBC mass.
D) Leukopenia and thrombocytopenia are common.
E) Physical examination usually shows decreased peripheral reflexes.

The answer is C: Polycythemia vera is a chronic myeloproliferative disorder that is associated with increased levels of hemoglobin concentration and increased RBC mass. The cause is unknown. The condition is associated with an increased production and turnover of RBCs. As many as one-fourth of those affected develop a reduction in the RBC life span, an associated anemia, and sometimes myelofibrosis.

Symptoms are associated with the increased viscosity and volume of blood and include headaches, visual disturbances, shortness of breath, weakness, and fatigue. Patients may also report generalized pruritus, particularly after bathing in warm water. Hepatosplenomegaly is common. Associated conditions include peptic ulcer disease, thrombosis, bone pain, renal lithiasis and gout.

The diagnosis should be considered when the hematocrit is >54% for men and >49% for women. Elevations in all three blood components, namely, RBCs, white blood cells, and platelets, are common. If the condition goes untreated, as many as 50% of those affected die within 1.5 years. Thrombosis is the most common cause of death, followed by complications of myeloid dysplasia, hemorrhage, and leukemia. With therapy, survival time is between 7 and 15 years.

Treatment involves phlebotomy (especially for pregnant women and individuals younger than 40 years) and, in some cases, myelosuppressive agents, including hydroxyurea. Hyperuricemia may also be treated with allopurinol.

Additional Reading: Polycythemia vera. In: Domino F, ed. *The 5-Minute Clinical Consult*. Wolters Kluwer; 2022.

8. A young patient is concerned as his previously quite healthy cousin was recently diagnosed with Hodgkin disease. Which one of the following statements about this disease is true?

A) Lymphocyte-depleted disease is the most common type.
B) Lymphocyte-predominant disease has a better prognosis than mixed cellularity type.
C) Stages A and B are distinguished by metastatic disease to regional lymph nodes.
D) The disease most commonly affects patients between 40 and 50 years of age.
E) Treatment for stages 1A and 2A involves chemotherapy.

The answer is B: Hodgkin disease is a type of lymphoma that involves the presence of Reed-Sternberg cells. This type of cell is a large, abnormal macrophagelike white cell with two prominent nuclei and surrounding halos that look like owl eyes. The disease has a bimodal distribution with a peak in individuals in their mid-20s and another peak in individuals older than 50 years.

Symptoms include fever, weight loss, night sweats, and occasionally pain associated with involved lymph nodes with the ingestion of alcohol. Most patients affected present with painless lymphadenopathy in the neck. Metastasis usually spreads to local lymph nodes, with hematogenous spread late in the course of the disease. Chest radiographs may show asymmetric mediastinal lymphadenopathy (compared with sarcoidosis, which usually involves symmetric lymphadenopathy). The disease is classified into four different types:

1. Lymphocyte predominant
2. Nodular sclerosis (most common type)
3. Mixed cellularity
4. Lymphocyte depleted

Once the diagnosis is made, the disease is staged as follows:

Stage 1: involvement of one lymph node region
Stage 2: involvement of two areas of lymph nodes on the same side of the diaphragm
Stage 3: lymph node involvement on both sides of the diaphragm
Stage 4: disseminated disease with bone marrow or liver involvement

Stage A: lack of constitutional symptoms
Stage B: weight loss, fever, and night sweats present

- Treatment of stages 1A and 2A involves radiation.
- Treatment of stages 3B and 4 involves combination chemotherapy.
- Treatment of stages 2B and 3A usually involves combined chemotherapy and radiotherapy.

The prognosis is variable. Those with localized disease have excellent prognoses, whereas those with disseminated disease have poorer prognoses. In addition, those who have lymphocyte-predominant and nodular-sclerosing type are far better than those with mixed-cellularity and lymphocyte-depleted forms.

Additional Reading: Hodgkin disease. In: Domino F, ed. *The 5-Minute Clinical Consult*. Wolters Kluwer; 2022.

9. A young man with von Willebrand disease presents to the emergency department with a severe nose bleed that he has been unable to stop with ice and direct pressure. Which one of the following products would best help to stop bleeding in this patient?

A) Cryoprecipitate
B) Fresh frozen plasma
C) Platelets
D) Protamine sulfate
E) Vitamin K

The answer is A: von Willebrand disease is an autosomal dominant transmitted disorder that can lead to abnormal bleeding tendencies. Men and women are equally affected. It is the most common congenital bleeding disorder. The disease is due to a lack of production of von Willebrand factor (type 1) or when the von Willebrand factor is not synthesized properly and is nonfunctional (type 2). The result is a decreased ability of platelets to adhere to collagen.

Symptoms include mild to moderate bleeding from small cuts, bruising, epistaxis, excessive menstrual blood loss, GI blood loss, and excessive bleeding during surgery.

Laboratory results show an increased bleeding time with a slightly prolonged partial thromboplastin time (PTT) if factor VIII is below 25% to 30%. In most cases, the prothrombin time, PTT, and platelet count are normal. Definitive diagnosis for von Willebrand disease type 1 is made by measuring the levels of (1) von Willebrand factor, (2) antibody response to von Willebrand antigen, (3) factor VIII, and (4) ristocetin cofactor activity. In patients with type 1 disease, all four measurements are decreased; in patients with type 2 disease, electrophoresis studies may be needed for the diagnosis.

Treatment involves the administration of cryoprecipitate, which replaces the von Willebrand factor and stops bleeding. Desmopressin acetate, a synthetic analogue of vasopressin, stimulates the release of von Willebrand factor from endothelial cells and can be used in the treatment of mild type 1 disease (but not of type 2). Oral contraceptives can also increase the levels of factor VIII and may be beneficial for women with menorrhagia.

Additional Reading: Diagnosis and management of Von Willebrand disease: guidelines for primary care. *Am Fam Physician*. 2009;80(11):1261-1268.

10. An elderly patient is receiving a blood transfusion following an operation to repair her fractured hip. The floor nurse reports that the patient is flushed and complaining of abdominal discomfort. Her temperature is 101 °F. The most appropriate management at this time would be which one of the following measures?

A) Administer acetaminophen 650 mg po and decrease the transfusion rate.
B) Administer diphenhydramine 50 mg po and decrease the transfusion rate.
C) Administer hydrocortisone 100 mg intravenously and decrease the transfusion rate.
D) Administer ranitidine 300 mg intravenously and order an abdominal x-ray.
E) Administer intravenous fluids and stop the transfusion.

The answer is E: Many hemolytic transfusion reactions are caused by human error in the laboratory during the matching process or during the administration of blood. Symptoms may include anxiety, dyspnea, tachycardia, flushing, headache, chest or abdominal pain, nausea, vomiting, and shock with an acute decrease in blood pressure. In most cases, the severity of symptoms and the prognosis depend on the amount of transfusion, rate of delivery, degree of incompatibility, and overall health of the patient.

The laboratory evaluation for hemolysis consists of measurements of serum haptoglobin, lactate dehydrogenase, and indirect bilirubin levels. The immune complexes that result in red blood cell (RBC) lysis can cause renal dysfunction and failure.

Treatment consists of stopping the transfusion as soon as possible, increasing intravenous fluids with vigorous diuresis using furosemide or mannitol, and possible dialysis if renal failure occurs. With multiple transfusions, the patient may develop antibodies to white blood cell antigens, which cause febrile reactions that are manifested by chills and temperatures higher than 100.4 °F. Using washed RBCs helps prevent these reactions.

Additional Reading: Transfusion of blood and blood products: indications and complications. *Am Fam Physician*. 2011;83(6):719-724.

11. Hypersplenism is associated with several disorders, including all of the following conditions, except which one?

A) Congestive heart failure
B) Hereditary spherocytosis
C) Infectious mononucleosis
D) Lymphoma
E) Polycythemia vera

The answer is A: Hypersplenism is associated with several disorders that lead to a reduction in one or more blood constituents, leading to leukopenia, thrombocytopenia, or a combination of both. Most cases of chronic hemolytic anemias are associated with splenomegaly.

Causes of splenomegaly include lymphoma, leukemia, polycythemia vera, myelofibrosis, mononucleosis, psittacosis, subacute bacterial endocarditis, tuberculosis, malaria, syphilis, kala-azar, brucellosis, sarcoidosis, amyloidosis, systemic lupus erythematosus, Felty syndrome, hereditary spherocytosis, thalassemias, cirrhosis, Gaucher disease, Niemann-Pick disease, Schüller-Christian disease, Letterer-Siwe disease, and thrombosis or compression of the portal or splenic veins.

Patients may exhibit bleeding disorders, palpable splenomegaly, left-upper abdominal discomfort, or splenic bruits. Management usually involves treatment of the underlying disorder; elective splenectomy is reserved for refractory cases. Asplenic patients are at increased risk for infection secondary to encapsulated bacteria and should receive pneumococcal immunization.

Additional Reading: Approach to the adult patient with splenomegaly and other splenic disorders. In: *UpToDate*. 2022.

12. Which one of the following findings is associated with chronic myelogenous leukemia (CML)?

A) Decreased vitamin B_{12} levels
B) Elevated leukocyte alkaline phosphatase level
C) Leukopenia
D) Philadelphia chromosome
E) Thrombocytopenia

The answer is D: CML is a myeloproliferative disorder that results in the overproduction of granulocytes from the bone marrow, liver, and spleen. The average age of onset is approximately 45 years. In most cases, CML has the potential to progress into an accelerated phase and final blast crisis but usually remains stable for years before transformation. Symptoms are usually nonspecific and include low-grade fever, weight loss, night sweats, fatigue, anorexia, and, in some cases, abdominal fullness secondary to splenomegaly.

Physical examination may show significant splenomegaly and generalized lymphadenopathy (ominous signs). Laboratory findings include significant elevation in the white blood cell (WBC) count (200,000 at the time of diagnosis) and thrombocytosis. Bone marrow studies show hypercellularity with a significant left shift and low leukocyte alkaline phosphatase value. Vitamin B_{12} levels and serum vitamin B_{12}–binding capacity are usually elevated as a result of increased granulocyte production of transcobalamin I, and there is almost always a Philadelphia chromosome (translocation of a part of chromosome 9 to chromosome 22) present. Treatment involves the use of chemotherapy medications such as hydroxyurea. In most cases, the patient may be kept asymptomatic for long periods while maintaining the WBC count at <50,000. True remission does not occur because of the persistence of the Philadelphia chromosome in the bone marrow. Median survival after the clinical onset is approximately 3 to 4 years. If a blast crisis occurs, the average survival is approximately 2 months but can be improved with adequate treatment. α-Interferon produces remission in 20% to 25%. Bone marrow transplantation has been shown to improve survival in select patients.

Additional Reading: Clinical manifestations and diagnosis of chronic myeloid leukemia. In: *UpToDate*. 2022.

CML is a myeloproliferative disorder that results in the overproduction of granulocytes. A Philadelphia chromosome (translocation of a part of chromosome 9 to chromosome 22) is almost always present.

13. A 67-year-old man presents complaining of back pain and generalized fatigue. A radiograph of his lumbar spine showed lytic lesions, and a subsequent workup revealed several abnormal laboratory findings, including anemia with Rouleau formation, a serum protein electrophoresis with a monoclonal spike and hypercalcemia. The most likely diagnosis to account for his presentation is which one of the following conditions?

A) Colon cancer
B) Metastatic prostate cancer
C) Multiple myeloma
D) Osteitis fibrosa cystica
E) Paget disease

The answer is C: Multiple myeloma is a malignancy associated with plasma cells and involves replacement of the bone marrow, bone destruction, and the formation of paraproteins that are found in the blood and urine. It is the most common primary malignancy that affects the spine. Affected patients are usually older than 60 years and present with anemia, bone pain, and an elevated sedimentation rate. Other manifestations include renal failure; spinal cord compression; or symptoms of hyperviscosity, including mucosal bleeding, vertigo, visual abnormalities, and alterations in mental status.

Laboratory abnormalities include an anemia with Rouleau formation, abnormal serum and urine protein electrophoresis with a monoclonal spike in the β or γ region, hypercalcemia as a result of bone destruction, and radiographs showing lytic lesions associated with the skeletal bones (bone scans are inferior to conventional radiographs). Diagnosis is made by bone marrow biopsy showing more than 10% of plasma cells in the bone marrow.

Treatment is aimed at palliation and involves chemotherapy and correction of hypercalcemia. Patients are at increased risk of infection caused by encapsulated organisms, such as *S pneumoniae* and *H influenzae*, because of impaired immune response. The median survival time is 3 to 5 years.

Additional Reading: Multiple myeloma. In: Domino F, ed. *The 5-Minute Clinical Consult*. Wolters Kluwer; 2022.

14. Anemia of chronic disease is a commonly seen problem. Which one of the following laboratory findings is associated with this condition?

A) Hemoglobin of 5 to 8 mg/dL
B) Increased serum ferritin levels
C) Increased total iron-binding capacity (TIBC) levels
D) Increased serum iron levels
E) Macrocytic, normochromic RBC morphology

The answer is B: Anemia of chronic disease symptoms include the typical complaints associated with anemia such as generalized fatigue, malaise, and decreased mentation. Additionally, patients will have symptoms associated with the primary disorder that is causing the anemia, which can include any of the following.

- Chronic infections: for example, osteomyelitis and SBE
- Chronic disorders: for example, RA, lupus, renal failure, sarcoidosis, and PMR
- Other disorders: for example, neoplasia, hepatic disease, and hypothyroidism

Laboratory tests show a mild, normocytic normochromic anemia, although microcytic indices are also possible; the hemoglobin is around 10 mg/dL. Serum ferritin is also usually increased, with a low TIBC and low serum iron levels.

The only therapy is treatment of the underlying disorder. The administration of iron, folic acid, or vitamin B_{12} is ineffective. Transfusion should only be considered in advanced cases in patients with severe symptoms.

Additional Reading: Anemia, chronic disease. In: Domino F, ed. *The 5-Minute Clinical Consult*. Wolters Kluwer; 2022.

15. Hereditary hemochromatosis is an autosomal recessive disorder that disrupts the body's regulation of iron. The best test to evaluate a patient with suspected hemochromatosis is which one of the following laboratory investigations?

A) Aspartate transaminase (AST)
B) Serum ferritin
C) Transferrin saturation
D) Total iron
E) Total iron-binding capacity

The answer is C: Hereditary hemochromatosis is the most common genetic disease in Whites. Men are more often affected than women. Persons who are homozygous for the *HFE* gene mutation C282Y comprise 85% to 90% of phenotypically affected persons. End-organ damage or clinical manifestations of hereditary hemochromatosis occur in approximately 10% of persons homozygous for C282Y.

Symptoms of hereditary hemochromatosis are nonspecific (eg, weakness, lethargy, arthralgias, and impotence) and typically absent in the early stages. Late manifestations include arthralgias, osteoporosis, cirrhosis, hepatocellular cancer, cardiomyopathy, dysrhythmia, diabetes mellitus, and hypogonadism.

Initial screening of individuals with suspected iron overload and those above the age of 20 years who are first-degree relatives of known cases of hereditary hemochromatosis should be done by obtaining a transferrin saturation measurement after an overnight fast. Simultaneous serum ferritin determination increases the predictive accuracy for diagnosis of iron overload. Transferrin saturation is also the test of choice for screening the general adult population for iron overload states.

Additional Reading: Hereditary hemochromatosis. *Am Fam Physician*. 2013;87(3):183-190.

16. The most common primary cancer of the bone in adults is which one of the following conditions?

A) Metastatic prostate cancer
B) Multiple myeloma
C) Osteosarcoma
D) Osteoid osteoma
E) Osteitis fibrosa cystica

The answer is B: Multiple myeloma is the malignant proliferation of plasma cells involving more than 10% of the bone marrow. Multiple myeloma is the most common primary cancer of the bones in adults. The median age at diagnosis of multiple myeloma is 62 years. Only 2% to 3% of cases are reported in patients younger than 30 years. African Americans in the United States are twice as likely to develop multiple myeloma as whites.

The multiple myeloma cell produces monoclonal immunoglobulins that may be identified on serum or urine protein electrophoresis. Bone pain related to multiple lytic lesions is the most common clinical presentation. However, up to 30% of patients are diagnosed incidentally while being evaluated for unrelated problems, and one-third of patients are diagnosed after a pathologic fracture, commonly of the axial skeleton.

Multiple myeloma must be differentiated from other causes of monoclonal gammopathy, including monoclonal gammopathy of undetermined significance, heavy chain disease, plasmacytoma, and Waldenström macroglobulinemia.

Routine laboratory workup may show pancytopenia, abnormal coagulation, hypercalcemia, azotemia, elevated alkaline phosphatase and erythrocyte sedimentation, and hypoalbuminemia. Examination may reveal proteinuria, hypercalciuria, or both. Urine dipstick tests may not indicate the presence of Bence Jones proteinuria. All patients with suspected multiple myeloma require a 24-hour urinalysis by protein electrophoresis to determine the presence of Bence Jones proteinuria and kappa or lambda light chains. Serum protein electrophoresis identifies an M protein as a narrow peak or "spike" in the γ, β, or $\alpha 2$ regions of the densitometer tracing.

Chemotherapy with melphalan and prednisone is the standard treatment for multiple myeloma. Other treatment modalities include polychemotherapy (thalidomide, immunomodulatory drugs, proteasome inhibitors) and bone marrow transplantation. Only 50% to 60% of patients respond to therapy. The aggregate median survival for all stages of multiple myeloma is 3 to 5 years.

Additional Reading: Multiple myeloma. In: Domino F, ed. *The 5-Minute Clinical Consult*. Wolters Kluwer; 2022.

Section X. Special Senses

Questions related to the special senses are a small part, about 2% of the American Board of Family Medicine certifying examination, yet cover sight, smell, hearing, taste, and touch! Remember, as this examination is for family physicians, the focus is on the primary care management of these conditions, and some are covered in Chapter 2, Care of Children and Adolescents and Chapter 6, Care of the elderly. As you study for the examination, ensure that you have a good overview of the following topics.

1. The eye
   - Know the differential diagnosis for red eye.
   - Appreciate an overview of glaucoma. (For example, acute angle-closure glaucoma is a medical emergency and is suspected in any patient above 50 years with a painful eye. Symptoms include nausea, vomiting, and halo around bright lights and can lead to blindness within 2 to 5 days. Treatment includes topical agents.)
   - Know the approach for both acute and chronic vision loss.
   - Appreciate the recommendations for pediatric vision screening.
   - Know the treatment for "lazy eye."
2. The ear
   - Appreciate an overview of hearing loss (eg, sensorineural vs conductive; sensorineural is most commonly related to aging (presbycusis) with high frequency loss initially; most common cause of conductive hearing loss is otosclerosis, an inherited disease).
   - Know the approach for dizziness/vertigo (eg, acute labyrinthitis follows otitis media or urinary tract infection and is a considered an irritation of the inner ear associated with dizziness and hearing loss and severe vertigo; Meniere disease—vertigo lasts hours with tinnitus; acute labyrinthitis is vertigo lasting days with hearing loss; vestibular neuronitis is vertigo often following a viral infection—treated with rest and antiemetics, lasting days with no hearing loss; positional vertigo is vertigo lasting for seconds associated with change in position).

Each of the following questions or incomplete statements is followed by suggested answers or completions. Select the ONE BEST ANSWER in each case.

1. A 63-year-old White woman presents with complaints that she has been seeing flashes of light and floaters in her right eye. She complains that her vision is a bit blurry as well. You suspect that she is suffering from a retinal detachment. In addition to her age, which one of the following is considered a risk factor for retinal detachment?

A) Diabetic retinopathy
B) Glaucoma
C) Hyphema
D) Myopia

The answer is D: Retinal detachment is relatively common after the age of 60. Risk factors for retinal detachment include advancing age, previous cataract surgery, myopia (near-sighted), and trauma. Other eye conditions such as hyphema (blood in the front chamber of the eye), glaucoma, and diabetic retinopathy are not considered risk factors for retinal detachment.

Retinal detachment occurs when fluid accumulates in the potential space between the neurosensory retina and the underlying retinal pigment epithelium. Retinal detachments are classified based on the mechanism of this subretinal fluid accumulation. There are three classifications:

Rhegmatogenous is the most common type of detachment and occurs when a tear in the retina leads to the subretinal fluid accumulation. The term rhegmatogenous is derived from the Greek word rhegma, which means a discontinuity or a break.

Exudative (or serous) retinal detachment results from the accumulation of serous and/or hemorrhagic fluid in the subretinal space because of hydrostatic factors (eg, severe acute hypertension), inflammation (eg, sarcoid uveitis), or neoplastic effusions.

Tractional retinal detachment occurs via centripetal mechanical forces on the retina, usually mediated by fibrotic tissue resulting from previous hemorrhage, injury, surgery, infection, or inflammation.

Patients typically present with symptoms such as light flashes, floaters, peripheral visual field loss, and blurred vision. Retinal tears may occur without symptoms, but often photopsia (light flashes) is noted; a result of vitreoretinal traction. When the retina tears, blood and retinal pigment epithelium cells may enter the vitreous cavity and are perceived as "floaters."

Immediate intervention can prevent retinal detachment. Patients with the acute onset of flashes or floaters should be referred to an ophthalmologist.

Additional Reading: Common eye emergencies. *Am Fam Physician*. 2013;88(8):515-519.

2. Glaucoma is the second-most common cause of legal blindness in the United States. Which one of the following statements is true regarding glaucoma?

A) Closed-angle glaucoma is an ophthalmologic emergency.
B) Glaucoma suspects have normal intraocular pressure.
C) Intraocular pressure is diagnostic for glaucoma.
D) Laser treatment is the treatment of choice once glaucoma is identified.

The answer is A: Glaucoma is the second-most common cause of legal blindness (after diabetic retinopathy) in the United States, and open-angle glaucoma is the most common form. Although most patients are asymptomatic, the condition results in a progressive optic neuropathy characterized by enlarging optic disc cupping and visual field loss, from a slow buildup of intraocular pressure due to poor drainage of the aqueous fluid.

Closed-angle glaucoma, also called acute glaucoma, occurs when the iris bows forward and completely blocks fluid access to the trabecular meshwork. Pressure builds, resulting in severe eye pain, and vision can be quickly lost. This is considered an ophthalmologic emergency.

Patients at increased risk for open-angle glaucoma include African Americans above 40 years and white Americans older than 65 years, with a personal history of diabetes or severe myopia (nearsighted) and a family history of glaucoma.

Elevated intraocular pressure is a risk factor for open-angle glaucoma, but it is not diagnostic. Some patients with glaucoma have normal intraocular pressure (ie, normal-pressure glaucoma), but other patients with elevated intraocular pressure do not have glaucoma (ie, glaucoma suspects).

Nonspecific β-blocker or prostaglandin analogue eye drops are generally the first-line treatment to reduce intraocular pressure. Laser treatment and surgery are usually reserved for patients in whom medical treatment has failed. Without urgent treatment, open-angle glaucoma can result in irreversible vision loss.

Additional Reading: Open-angle glaucoma: epidemiology, clinical presentation, and diagnosis. In: *UpToDate*. 2022.

3. A 59-year-old postal worker presents complaining of left eye pain and blurred vision. The patient also reports seeing halos around light sources as well as nausea, abdominal pain, and vomiting. On examination, his left eye is red and the pupil is dilated. The most likely diagnosis to explain this presentation is which one of the following conditions?

A) Angle-closure glaucoma
B) Graves disease
C) Digoxin toxicity
D) Hyphema
E) Atropine poisoning

The answer is A: Glaucoma is classified into two types: open-angle and angle-closure.

- *Open-angle glaucoma* (90% of cases) results when the rate of aqueous fluid outflow is decreased and the ocular pressure is consistently increased, giving rise to optic atrophy with loss of vision. The disease usually is bilateral, affects African Americans more commonly than white Americans, and appears to have genetic predisposition. Examination may show optic disc cupping and an increase in intraocular pressure (normal: 10-21 mm Hg). The diagnosis should not be based on one reading. Treatment involves the use of intraocular β-blockers, such as timolol and pilocarpine. Surgical therapy may be necessary for patients whose conditions do not respond appropriately to medical treatment.
- *Angle-closure glaucoma* is less common, often more acute in onset, and is associated with a narrow anterior chamber and pupillary dilation that obstructs the normal flow of aqueous fluid. The condition constitutes an ophthalmologic emergency and is sometimes triggered by stress, dark rooms, and pupillary dilation from medication used to perform eye examinations. Most patients experience pain and blurred vision with halos around lights. They may also present with abdominal pain and vomiting. Physical examination shows an eye that is red with the pupil dilated and unresponsive to light. Untreated, the condition can lead to blindness in 2 to 5 days. Treatment involves medication (miotics and carbonic anhydrase inhibitors) and laser peripheral iridectomy. Patients older than 65 years should be screened for glaucoma every 1 to 2 years, or every year if there is a strong family history for glaucoma. African American individuals should be screened at an earlier age (40 years). The report of the U.S. Preventive Services Task Force does not recommend the routine performance of tonometry by primary care physicians. Instead, primary care physicians are encouraged to refer to an eye specialist for screening.

Additional Reading: Angle-closure glaucoma. In: *UpToDate*. 2022.

Angle-closure glaucoma often presents acutely with pain, blurred vision, and halos around lights. The eye is red with a dilated pupil and unresponsive to light. Untreated, the condition can lead to blindness in 2 to 5 days.

4. After a stroke, it is observed that a patient can no longer recognize objects by his sense of touch. Which one of the following terms refers to this loss of the ability to recognize objects by touching them?

A) Agnosia
B) Aphasia
C) Apraxia
D) Astereognosis

The answer is D: *Astereognosis* is the loss of the ability to recognize objects by the sense of touch.

- *Apraxia* is the loss of the ability to carry out movements in the absence of paralysis or sensory deficits.
- *Agnosia* is the inability to recognize sensory stimuli—subgroups include auditory, visual, olfactory, gustatory, and tactile agnosias.
- *Aphasia* is the loss of the ability to express oneself by speech or written language.

Additional Reading: *Aphasia, agnosia, apraxia, and amnesia.* In: *Massachusetts General Hospital Handbook of Neurology*. Lippincott Williams & Wilkins; 2007.

5. A 20-year-old student jumped off the high diving board at a local swimming pool and presented to your office complaining of severe left-sided ear pain. He reported landing awkwardly in a sideways fashion when he hit the water and you diagnosed him with a perforated tympanic membrane (TM), when he was first seen 3 months ago. He returns today and a small TM perforation remains. There is no erythema and no discharge. Appropriate treatment at this time would be which one of the following?

A) Continue observation and schedule follow-up in a month.
B) Obtain an audiogram to assess hearing.
C) Prescribe steroid eardrops.
D) Prescribe antibiotic eardrops.
E) Refer to an ear-nose-throat specialist.

The answer is E: Rupture of the TM can be caused by placing objects in the ear canal, excessive positive pressure applied to the ear (eg, an explosion), swimming, diving, or excessive negative pressure (eg, a kiss over the ear).

Symptoms of traumatic rupture include a sudden severe pain and occasionally bleeding from the ear. Hearing loss and tinnitus are also usually present. Vertigo suggests damage to the inner ear.

Treatment involves gentle removal of debris and blood from the ear canal and the use of earplugs to provide protection when bathing or shampooing.

Antibiotic eardrops are indicated only if there has been contamination by dirty water or debris. Oral antibiotics can be used prophylactically to prevent infection but are generally unnecessary.

Pain medication may be necessary for the first few days. Persistent perforation for more than 4 to 6 weeks is an indication for otolaryngology referral. An audiogram should be performed after treatment to document the return of hearing.

Additional Reading: Barotrauma. In: Domino F, ed. *The 5-Minute Clinical Consult*. Wolters Kluwer; 2022.

6. Diabetic retinopathy is the leading cause of blindness in middle-aged Americans. All of the following statements about diabetic retinopathy are true, except which one?

A) Persons with diabetes should have eye examinations every year.
B) Proliferative retinopathy is associated with neovascularization.
C) Proliferative retinopathy is associated with a poorer prognosis than nonproliferative retinopathy.
D) Symptoms of retinopathy usually begin with eye pain.

The answer is D: Diabetic retinopathy is the leading cause of blindness in middle-aged Americans, and the degree of retinopathy is correlated with the duration of the diabetes. Therefore, diabetics should be encouraged to have yearly eye examinations. The disease process is categorized as proliferative or nonproliferative.

Nonproliferative retinopathy: Characterized by dilated retinal veins, retinal hemorrhages, microaneurysms, retinal edema, and soft exudates (cotton-wool spots). Hard exudates are usually yellow in appearance and caused by chronic edema. Visual symptoms generally do not occur in the early stages of nonproliferative retinopathy.

Proliferative retinopathy: Associated with neovascularization and proliferation of blood vessels into the vitreous with resulting fibrosis and retinal detachment and hemorrhage. The prognosis of proliferative retinopathy is worse than that of nonproliferative retinopathy.

Symptoms of diabetic retinopathy usually begin with a decrease in visual acuity. Diagnosis can be made with ophthalmologic examination and fluorescein angiography. Treatment involves panretinal laser coagulation and vitrectomy, as well as active management to control the diabetes and, if present, hypertension.

Additional Reading: Vision loss in older adults. *Am Fam Physician*. 2016;94(3):219-226.

7. A 63-year-old woman presents complaining of a pressure sensation in her right ear and a loss of hearing for the past couple of days. She has been in good health, and her physical examination, including your neurologic examination, is normal. Although both tympanic membranes are normal, a vibrating tuning fork in the midline of the forehead reveals sound lateralizing to the left ear. Her audiogram shows a 30-dB hearing loss at three consecutive frequencies in the right ear, with normal hearing on the left. Which one of the following would be most appropriate for this patient at this point?

A) Prescribe oral nifedipine (Procardia).
B) Prescribe oral acyclovir (Zovirax).
C) Prescribe oral corticosteroids.
D) Obtain a computed tomographic (CT) scan of the head.
E) Send her to the laboratory for a complete blood count, metabolic profile, and thyroid studies.

The answer is C: Sudden hearing loss is defined as the loss of 30 dB or more of hearing ability over several hours or days, with no other cause indicated from the examination. Normal conversation is 60 dB. Ninety percent of the time the loss only affects one ear, and the cause is unknown.

It is important to distinguish between a sensorineural or a conductive hearing loss when a patient presents with sudden hearing loss. Patients should be asked about previous episodes, and the workup should include an assessment for bilateral hearing loss and a neurologic examination.

Routinely prescribing antiviral agents, thrombolytics, vasodilators, vasoactive substances, or antioxidants is not recommended. However, oral corticosteroids may be offered as initial therapy, and hyperbaric oxygen therapy may be helpful within 3 months of diagnosis.

Guidelines recommend against routine laboratory tests or CT of the head as part of the initial evaluation as such testing is unlikely to be helpful. If there is a concern for retrocochlear pathology, a workup may include obtaining an auditory brainstem response, magnetic resonance imaging, or follow-up audiometry.

Additional Reading: AAO-HNS releases guideline on sudden hearing loss. *Am Fam Physician*. 2013;87(5):377-380.

8. A 24-year-old woman with poorly controlled diabetes presents to the emergency department with a fever, pain, and dyspnea. She is diagnosed with diabetic ketoacidosis (DKA), and on examination she is noted to have a purulent nasal discharge and a black eschar formation on his nasal septum. The most likely diagnosis to explain this finding is which one of the following conditions?

A) Cocaine use
B) Sinusitis maligna
C) Mucormycosis
D) *Pseudomonas* infection
E) *Staphylococcus* infection

The answer is C: Mucormycosis (phycomycosis) is a fungal infection that can be fulminant and lethal. It affects the nose, sinus, and orbit and is seen in patients with poorly controlled diabetes, DKA, or immunodeficiency. Symptoms include dull sinus pain, fever, orbital cellulitis, proptosis, nasal congestion and purulent or bloody nasal discharge, and gangrenous destruction of the nasal septum, orbits, or palate. In many cases, a black eschar is formed in the nasal area.

If the fungus invades the cerebral vessels, then convulsions, blindness, and death can result. Diagnosis almost always involves biopsy. Computed tomography or magnetic resonance imaging can help evaluate the extent of the disease. Treatment is accomplished with diabetic control, amphotericin B, and surgical debridement. The prognosis is poor, with up to a 50% mortality rate in disseminated cases.

Additional Reading: *Mucormycosis (Zygomycosis)*. www.cdc.gov/fungal/mucormycosis

9. A patient is in with concern over a red growth in his eye, which has been slowly enlarging. After examination, you diagnose him with a pterygium. This finding is associated with which one of the following?

A) An increased risk of glaucoma
B) Improvement with the use of topical anesthetics
C) Involvement of the pupillary area, which may require surgical excision
D) Macular degeneration
E) Trauma to the retina

The answer is C: Pingueculae are hyaline, elastic nodules that appear yellow and affect both sides of the cornea but usually more on the nasal side. Occasionally, they become inflamed and require treatment with topical steroids. However, in most cases no treatment is required. Pterygium is a fleshy, triangular growth of a pinguecula that involves the cornea. In some cases, it may involve the pupillary area and requires surgical removal. The causes include irritation from ultraviolet sunlight, allergens, and excessive drying, sandy, or windy conditions that cause chronic irritation. In most cases, treatment is supportive with topical vasoconstrictors, saline drops, and protection from sunlight. Surgery is reserved for more severe cases in which vision is compromised.

Additional Reading: Painless red eye. *Am Fam Physician.* 2013;88(8):533-534.

10. A 57-year-old truck driver presents with a complaint of ringing in his ears. It is a buzzing type of sound and has been slowly worsening over the past few months. You diagnose him with tinnitus and indicate that the most common cause for this condition is which one of the following?

A) Acoustic neuroma
B) Long-term use of salicylates
C) Hypertension
D) Infection (otitis media)
E) Sensorineural hearing loss

The answer is E: Tinnitus is a common condition that is characterized by a ringing, roaring, rushing, buzzing, or whistling sound in the ears. The condition may be continuous or pulsatile with each heartbeat. In most cases, there is an associated hearing loss, and the major cause of tinnitus is a sensorineural hearing loss.

The list of associated conditions is extensive and includes obstruction of the canals, eustachian tube dysfunction, otosclerosis, Meniere disease, aminoglycoside toxicity, long-term use of salicylates, anemia, hypertension, hypothyroidism, hyperlipidemia, noise-induced hearing loss, and tumors associated with the inner ear (eg, acoustic neuroma).

The evaluation of a patient with tinnitus includes an audiogram and computed tomographic scan or magnetic resonance imaging of the head, with special emphasis given to the temporal area, if the audiogram is not supportive of the diagnosis. Pulsatile tinnitus may require vascular studies to rule out aneurysm formation. Treatment depends on the diagnosis, but in most cases if the underlying disease is controlled, the tinnitus disappears. If no underlying disease process is present, background music or amplification may help to relieve symptoms.

Additional Reading: Tinnitus. In: Domino F, ed. *The 5-Minute Clinical Consult.* Wolters Kluwer; 2022.

11. Macular degeneration associated with aging is a leading cause of blindness in the elderly. Which one of the following statements about this condition is true?

A) It typically affects only peripheral vision.
B) Neovascularization is typically associated with drusen and the dry form.
C) The wet form is usually more severe than the dry form.
D) The condition is more common in African American individuals.
E) The condition is rarely progressive.

The answer is C: Macular degeneration is more common in White Americans, appears to be hereditary, and is associated with atrophy or degeneration of the macular disc. There are basically two types: atrophic or dry and exudative or wet. Both types usually occur bilaterally and are progressive. The dry form usually progresses slowly and affects the outer retina, retinal pigment epithelium, choriocapillaris, and Bruch membrane.

The wet form of macular degeneration is more severe and progressive, usually affects the eyes sequentially, and is responsible for approximately 90% of blindness in those affected with macular degeneration. The wet form occurs when there is drusen (ie, degeneration of the pigment epithelium and Bruch membrane) and an accumulation of serous fluid or blood in the retina that produces elevation of the retinal pigment membrane from Bruch membrane. Neovascularization may then occur, giving rise to a subretinal neovascular membrane that causes permanent vision loss.

There is no specific treatment for macular degeneration; however, laser photocoagulation may help stop neovascularization in select cases, and vision aids may help acuity. Macular degeneration affects central vision and does not affect peripheral vision.

Additional Reading: Vision loss in older adults. *Am Fam Physician.* 2016;94(3):219-222.

Macular degeneration associated with aging is a leading cause of blindness in the elderly.

12. A previously healthy 37-year-old school teacher presents with complaints of dizziness that comes on suddenly when she turns her head to look up at her chalk board. If she waits for a few seconds, the sensation goes away, and now she is having some associated nausea. Given her presentation, your diagnosis includes benign positional vertigo. Which one of the following diagnostic procedures would confirm your suspicion?

A) An audiogram
B) Cold/warm-water caloric testing
C) Dix-Hallpike maneuvers
D) Orthostatic blood pressures
E) The cover-uncover test

The answer is C: Benign positional vertigo is a condition characterized by severe episodes of vertigo that usually last less than 1 minute and are precipitated by certain head positions. The vertiginous symptoms are accompanied by nystagmus, and there is no tinnitus or hearing loss (as seen in Meniere disease).

The diagnosis is usually based on the history and reproduction of symptoms by the Dix-Hallpike maneuver: The patient's head is turned to the side and the patient goes from a sitting to a lying position with the head positioned beneath the level of the bed. A positive response is noted when the patient reports vertigo (recurrence of her symptoms) and there is evidence of nystagmus.

Most cases are self-limited, and repeating the position that causes the vertigo usually fatigues the vertiginous response. Vestibular-type exercises performed several times daily may help eliminate the symptoms, especially for younger patients. Labyrinthine sedatives are of little help for this condition. Canalith repositioning can also be attempted and is beneficial for select patients. If fatigability of symptoms does not occur, further workup may be indicated to rule out a central cause for the vertigo.

Additional Reading: Dizziness: approach to evaluation and management. *Am Fam Physician.* 2017;95(3):154-162.

13. A 59-year-old man presents to your office with complaints of a runny nose. This has been occurring for a couple of weeks and has been clear. He has no fever or other symptoms and is concerned that his allergies are acting up. Which one of the following classes of medications would treat this symptom but would not be effective against other symptoms of allergic rhinitis?

A) Oral antihistamines
B) Topical corticosteroids
C) Topical anticholinergics
D) Topical antihistamines
E) Topical decongestants

The answer is C: Allergic rhinitis may be seasonal or perennial. Seasonal allergic rhinitis is caused by seasonal allergens. Perennial allergic rhinitis may be caused by dust mites, molds, animal allergens, occupational allergens, or pollen. Risk factors for allergic rhinitis include a family history of atopy, serum immunoglobulin E (IgE) levels greater than 100 IU/mL before 6 years of age, higher socioeconomic class, and a positive allergy skin prick test. The diagnosis of rhinitis includes a history of symptoms and a physical examination. Skin testing for specific IgE antibody is the preferred diagnostic test to provide evidence of an allergic cause of the patient's symptoms.

There are numerous topical (intranasal) and oral agents available to treat allergic rhinitis such as antihistamines, decongestants, corticosteroids, and anticholinergics. Ipratropium (Atrovent) is a topical anticholinergic that reduces rhinorrhea but not the other allergic rhinitis symptoms. It is recommended for episodic rhinitis because of its rapid onset of action and minimal side effects, although dryness of nasal membranes may occur.

Additional Reading: Treatment of allergic rhinitis. *Am Fam Physician.* 2015;92(11):985-992.

14. Human immunodeficiency virus (HIV) syndrome can affect many different organ systems, including the eye. Which one of the following is a common ophthalmologic finding in patients with HIV infection?

A) Cataracts
B) Conjunctivitis
C) Glaucoma
D) Retinitis
E) Retinal tears

The answer is D: Ophthalmologic findings include toxoplasmic and cytomegalovirus retinitis, herpes infections, syphilis, and *Pneumocystis* infections of the eye. The most common ophthalmologic finding is cotton-wool spots caused by retinal ischemia secondary to microvascular disease. All patients with HIV should undergo complete eye examinations to rule out associated conditions.

Additional Reading: Pathogenesis, clinical manifestations, and diagnosis of AIDS-related cytomegalovirus retinitis. In: *UpToDate.* 2022.

15. Vertigo with hearing loss and tinnitus are considered classic findings for which one of the following conditions?

A) Acoustic neuroma
B) Benign positional vertigo
C) Cholesteatoma
D) Meniere disease
E) Vestibular neuronitis

The answer is D: Meniere disease is a peripheral cause of vertigo. Symptoms include the hallmark findings of recurrent vertigo, tinnitus, and hearing loss. The cause is thought to arise from endolymphatic hydrops. In most cases, the vertigo lasts for several hours, up to an entire day. Although, at first, hearing may be little affected, over time, it deteriorates. Tinnitus is usually constant and may become worse during the acute attacks. Vertigo may be severe and accompanied by nausea and vomiting.

Treatment consists of salt restriction (ie, no more than 2 g/d) and the use of hydrochlorothiazide, anticholinergics, antihistamines, and antiemetics. Resistant cases may require referral to an otolaryngologist.

An acoustic neuroma is a slow-growing benign tumor of the vestibular cochlear nerve. The symptoms vary, based on the size and location of the tumor, but common symptoms are similar and include vertigo, hearing loss, and tinnitus in the affected ear, and should be considered in the differential diagnosis; however, the symptoms are usually less severe and come on gradually over time.

Cholesteatoma is a type of skin cyst that is located in the middle ear and mastoid bone in the skull. It can usually be visualized on otoscopy, and symptoms, such as hearing loss, are late findings.

Vestibular neuritis is an inflammation of the vestibular portion of the vestibulocochlear nerve, which is also associated with sudden, severe vertigo. Hearing loss and tinnitus are not usually reported.

Additional Reading: Dizziness: approach to evaluation and management. *Am Fam Physician.* 2017;95(3):154-162.

16. A 43-year-old waitress presents with a complaint of "pink eye." She reports that when she awoke this morning that her right eye was stuck shut and now is red and has been draining. You diagnose her bacterial conjunctivitis and note that the most common pathogen in American adults is which one of the following organisms?

A) *Chlamydia trachomatis*
B) *H influenzae*
C) *Klebsiella*
D) *S aureus*
E) *S pneumoniae*

The answer is D: The conjunctiva is a thin, translucent, relatively elastic tissue layer with bulbar (outer aspect of the globe) and palpebral (inside of the eyelid) portions. Underneath the conjunctiva lie the episclera, sclera, and uveal tissue layers. Conjunctivitis is the most common cause of red eye. Most frequently, acute conjunctivitis is caused by a bacterial or viral infection.

The three most common pathogens in bacterial conjunctivitis are *S pneumoniae*, *H influenzae*, and *S aureus*. Infections with *S pneumoniae* and *H influenzae* are more common in children, whereas *S aureus* most frequently affects adults. Childhood immunizations for *H influenzae* and *S pneumoniae* further decrease the incidence of these causative organisms. Sexually transmitted diseases such as chlamydia and gonorrhea are less common causes of conjunctivitis.

In persons with suspected, but not confirmed, bacterial conjunctivitis, empiric treatment with topical antibiotics may be beneficial. However, this benefit is marginal, so it is advisable to recommend good eyelid hygiene and suggest that patients take antibiotics only if symptoms do not resolve after 1 to 2 days.

Adenovirus is by far the most common cause of viral conjunctivitis, although other viruses can also cause the condition. Viral conjunctivitis often occurs in community epidemics, with the virus transmitted in schools, workplaces, and physicians' offices. The usual modes of transmission are contaminated fingers, medical instruments, and swimming pool water. Patients with viral conjunctivitis typically present with an acutely red eye, watery discharge, conjunctival swelling, a tender preauricular node, and, in some cases, photophobia and a foreign body sensation. Both eyes may be affected simultaneously, or the second eye may become involved a few days after the first eye. Some patients have an associated upper respiratory tract infection. Patients should be instructed to avoid direct contact with other persons for at least 1 week after the onset of symptoms. Treatment is supportive. Cold compresses and topical vasoconstrictors may provide symptomatic relief. Topical antibiotics are rarely necessary because secondary bacterial infection is uncommon.

Allergic conjunctivitis is distinguished by severe itching and allergen exposure. This condition is generally treated with topical antihistamines, mast cell stabilizers, or anti-inflammatory agents.

Pain and photophobia are not typical features of a primary conjunctival inflammatory process. If these features are present, the physician should consider more serious underlying ocular or orbital disease processes, including uveitis, keratitis, acute glaucoma, and orbital cellulitis. Similarly, blurred vision that fails to clear with a blink is rarely associated with conjunctivitis. Patients with pain, photophobia, or blurred vision should be referred to an ophthalmologist.

Additional Reading: Bacterial conjunctivitis. *Am Fam Physician.* 2010;82(6):665-666.

17. A 77-year-old patient presents acutely complaining of flashes of light and blurred vision in his right eye. He reports no pain, and your examination reveals no obvious findings other than decreased vision in that eye. Appropriate management for this patient would be which one of the following actions?

A) Order a carotid ultrasonography
B) Patch the affected eye
C) Prescribe a course of oral steroids
D) Refer for an urgent ophthalmology evaluation
E) Start aspirin therapy

The answer is D: Retinal detachment is painless, but early symptoms can include dark or irregular vitreous floaters, flashes of light, or blurred vision. Retinal detachment can occur as the result of a retinal tear (occurs more frequently in myopia, after cataract surgery, or after ocular trauma) by detachment without a tear as a result of vitreal traction (seen in proliferative retinopathy of diabetes or sickle cell disease) or by transudation of fluid into the subretinal space (eg, severe uveitis or primary or metastatic choroidal tumors). As the detachment progresses, the patient notices a curtain or veil in the field of vision. If the macula is involved, central visual acuity is significantly affected.

Direct ophthalmoscopy may show retinal irregularities and a retinal elevation with darkened blood vessels. Indirect ophthalmoscopy, including scleral depression, is necessary for detecting peripheral breaks and detachment. If a vitreous hemorrhage obscures the retina, especially in myopia, postcataract extraction, or eye injury, retinal detachment should be suspected and B-scan ultrasonography performed.

Although often localized, retinal detachments due to retinal tears can expand to involve the entire retina if not treated promptly. Any patient with a suspected or established retinal detachment should be seen urgently by an ophthalmologist.

Additional Reading: Common eye emergencies. *Am Fam Physician.* 2013;88(8):515-519.

Retinal detachment is painless, but early symptoms can include dark or irregular vitreous floaters, flashes of light, or blurred vision.

18. Oral hygiene is an important component of medical health and if not tended to results in the buildup of bacterial plaque, which leads to chronic gingivitis. If not treated, the disease will progress to which one of the following problems?

A) Dental caries
B) Glossitis
C) Oropharyngeal cancer
D) Oropharyngeal candidiasis
E) Periodontitis

The answer is E: Periodontitis is a consequence of untreated chronic gingivitis and is the most common cause of tooth loss. Signs include deepening of the gingival pockets between the teeth with the accumulation of calculus deposits. The gums soon lose their attachment to the tooth, and bone loss occurs. Later in the course of the disease, the gums recede and eventually tooth loss occurs due to loss of the bone support around the tooth root. Treatment involves dental referral and, in severe cases, surgery. Regular dental visits twice yearly and proper brushing and flossing techniques help prevent plaque buildup.

Additional Reading: Common dental infections in the primary care setting. *Am Fam Physician.* 2008;77(6):797-802.

19. A 42-year-old bookkeeper presents with a complaint of a painful, red eye and she feels like there is something in her eye. She has also noted a discharge and her vision has been blurry. She wears contact lenses. And on examination her pupils are equal, round, and reactive to light, but her right eye has diffuse injection and she complains of photophobia on ophthalmic examination. You perform fluorescein staining, which reveals an area of focal corneal uptake. Which one of the following is the most likely diagnosis?

A) Acute angle-closure glaucoma
B) Corneal abrasion
C) Herpes zoster ophthalmicus
D) Subconjunctival hemorrhage
E) Uveitis

The answer is B: With corneal abrasion there is usually a history of an injury involving a foreign object or from direct trauma as can happen with contact lens wearers. Signs and symptoms include severe eye pain; red, watery eyes; photophobia; and a foreign body sensation. Vision is usually normal and pupils are equal and reactive to light. Fluorescein staining will usually reveals an area of focal corneal uptake, revealing the area of abrasion.

Pain can be treated with topical nonsteroidal anti-inflammatory drugs or oral medications (eg, ibuprofen). Patching is not recommended because it does not improve pain and can delay healing. Topical antibiotics are commonly prescribed to prevent bacterial infection, and contact lens–related abrasions should be treated with antipseudomonal topical antibiotics.

Acute angle-closure glaucoma causes an acute loss of vision, with dilated pupils that do not react normally to light. Symptoms include severe pain and watery eyes, with halos around lights. Patients may also report nausea and vomiting.

Herpes zoster ophthalmicus is associated with a vesicular rash, keratitis, and uveitis. The rash is preceded by pain and a tingling sensation. Findings include conjunctivitis and dermatomal involvement, which are usually unilateral.

Subconjunctival hemorrhage is painless and does not interfere with vision, whereas uveitis presents with a red eye, loss of vision, and photophobia. It is associated with autoimmune diseases, including reactive arthritis, ankylosing spondylitis, and inflammatory bowel disease.

Additional Reading: Evaluation and management of corneal abrasions. *Am Fam Physician.* 2013;87(2):114-120.

20. A 27-year-old carpenter complains of a sense of irritation in his left eye over the past couple of days. On ophthalmic examination, you detect a small foreign body on the periphery of his cornea, which you remove, although an area of tan discoloration remains where the foreign body had been. Which one of the following is most appropriate in this situation?

A) Advise care to avoid further injury and reassess the next day.
B) Irrigate the eye with a normal saline solution with light pressure.
C) Prescribe an antibiotic ointment and patch the eye.
D) Refer for an urgent ophthalmology evaluation.
E) Scrap the area lightly with a scalpel.

The answer is D: When metal foreign bodies are present on the cornea for more than 24 hours, a rust ring will often develop in the superficial layer of the cornea. This material is toxic to the cornea and should be removed within 24 to 48 hours. The proper removal of a rust ring requires the use of a slit lamp and specialized ophthalmic equipment; thus, an urgent referral to an eye specialist is the best management in this case.

Additional Reading: Evaluation and management of corneal abrasions. *Am Fam Physician.* 2013;87(2):114-120.

Section XI. Nonspecific System

Although the American Board of Family Medicine reports examination results based on major organ systems, many common conditions are not easily characterized as primarily affecting an organ. Many of these are infections, cancers, or other exposures. Remember, as this examination is for family physicians, the focus is on the primary care management of such conditions. The questions in this section are to remind you of key areas to review. If you are struggling with a question, find the suggested "Additional Reading" to review. The majority of these readings were selected specifically as easy-to-access primary care–focused resources for you to use as a means to solidify your knowledge. Good luck as you complete this final section relating primarily to adult medicine topics!

Each of the following questions or incomplete statements is followed by suggested answers or completions. Select the ONE BEST ANSWER in each case.

1. A 27-year-old auto mechanic is brought to the emergency department with slurred speech, confusion, and ataxia. He appears intoxicated and has a history of binge drinking, but he denies recent alcohol intake and no odor of alcohol is noted on his breath and his blood alcohol level is zero. Abnormal laboratory test results include a low carbon dioxide 10 mmol/L (N 20-30) with an arterial pH of 7.25. His urinalysis shows calcium oxalate crystals and red blood cells (10-20/HPF). Which one of the following would be the most appropriate steps to take for this patient?

A) Administer activated charcoal.
B) Administer fomepizole (Antizol) intravenously.
C) Begin immediate hemodialysis.
D) Place a nasogastric tube for gastric lavage.

The answer is B: This patient is suffering from ethylene glycol poisoning, a substance found in automotive antifreeze, deicing solutions, carpet cleaners, and other industrial compounds. This diagnosis should be considered in a patient who appears intoxicated but does not have an odor of alcohol and on investigation has a metabolic acidosis of unknown cause (anion gap acidosis), along with hypocalcemia, urinary crystals, and nontoxic blood alcohol levels. Ingestion of 100 mL of ethylene glycol by an adult can result in toxicity.

Treatment with intravenous fomepizole (Antizol) has a specific indication for ethylene glycol poisoning and should be initiated immediately when such poisoning is suspected. If ethylene glycol poisoning is treated early, hemodialysis may be avoided, but once severe acidosis and renal failure have occurred, hemodialysis is necessary.

Ethylene glycol is rapidly absorbed, and the use of ipecac or gastric lavage is therefore not effective. Large amounts of activated charcoal will only bind to relatively small amounts of ethylene glycol, and the therapeutic window for accomplishing this is less than 1 hour.

Additional Reading: Methanol and ethylene glycol poisoning. In: *UpToDate*. 2022.

2. Tumor markers are often used to track response to therapy and evaluate for recurrence after treatment. Which one of the following tumor markers is correct for the related condition?

A) α-fetoprotein (AFP) for ovarian carcinoma
B) β-human chorionic gonadotropin (β-hCG) for ovarian cancer
C) CA (cancer antigen) 19-9 for pancreatic cancer
D) CA 27.29 for metastatic cervical cancer
E) CA 125 for hepatic carcinoma

The answer is C: Recognized tumor markers are most appropriate for monitoring response to therapy and detecting early recurrence. Although all of the markers listed are tumor markers, only CA 19-9 is correctly linked. It is useful in diagnosing pancreatic abnormalities. Levels >1000 U/mL are correlated with pancreatic cancer. Benign conditions such as cirrhosis, cholestasis, cholangitis, and pancreatitis can also result in CA 19-9 elevations, although values are usually <1000 U/mL.

AFP is a marker for hepatocellular carcinoma. It is used to screen highly selected populations and to assess hepatic masses in patients at particular risk for developing hepatic malignancy.

The β-hCG is used in the diagnosis and management of gestational trophoblastic disease. Combined AFP and β-hCG testing is an essential adjunct in the evaluation and treatment of nonseminomatous germ cell tumors and in monitoring the response to therapy. AFP and β-hCG are useful in evaluating potential origins of poorly differentiated metastatic cancer.

CA 27.29 is most often used to follow response to therapy in patients with metastatic breast cancer. CA 27.29 is highly associated with breast cancer, although levels are elevated in several other malignancies (colon, gastric, hepatic, lung, pancreatic, ovarian, and prostate cancers). CA 27.29 also can be found in patients with benign disorders of the breast, liver, and kidney and in patients with ovarian cysts. CA 27.29 levels higher than 100 units/mL are rare in benign conditions.

CA 125 is useful for evaluating pelvic masses in postmenopausal women, monitoring response to therapy in women with ovarian cancer, and detecting recurrence of ovarian carcinoma. Postmenopausal women with asymptomatic palpable pelvic masses and CA 125 levels >65 units/mL likely have ovarian cancer. Because premenopausal women have more benign causes of elevated CA 125 levels, testing for the marker is less useful in this population.

Additional Reading: Diagnosis and management of pancreatic cancer. *Am Fam Physician.* 2014;89(8):626-632.

3. Desensitization immunotherapy is used in various allergic conditions and commonly is utilized in the treatment of which one of the following conditions?

A) Atopic dermatitis
B) Chronic urticaria
C) Hymenoptera allergies
D) Milk allergy
E) None of the above

The answer is C: Desensitization immunotherapy is used in the treatment of severe allergic rhinitis and beesting (hymenoptera) allergies. The patient is given gradually increasing concentrations of the allergen over an increasing period. Typically, there is a decrease in the mast cell response with a decrease in histamine production when the patient is exposed to the allergen. In addition, immunoglobulin E levels decrease. In most cases, the injections are continued year-round and may be spaced out as the desired response occurs.

Injections should always be given in the presence of a physician, and appropriate equipment must be available to treat potential anaphylaxis. Patients must be observed for at least 30 minutes after administration of the injections.

Desensitization immunotherapy is not appropriate for the treatment of chronic urticaria, milk allergies, or atopic dermatitis.

Additional Reading: Subcutaneous immunotherapy for allergic disease: indications and efficacy. In: *UpToDate*. 2022.

4. Patients use various vitamins, herbs, and other supplements to improve health and treat illness. Black cohosh has been advocated to treat which one of the following conditions?

A) Depression
B) Menopausal symptoms
C) Musculoskeletal pain
D) Osteoporosis
E) The common cold

The answer is B: The herb black cohosh, or *Actaea racemosa*, is native to North America. The roots and rhizomes of this herb are widely used in the treatment of menopausal symptoms and menstrual dysfunction. Although the clinical trials on black cohosh are of insufficient quality to support definitive statements, this herbal medicine may be effective in the short-term treatment of menopausal symptoms. The mechanism of action is unclear, and early reports of an estrogenic effect have not been proved in recent studies. Although black cohosh may be useful in treating some menopausal symptoms, there is currently no evidence regarding any protective effect of black cohosh against the development of osteoporosis. Adverse effects are uncommon, and there are no known significant adverse drug interactions.

Additional Reading: Hormone therapy and other treatments for symptoms of menopause. *Am Fam Physician.* 2016;94(11):884-889.

5. Lyme disease is a bacterial illness, which has become more prominent in the United States. Which one of the following statements is true of Lyme disease?

A) The disease is transmitted by the bite of a common wood tick.
B) The second stage may be characterized by fever, malaise, a stiff neck, back pain, and erythema chronicum migrans.
C) The first stage may involve carditis with atrioventricular (AV) block or pericarditis, peripheral neuropathies, and meningitis.
D) Treatment may be accomplished with doxycycline or amoxicillin.
E) The disease is most predominant in the Western regions of the United States.

The answer is D: Caused by the spirochete *B burgdorferi*, Lyme disease is transmitted by the bite of the deer tick (*Ixodes dammini*). Although reported in most states, it appears to be predominant in the Great Lakes area and the Western and Northeastern United States. The symptoms occur in three stages:

First stage. This stage usually begins with malaise, fever, headache, stiff neck, and back pain. Generalized lymphadenopathy with splenomegaly occurs, and a large annular erythematous lesion forms at the bite site and shows central clearing (erythema chronicum migrans). Multiple lesions may occur and affect other areas of the body. The lesions are warm but not often painful. As many as 25% may not exhibit skin manifestations. These symptoms usually appear within a few days to up to 1 month after the tick bite.

Second stage. This is the disseminated stage. Complications include carditis with AV block, palpitations, dyspnea, chest pain, and syncope. Pericarditis may also occur. Neurologic manifestations, including peripheral neuropathies and meningitis, are sometimes present. Large joint arthritis is also common.

Chronic phase. After the second stage, a chronic phase may result, although this is controversial. This phase is predominantly characterized with intermittent attacks of oligoarthritis lasting weeks to months. Other symptoms include subtle neurologic abnormalities (eg, memory problems and mood or sleep disorders). Diagnosis is usually made by the clinical presentation; however, an enzyme-linked immunosorbent assay followed by Western blot for positive results can help in the diagnosis but is somewhat unreliable.

Treatments for early disease include doxycycline, amoxicillin, and cefuroxime. A single dose of doxycycline has been shown to reduce the likelihood of Lyme disease after a deer tick bite.

Additional Reading: Lyme disease. In: Domino F, ed. *The 5-Minute Clinical Consult*. Wolters Kluwer; 2022.

6. The condition leishmaniasis refers to various clinical syndromes caused by a protozoa infection. The treatment of choice for leishmaniasis is which one of the following?

A) Antimonial compound
B) Ciprofloxacin
C) Doxycycline
D) Mebendazole
E) Quinine

The answer is A: Leishmaniasis is endemic to many regions of the tropics, the subtropics, and southern Europe. It is typically a vector-borne disease, with rodents and canids as common reservoir hosts and humans as incidental hosts. In humans, visceral, cutaneous, and mucosal leishmaniasis results from infection of macrophages throughout the reticuloendothelial system, in the skin, and in the nasal and oropharyngeal mucosa.

Leishmania parasites are transmitted by the bite of female sandflies. The transmission of *Leishmania* species typically is localized because of the limited area that sandflies inhabit.

The primary lesion at the site of an infected sandfly bite is small and usually not noticed. Parasites travel from the skin through the bloodstream to the lymph nodes, spleen, liver, and bone marrow.

Clinical signs develop gradually after 2 weeks up to 1 year later. The typical syndrome consists of fevers, hepatosplenomegaly, pancytopenia, and polyclonal hypergammaglobulinemia with reversed albumin/globulin ratio. In up to 10% of patients, twice-daily temperature spikes occur. Death can occur within 1 to 2 years in a majority of untreated symptomatic patients. A subclinical form with vague minor symptoms resolves spontaneously in a majority of patients and can progress to full-blown visceral leishmaniasis in one-third of cases. Those infected are resistant to further attacks, unless they are immunocompromised. One to two years after apparent cure, some patients develop nodular cutaneous lesions full of parasites, which can last for years and is often treated as folliculitis.

Treatment consists of a regimen of antimonial compounds. Toxicity, including myalgia, arthralgia, fatigue, elevated liver function tests, pancreatitis, and electrocardiographic abnormalities, is more common as the length of treatment progresses but usually does not limit treatment and is reversible. Alternatives include amphotericin B and pentamidine.

Additional Reading: *Parasites—Leishmaniasis*. Center for Disease Control and Prevention. www.cdc.gov/parasites/leishmaniasis/health_professionals/index.html#tx

7. Acetaminophen is utilized in various over-the-counter and prescription medication, and overdose is not uncommon. Which one of the following statements about acetaminophen overdose is correct?

A) Blood levels obtained 4 hours after ingestion determine treatment.
B) Elevations in liver tests peak 3 to 4 hours after ingestion.
C) Most cases involve adolescents and the elderly.
D) Symptoms include extremity pain with physical findings of peripheral neuropathy.
E) Treatment involves the use of deferoxamine.

The answer is A: Most cases of acetaminophen overdose involve children younger than 6 years, with toxic effects occurring when the dose exceeds 140 to 150 mg/kg or a total dose of 7.5 g. The drug primarily affects the liver by depleting glutathione stores 24 to 72 hours after ingestion and causing hepatocellular necrosis.

Symptoms include nausea, vomiting, and right-upper quadrant abdominal pain. Treatment, including emesis induced by syrup of ipecac, gastric lavage, and administration of activated charcoal, should be initiated as soon as possible.

Acetaminophen levels should be checked 4 hours after ingestion and plotted on the Rumack-Matthew nomogram. A 4-hour acetaminophen level greater than 150 μg/mL requires administration of the antidote acetylcysteine (Mucomyst). For maximal therapeutic effect, N-acetylcysteine should be administered within 8 hours of acetaminophen ingestion.

Peak aspartate aminotransferase, alanine transaminase, bilirubin, and PT values are seen 3 to 4 days after ingestion.

Additional Reading: Management of acetaminophen (paracetamol) poisoning in children and adolescents. In: *UpToDate*. 2022.

8. Chronic fatigue syndrome is a poorly understood condition that presents with a constellation of symptoms. Which one of the following statements about chronic fatigue syndrome is true?

A) Antibiotics may be beneficial.
B) Antidepressants may be beneficial.
C) Bed rest is usually beneficial.
D) Symptoms rarely improve.
E) The disease is most likely linked to the Epstein-Barr virus (EBV).

The answer is B: Chronic fatigue syndrome is a poorly understood constellation of symptoms that includes generalized fatigue, sore throat, tender lymphadenopathy, headaches, and generalized myalgias. The disease does not appear to be associated with chronic infections of EBV or Lyme disease. It does appear to be associated with underlying psychiatric disorders, such as somatization disorder, depression, and anxiety.

Chronic fatigue syndrome has no pathognomonic features and remains a constellation of symptoms and a diagnosis of exclusion. Patients with this constellation of symptoms should receive supportive therapy and be encouraged to gradually increase their exercise program within their limits and participate in their usual activities. Alternative medicines and vitamins are popular with many chronic fatigue syndrome patients but generally are not helpful. The use of antibiotics or antiviral agents is contraindicated. In some cases, patients may respond to antidepressant medications. Given enough time, most patients show improvement in symptoms.

Additional Reading: Chronic fatigue syndrome: diagnosis and treatment. *Am Fam Physician*. 2012;86(8):741-746.

9. Hereditary angioedema is an autosomal dominant transmitted genetic disorder, which can be life-threatening. Which one of the following statements about this condition is true?

A) Attacks are triggered by antihistamines.
B) It is related to excessive amyloid deposition.
C) It is caused by a deficiency of the C1 esterase inhibitor.
D) Treatment involves dehydroepiandrosterone administration.

The answer is C: Hereditary angioedema is an autosomal dominant transmitted genetic disorder that is related to a deficiency of C1 esterase inhibitor or, less commonly, to inactive C1 esterase inhibitor that is involved in the first step of complement activation. Symptoms include pruritus, urticarial rashes, abdominal pain, and, in severe cases, bronchoconstriction, which can be life-threatening. Attacks are usually triggered by stress, trauma, or illnesses. Diagnosis is made by detection of low C4 levels or deficiency of the C1 esterase inhibitor by immunoassay.

Treatment involves the use of antihistamines, glucocorticoids, and epinephrine (in severe cases). Fresh frozen plasma given before procedures can be used for short-term prophylaxis. Other medications used to prevent attacks include the androgens: methyltestosterone, danazol, and stanozolol. In addition, the C1 esterase inhibitor concentrate may be given directly in life-threatening cases.

Additional Reading: Angioedema. In: Domino F, ed. *The 5-Minute Clinical Consult*. Wolters Kluwer; 2022.

10. Aspirin and acetaminophen are marketed for various conditions and are available over the counter and in prescription therapies. Although they have many similar effects, which one of the following effects is provided by aspirin, but not acetaminophen?

A) Analgesic properties
B) Antipyretic properties
C) Anti-inflammatory properties
D) Amnestic properties
E) Antipruritic properties

The answer is C: Nonsteroidal anti-inflammatory drugs like Aspirin (acetylsalicylic acid) are the drug of choice for mild to moderate pain. It has antipyretic and anti-inflammatory properties (unlike acetaminophen, which has no anti-inflammatory properties). The major side effect is gastric irritation, which can be reduced by using an enteric-coated aspirin and taking the medication with meals. Tinnitus has also been associated with long-term aspirin use.

Aspirin's mode of action is accomplished by the inhibition of prostaglandin synthesis by permanently acetylating cyclooxygenase. Because platelet function is irreversibly inhibited, bleeding times are prolonged as much as 1 to 2 weeks. Aspirin can evoke an anaphylactic response in some individuals, especially in those with a history of asthma and nasal polyps, and thus should be avoided. Aspirin use should also be avoided in children and teenagers with viral febrile illnesses (eg, chickenpox, infectious mononucleosis, and viral influenza) because of the risk of Reye syndrome.

Additional Readings:
1. Drugs for pain. *Treat Guidel Med Lett.* 2013;11(128):31-42.
2. Pharmacologic therapy for acute pain. *Am Fam Physician.* 2021;104(1):63-72.

Aspirin has antipyretic and anti-inflammatory properties. Acetaminophen has no anti-inflammatory properties.

11. In caring for patients with human immunodeficiency virus (HIV) infection, it is important to follow CD4 counts as markers of disease and for treatment protocols to prevent opportunistic infections. A 30-year-old man was recently diagnosed with HIV infection and is found to have a CD4 cell count of 150 cells/mm^3 should have which one of the following?

A) Additional follow-up tests in 1 month
B) Additional follow-up tests in 3 months
C) Additional follow-up tests in 6 months
D) Tests repeated in 1 year
E) Antiviral medication prescribed now

The answer is E: The CD4 cell count is a marker for T-helper cells and is used in the treatment of HIV. Once the patient has been diagnosed with HIV, the CD4 cell count should be measured and followed. Typically, there is a diurnal variation in the CD4 cell count; therefore, it should be measured at the same time of the day, with each determination.

Plasma HIV viral load is used to determine response to treatment in HIV and is no longer used when considering initiation of antiretroviral drug therapy (ART). ART is recommended for all HIV-infected individuals to reduce the risk of disease progression and for the prevention of transmission of HIV. Patients starting ART should be willing and able to commit to treatment and understand the benefits and risks of therapy and the importance of adherence. Patients may choose to postpone therapy, and providers, on a case-by-case basis, may elect to defer therapy on the basis of clinical and/or psychosocial factors.

Without treatment, the vast majority of HIV-infected individuals will eventually develop progressive immunosuppression (as evident by CD4 count depletion), leading to acquired immunodeficiency syndrome (AIDS)-defining illnesses and premature death. The primary goal of ART is to prevent HIV-associated morbidity and mortality. This goal is best accomplished by using effective ART to maximally inhibit HIV replication so that plasma HIV RNA levels (viral load) remain below that detectable by commercially available assays. Durable viral suppression improves immune function and quality of life, lowers the risk of both AIDS-defining and non–AIDS-defining complications, and prolongs life. Furthermore, high-plasma HIV RNA is a major risk factor for HIV transmission, and the use of effective ART can reduce viremia and transmission of HIV to sexual partners.

Regardless of CD4 count, the decision to initiate ART should always include consideration of any comorbid conditions, the willingness and readiness of the patient to initiate therapy, and the availability of resources. In settings where resources are not available to initiate ART in all patients, treatment should be prioritized for patients with the lowest CD4 counts and those with the following clinical conditions: pregnancy, CD4 count <200 cells/mm^3 (as in this patient), or history of an AIDS-defining illness, including HIV-associated dementia, HIV-associated nephropathy, hepatitis B virus, and acute HIV infection.

Additional Reading: Initial management of patients with HIV infection. *Am Fam Physician.* 2016;94(9):708-716.

12. Which of the following tests is most helpful in distinguishing fever of unknown origin from factitious fever?

A) Blood cultures
B) Chest x-ray
C) Rheumatoid factor
D) Sedimentation rate
E) Urinalysis

The answer is D: Fever of unknown origin is defined as a fever higher than 101 °F (38.3 °C) on at least three occasions, accompanied by an illness that lasts longer than 3 weeks, and the diagnosis is uncertain after 3 days of hospitalization, although most workups are now done in the outpatient setting. Causes include infection, neoplasm, drugs, collagen vascular disease, vasculitis, and factitious fever.

Laboratory tests include complete blood count, urinalysis with culture, blood cultures, chest radiography, human immunodeficiency virus testing, serum protein electrophoresis, sedimentation rate, serology tests, antinuclear antibody, rheumatoid factor, and thyroid tests. The erythrocyte sedimentation rate may be helpful in distinguishing real disease from a factitious fever.

A good history and physical examination are imperative in the evaluation of a patient with fever of unknown origin and help direct further testing. Observing the temperature pattern can be helpful. Disease states such as malaria, babesiosis, Hodgkin disease, and cyclic neutropenia have patterns, whereas factitious fever often has no pattern.

Additional Reading: Approach to the adult with fever of unknown origin. In: *UpToDate*. 2022.

13. Third-generation cephalosporins differ from first-generation cephalosporins in their increased effectiveness against which one of the organisms?

A) Anaerobic bacteria
B) Gram-positive bacteria
C) Gram-negative bacteria
D) Parasites
E) Fungi

The answer is C: Cephalosporins are antibiotics with chemical structure similar to the penicillins. They are bactericidal and cover gram-positive bacteria; second-generation and third-generation cephalosporins also cover gram-negative bacteria. As a group, the cephalosporins' mechanism of action is the inhibition of cell wall synthesis. Inflammation increases their absorption, and they are active against a wide spectrum of organisms with relatively few side effects. Some of the cephalosporins, especially third-generation ones, are concentrated enough in the cerebrospinal fluid to treat meningitis.

Because of their similarity to penicillin, there is a 2% to 3% cross-reactivity in those allergic to penicillin. Unfortunately, there are no predictable skin tests that can test for allergic reactions. Therefore, the use of cephalosporins in patients with penicillin allergies should be monitored closely.

Additional Reading: Drugs for bacterial infections. *Treat Guidel Med Lett*. 2013;11(131):65-74.

14. Mononucleosis is a common infection among adolescents and young adults. The best treatment for uncomplicated case is which one of the following?

A) Empiric antibiotic treatment
B) Intravenous antiviral medication
C) Oral antiviral therapy (acyclovir or ganciclovir)
D) Oral steroids
E) Symptomatic treatment only

The answer is E: The mainstay of treatment for individuals with uncomplicated mononucleosis is supportive care. Acetaminophen or nonsteroidal anti-inflammatory drugs are recommended for the treatment of fever, throat discomfort, and malaise. Provision of adequate fluids and nutrition is also important. It is prudent to get adequate rest, although complete bed rest is unnecessary.

The incidence of mononucleosis is highest in young adults 15 to 35 years of age. Asymptomatic infections are common, and most adults are seropositive to the Epstein-Barr virus. Symptoms include fever, headache, generalized fatigue, and malaise. Signs include lymphadenopathy (especially the posterior cervical chain), splenomegaly, hepatomegaly, jaundice, periorbital edema, exudative pharyngitis, palatine petechiae, and rash.

Laboratory findings show a lymphocytosis with 20% or more atypical lymphocytes (Downey lymphocytes), a positive heterophile agglutination (Monospot) test after the second week of illness, and a heterophile titer greater than 1:56. Liver function test results are usually elevated. Other laboratory findings may include granulocytopenia, thrombocytopenia, and hemolytic anemia in complicated cases.

No specific treatment is recommended for mild cases, and symptoms usually improve in 2 to 4 weeks. In severe cases in which pharyngitis threatens to obstruct the patient's airway, a 5-day course of steroids may be beneficial. Specific antiviral therapies (acyclovir or ganciclovir) do not appear to be clinically beneficial. Treatment with amoxicillin or ampicillin may lead to a severe maculopapular rash and should be avoided. If the patient has evidence of splenomegaly, contact sports should be avoided until the splenomegaly has resolved.

Additional Reading: Infectious mononucleosis in adults and adolescents. In: *UpToDate*. 2022.

15. Which one of the following drugs is associated with drug-induced lupus erythematosus (LE)?

A) Azithromycin
B) Digoxin
C) Hydralazine
D) Metoprolol
E) Penicillin

The answer is C: Drug-induced LE is associated with the use of procainamide (most common), hydralazine, isoniazid, penicillamine, sulfonamides, quinidine, thiouracil, methyldopa, and cephalosporins. All patients with drug-induced LE have positive reactions to antinuclear antibody testing; however, they usually do not have positive reactions to antibodies to double-stranded DNA. Other laboratory findings supporting drug-induced lupus include anemia, leukopenia, thrombocytopenia, positive rheumatoid factor, positive cryoglobulins, positive lupus anticoagulants, false-positive Venereal Disease Research Laboratory test results, and positive results on a direct Coombs test.

Signs and symptoms include polyarthralgias, fever, butterfly rash affecting the facial area, alopecia, photosensitivity, pleurisy, proteinuria, and glomerulonephritis. In most cases, the symptoms disappear when the medication is discontinued. Steroids may be necessary for severe cases.

Additional Reading: Lupus erythematosus. In: Domino F, ed. *The 5-Minute Clinical Consult*. Wolters Kluwer; 2022.

16. Bacteria are increasingly developing resistance to commonly used antibiotics, and there has been an increasing incidence of Methicillin-resistant *S aureus* (MRSA) infection. The drug of choice to treat a serious MRSA skin infection would be which one of the following antibiotics?

A) Cefuroxime
B) Dicloxacillin
C) Metronidazole
D) Penicillin
E) Vancomycin

The answer is E: MRSA is the predominant cause of suppurative skin infection in the United States. Community-associated MRSA (CA-MRSA) usually causes furunculosis, cellulitis, and abscesses, but necrotizing fasciitis and sepsis can occur. CA-MRSA strains are usually susceptible to trimethoprim-sulfamethoxazole, clindamycin, and tetracyclines. Patients with serious skin and soft tissue infections suspected to be caused by MRSA should be treated empirically with vancomycin, linezolid, or daptomycin.

Isolates are usually resistant to all the cillin-type antibiotics and the cephalosporins. Duration of therapy is based on the patient's response but is usually 2 to 4 weeks. Colonization occurs in approximately 50% of treated patients. The most common reservoir for chronic infections is the nasal mucosa and oropharynx. Asymptomatic colonization with MRSA does not require systemic treatment.

Additional Reading: Skin and soft tissue infections. *Am Fam Physician*. 2015;92(6):474-483.

17. A 27-year-old man is on a routine examination and he reports that he is in a monogamous sexual relationship with another man. He works full-time as a clerk in a clothing store and is in good health. You have cared for him since he was a preteen and his immunizations are current. Based on expert consensus, which one of the following would be most appropriate at this visit?

A) Preexposure human immunodeficiency virus (HIV) prophylaxis
B) Screening for sexually transmitted infections now and every 3 months
C) Meningococcal vaccine
D) Hepatitis B surface antigen (HBsAG) testing

The answer is D: Men who have sex with men but are in a monogamous relationship need not be offered preexposure or postexposure HIV prophylaxis, unlike men with multiple or anonymous sexual partners. Likewise, because this patient is in a monogamous relationship, screening for sexually transmitted infections once a year is adequate.

Screening for hepatitis B (HBsAG testing), as well as testing for hepatitis C infection, at this visit is recommended. Meningococcal vaccine is not indicated, unless there are other risk factors.

Additional Reading:

1. *Final Recommendation Statement: Hepatitis B Virus Infection: Screening*. US Preventive Services Task Force; 2014.
2. Preventive health care for men who have sex with men. *Am Fam Physician*. 2015;91(12):844-851.

18. A 42-year-old construction worker is brought to the emergency department by his coworkers. He has been working in the sun all day and, on arrival, he is hyperventilating and sweating profusely. On examination, his blood pressure (BP) is 90/54, and his oral temperature is 99.4 °F. The most likely diagnosis to account for these findings is which one of the following diagnosis?

A) Heat exhaustion
B) Heat stroke
C) Hypothermia
D) Thyroid storm
E) Organophosphate poisoning

The answer is A: Heat exhaustion is seen with prolonged exposure in hot conditions, and individuals usually exhibit hyperventilation, profuse sweating with substantial bodily fluid loss, and low BP. Body temperature is usually normal and, when elevated, does not exceed 40 °C. Mental status is usually normal, unlike in with heat stroke.

Heat stroke is a medical emergency. Symptoms include headache, vertigo, fatigue, and increased body temperature (>40 °C). Sweating is usually absent. The skin is hot and dry. Patients may exhibit bizarre and confused behavior, hallucinations, loss of consciousness, and seizures. Other manifestations include tachycardia and tachypnea; BP is usually preserved. If circulatory collapse occurs, patients may suffer brain damage and even death.

Patients should immediately be treated with cool water or wet dressings. Careful monitoring of body core temperature should be instituted to avoid conversion of hyperpyrexia to hypothermia. Once hospitalized, fluid replacement and further temperature management can be instituted. Complications include renal failure, cardiac failure, and the development of disseminated intravascular coagulopathy. Treatment for heat exhaustion is similar to heat stroke and consists mainly of fluid resuscitation.

Additional Reading: Heat-related illness. *Am Fam Physician*. 2011;83(11):1325-1330.

Heat stroke is a medical emergency. Symptoms include headache, vertigo, fatigue, and increased body temperature (>40 °C). Sweating is usually absent, and the skin is hot and dry.

19. An 18-year-old woman brought in to the emergency department by paramedics after she fainted at a rock concert. On examination, you notice that she has circumoral paresthesias and is exhibiting carpopedal spasms. The most likely diagnosis to account for her condition is which one of the following?

A) Cardiac arrhythmia
B) Cocaine overdose
C) Heat exhaustion
D) Hyperventilation
E) Seizure disorder

The answer is D: Hyperventilation can lead to a significant respiratory alkalosis and is frequently the result of anxiety or extreme excitement. Other less common causes include drug effects, central nervous system dysfunction, alcohol withdrawal, asthma, heart failure, pulmonary embolus, exposure to high altitudes, intense exercise, and chronic pain.

Symptoms include circumoral and extremity paresthesias, lightheadedness, giddiness, and sometimes syncope. Carpopedal spasm occurs when acute hypocarbia causes reduced ionized calcium and phosphate levels, resulting in involuntary contraction of the hands and occasionally the feet. Blood gases usually show low CO_2 (20-25 mm Hg) and elevated pH (respiratory alkalosis).

Treatment can be accomplished by breathing into a paper bag. Other efforts should be directed at the treatment of anxiety or underlying contributing factors; relaxation training may be beneficial.

Additional Reading: Hyperventilation syndrome, emergency medicine. In: *The 5-Minute Clinical Consult*. Wolters Kluwer; 2022.

20. Which one of the following statements regarding aminoglycoside antibiotics is true?

A) Liver function should be followed closely during administration.
B) Lupuslike syndrome can occur with prolonged use.
C) Nephrotoxic effects can occur with administration.
D) Respiratory depression is not associated with aminoglycosides.
E) Volume of distribution is increased in obese patients.

The answer is C: Toxicity associated with the use of aminoglycosides (eg, gentamicin) includes ototoxicity with clinically apparent hearing loss (<1% of cases), tinnitus, and vertigo, as well as nephrotoxic effects (5%-10% of adults who receive therapy for 10-14 days), including renal failure. Rarely, respiratory depression can occur.

Drug levels should be followed after a steady state is achieved—every 3 to 5 days or more often if increases in serum creatinine are noted. Patients with decreased renal function may need an adjustment of medication on the basis of their creatinine clearance. Some data suggest that once-daily administration may cause less nephrotoxicity.

Aminoglycosides have low solubility in lipids; therefore, the volume of distribution is decreased in obese patients. Patients with trauma, burns, cancer, and postoperative septic shock have increased volumes of distribution. Neuromuscular depression from aminoglycosides is caused by reduced acetylcholine activity at postsynaptic membranes and can result in rare but severe respiratory depression. This can be largely avoided if the aminoglycoside is given intravenously over 30 minutes or by an intramuscular injection. If respiratory depression does occur, it can be reversed by the administration of calcium.

Additional Reading: Drugs for bacterial infections. *Treat Guidel Med Lett*. 2013;11(131):65-74.

21. *Babesia* infections range from subclinical presentations to severe complications. Which one of the following statements about babesiosis is true?

A) Affected patients without spleens usually have a better prognosis.
B) Diagnosis is made with a peripheral blood smear.
C) Generalized paralysis occurs in those affected.
D) The disease is transmitted by fecal-oral contamination.
E) The disease is caused by a rickettsial organism.

The answer is B: Babesiosis is a tick-borne disease caused by *Babesia microti*. Symptoms of symptomatic babesiosis develop within a few weeks or months after exposure but may first appear or recur many months later, particularly in persons who are or become immunosuppressed. Clinically manifest *Babesia* infection is characterized by the presence of hemolytic anemia and nonspecific flulike symptoms (eg, fever, chills, body aches, weakness, and fatigue). Some patients have splenomegaly, hepatomegaly, or jaundice.

Risk factors for severe babesiosis include asplenia, advanced age, and other causes of impaired immune function (eg, human immunodeficiency virus, malignancy, and corticosteroid therapy). Some immunosuppressive therapies or conditions may affect the clinical manifestations (eg, the patient might be afebrile). Severe cases can be associated with marked thrombocytopenia, disseminated intravascular coagulation, hemodynamic instability, acute respiratory distress, myocardial infarction, renal failure, hepatic compromise, altered mental status, and death.

If the diagnosis of babesiosis is being considered, a manual review of the peripheral blood smear should be requested to look for the parasite. In symptomatic patients with acute infection, *Babesia* parasites typically can be detected by light microscopic examination of blood smears, although multiple smears may need to be examined.

When symptomatic, babesiosis is treated for 7 to 10 days with a combination of two medications:

- Atovaquone *plus* azithromycin *or*
- Clindamycin *plus* quinine

Additional Reading: *Parasites—Babesiosis.* Center for Disease Control and Prevention. www.cdc.gov/parasites/babesiosis/health_professionals/index.html

22. A 31-year-old florist with no history of allergy to beestings presents to the ED after being stung by a yellow jacket. Other than local swelling at the site, she has no other symptoms. The most appropriate treatment involves which one of the following?

A) Administration of epinephrine and antihistamine as well as hospitalization
B) Administration of steroids, epinephrine, intravenous hydration, and β2-agonist
C) Ice therapy, administration of antihistamine, and observation at home
D) Immediate removal of the stinger using tweezers
E) Meat tenderizer sprinkled over the sting site, warm-water soaks, and aspirin

The answer is C: Stings by a hymenopteran (eg, bees, wasps, yellow jackets, hornets, and ants) may be fatal in a hypersensitive patient. Indeed, each year in the United States, more patients die of beestings than of snakebites.

Individuals with no history of hypersensitivity may be treated by application of ice to the sting, administration of oral antihistamine, and observation at home. Large local reactions may be treated with glucocorticoids. Removal of the stinger by tweezers is usually avoided because of the possibility of injecting further venom at the site. Application of meat tenderizer containing papain is of no proven value.

Patients with a history of hypersensitivity may experience severe swelling at the site of the sting with the development of shock, often within minutes. Treatment should be immediate and includes application of ice to the sting site, administration of intramuscular epinephrine and oral antihistamine, and prompt transfer to the hospital. All patients with Hymenoptera-sting hypersensitivity should receive a prescription for an epinephrine kit and carry this with them whenever they are outdoors. Patients should also be counseled to receive hymenoptera desensitization immunotherapy.

Additional Reading: Bites and stings, sports medicine. In: *The 5-Minute Clinical Consult.* Wolters Kluwer; 2022.

23. A 27-year-old farmer is brought to the emergency department by his spouse, as he has been vomiting with diarrhea. You notice that he is sweaty and excessively salivating, with breath that has a garlic odor. On examination, he has miosis and is wheezing. The most likely diagnosis to account for this presentation is which one of the following conditions?

A) Alcohol overdose
B) Cocaine overdose
C) Cyanide ingestion
D) Diabetic ketoacidosis
E) Organophosphate poisoning

The answer is E: Organophosphate insecticides are inhibitors of acetylcholinesterase and result in an accumulation of acetylcholine at the synaptic junction. Organophosphate poisoning is characterized by miosis (pupillary constriction), bronchoconstriction, sweating, salivation, headache, vomiting, diarrhea, muscle weakness, and convulsions. The patient's breath typically has a garlic odor.

Treatment involves gastric lavage followed by activated charcoal or aggressive cleansing if skin exposure had occurred. Parasympathetic stimulation can be counteracted by the administration of atropine sulfate until symptoms disappear or until signs of atropine use occur (eg, dilated pupils and dry mouth). In addition, pralidoxime helps remove the organophosphate from the cholinesterase.

Additional Reading: Organophosphate and carbamate poisoning. In: *UpToDate.* 2022.

24. Which one of the following medications is the most appropriate to use in the emergent treatment of a patient suffering from an anaphylactic reaction?

A) Atropine
B) Diphenhydramine
C) Epinephrine
D) Isoproterenol
E) Prednisone

The answer is C: Anaphylaxis may be caused by various factors, including ingestion of certain foods, insect bites or stings, drugs, and contrast dyes. Symptoms include urticaria, angioedema, dyspnea, cough, hoarseness, wheezing, a sense of impending doom, abdominal pain, hypotension, and syncope. Death occurs in 3% of patients. The cause is a massive immunoglobulin E–mediated response, which results in the release of large amounts of histamine from mast cells. Treatment must be prompt and includes securing the patient's airway and administering epinephrine, 0.2 to 0.5 mL of 1:1000 subcutaneously, every 15 to 20 minutes, repeated three times if the patient is stable; if the patient is unstable, epinephrine should be administered intravenously.

At the time of epinephrine administration, intravenous fluids should be started, and after the administration, diphenhydramine (H1 receptor blocker) should also be given. All patients with anaphylaxis should be hospitalized and monitored for 24 hours.

Corticosteroids have no role in the short-term treatment of anaphylaxis but should be initiated to prevent a late-phase reaction. Bronchodilators such as albuterol should also be used if the patient is wheezing or short of breath.

Additional Reading: Anaphylaxis. In: *UpToDate*. 2022.

25. Ingestion of toxins can cause a multitude of symptoms and some toxins cause specific symptoms, which can be helpful in identifying a toxic exposure. Which one of the following toxins causes the associated listed symptom?

A) Chromate and cocaine—nasal septal perforations
B) Iron, lithium, and lead—pulmonary fibrosis
C) Mercury, lead, and pesticides—acro-osteolysis
D) Vinyl chloride—behavioral changes

The answer is A: Ingestion of toxins can cause a multitude of symptoms; however, there are specific symptoms particularly associated with specific toxins. The following are some toxins and their common identifiable symptoms:

Toxin Exposure	Symptom
Chromate and cocaine	Nasal septal perforations
Asbestos exposure	Pulmonary fibrosis
Mercury, lead, pesticides	Behavior change
Vinyl chloride	Acro-osteolysis (resorption of the distal bony phalanges)

Additional Reading: Pulmonary complications of cocaine abuse. In: *UpToDate*. 2022.

26. A 47-year-old florist presents to your office complaining of a nontender nodule that formed on his hand, then enlarged, and finally ulcerated. In the days that followed, the patient developed similar nodules in the area of the axillary lymphatics. Otherwise he has had no other symptoms. The most likely diagnosis to account for these findings is which one of the following infections?

A) Blastomycosis
B) Cat scratch fever
C) Histoplasmosis
D) Sporotrichosis
E) Tuberculosis

The answer is D: Sporotrichosis is a disease caused by inoculation of the plant *Sporothrix schenckii* when patients prick themselves with a thorn. The condition is associated with the formation of nodules, ulcers, and abscesses affecting the skin and lymphatic system. Farm workers and those who work around plants (ie, florists, gardeners, nursery workers, and horticulturists) such as sphagnum moss, rosebushes, and barberry bushes are the most likely to be affected.

Most patients present with a nontender nodule that forms on an arm or hand. The nodule enlarges, becomes erythematous (blush red), and finally ulcerates. In the following days, other nodules may form in the area of the draining lymphatics. Local pain and constitutional symptoms are usually absent. Other areas such as lungs, spleen, liver, kidney, genitalia, muscle, joints, and eyes may become involved.

Diagnosis is usually achieved by culturing the organism from the nodules. Treatment is accomplished with itraconazole and extended courses of saturated solution of potassium iodide; in severe disseminated cases, intravenous amphotericin B or ketoconazole (less effective) is used.

Blastomycosis refers to an infection with the fungus *Blastomyces*. The symptoms of blastomycosis are often similar to the symptoms of flu.

Cat scratch fever is usually a benign infectious disease caused by the bacterium *Bartonella henselae*, following a scratch or bite from a cat. Cat scratch disease commonly presents as tender, swollen lymph nodes near the site of the inoculating bite or scratch or on the neck.

Histoplasmosis is a disease caused by the fungus *Histoplasma capsulatum*. Symptoms of this infection vary, but the disease primarily affects the lungs. It is an opportunistic infection, seen in immunocompromised individuals.

Additional Reading: Sporotrichosis. In: Domino F, ed. *The 5-Minute Clinical Consult*. Wolters Kluwer; 2022.

27. Toxins are often treated using an "antidote" to counter the adverse effects of the toxic agent. Which one of the following toxin-antidote associations is correct?

A) Cyanide-calcium carbonate antidote
B) Ethylene glycol-ethanol and pyridoxine antidotes
C) Magnesium-amyl nitrite antidote
D) Organic phosphates-epinephrine antidote

The answer is B: Toxin exposure is often treated by family physicians. The following are the drugs of choice for treating the associated toxin exposures:

Toxin	Antidote
Cyanide	Amyl nitrite
Ethylene glycol	Ethanol and pyridoxine
Magnesium	Calcium carbonate
Organic phosphates	Atropine

Additional Reading: General approach to drug poisoning in adults. In: *UpToDate*. 2021.

28. A 32-year-old woman reports a previous allergic reaction to penicillin. As a smoker, she has had recurrent sinus and respiratory tract infections that frequently require antibiotic treatment and has a recurrent episode of sinusitis. Appropriate management for this situation would consist of which one of the following actions?

A) Administer diphenhydramine with any penicillin.
B) Prescribe a cephalosporin if the patient has had a previous anaphylactoid reaction.
C) Prescribe amoxicillin instead of penicillin.
D) Prescribe imipenem instead of penicillin.
E) Test the patient for penicillin allergies.

The answer is E: An allergy to penicillin is related to penicilloic acid—a breakdown product—and other degradation products that are involved in the metabolism of penicillin. All penicillins are cross-reactive and cross-sensitizing. The incidence of penicillin allergy is approximately 1% to 10% of adults. However, studies have shown that 80% to 90% of patients who report a penicillin allergy are not actually allergic to the drug.

The decision to use penicillin in patients with previous reactions should be based on the severity of previous reactions. If the patient has had a severe anaphylactic reaction in the past, penicillins should be avoided. In addition, there is a 2% cross-reactivity between cephalosporins in patients with penicillin allergies; thus, cephalosporins should be avoided in patients who have had an immediate reaction to penicillin. The same is true for imipenem. Skin tests that use penicilloyl-polylysine and undegraded penicillin may be used to detect patients who have true penicillin allergies.

Additional Reading: *Don't Overuse Non-Beta Lactam Antibiotics in Patients with a History of Penicillin Allergy, Without an Appropriate Evaluation*. www.aafp.org/afp/recommendations/viewRecommendation.htm?recommendationId=197

29. Which one of the following is associated with chronic fatigue syndrome?

A) A recent Epstein-Barr virus (EBV) infection
B) Associated psychiatric disorders
C) Minimal impairment of normal activity
D) Muscle weakness
E) Temporal artery tenderness

The answer is B: Fatigue is a common complaint heard in a family physician's office. Broadly defined, the chronic fatigue syndrome is described as long-standing severe fatigue without substantial muscle weakness and without proven psychological or physical causes. Various criteria have been published. The Centers for Disease Control and Prevention Diagnostic Criteria for Chronic Fatigue Syndrome include severe fatigue for longer than 6 months and at least four of the following symptoms:

1. Headache of new type, pattern, or severity
2. Multijoint pain without swelling or erythema
3. Muscle pain
4. Postexertional malaise for longer than 24 hours
5. Significant impairment in short-term memory or concentration
6. Sore throat
7. Tender lymph nodes
8. Unrefreshing sleep

Symptoms may develop acutely. Typically, there are no signs of muscle weakness, arthritis, neuropathy, or organomegaly. Women are more often affected than men. The syndrome has not been proven to be associated with EBV; however, some believe that it may be linked to a viral infection.

Persons with chronic fatigue should be evaluated with a comprehensive history and physical examination. Initial laboratory testing would include urinalysis, complete blood count, comprehensive metabolic panel, thyroid-stimulating hormone, C-reactive protein, and phosphorus levels.

There appears to be a high incidence of associated psychiatric disorders, and patients with chronic fatigue syndrome should be evaluated for concurrent depression, pain, and sleep disturbances. Persons diagnosed with chronic fatigue syndrome should be treated with cognitive behavior therapy, graded exercise therapy, or both. Cognitive behavior therapy and graded exercise therapy have been shown to improve fatigue, work and social adjustment, anxiety, and postexertional malaise.

Although no placebo-controlled trials have supported the treatment, antidepressants have shown some anecdotal benefits in those affected. Antiviral medication, immunologic treatments (steroids, immunoglobulin, interferon), and vitamin therapy are used, but their effectiveness has not been proved.

Additional Reading: Chronic fatigue syndrome: diagnosis and treatment. *Am Fam Physician*. 2012;86(8):741-746.

30. A 52-year-old man is seen because he has been having fevers and weight loss over the past couple of months. His chest radiograph shows mediastinal lymphadenopathy, and his laboratory results include hypercalcemia, elevated alkaline phosphatase, and an elevated angiotensin-converting enzyme (ACE) level. The most likely diagnosis that would account for his presentation is which one of the following conditions?

A) Asbestosis
B) Histoplasmosis
C) Pulmonary tuberculosis
D) Sarcoidosis
E) Small cell carcinoma of the lung

The answer is D: Sarcoidosis is a systemic granulomatous disease of unknown cause, which is characterized by noncaseating granulomas that may affect multiple organ systems. The condition occurs mainly in individuals aged 20 to 40 years and is most common in Northern Europeans and African Americans.

Symptoms are variable and the condition usually presents with fever, weight loss, arthralgias, and erythema nodosum. Cough and dyspnea may be minimal or absent. Other manifestations include mediastinal lymphadenopathy seen on chest radiograph, hepatic granulomas, granulomatous uveitis, polyarthritis, cardiac symptoms (including angina, congestive heart failure, and conduction abnormalities), cranial nerve palsies, and diabetes insipidus.

Laboratory findings include leukopenia, hypercalcemia, hypercalciuria, and hypergammaglobulinemia (particularly in African American patients). Other abnormalities include elevated uric acid, elevated alkaline phosphatase, elevated gamma glutamyl transpeptidase, and elevated levels of ACE. Pulmonary function tests (PFTs) show restriction and impaired diffusing capacity, and serial PFTs are important for assessing disease progression and guiding treatment.

Diagnosis can be made with a biopsy of peripheral lesions or fiber-optic bronchoscopy for central pulmonary lesions. Whole-body gallium scans can be used to show useful sites for biopsy and, in some cases, to follow disease progression.

The prognosis depends on the severity of the disease. Spontaneous improvement is common; however, significant disability can occur with multiorgan involvement. Treatment for symptomatic patients consists of corticosteroids, methotrexate, and other immunosuppressive medications if steroid therapy is not helpful. Pulmonary fibrosis is the leading cause of death.

Additional Reading: Sarcoidosis. In: Domino F, ed. *The 5-Minute Clinical Consult*. Wolters Kluwer; 2022.

Sarcoidosis is a systemic granulomatous disease of unknown cause, which is characterized by noncaseating granulomas that may affect multiple organ systems, but primarily the lungs.

31. Patients suffering from acquired immunodeficiency syndrome (AIDS) are at risk for various opportunistic infections, including cytomegalovirus (CMV). When an AIDS patient is suffering from a CMV infection, the most appropriate treatment is to prescribe which one of the following agents?

A) Amphotericin B
B) Amantadine
C) Ciprofloxacin
D) Ganciclovir
E) Metronidazole

The answer is D: CMV is a viral infection that may occur congenitally or at any age. The severity of the infection varies. The virus is a variant of the herpes virus and is ubiquitous. Patients with AIDS or immunocompromised conditions such as transplant patients and those living in institutions (such as nursing homes) or attending day care centers are at increased risk of disease complications.

The infection is common (as much as 90% of the population is affected) and in most cases is represented by mild symptoms. More severe cases can produce a mononucleosis-type illness, retinitis, or pneumonitis in adults.

Diagnosis is achieved with the detection of the virus by immunofluorescence with monoclonal antibodies. Treatment is usually supportive; however, ganciclovir can be used in more severe cases and particularly in AIDS patients. Foscarnet sodium (Foscavir) is also effective, especially in ganciclovir-resistant cases.

Additional Reading: Antiviral drugs. *Treat Guidel Med Lett*. 2013;11(127):19-30.

32. A homeless man is brought to the emergency department, suffering from hypothermia. An electrocardiogram (ECG) is obtained and his ECG would be expected to have which one of the following findings?

A) A "J wave" (Osborne wave)
B) Atrioventricular (AV) dissociation
C) A first-degree AV block
D) Atrial fibrillation
E) Tachycardia

The answer is A: Hypothermia is caused by prolonged exposure to a cold environment, causing the body's core temperature to fall below 35 °C (or 95 °F). Infants, the elderly, and those with altered mental status or debilitating illnesses are at increased risk. Others at increased risk include trauma and burn victims and those with malnutrition.

Symptoms include shivering, decreased mental status with confusion, impaired coordination, drowsiness, bradycardia, and, in more severe cases, loss of the shivering reflex and coma. ECG tracings may show a characteristic positive deflection after the QRS complex in the lateral leads, known as a J or Osborne wave.

Treatment involves slow central body warming (over 2-3 hours to prevent shock) with warmed intravenous fluids, warmed oxygen, and warming blankets or warm baths. Life-sustaining measures should always be continued until the normal core body temperature is achieved. Death can result from the progression of severe bradycardia to ventricular fibrillation.

Additional Reading: Hypothermia. In: Domino F, ed. *The 5-Minute Clinical Consult*. Wolters Kluwer; 2022.

33. Hypersensitivity reactions to cephalosporins may occur and include rash, urticaria, and, in severe cases, anaphylaxis. To avoid such reactions, cephalosporins are contraindicated for which one of the following groups?

A) Patients allergic to eggs
B) Patients who have had a mild rash following penicillin administration
C) Patients with glucose-6-phosphate dehydrogenase deficiency
D) Patients suspected of bacterial meningitis
E) None of the above

The answer is E: Because of the similar chemical structure, there is a small proportion (<2%) of patients with penicillin allergy who cross-react with cephalosporins. Therefore, cephalosporins should be avoided in patients with a history of an immediate reaction to penicillin. Cephalosporins can be used in patients with a history of a mild reaction to penicillins. The other listed conditions are not related to cephalosporin sensitivity.

Additional Reading: Cephalosporins for patients with penicillin allergy. *Med Lett Drugs Ther*. 2012;54(1406):101.

34. A mother brings her 10-year-old son with a fever and rash, which developed a few days after they had been hiking in the mountains with friends. A friend thought that the rash looked like Rocky Mountain spotted fever. Which one of the following statements best describes the rash associated with this condition?

A) The rash develops on the extremities and then spreads centrally.
B) The rash eruption develops on the trunk and spreads to the extremities.
C) The rash typically only affects the face.
D) The rash consists of bull's-eye lesions with central clearing.
E) The rash consists of erythematous, raised papules that are intensely pruritic.

The answer is A: The causative agent of Rocky Mountain spotted fever is *Rickettsia rickettsii*, which is transmitted by the bite of the wood tick or the dog tick. The disease is usually found in the southern United States and is more commonly seen during the summer months. It is the most common rickettsial disease in the United States. The wood tick (*Dermacentor andersoni*) is the principal vector in the Western United States, whereas the dog tick (*Dermacentor variabilis*) is the most common vector in the eastern and southern United States. Transmission from person to person is not thought to occur.

The incidence of Rocky Mountain spotted fever is highest in children 5 to 9 years of age. A tick bite is recalled by only 50% to 70% of patients. The onset of symptoms of Rocky Mountain spotted fever usually begins 5 to 7 days after inoculation. Common symptoms include generalized malaise, myalgias (especially in the back and leg muscles), fever, frontal headaches, nausea, and vomiting. Other symptoms may include nonproductive cough, sore throat, pleuritic chest pain, and abdominal pain.

The classic presenting symptoms include sudden onset of headache, fever, and chills accompanied by an exanthem appearing within the first few days of symptoms. Initially, lesions appear on the palms, soles, wrists, ankles, and forearms. The lesions are pink and macular and fade with applied pressure. The rash then extends to the axilla, buttocks, trunk, neck, and face, becoming maculopapular and then petechial. The lesions may then coalesce to form large areas of ecchymosis and ulceration.

Diagnosis is based primarily on clinical signs and symptoms. If a rash is present, the use of skin biopsy and immunofluorescent staining for *Rickettsia* is highly specific, although with only slightly more than 60% sensitivity. Laboratory testing is of limited usefulness but may include thrombocytopenia and hyponatremia. Elevation of specific enzyme-linked immunosorbent assay and latex agglutination titers is usually delayed until the convalescence period. Fever and headache during peak months of tick exposure in endemic areas should suggest Rocky Mountain spotted fever. Rash, thrombocytopenia, and hyponatremia make immediate treatment imperative.

Doxycycline is the recommended treatment for Rocky Mountain spotted fever, given for a minimum of 7 days. For optimal effect, it is critical to treat patients early in the course of their illness. Treatment should not be delayed until laboratory confirmation is obtained. Respiratory and circulatory failure, as well as neurologic compromise, may occur. Patients with glucose-6-phosphate dehydrogenase deficiency are at especially high risk for complications and poor outcomes. Mortality rates for the elderly can approach 70%, whereas mortality rates for children are less than 20%.

Additional Reading: Rocky mountain spotted fever. In: Domino F, ed. *The 5-Minute Clinical Consult.* Wolters Kluwer; 2022.

Rocky Mountain spotted fever presents with pink, macular lesions on the palms, soles, wrists, ankles, and forearms. The rash then extends to the axilla, buttocks, trunk, neck, and face, becoming maculopapular and then petechial. The lesions may then coalesce to form large areas of ecchymosis and ulceration.

35. Amyloidosis affects several body systems. Which one of the following conditions is often the first sign of amyloidosis?

A) Congestive heart failure
B) Cardiac arrhythmias
C) Night blindness
D) Proteinuria
E) Rheumatoid arthritis

The answer is D: Amyloidosis is a condition characterized by excessive protein deposition in tissues, which interferes with normal organ functioning. Common forms include the following:

Primary idiopathic amyloidosis is associated with multiple myeloma. This condition is also referred with the designation *AL*, which denotes amyloidosis involving Ig light chains. Fewer than 20% of patients with AL have myeloma and about 20% of patients with myeloma have amyloidosis.

Secondary amyloidosis (designated *AA*, reactive or acquired amyloidosis) is associated with chronic inflammatory diseases such as tuberculosis, osteomyelitis, and leprosy. It more commonly affects the liver, spleen, kidneys, adrenal glands, and lymph nodes. Vascular involvement may be widespread.

Effective treatment of the underlying chronic inflammatory disease has reduced the incidence in developed countries. Diagnosis is usually accomplished after the point of irreversible organ damage and involves biopsy of the abdominal fat or rectal mucosa. Tissue is then examined under a polarizing microscope using Congo red stain to look for a characteristic green birefringence of amyloid. Proteinuria is often the first symptom associated with systemic amyloidosis, particularly the AA and AL types. Nephrotic syndrome may be severe and lead to renal failure. Myocardial amyloidosis–causing arrhythmias and congestive heart failure are two common forms of death in those affected with amyloidosis.

Generalized amyloidosis is usually a slowly progressive disease that leads to death in several years, but, in some instances, prognosis is improving. The most effective form of treatment (for the AL form) is stem cell transplantation and immunosuppressive drugs (melphalan). Cardiac transplantation has also been used.

Additional Reading: Amyloidosis. In: Domino F, ed. *The 5-Minute Clinical Consult.* Wolters Kluwer; 2022.

36. Acyclovir is a purine compound used as an antiviral agent against the herpes virus. Which one of the following statements is true regarding the use of acyclovir?

A) The medication is not effective for the treatment of herpes zoster.
B) The drug effectively prevents the transmission of herpes from those affected.
C) Topical acyclovir is less effective than oral acyclovir.
D) The medication is most effective after the onset of vesicles.
E) Seizures are not associated with the use of acyclovir.

The answer is C: Acyclovir is incorporated into viral DNA and inhibits DNA polymerase, thus preventing replication of the virus. Available in topical, oral, and intravenous (IV) formulations, acyclovir is used to treat herpes simplex virus (HSV) and varicella zoster virus infections. Topical acyclovir cream reduces the duration of orolabial herpes by about 0.5 day. Oral acyclovir can shorten the duration of symptoms in primary orolabial, genital, and anorectal HSV infections and, to a lesser extent, in recurrent orolabial and genital HSV infections.

Oral acyclovir suspension is an effective treatment for children with primary herpetic gingivostomatitis. Oral acyclovir, valacyclovir, and famciclovir are effective in treating acute recurrence of herpes labialis (cold sores). Recurrences may be diminished with daily oral acyclovir or valacyclovir. Topical acyclovir, penciclovir, and docosanol are optional treatments for recurrent herpes labialis, but they are less effective than oral treatment.

Oral acyclovir began within 24 hours after the onset of rash decreases the severity of primary varicella infection and can also be used to treat localized zoster. Suppression with acyclovir for 1 year reduced varicella zoster virus reactivation in immunocompromised patients. Intravenous acyclovir is the drug of choice for treatment of HSV infections that are visceral, disseminated, or involve the central nervous system and for serious or disseminated varicella zoster virus infections.

The medication is generally well tolerated but should be used with caution in patients with underlying renal disease or dehydration. Adverse reactions include headache, encephalopathic signs (eg, lethargy, obtundation, hallucinations, and seizures), hypotension, rash, pruritus, nausea, vomiting, diarrhea, renal dysfunction, and arthralgias. The patient must be informed that the medication helps decrease the number and severity of occurrences but does not cure the virus. Patients should also be counseled that there is risk of herpes transmission even when there is no visible evidence of the virus.

Additional Reading: Nongenital herpes simplex virus. *Am Fam Physician.* 2010;82(9):1075-1082.

37. Mucormycosis infections are usually fulminant and can be fatal. The treatment of choice for mucormycosis is which one of the following?

A) Amphotericin
B) Clotrimazole
C) Ketoconazole
D) Miconazole

The answer is A: Mucormycosis is a serious fungal infection that will present with necrotic lesions on the nasal mucosa or palate. Vascular invasion by hyphae leads to progressive tissue necrosis that may involve the nasal septum, palate, and bones surrounding the orbit or sinuses. Findings include pain, fever, orbital cellulitis, proptosis, purulent nasal discharge, and mucosal necrosis. Extension of the infection to involve the brain can cause cavernous sinus thrombosis, convulsions, aphasia, or hemiplegia.

Patients with diabetic ketoacidosis are most commonly affected, but opportunistic infections may also develop in chronic renal disease or with immunosuppression, particularly with neutropenia or high-dose corticosteroid therapy. Pulmonary infections resemble invasive aspergillosis.

Diagnosis requires a high index of suspicion and careful examination of tissue samples for large nonseptate hyphae with irregular diameters and branching patterns because much of the necrotic debris contains no organisms. Cultures usually are negative, even when hyphae are clearly visible in tissues. Computed tomographic scans and x-rays often underestimate or miss significant bone destruction.

Effective antifungal therapy requires that diabetes be controlled or, if at all possible, immunosuppression reversed. An antifungal medication, usually amphotericin B, posaconazole, or isavuconazole, is typically used. Surgical debridement of necrotic tissue may be needed because amphotericin cannot penetrate into such avascular areas.

Additional Reading: *Treatment for Mucormycosis*. www.cdc.gov/fungal/diseases/mucormycosis/treatment.html

38. A 27-year-old hiker was bitten by a venomous snake while preparing for a hike in the parking lot. Which one of the following is considered an acceptable treatment in this situation?

A) Apply an ice pack.
B) Apply an arterial tourniquet.
C) Apply a lymphatic tourniquet.
D) Incise the wound and force bleeding.
E) None of the above.

The answer is C: Poisonous snakebites, although rare, are potentially a life-threatening emergency in the United States. Rattlesnakes are responsible for most snakebites and related fatalities. Venomous snakes in the United States can be classified as having hemotoxic or neurotoxic venom. Associated signs and symptoms ranging from fang marks, with or without local pain and swelling, to life-threatening coagulopathy, renal failure, and shock are seen.

First aid techniques such as arterial tourniquets, application of ice, and wound incisions are ineffective and can be harmful. However, suction with a venom extractor within the first 5 minutes after the bite may be useful as are conservative measures, such as immobilization and lymphatic constriction tourniquets, until emergency care can be administered. A lymphatic constriction device is a blood pressure (BP) cuff inflated to the diastolic BP level so that the blood can flow past the cuff but lymph flow is obstructed. Surgical intervention with fasciotomy is reserved for rare cases. Snakebite prevention should be taught to patients.

Additional Reading: Envenomations: an overview of clinical toxicology for the primary care physician. *Am Fam Physician*. 2009;80(8):793-802.

39. Low-carbohydrate diets restrict caloric intake by reducing the consumption of carbohydrates to 20 to 60 g/d (<20% of caloric intake). Which one of the following statements is true regarding such diets?

A) They may be more effective than low-fat diets in helping patients lose weight in the short term.
B) They cause adverse changes in lipid values.
C) They are often effective years after initiation.
D) They invariably lead to longer healthier lives.

The answer is A: When utilizing a low-carbohydrate diet, the consumption of protein and fat is increased to compensate for the calories that formerly came from carbohydrates. The Atkins diet is the original low-carbohydrate diet, whereas others such as the Zone diet and the South Beach diet restrict carbohydrates to <40% of calories and focus more on the glycemic index of foods than does the Atkins diet.

Low-carbohydrate diets appear to be slightly more effective than low-fat diets for initial, short-term weight loss (3-6 months), but they are no more effective after 1 year. Low-carbohydrate diets do not adversely affect lipid profiles, but evidence of their effect on long-term cardiovascular health is lacking. Because long-term data on patient-oriented outcomes are lacking for many diets, it is not possible to clearly endorse one diet over another.

Additional Reading: Low-carbohydrate diet better than low-fat diet to reduce cardiovascular risk factors and cause weight loss. *Am Fam Physician*. 2015;91(4):262.

40. A 42-year-old indigent patient is found to have secondary syphilis, and treatment is started. Two hours after his first dose of antibiotics, he is noted to have low-grade fever, chills, myalgias, headache, tachypnea, and tachycardia. Appropriate management at this point consists of which one of the following?

A) Stopping all antibiotics
B) Ordering electrocardiogram, chest x-ray, blood cultures, and urinalysis
C) Starting intravenous dexamethasone
D) Administering acetaminophen for symptomatic treatment
E) Administering diphenhydramine and epinephrine

The answer is D: This presentation is consistent with a Jarisch-Herxheimer reaction, which can be seen after initiating treatment for syphilis or other spirochete-related illness. The reaction is usually mild, consisting of an acute, transient low-grade fever, chills, myalgias, and headache. The patient has vasodilation with mild hypotension, tachycardia, and an increased respiratory rate. Laboratory test results will reveal a mild increased neutrophil count (average white blood cell count 12,500 per μL). The pathogenesis of this reaction is undefined, although it is likely secondary to the induction of inflammatory mediators such as tumor necrosis factors by treponemal lipoproteins.

This reaction occurs in approximately 50% of patients with primary syphilis, 90% of those with secondary syphilis, and 25% of those with early latent syphilis. The onset comes within 2 hours of treatment, the temperature peaks at approximately 6 hours, and defervescence takes place within 12 to 24 hours. The reaction is more delayed in neurosyphilis, with fever peaking after 12 to 14 hours. In patients with secondary syphilis, erythema and edema of the mucocutaneous lesions increase; occasionally, subclinical or early mucocutaneous lesions may first become apparent during the reaction.

Patients should be warned to expect such symptoms, which can be managed by symptomatic treatment.

Additional Reading: *Syphilis – CDC Fact Sheet*. www.cdc.gov/std/syphilis/stdfact-syphilis.htm

41. The main difference between vegan diets and traditional vegetarian diets is in which one of the following ways?

A) Vegan diets avoid all animal products.
B) Vegan diets allow for the consumption of eggs and their products.
C) Vegetarian diets are less likely to satisfy nutritional needs.
D) Vegetarian diets are more likely to lead to iron deficiency.

The answer is A: Vegetarian diets differ according to the degree of avoidance of foods of animal origin. According to the traditional definition, a vegetarian diet consists primarily of cereals, fruits, vegetables, legumes, and nuts; animal foods, including milk, dairy products, and eggs, are generally excluded. However, less restrictive vegetarian diets may include animal foods, such as eggs, milk, and dairy products.

Vegan diets are more rigid in that all animal products, including eggs, milk, and milk products, are excluded from the diet. Some vegans do not use honey and may refrain from using animal products such as leather or wool. They also may avoid foods that are processed or not organically grown. Vegetarian diets usually satisfy nutritional needs for growth and development if they are carefully planned with attention to the following possible limiting nutrients: energy, protein, iron, zinc, calcium, vitamin D, vitamin B_{12} (cyanocobalamin), and dietary fiber.

Additional Reading: *Vegetarian Diet*. National Library of Medicine. www.nlm.nih.gov/medlineplus/vegetariandiet.html

42. A 23-year-old returns from a camping trip early, as she was having dull numbness affecting her upper left arm. The patient now describes a cramping pain and stiffness of her back and chest area. She is also nauseous and has vomited. She believes that she had a bug bite on her arm before the development of symptoms and now has a red, indurated area on the distal left arm. On examination, you note profuse sweating and dyspnea. The likely diagnosis to account for her presentation is which one of the following?

A) Lyme disease
B) Tick paralysis
C) Malaria
D) Rocky Mountain spotted fever
E) Black widow spider envenomation

The answer is E: Black widow spider bites are associated with a sharp, pinpricklike pain, followed by a dull, sometimes numbing pain in the affected extremity and by cramping pain and muscular rigidity in the abdomen or the shoulders, back, and chest. Associated manifestations may include severe abdominal pain, restlessness, anxiety, sweating, headache, dizziness, ptosis, eyelid edema, rash and pruritus, respiratory distress, nausea, vomiting, salivation, weakness, and increased skin temperature over the affected area. Blood pressure and cerebrospinal fluid pressure are usually elevated in more severe cases in adults.

An ice cube may be placed over a black widow spider bite to reduce pain. Patients younger than 16 years or older than 60 years, those with hypertensive cardiovascular disease or those with symptoms and signs of severe envenomation should be hospitalized and when symptomatic treatment is unsuccessful should be given antivenin. Antivenin must be given within 30 minutes, and the manufacturer recommends skin testing before administration (however, skin testing does not always predict anaphylaxis). Children may require respiratory assistance. Vital signs should be checked frequently during the 12 hours after the bite. In the elderly, acute hypertension may require treatment. For muscle pain and spasms, intravenous calcium gluconate may be given slowly and requires cardiac monitoring. Several doses at 4-hour intervals may be necessary.

Additional Reading: Arthropod bites. *Am Fam Physician*. 2013;88(12):841-847.

43. A 29-year-old scuba diver presents to the emergency department after a long dive, complaining of severe back pain, loss of sensation around the trunk, and numbness of the legs. Appropriate management at this time consists of which one of the following measures?

A) Administration of acetazolamide
B) Administration of furosemide (Lasix) and fluid restriction
C) Administration of prednisone and pain medication
D) Intravenous steroid bolus
E) Transfer to a facility with a recompression chamber

The answer is E: Recreational scuba diving, which is defined as pleasure diving without mandatory decompression to a maximum depth of 130 ft, has become a popular activity since the mid-1980s. Although divers are concentrated along coastal regions, many others dive in inland lakes, streams, quarries, and reservoirs, or fly to distant dive sites. Physicians practicing almost anywhere in the United States may see a patient with a dive-related injury or complaint. Injuries related to diving are usually mild and often include ear-related complaints.

However, the most severe illness related to diving is decompression illness (the "bends"). Neurologic decompression sickness can present with a wide spectrum of symptoms. A prodrome of malaise, fatigue, anorexia, and headache is common. The most severe presentation is partial myelopathy referable to the thoracic spinal cord. Patients complain of paresthesias and sensory loss in the trunk and extremities, a tingling or constricting sensation around the thorax, ascending leg weakness ranging from mild to severe pain in the lower back or pelvis, and loss of bowel and/or bladder control.

Neurologic examination often reveals monoparesis or paraparesis and sphincter disturbances. However, neurologic examination may also be normal. The diagnosis of neurologic decompression sickness is clinical and should be suspected in any patient with a recent history of diving who has a consistent presentation. Flying shortly after a dive can precipitate symptoms.

The initial management of neurologic decompression sickness requires transport to a recompression facility. The majority of recreational divers with neurologic decompression sickness have an excellent recovery after prompt recompression therapy.

Additional Reading: Decompression sickness. In: Domino F, ed. *The 5-Minute Clinical Consult*. Wolters Kluwer; 2022.

44. An 18-year-old gay male patient presents to clinic today to follow up on asymptomatic sexually transmitted infection testing. Unfortunately, he tested positive for rectal chalmydia but tested negative for all other infections including human immunodeficiency virus. In addition to offering to start the patient on pre-exposure prophylaxis what is the first-line treatment for his current infection?

A) Doxyclyine 100 mg orally twice daily for 1 week
B) Doxycyline 100 mg orally twice daily for 1 week plus ceftriaxone intramuscularly (IM) once
C) Azithromycin 1 g orally once
D) Benzathine penicillin G 2.4 million units IM in a single dose

The answer is A: The Centers for Disease Control and Prevention guidelines changed in 2022. Infections caused by *C trachomatis* and *Neisseria gonorrhoeae* are increasing in the United States. Because most infections are asymptomatic, screening is key to preventing complications such as pelvic inflammatory disease and infertility and decreasing community and vertical neonatal transmission. All sexually active people with a cervix who are younger than 25 years and older people with a cervix who have risk factors should be screened annually for chlamydial and gonococcal infections. Sexually active men who have sex with men should be screened at least annually. Physicians should obtain a sexual history free from assumptions about sex partners or practices. Acceptable specimen types for testing include vaginal, endocervical, rectal, pharyngeal, and urethral swabs, and first-stream urine samples. Uncomplicated gonococcal infection should be treated with a single 500-mg dose of intramuscular ceftriaxone in people weighing less than 331 lb (150 kg). Preferred chlamydia treatment is a 7-day course of doxycycline, 100 mg taken by mouth twice per day. Azithromycin is now reserved for patients who may have difficulty adhering to 7 day course of doxycycline due to rise of gonococcal resistance.

Additional Reading: Chlamydial and gonococcal infections: screening, diagnosis, and treatment. *Am Fam Physician.* 2022;105(4):388-396.

CHAPTER 2

Care of Children and Adolescents

To help with your Board Prep study, we have grouped the questions primarily by "system" so that you can focus your studying on one system at a time. Although not all questions easily fall into one specific study section, they will generally provide similar additional readings, and as noted previously, the readings are not listed to be specific references for the question and answer, rather to provide you with a family medicine–focused overview of the general topic area. As you go through these questions, you may identify particular areas or systems that you will want to study in a more focused manner as you continue to prepare for the American Board of Family Medicine certification/recertification examination and that is where the additional readings should prove useful.

Section I. Integumentary System

Each of the following questions or incomplete statements is followed by suggested answers or completions. Select the ONE BEST ANSWER in each case.

1. A 14-year-old boy presents to your office with a mildly pruritic rash that involves his chest and back. He reports that it began with a single lesion on his back that subsequently spread to involve his entire back and chest. On examination, you note the presence of multiple secondary lesions that appear to follow skin cleavage lines. The most likely diagnosis to account for this presentation is which one of the following conditions?

A) Herpes zoster
B) Pityriasis rosea
C) Rhus dermatitis
D) Tinea versicolor
E) Varicella

The answer is B: Pityriasis rosea typically occurs in children and young adults and chiefly involves the trunk. It is characterized by an initial herald patch, followed within 2 weeks by the development of a diffuse papulosquamous rash. The herald patch can be mistaken for nummular eczema or tinea corporis. Pityriasis rosea is easier to identify when the general eruption appears with smaller secondary lesions that follow Langer lines (cleavage lines) in a "Christmas tree–like pattern" on the back. The appearance of the exanthem may differ in persons of color. Many diseases can mimic pityriasis rosea, including drug exanthems, but the most worrisome condition to be ruled out is secondary syphilis. Low-potency topical steroids and antihistamines are often used to relieve itching. Asymptomatic lesions do not require treatment.

Herpes zoster presents as grouped vesicles with an erythematous base arising in a unilateral dermatomal distribution.

Tinea versicolor presents with small, scaly patches of varied colors on the chest or back.

Varicella presents with a generalized pruritic vesicular rash that appears on the face, spreads to the rest of the body, and is often preceded by a prodrome of fever, malaise, and anorexia. Individual lesions appear as a clear vesicle on an erythematous base ("dewdrop on a rose petal"). The rash may be atypical in vaccinated individuals with breakthrough infections.

Rhus dermatitis is associated with an intensely pruritic and erythematous, rash often presenting with papules, plaques, vesicles, or bullae arranged in a pattern consistent with where the patient had contact with the inciting plant.

Additional Reading: Pityriasis rosea: diagnosis and treatment. *Am Fam Physician*. 2018; 97(1):38-44.

2. The local elementary school has reported two students with head lice infestations, and your office has received calls from worried parents. You inform them of all of the following statements regarding head lice infestations, except which one?

A) African Americans are less likely to be affected.
B) Recurrence is rare when treated with pyrethrin.
C) Head lice can live off the body for up to 1 month.
D) Dogs are not usually vectors for head lice.
E) The hallmark presentation includes pruritus.

The answer is B: Head louse infection (pediculosis capitis) is an infestation of lice in the scalp hair that feeds on human blood and rarely affects African Americans. Transmission occurs through head-to-head contact and less commonly fomites. Head lice require a blood meal several times a day to survive and will die in 1 to 2 days off of the host. The hallmark of all types of pediculosis is pruritus.

The treatment of choice for head lice is malathion 0.5% in isopropanol, because there is known resistance to pyrethroids. The medication is applied to dry hair and scalp until wet and allowed to air-dry. Medication should be left on the hair for 8 to 12 hours. After this period, thoroughly shampoo the hair, then use a fine-tooth comb to remove lice. Reapplication 7 to 9 days after initial treatment may be necessary if infestation persists. All household members should be treated at the same time and advised that clothing and bed linens be washed or dry-cleaned. Brushes and combs used during infestation or treatment should be soaked in hot water for 5 to 10 minutes. Children can return to school after the initial treatment even if nits remain attached to the hair shaft. "No nit" school attendance policies should be discouraged. Malathion is approved for children 6 years of age and older. Alternatives for younger children include benzoyl alcohol lotion 5%, ivermectin lotion 5%, and spinosad 0.9% topical suspension.

Additional Reading: Centers for Disease Control, Lice-Head Lice.

3. A concerned mother brings her 4-year-old daughter to your office reporting that the girl's head has been itchy, and her hair has been falling out. Inspection of the scalp shows short broken hair shafts just above the skin, and scaly, pruritic, mildly inflamed gray patches on the skin. Scrapings of the area show the presence of hyphae. Which one of the following is considered the treatment of choice?

A) Oral antifungals
B) Permethrin cream
C) Topical antifungals
D) Topical hydrocortisone cream
E) Shave the hair off at the scalp and let it regrow

The answer is A: Tinea capitis is a contagious fungal infection of the scalp affecting infants and young children. The etiologic fungi include *Trichophyton*, *Microsporum*, and *Epidermophyton*. Infected lesions are pruritic, scaly, gray patches and may be accompanied by areas of hair loss and a black dot appearance of broken hair shafts just above the scalp. Extreme inflammation may result in kerions, exudative pustular nodulations. Microscopic examination of scrapings treated with 10% potassium hydroxide reveals fungal hyphae. Culture is the gold standard for diagnosis. In cases of infection with *Microsporum*, black light examination of hair demonstrates green-yellow fluorescence.

Although treatment for most tinea infections is topical antifungals, tinea capitis requires oral antifungals, such as terbinafine or griseofulvin. Additionally, systemic or intralesional steroids may be beneficial in severely inflamed lesions. Until tinea capitis infection is cleared, it is also recommended to use a selenium sulfide 1% or 2.5% or ketoconazole 2% shampoo twice weekly for 2 weeks to prevent the spread, especially to other children. Children may attend school during treatment because there is low risk of transmission.

Additional Reading: *Pediatric Dermatology, A Quick Reference Guide*. 4th ed.

4. A 14-year-old girl presents with her mother, as they are concerned over acne, which has been flaring lately, and she is worried about developing facial scarring. Which one of the following is associated with facial acne?

A) Consumption of chocolate
B) Ingestion of fatty foods
C) Poor hygiene
D) Presence of *Propionibacterium acnes*
E) Presence of *Staphylococcus aureus*

The answer is D: Acne often presents among adolescent patients between 12 and 25 years of age and is associated with increasing androgen production. It arises when greater sebum production and bacterial proliferation result in keratinization of blocked follicular canals. The plugged pilosebaceous unit can be closed, known as a whitehead, or open when the sebum becomes oxidized resulting in a blackhead. *P acnes* is the typical bacterial etiologic agent that proliferates and releases chemotactic factors that attract leukocytes. Acne is diagnosed clinically by the presence of characteristic lesions on the face, chest, shoulders, and back. In females, lesions can worsen before or during menses.

Acne is not the result of poor hygiene, dietary choices (eg, chocolate, pizza, soda), or stress. Although the exact influence of cosmetic use on acne remains unclear, hair products and tanning lotions tend to worsen acne, and oil-free and noncomedogenic products are recommended. Mechanical trauma from picking at lesions can increase inflammation and worsen acne. Lesions cannot be scrubbed off, and alcohol-based astringents can dry and irritate the skin.

Additional Reading: Acne vulgaris: treatment guidelines from the AAD. *Am Fam Physician*. 2017;95(1):740-741.

5. Which one of the following statements is true regarding oral medications used in the treatment of acne?

A) An oral contraceptive can be helpful in the treatment of mild acne.
B) Doxycycline, tetracycline, and minocycline are contraindicated before the age of 18 years.
C) Lipid values must be monitored when using isotretinoin.
D) When administering isotretinoin, oral contraceptives are sufficient to prevent pregnancy.

The answer is C: Topical agents are usually the first-line treatment for acne, but oral agents are often needed as well. A 6-month course of oral doxycycline, tetracycline, or minocycline can be prescribed in patients with moderate to severe inflammatory acne. Due to safety concerns and lack of superiority to doxycycline, 2015 Canadian clinical practice guidelines for management of acne prefer doxycycline or tetracycline. A combined oral contraceptive pill or spironolactone is also effective in women with moderate to severe acne.

Isotretinoin is reserved for use in the treatment of the most severe or refractory cases of inflammatory cystic type acne. Isotretinoin is teratogenic and has a poor side effect profile; therefore, it must be prescribed by a physician who is registered with an U.S. Food and Drug Administration–approved monitoring program. Serious side effects include hepatitis, hypertriglyceridemia, intracranial hypertension, arthralgia, myalgias, night blindness, and hyperostosis. Serum liver function tests and triglyceride levels must be monitored monthly. The link between isotretinoin and depression remains unclear.

Teratogenicity leads to severe fetal anomalies of many organ systems; thus, two forms of contraception must be implemented for 1 month before, during, and after isotretinoin treatment has ceased. To ensure that female patients are not pregnant when the treatment is initiated, two negative urine pregnancy tests are required. Monthly follow-up appointments should also include testing for pregnancy.

Additional Reading: Acne vulgaris: diagnosis and treatment. *Am Fam Physician*. 2019;100(8):475-484. (2) *Pediatr Rev*. 2019;40(11):577-589.

6. A 6-month-old infant is brought to the office by his concerned mother. He has an erythematous diaper rash with small satellite lesions that have not improved with application of petroleum jelly. What is the most appropriate topical treatment?

A) Clotrimazole (Lotrimin) ointment
B) Hydrocortisone cream
C) Mupirocin (Bactroban) ointment
D) Neosporin ointment
E) Zinc oxide

The answer is A: Diaper dermatitis secondary to *Candida albicans* infection is an intensely, beefy red rash that involves the perineal area. The rash may be well demarcated and possesses vesicles that weep, pustules, and papules with characteristic satellite lesions.

Treatment consists of antifungal ointment (ie, clotrimazole or nystatin) and, if severe, short-term use of 1% hydrocortisone cream. Use of higher-potency topical steroid creams/ointments should be avoided. Soothing creams or ointments (eg, vitamins A and D, zinc oxide) can also be applied on top of the antifungal ointment. Keeping the area dry minimizes the development of yeast dermatitis.

Additional Reading: *Pediatric Dermatology, A Quick Reference Guide*. 4th ed.

7. A 14-year-old boy presents with tenderness in the right breast. There are no other findings, and his testicular examination is unremarkable. Which one of the following should be done as the next appropriate step in his management?

A) Biopsy of the breast
B) Genetic testing
C) Mammogram of his breast
D) Reassurance and continued observation
E) Ultrasonography of his breast

The answer is D: Benign gynecomastia of adolescence is a common finding among boys in middle to late puberty. The breast tissue enlargement is usually asymmetric and often tender to palpation. Provided the history and physical examination, including palpation of the testicles, are unremarkable, reassurance and periodic reevaluation are sufficient because most cases resolve in 1 to 2 years.

Benign gynecomastia does not require further evaluation. However, if there is evidence of hypogonadism, further workup should ensue. Familial gynecomastia is a common genetic disorder transmitted as an X-linked recessive trait or a sex-limited dominant trait causing limited breast development around the time of puberty. Rarely, those with severe gynecomastia require cosmetic surgery.

Pathologic gynecomastia occurs in Klinefelter syndrome, prolactin-secreting adenomas, and many different types of drug use, including marijuana and phenothiazines.

Additional Reading: Gynecomastia. *Am Fam Physician*. 2012;85(7):716-722.

➔ **Benign gynecomastia of adolescence is a common finding among boys during puberty, and most cases resolve in 1 to 2 years.**

8. A 6-year-old boy presents with his father with impetigo of his right ankle. No other areas are involved, and he appears otherwise well. Which one of the following treatments would be the most appropriate treatment to recommend at this time?

A) Oral cephalexin
B) Topical mupirocin
C) Topical bacitracin
D) Topical neomycin
E) Topical polymyxin B

The answer is B: Impetigo is a contagious superficial skin infection most commonly seen in children, with a peak incidence between the ages of 2 and 6 years. It is the most common skin infection among children. Causative agents include group A β-hemolytic streptococci (GABHS) and *S aureus*. The infection is transmitted via direct contact with an infected lesion. Complications result from spread of infection and rarely lead to cellulitis, lymphangitis, and septicemia.

Antibiotic administration is the mainstay of therapy. If there is a limited area of infected skin, as in this scenario, topical mupirocin is recommended. The other topical antibiotics listed (neomycin, bacitracin, polymyxin B, and gentamicin) are less effective. Oral antibiotics may provide greater coverage for patients with extensive disease; and if needed, choices would include cephalosporins, for example, cephalexin, amoxicillin-clavulanate, or dicloxacillin. Streptococcal infections can be treated with penicillin. Oral antibiotics have greater side effects, particularly gastrointestinal disruptions, compared with topical agents.

Additional Reading: Impetigo: diagnosis and treatment. *Am Fam Physician*. 2014;90(4):229-235.

9. A mother is concerned because her newborn daughter has a large bump in her umbilicus. It does not seem to be bothering her—she is nursing easily and moving her bowels regularly. You tell the mother that which one of the following recommendations is the most appropriate management of an asymptomatic umbilical hernia for her newborn?

A) Immediate surgical correction should be scheduled.
B) Reassure that most hernias resolve within 6 to 8 weeks.
C) Surgical correction is indicated if the hernia does not resolve before school age.
D) Apply an elastic support to his mid-abdomen.
E) None of the above.

The answer is C: The umbilical ring is a fascial opening that exists to allow passage of the umbilical vessels. After birth, it spontaneously closes with the growth of the rectus abdominis muscles toward one another and ultimate fusion of peritoneal and fascial layers. Closure of the umbilical ring is achieved in most children by 5 years of age, although closure can continue into adolescence in some children. Spontaneous closure is less likely to occur in patients who have an opening that is >1.5 cm, with a significant amount of protruding skin or have an underlying predisposing condition such as Ehlers-Danlos syndrome, hypothyroidism, Down syndrome, and Beckwith-Wiedemann syndrome. Surgery prior to 4 years of age is not recommended due to the risk of recurrence.

Indications for surgical repair include incarcerated or strangulated hernia; large, trunklike hernias that do not decrease in size in the first 2 years of life in children; and hernias associated with genetic syndromes, hypothyroidism, and other syndromes.

"Taping" a hernia is of no benefit, and the adhesive may result in skin maceration.

Additional Reading: Care of the umbilicus and management of umbilical disorders. In: *UpToDate*. 2022.

10. A mother calls panicked that her son brought home a note that a child in his class is being treated for head lice. You inform her that which one of the following is important to consider in the management of head lice?

A) Children should not attend school until nits cannot be seen.
B) Cleaning of bedding does not significantly contribute to head lice eradication.
C) Head lice programs significantly lower the incidence of head lice.
D) Household contacts should be treated if live lice or eggs are noted within 1 cm of the scalp.
E) The health of those exposed is more important than the confidentiality of the child affected.

The answer is D: If a case of head lice is identified, check all household members and treat only those with live lice or eggs within 1 cm of the scalp. Family members who share a bed with the person infected should be treated, and ensure that hair care items and bed linens are thoroughly cleaned. A child with active head lice has likely had the infestation for at least 1 month and poses little risk to others. There is no association of infestation with underlying health or hygiene. The child can return to school after proper treatment. Head lice screening programs have not been proven effective.

Additional Reading: Centers for Disease Control, Lice-Head Lice.

11. You are seeing a 12-year-old boy with small flesh-colored papules with central umbilication on his arms. You diagnose him with molluscum contagiosum (MC). All of the following are considered as suitable treatments for MC, except which one?

A) 5-Fluorouracil
B) Curettage
C) Cryotherapy
D) Imiquimod (Aldara)
E) Trichloroacetic acid

The answer is A: MC is a benign superficial eruption resulting from viral infections of the skin. MC eruptions are usually self-limited and without sequelae; however, they can be more extensive especially in immunocompromised persons. In patients with human immunodeficiency virus (HIV), MC infection frequently can be extensive and disfiguring. MC may serve as a cutaneous marker of severe immunodeficiency and may be the first indication of HIV infection.

After a period of inflammation and minor tenderness, MC lesions may spontaneously regress without residual scarring. Autoinoculation is associated with scratching of the lesions, and transmission to others can occur. Although lesions usually spontaneously disappear in 1 year, treatment with local destruction or immunologic modulation can shorten the disease course.

Lesion destruction may be mechanical (curettage, laser, or cryotherapy with liquid nitrogen or nitrous oxide cryogun), chemical (trichloroacetic acid, tretinoin), or immunologic (imiquimod). Imiquimod therapy has minimal side effects and easy application. 5-Fluorouracil is used as a topical treatment for skin cancer.

Additional Reading: Common skin rashes in children. *Am Fam Physician*. 2015;92(3):211-216.

12. An infant is brought in by his mother because he has thick, yellow, crusted scalp lesions, consistent with cradle cap. All of the following have been found to be effective in treating this condition, except which one?

A) Hydrocortisone cream
B) Ketoconazole cream
C) Moisturizing ointments
D) Topical use of vegetable oils
E) Vitamin E supplements

The answer is E: Cradle cap refers to seborrheic dermatitis that is commonly seen in newborns. It presents with thick, yellow, greasy scales on the scalp and flexural areas behind the ears; frequently, red facial papules and an irritated diaper rash are also present. Treatment for infants includes the application of baby oil or mineral oil to the scalp prior to shampooing to facilitate removal of the scale via gentle brushing. Selenium sulfide or ketoconazole shampoos may be used as needed. If inflammation is present, a low-potency topical steroid can be uses. Vitamin E supplements do not help to alleviate cradle cap.

Additional Reading: *Pediatric Dermatology, A Quick Reference Guide*. 4th ed.

13. A 4-month-old infant is brought to the office with an erythematous perineal rash that spares the skinfolds of the groin area. Which one of the following is the most likely diagnosis?

A) Childhood eczema
B) Diaper dermatitis
C) Heat rash
D) Varicella
E) Yeast dermatitis

The answer is B: Diaper dermatitis, also known as "primary irritant dermatitis," results from skin irritation that arises from long-term exposure to urine and feces. The rash is shiny and erythematous, classically sparing the skinfolds in the groin area. In severe cases, the skin may ulcerate.

Treatment involves maintaining adequate ventilation to keep the affected area dry, frequent diaper changes, and application of petroleum jelly or zinc oxide-containing diaper creams. Also consider hydrocortisone 1 or 2.5% for inflammation but avoid potent topical steroids. If the condition persists for more than a few days, consider candidiasis. Avoid rubber or plastic pants that hinder moisture evaporation and reduce airflow.

Additional Reading: *Pediatric Dermatology, A Quick Reference Guide*. 4th ed.

14. A 7-year-old boy is brought in by his mother because he has recurring episodes of a rash, which breaks out behind his knees and occasionally on other areas of his skin. The rash is itchy and red, sometimes with a slight scaly appearance. Which one of the following conditions is the most likely diagnosis in this situation?

A) Atopic dermatitis
B) Cushing disease
C) Hereditary angioedema
D) Lyme disease
E) *Rhus* dermatitis

The answer is A: Atopic dermatitis is characterized by chronic relapsing, superficial inflammation of the skin. It is the most common chronic pediatric skin disorder. It is characterized by pruritus with resultant scratching that can lead to excoriations and lichenification.

The appearance of the lesions varies across the life span and may appear differently in persons of color.

In infants and toddlers, extensive involvement is common, affecting the face, trunk, and extensor extremities.

In childhood, lesions are concentrated in flexural areas such as the popliteal and antecubital fossae, the wrists, and ankles.

Adolescents continue to have lesions in the flexural areas but also have involvement of the hands, face, and neck.

The condition has a strong genetic predisposition and is associated with atopic conditions. Affected skin may become colonized with *S aureus*. Treatment involves hydration of the skin daily, in a warm (not hot) bath for less than 10 minutes with avoidance of soap. Nonsoap cleansers should be used sparingly. Immediately after bathing, an emollient should be applied. Creams and ointments are generally more effective moisturizers than lotions. Disease flares are treated with topical steroids applied twice daily, preferably in an ointment vehicle. Pruritus can be controlled with a bedtime dose of a first-generation antihistamine. Secondary bacterial infection of affected skin is not uncommon and can be treated with topical antibiotics (mupirocin) or oral antibiotics. Bleach baths 1 to 2 times weekly can reduce bacterial skin colonization.

Additional Reading: *Pediatric Dermatology, A Quick Reference Guide*. 4th ed.

15. Atopic dermatitis is a chronic inflammatory condition of the skin; however, patients affected by this disorder frequently also suffer from which one of the following conditions?

A) Asthma
B) Dysplastic nevus syndrome
C) Immunoglobulin A gammopathy
D) Retinitis pigmentosa
E) Vasomotor rhinitis

The answer is A: Atopic dermatitis is a chronic inflammatory condition of the skin that is common among children and often associated with asthma. The condition is characterized by intense pruritus, associated with exacerbations and remissions. Atopic dermatitis affects as many as 10% of children. More than 50% of patients with atopic dermatitis have or develop asthma or allergic rhinitis. Most patients have a positive family history of atopy. Most cases resolve by adolescence, but few can persist into adulthood; although even if atopic dermatitis resolves with age, the predisposition for asthma and rhinitis persists. Poor prognostic features include a family history of the condition, early disseminated infantile disease, female sex, and coexisting allergic rhinitis and asthma.

Diagnosis of atopic dermatitis is based on the findings of the history and physical examination. There are no specific laboratory findings or histologic features that define atopic dermatitis. Food allergies should be considered in children with moderate to severe disease who do not respond to standard therapies, especially infants with widespread involvement.

Additional Reading: *Pediatric Dermatology, A Quick Reference Guide*. 4th ed.

16. A 16-year-old patient is in for follow-up of her acne, and she reports that she has decided to do a report on acne for her biology class. She has questions about her condition, and you inform her that all of the following factors are involved in the development of acne, except which one?

A) Accumulation of lipids and cellular debris
B) Bacterial colonization
C) Excessive sebum production
D) High-fat diets
E) Hyperkeratinization with development of microcomedones

The answer is D: Acne is associated with the pilosebaceous units in the skin and has not been definitively associated with diet. Development of acne is due to the following four factors:

1. Excessive sebum production secondary to sebaceous gland hyperplasia.
2. Subsequent hyperkeratinization of the hair follicle prevents normal shedding of the follicular keratinocytes, which then obstruct the follicle and form microcomedones.
3. Lipids and cellular debris accumulate within the blocked follicle.
4. This microenvironment encourages colonization of the bacteria *P acnes*, which provokes an immune response through the production of numerous inflammatory mediators. Inflammation is further enhanced by follicular rupture and subsequent leakage of lipids, bacteria, and fatty acids into the dermis.

Additional Reading: Acne vulgaris: treatment guidelines from the AAD. *Am Fam Physician*. 2017;95(1):740-741.

17. You receive a call from the school nurse at the local elementary school, who is concerned that three children have been diagnosed with lice infections. You tell them all the following statements are true about the characteristics of lice infestations, except which one?

A) Head and pubic lice do not cause systemic disease.
B) Lice are obligate human parasites.
C) Lice can jump or hop from host to host.
D) Person-to-person contact is necessary for lice transmission.
E) The incidence of head lice is increasing.

The answer is C: The three lice species that infest humans are *Pediculus humanus capitis* (the head louse), *Phthirus pubis* (the crab or pubic louse), and *Pediculus humanus corpus* (the body louse). All three species are obligate human parasites. Contrary to popular belief, these insects do not hop, jump, or fly. Instead, the lice are transmitted by person-to-person contact. Despite the introduction of new treatments, the frequency of lice infestation is increasing. This trend could be attributed to the development of resistance to existing treatments. Head and pubic lice do not transmit systemic disease. Treatment is directed at relieving symptoms and preventing reinfestation and transmission to others.

Additional Reading: Pediculosis and scabies: a treatment update. *Am Fam Physician*. 2012;86(6):535-541.

18. An 8-year-old boy is brought in by his father. He had been bitten on the arm by the neighbor's dog a couple of days ago, and the area has become red and swollen. You are concerned that the bite has become infected and prescribe which one of the following antibiotics?

A) Amoxicillin
B) Amoxicillin-clavulanate
C) Azithromycin
D) Cephalexin
E) Penicillin

The answer is B: Almost one-half of all dog bites involve an animal owned by the victim's family or neighbor. Most dog-bit victims are children. Although some breeds of dogs are considered to be more aggressive than other breeds, any dog may attack when threatened. All dog bites carry a risk of infection, but immediate copious irrigation can significantly decrease that risk. Only 15% to 20% of dog bite wounds become infected. Crush injuries, puncture wounds, and hand wounds are more likely to become infected than are scratches or tears.

Most infected dog bite wounds yield polymicrobial organisms. *Pasteurella multocida* and *S aureus* are the most common aerobic organisms. Amoxicillin-clavulanate, in a formulation of amoxicillin-to-clavulanate ratio of 4:1 given tid or 7:1 given bid, should be used for an infected dog bite. For patients with an allergy to penicillin, doxycycline is an acceptable alternative. Assess every dog bite situation for the risk of tetanus and rabies virus infection. The dog bite injury should be documented with photographs and diagrams when appropriate. Patients who have been bitten by a dog should be instructed to elevate and immobilize the involved area and should have the wound reexamined within 24 to 48 hours after injury, especially if the bite affects the hands. In some states, health care providers are mandated to report dog bites. Family physicians should educate parents and children on the ways to prevent dog bites.

Additional Reading: Dog and cat bites. *Am Fam Physician*. 2014;90(4):239-243.

19. You are evaluating a young child with a rash, who has just returned from a visit abroad with his parents. His parents had refused the measles-mumps-rubella (MMR) immunization during his routine well-child checks over a concern for vaccine safety. You suspect that he has a measles (rubeola) infection. In making the diagnosis, you would expect to see which one of the following physical findings?

A) A rash with associated joint pain and swelling
B) A rash with associated small erythematous ulcerations on the tongue
C) A maculopapular rash that developed on the face and then spread to his body
D) A petechial rash that developed on his trunk and then spread to his extremities
E) Signs consistent with a disseminated intravascular coagulopathy

The answer is C: Measles is a highly contagious infectious disease that was common until the advent of immunization. It is caused by paramyxovirus and spreads via respiratory secretions. Most measles cases are self-limited, yet life-threatening complications can occur. Symptoms include the 3 C's (cough, coryza, and conjunctivitis), high fever, and a maculopapular rash. Pathognomonic Koplik spots appear on the buccal mucosa, opposite the first and second upper molar 1 to 2 days prior to the rash.

The incubation period of measles is approximately 11 to 14 days and is most communicable 2 to 4 days before the onset of the rash, which characteristically develops first at the hairline, followed by the face then spreads to the entire body. Within the first 3 to 5 days, the fever and rash subside and the patient shows improvement. Complications include pneumonia, secondary bacterial infection, acute thrombocytopenic purpura, and encephalitis. Subacute sclerosing panencephalitis develops years after infection and is characterized by progressive neurological deterioration and death. Treatment for measles is supportive, with vitamin A administered in severe cases, such as hospitalized children.

Children should be immunized with the live attenuated MMR vaccination at 12 to 15 months and again at age 4 to 6 years. Measles vaccine is not recommended for pregnant women, immunocompromised patients, or human immunodeficiency virus patients.

Additional Reading: Measles (Rubeola). Centers for Disease Control and Prevention. www.cdc.gov/measles/index.html

20. A female child appears to have swelling of the dorsal hands and feet, and of the skin over the posterior aspect of the neck. On examination, the swelling appears because of lymphedematous changes and the child has a low hairline on the back of the neck, ptosis, and a broad chest with widely spaced nipples. A follow-up ultrasonography for the systolic murmur that you hear reveals coarctation of the aorta. Which one of the following syndromes would most likely account for these findings?

A) Down syndrome
B) Klinefelter syndrome
C) Marfan syndrome
D) Prader-Willi syndrome
E) Turner syndrome

The answer is E: Turner syndrome occurs in 1 of every 2500 to 3000 live female births. The syndrome is characterized by the partial or complete absence of one X chromosome (45,X karyotype). Newborns with Turner syndrome may present with excessive dorsal lymphedema of the hands and feet, and with lymphedema or loose folds of skin over the posterior aspect of the neck. However, many female children with Turner syndrome are only mildly affected.

Typical findings include short stature, webbing of the neck, low hairline on the back of the neck, ptosis, a broad chest with widely spaced nipples, multiple pigmented nevi, short fourth metacarpals and metatarsals, prominent finger pads, hypoplasia of the nails, coarctation of the aorta, bicuspid aortic valve, and increased carrying angle at the elbow. Renal anomalies and hemangiomas are common. Occasionally, telangiectasia of the gastrointestinal tract presents with intestinal bleeding.

Intellectual disability is unusual; however, there tends to be diminution of certain perceptual abilities and thus affected individuals tend to score poorly on performance tests and in mathematics. Verbal intelligence quotient tests tend to demonstrate average or above-average performance.

Most patients have gonadal dysgenesis, with failure to go through puberty, develop breast tissue, or menstruate. Menarche can be attained with hormone replacement. Ovaries are replaced by bilateral streaks of fibrous stroma and tend to lack developing ova. However, 5% to 10% of affected girls undergo spontaneous menarche and rarely retain fertility.

Additional Reading: Turner syndrome: diagnosis and management. *Am Fam Physician*. 2007;76(3):405-417.

Section II. Special Sensory Systems

Each of the following questions or incomplete statements is followed by suggested answers or completions. Select the ONE BEST ANSWER in each case.

1. A 16-month-old girl presents to the office with her father, who is concerned that she has been having difficulty hearing. The patient has had sneezing and nasal congestion for the past week, and she has been rubbing her left ear over the past 2 days. On examination, you note decreased eardrum motility with moderately bulging tympanic membrane. What is the next step in management?

A) Amoxicillin
B) Amoxicillin-clavulanate
C) Azithromycin
D) Ceftriaxone
E) Cefuroxime

The answer is A: Suspect acute otitis media in a young patient (6-24 months) with the acute onset of ear pain and difficulty hearing in the setting of viral upper respiratory tract infection symptoms. Bacterial infection has likely occurred secondary to the viral infection causing eustachian tube dysfunction. Although there are several infectious etiologies, *Streptococcus pneumoniae* is the most common. Empirically begin high-dose amoxicillin (80-90 mg/kg/d divided bid), unless the patient has received amoxicillin within the past 30 days or has concurrent purulent conjunctivitis. In children who have taken amoxicillin in the past 30 days or have concurrent conjunctivitis, therapy should be initiated with amoxicillin-clavulanate (90 mg/kg/d of amoxicillin, with the ratio of amoxicillin to clavulanate 14:1, given in 2 divided doses, which is less likely to cause diarrhea than other amoxicillin-clavulanate preparations).

Alternative antibiotics include cefdinir (14 mg/kg/d in 1 or 2 doses), cefpodoxime (10 mg/kg/d in 2 divided doses), or ceftriaxone (50 mg/kg/dose, intramuscularly),

For penicillin-allergic patients, the degree of cross-reactivity between penicillin and second- and third-generation cephalosporins is negligible.

Macrolides such as azithromycin have limited efficacy against *Haemophilus influenzae* and *S pneumoniae*.

Additional Reading: Acute otitis media in children. *Am Fam Physician*. 2017;95(2):109-110.

2. You are seeing a 4-month-old child for a well-child check, and her mother notes that she has been sleeping through the night with a bottle. You inform her that bottle-feeding at bedtime puts her infant at increased risk for developing which of the following conditions?

A) Aspiration pneumonia
B) Dental caries
C) Hiatal hernia
D) Nasal polyps
E) Oral candidiasis

The answer is B: Baby bottle tooth decay can occur after a child repeatedly falls asleep with a bottle in their mouth. This practice tends to be more common among families of lower socioeconomic status and can lead to major dental complications including the development of caries. Dental caries occur when oral bacteria, primarily *Streptococcus mutans*, ferment carbohydrates into organic acids that demineralize tooth enamel and subsequently cause enamel cavitation. Prevention of bedtime bottle-feeding is focused on educating the parents about the risk for dental caries so that they can adjust this practice.

Additional Reading: A practical guide to infant oral health. *Am Fam Physician*. 2004; 70(11):2113-2120.

3. Which one of the following is a known risk factor for the development of acute otitis media (AOM) in children?

A) Presence of pets in the home
B) Low birth weight
C) Low socioeconomic class
D) Day care attendance
E) Premature birth

The answer is D: AOM usually results as a complication of a viral upper respiratory infection. It is particularly common in children of 6 months to 3 years of age. The most common bacterial etiologic agents are *S pneumoniae*, *H influenzae*, and *Moraxella (Branhamella) catarrhalis*. In newborns, *Escherichia coli* and *S aureus* predominate. Viral etiologies include respiratory syncytial virus, parainfluenza virus, influenza virus, enterovirus, and adenovirus and coronavirus.

Risk factors include attending day care bottle-propping, cleft palate and craniofacial anomalies, trisomy 21 and other genetic syndromes, immunocompromising conditions and ciliary dysfunction, and atopy. Low birth weight, young gestational age, and the presence of pets in the home are not significantly associated with an increased risk of AOM.

Symptoms of AOM include otalgia, nausea, hearing loss, difficulty sleeping, and fussiness. Otorrhea is seen if a perforation is present. Fever is present in 66% of those affected. The combination of a "cloudy," bulging tympanic membrane with impaired mobility is the best predictor of acute otitis media. Eardrum motion is best assessed by looking at the pars flaccida, in the superior part of the drum. Crying children can present with a red drum and normal mobility, but this is not diagnostic of acute bacterial infection. The first-line treatment for AOM is amoxicillin, and if no improvement is seen within 48 to 72 hours, reexamine and add the second-line agent amoxicillin-clavulanate. If patient has a penicillin allergy, use a cephalosporin. Complications include mastoiditis, labyrinthitis, conductive and sensory neural hearing loss, and meningitis.

Additional Reading: Acute otitis media in children. *Am Fam Physician*. 2017;95(2):109-110.

4. When a child is screened for lead exposure and the blood lead level (BLL) is found to be elevated, she is at greatest risk for developing which of the following?

A) A decline in intelligence quotient (IQ)
B) Progressively worsening visual deficits
C) Clear cell carcinoma of the vagina in girls
D) The development of a personality disorder
E) Worsening hyperactivity disorder

The answer is A: BLL > 3.5 μg/dL is associated with a decline in IQ, and a significant number of preschool-age children in the United States are affected. The Centers for Disease Control and Prevention advises universal blood lead screening between ages 9 and 12 months, at ages 2 and 3 years, and again at 4 years of age for populations at higher risk. Venous specimens are more accurate and are preferred. Efforts to remove lead from gasoline and paint have helped reduce exposure and consequently elevated lead levels in children. Secondary prevention includes lead paint removal in homes built before 1978, which are most likely to contain lead paint.

Management of elevated blood levels in children is guided by the results in micrograms per deciliter. For any result 20 μg/dL or higher, management should be coordinated with a pediatric environmental health specialty unit. Chelation therapy may be indicated when blood lead levels are very high.

Additional Reading: Centers for Disease Control, Childhood Lead Poisoning Prevention Program.

5. A young child is brought in by his mother because her day care provider thought the child had amblyopia. Which of the following conditions is consistent with amblyopia?

A) Congenital cataracts that are noted at birth
B) Irregular pupillary size
C) Increased distance between the medial and lateral canthus
D) Retinal detachment seen in premature children
E) Subnormal visual acuity in one or both eyes despite correction of refractive error

The answer is E: Amblyopia is a subnormal visual acuity in one or both eyes despite correction of a refractive error. It results when the child suppresses the vision of one eye to avoid seeing double (diplopia). Amblyopia is frequently asymptomatic and detected only by screening programs. It is more difficult to treat with increasing age; therefore, children should be screened and treated early. If history and examination do not suggest amblyopia, consider other causes of visual disturbance (neurologic, psychological).

Treatment includes correction of refraction error and then forced use of the amblyopic eye by patching the normal eye. For those children unable to tolerate the patch, the normal eye can be blurred with glasses or drops (penalization therapy) so that the more severely affected eye can be stimulated to develop. If the child is found to have an underlying cataract to account for the visual disturbance, surgery to remove the cataract is indicated.

Additional Reading: Identification and treatment of amblyopia. *Am Fam Physician*. 2013;87(5):348-352.

6. Which one of the following conditions may be associated with leukocoria?

A) Infection
B) Leukemia
C) Pyuria
D) Pregnancy
E) Retinoblastoma

The answer is E: Leukocoria (white pupil) refers to an abnormal pupillary light reflex, in which the pupil appears white, and may indicate a disorder anywhere within the eye. Often, this condition is noted when photographs are taken of a child and only one pupil has a red reflex, the other being white. Clinicians should assess the red reflex during well-child visits with a direct ophthalmoscope in the first years of life. Causes include cataracts, retinoblastoma, Coats disease (retinal telangiectasias and subretinal exudation leading to retinal detachment), persistent fetal vasculature, vitreous hemorrhage, ocular toxocariasis, hereditary retinal dysplasia, retinal detachment, coloboma, and astrocytic hamartoma.

The most serious diagnosis is retinoblastoma, a malignancy of the retina that likely arises from retinal germ cells that have a loss-of-function mutation of the *Rb1* gene. Retinoblastoma may be hereditary, and a family history of bilateral retinoblastoma or enucleation should be noted.

Treatment of retinoblastoma is determined by risk and may involve systemic chemotherapy, intra-arterial chemotherapy, laser photocoagulation, and in some cases surgical enucleation. Retinoblastoma is fatal if untreated. With prompt diagnosis and treatment, the cure rate is greater than 90%, and most children do not require enucleation.

Additional Reading: Approach to the child with leukocoria. In: *UpToDate*. 2022.

The lack of a red reflex in the eye on examination or in a photograph is referred to as leukocoria, and the child should be evaluated to ensure that he or she does not have retinoblastoma or other underlying conditions.

7. You are seeing a 6-year-old child who has failed a course of amoxicillin that was prescribed to treat an episode of acute otitis media (AOM) and you consider prescribing another antibacterial agent. Which one of the following medications would be the recommended second-line treatment of otitis media in a young child?

A) Azithromycin
B) Cefaclor
C) Cefixime
D) Amoxicillin-clavulanate
E) Erythromycin

The answer is D: Of the antibiotics listed, amoxicillin-clavulanate (90 mg/kg/d of amoxicillin, with 6.4 mg/kg/d of clavulanate in 2 divided doses) is the recommended first-line treatment after a failed initial antibiotic treatment. Alternative treatments include ceftriaxone and 3 days of clindamycin (30-40 mg/kg/d in 3 divided doses) with or without a third-generation cephalosporin.

Additional Reading: Acute otitis media in children. *Am Fam Physician*. 2017;95(2):109-110.

8. Differentiating between normal developmental dysfluency and stuttering can be difficult when a child has language issues. What is the major difference between stuttering and developmental dysfluency?

A) Those affected with developmental dysfluency are more easily frustrated.
B) Those with developmental dysfluency may display inappropriate articulating postures.
C) Stuttering involves repetition of word parts and prolongation of sounds.
D) Stuttering involves repetition of whole words and phrases.
E) Stuttering involves slower speech compared with those with developmental dysfluency.

The answer is C: Differentiating between normal developmental dysfluency and stuttering can be done with examination of speech patterns. Developmental dysfluency involves the repetition of whole words and phrases, whereas stuttering involves the repetition of word parts and the prolongation of sounds. Those who stutter frequently speak at a faster tempo, display silent pauses, have inappropriate articulating postures, become more dysfluent in response to stress, and are more easily frustrated.

The majority of stuttering cases are classified as a developmental disorder; however, stuttering can further be considered a neurologic or psychogenic problem. A person who stutters has difficulty coordinating airflow, articulation, and resonance. They may also have small asynchronies identifiable in their fluent speech.

Boys are more frequently affected, and a genetic risk may exist. Generally, there is cause for concern if a patient has five or more breaks per 100 words of speech. Almost 80% of children who stutter recover fluency by the age of 16 years. Mild stuttering is self-limited. More severe stuttering requires speech therapy, the mainstay of treatment. Delayed auditory feedback and computer-assisted training are used to help slow speech and enable control of other speech mechanisms. Pharmacologic therapy is seldom used; however, haloperidol may help.

Additional Reading: Stuttering: an overview. *Am Fam Physician*. 2008;77(9):1271-1276.

9. Which one of the following antibiotics could be used to treat penicillin-resistant *S pneumoniae* otitis media?

A) Azithromycin
B) Amoxicillin-clavulanate
C) Cefaclor
D) Cephalexin
E) Clarithromycin

The answer is B: Only three antibiotics have demonstrated efficacy in the treatment of acute otitis media caused by penicillin-resistant *S pneumoniae*—high-dose amoxicillin (80-90 mg/kg/d), amoxicillin-clavulanate, cefuroxime, and ceftriaxone.

Additional Reading: Acute otitis media in children. *Am Fam Physician*. 2017;95(2):109-110.

10. A 4-year-old boy presents to your office with his mother who is concerned that he has recurrent ear infections. In the past year, he has had seven ear infections. What is the next best step in management?

A) Prescribe a single-dose prophylactic antibiotic at bedtime.
B) Prescribe long-term use of an antihistamine-decongestant preparation.
C) Refer for a tonsillectomy and adenoidectomy.
D) Refer for surgical evaluation of possible tympanostomy tube placement.
E) Continue observation, with a follow-up visit in 6 weeks.

The answer is D: Chronic otitis media results from acute otitis media and eustachian tube dysfunction. Despite short courses of antibiotics, affected children have recurrent infections, which occur more often in the winter months. Persistent chronic otitis media can lead to hearing deficits.

Tympanostomy tubes have been shown to reduce the number of episodes of acute otitis media by 1.5 episodes in the 6 months after surgery. In one nonrandomized study, large improvements were seen in a disease-specific quality-of-life instrument that measured psychosocial domains of physical suffering, hearing loss, speech impairment, emotional distress, and activity limitations.

Additional Reading: Acute otitis media in children. *Am Fam Physician*. 2017;95(2):109-110.

11. In children, conductive hearing loss may be a consequence of which one of the following conditions?

A) Chronic eustachian tube dysfunction
B) Long-term exposure to loud noises
C) Intracranial hemorrhage
D) Meningitis
E) Medication side effect

The answer is A: Signs of hearing loss may include delayed speech development, behavioral problems, and impaired comprehension. Hearing loss can be conductive or sensorineural. Conductive hearing loss refers to a loss of effective sound conduction from the outer ear canal to the cochlea. It is usually caused by acute otitis media or otitis media with effusion but may also result from the presence of foreign bodies in the ear, cerumen impaction, otitis externa, cholesteatoma, disorders of auditory ossicles, tympanic membrane perforations, and malformations of the outer ear or ear canal. Sensorineural hearing refers to decreased hearing that has resulted from damage to the cochlear hair cells in the inner ear. It can result from meningitis or congenital infection, congenital defect, intracranial hemorrhage, long-term noise exposure, ototoxic medication, or trauma.

Hearing screening is part of the Bright Futures Recommendations for Preventative Pediatric Health Care. Screening is recommended to be conducted at 4, 5, 6, 8, and 10 years of age and once between 11 and 13 years of age, 15 and 17 years of age, and 18 and 21 years of age. Absolute indications for audiologic evaluation include premature birth (birth weight < 2500 g or birth weight > 2500 g with asphyxia, seizures, intracranial hemorrhage, hyperbilirubinemia, persistent fetal circulation, and assisted ventilation); intrauterine infection; bacterial meningitis; anomalies of the first or second branchial arch; anomalies of the neural crest or ectoderm; a family history of hereditary or unexplained deafness; parental concern; and delayed speech or language development, or other disabilities including intellectual disability, autism spectrum disorder, cerebral palsy, and blindness.

Newborn hearing screening is mandated in many states. Infants are tested using either otoacoustic emissions or automated auditory brainstem evoked response. The auditory brainstem evoked response uses external scalp electrodes to detect waveforms that occur in predictable patterns after an auditory stimulus. The prompt recognition of disordered hearing in children can help prevent delays in language development.

Additional Reading: Hearing loss in children: screening and evaluation. In: *UpToDate*. 2022.

12. Which condition is most likely to result in retinopathy of prematurity (ROP)?

A) Development of congenital cataracts
B) Excessive oxygen administration
C) Gestational diabetes
D) Maternal hypothyroidism
E) Maternal rubella infection

The answer is B: ROP refers to a developmental vascular proliferative disorder that occurs in the retina of preterm infants who have incomplete retinal vascularization at birth. The pathogenesis is thought to involve an initial hypoxic, hyperoxic, or hypotensive injury to the developing blood vessels resulting in free radical formation which leads to vascular injury and disruption of normal angiogenesis. If the neovascularization is mild, the abnormal vessels may spontaneously regress, preserving vision. The most important risk factor for ROP is the degree of prematurity, but over 50 separate risk factors have been identified including low birth weight, assisted ventilation for greater than 1 week, and elevated arterial oxygen tension. Breast milk feeding, docosahexaenoic acid supplementation, and interventions to reduce the risk of development of bronchopulmonary dysplasia have been shown to be protective.

Treatment consists of retinal ablative therapy with laser photocoagulation or intravitreal injection of anti–vascular endothelial growth factor. All infants with a birth weight less than 1500 g or gestational age less than 30 weeks should be evaluated by an ophthalmologist, generally at 30 weeks of postmenstrual age.

Additional Reading: Retinopathy of prematurity: pathogenesis, epidemiology, classification, and screening. In: *UpToDate*. 2022.

➜ ROP is secondary to oxygen administration in premature infants.

13. A 2-year-old child is brought to your office by his mother because she has noted a greenish-yellow, malodorous, bloody discharge coming from his left nostril. What is the most likely diagnosis to account for his presentation?

A) Acute sinusitis
B) Cerebrospinal fluid leak
C) Chronic tonsillitis
D) Foreign body in the nose
E) Wegener granulomatosis

The answer is D: Young children are at risk of lodging foreign bodies within their nasal cavities. Symptoms include unilateral purulent, malodorous, and often bloody nasal discharge. Other symptoms include nasal congestion and abnormal nasal sounds. Some children with a foreign body may have clear nasal discharge or mild sinus congestion.

It is important to also inspect the unaffected side and both ears to fully assess the potential involvement of other sites. Radiographs of the nasal area and sinuses may help with object localization. Lavage is not recommended because of the risk of pushing a foreign body deeper into the nasal cavity. Foreign bodies should be removed anteriorly using alligator forceps, ear curettes, probes, or a Fogarty catheter (which can slip behind the foreign body, inflate, and be pulled out, bringing the foreign body). The forced exhalation method utilizes either a bag valve mask or a parent's mouth to create a tight seal over the child's mouth. While occluding the unobstructed nare, air is forcibly blown into the child's mouth in the hopes of expelling the object. Otolaryngologists should be consulted in cases in which removal is difficult or unsuccessful.

Additional Reading: Foreign bodies in the ear, nose, and throat. *Am Fam Physician*. 2007;76(8):1185-1189.

14. Which one of the following conditions is associated with congenital cataracts?

A) Acromegaly
B) Congenital hypothyroidism
C) Fetal hydrops
D) Maternal rubella infection
E) Maternal varicella infection

The answer is D: Cataract refers to a proteinaceous opacity of the lens of the eye. Causes of congenital cataracts include ocular trauma, maternal rubella, diabetes mellitus, and galactosemia. Presenile cataracts may be seen in individuals with Marfan syndrome and Down syndrome.

Monocular cataracts should be corrected immediately, within the first 3 months of birth, to ensure proper development of vision. Treatment of the amblyopia may be the most demanding and difficult step in the visual rehabilitation of infants and children with cataracts.

Additional Reading: *Rubella (German Measles, Three-Day Measles)*. Centers for Disease Control and Prevention. www.cdc.gov/rubella/index.html

15. Oral health is an important component of children's care. Dental caries can be prevented with adequate daily tooth hygiene targeted at keeping the teeth and gums clean; however, caries are the consequences of bacterial activity. Which organism is most likely to cause dental caries in children?

A) *Bacteroides fragilis*
B) *Eikenella corrodens*
C) *P multocida*
D) *S aureus*
E) *S mutans*

The answer is E: The mutans streptococci (ie, *S mutans* and *Streptococcus sobrinus*) have been reported as the principal bacteria responsible for the initiation of dental caries in humans.

Additional Reading: Common dental infections. *Am Fam Physician*. 2018;98(11):online.

16. A mother has expressed concern that her toddler has "crossed eyes" at her 18-month well-child check. On examination, you suspect pseudostrabismus. Which one of the following would be the most useful to confirm this diagnosis?

A) A slit-lamp examination
B) A Snellen eye chart
C) The cover/uncover test
D) The corneal light reflex test
E) The funduscopic examination

The answer is D: Strabismus is the most common cause of amblyopia, which refers to a decrease in visual acuity in one eye. Strabismus refers to one eye turning in a different direction than the other and occurs when one of the two eyes does not aim at the same spot the other is focusing on to see. Pseudostrabismus refers to the situation when a child has a wide nasal bridge and prominent epicanthal folds so that it appears that the eyes are not looking in the same direction; yet when the eyes are closely examined for the corneal light reflex, it is found to be symmetric. No strabismus exists and no treatment is needed.

In a corneal light reflex test, the child's attention is attracted to look at a specific target (a picture or bright object) while the light from the ophthalmoscope is directed at the child's eyes. Normally, the light will be reflected symmetrically in each pupil by 6 months of age. A wide nasal bridge or epicanthal folds may give the appearance of eye deviation; however, the light reflection will be found to be symmetric.

In the cover-uncover test, a cover (a piece of paper or cardboard is commonly used) is placed in from of one eye while the child's attention is drawn to a target such as a picture or bright object. The cover is then removed rapidly, and the previously covered eye is observed for any movement from a deviated position back to fixation on the target. If this is seen, it is a sign of phoria, also called latent strabismus. Minimal phoria is a normal variant.

Most cases of strabismus develop between 18 months and 6 years of age. All infants should have consistent, synchronized eye movement by 5 to 6 months of age. Strabismus often results from an altered reflex arc in the central nervous system or less commonly due to cranial nerve palsies, neuromuscular disorders, or structural abnormalities.

Strabismus is categorized as medial deviation (esotropia), lateral deviation (exotropia), or vertical deviation (hypertropia). Vertical deviation is the least common type. Deviations that are always manifested are called *tropias*, whereas those that are only elicited by provocative testing are called *phorias*.

Amblyopia (vision loss in one eye) is not necessarily related to the degree of strabismus because even small deviations can result in significant vision loss. Amblyopia is treated by placing a patch over the better eye. The patch is removed for 1 to 2 waking hours each day to reduce the risk of a deprivation amblyopia in the good eye. Once the visual goal is achieved, part-time patching prevents relapse and is often continued for many months to years. Prognosis improves with a shorter duration of amblyopia and later age of onset.

Visual acuity improves as children become older. All children older than 8 years should be able to achieve 20/20 visual acuity using eyeglass correction. Younger children should be referred to an ophthalmologist if there is a difference between the right and left eyes of two or more lines on a Snellen chart visual evaluation.

Additional Reading: Amblyopia: detection and treatment. *Am Fam Physician*. 2019;100(12):745-750.

17. Which of the following statements about otitis media caused by *M catarrhalis* is true?

A) Analgesic medications are not usually beneficial.
B) *M catarrhalis* is not susceptible to amoxicillin.
C) Younger children tend to have milder clinical courses.
D) Treatment regimen includes antibiotics and antihistamines.
E) *M catarrhalis* is an uncommon cause of otitis media.

The answer is B: Otitis media is common and often presents in the winter months. Bottle-fed infants, particularly those put to bed with bottles, are more frequently affected compared with those infants who are not. Boys are more prone to otitis media more often than girls, as well as premature infants or those enrolled in frequent day care. Infants with cleft palate or Down syndrome are also at increased risk. Common etiologic agents for otitis media include the following:

- *S pneumoniae*
- *M catarrhalis*
- Nontypeable *H influenza*

Newborns are more likely to be affected with *E coli* and *S aureus*. Children older than 5 years are less frequently affected. *Klebsiella pneumoniae* and *Bacteroides* rarely cause otitis media. Viruses including respiratory syncytial virus, rhinovirus, and adenovirus cause otitis media and are often complicated with secondary bacterial organisms.

Eustachian tube dysfunction and anatomic immaturity are major factors contributing to otitis media. This finding results from a reflux communication of fluid and bacteria with the middle ear. Symptoms of otitis media include pain, fever, and purulent drainage if the tympanic membrane has ruptured. Younger children may be fussy and irritable, and show decreased appetite or sleep disturbances. Pulling at the ears may also be a sign of otitis media.

Physical examination usually shows a bulging erythematous tympanic membrane with a loss of tympanic landmarks and lack of mobility with pneumatoscopy.

Treatment includes analgesics and, in severe cases, high-dose amoxicillin, 80 to 90 mg/kg/d divided bid. In cases of treatment failure, amoxicillin-clavulanate (90 mg/kg/d, divided bid) is the preferred antibiotic.

Up to 60% of *S pneumoniae* and close to 100% of *M catarrhalis* strains produce β-lactamase that makes them resistant to amoxicillin. Antihistamines and decongestants are not recommended.

Additional Reading: Acute otitis media in children. *Am Fam Physician*. 2017;95(2):109-110.

The American Academy of Pediatrics and the American Academy of Family Physicians published treatment guidelines with the option of "watching and waiting" for nonsevere cases of otitis media. That includes those with only mild ear pain and without a high fever in children 2 years of age and older.

18. Which one of the following organisms would be the most likely pathogen causing periorbital cellulitis in a vaccinated child with no recent trauma?

A) *H influenzae* type B (Hib)
B) *M catarrhalis*
C) *Pseudomonas aeruginosa*
D) *S pneumoniae*
E) *S aureus*

The answer is D: Periorbital and orbital cellulitis may be caused by trauma (wound, insect bite), an associated infection (sinusitis), or seeding from bacteremia. Before widespread immunization, Hib was the most common cause secondary to bacteremia (about 80% of cases) and remains the most common etiologic agent among nonimmunized populations. *S pneumoniae* accounted for most of the remaining cases and is the most likely agent in Hib-vaccinated patients when sinusitis is present.

The most common pathogens associated with trauma are *S aureus* and *Streptococcus pyogenes*; however, these are seldom isolated from the blood. Fewer than one-third of patients with periorbital cellulitis have an organism present in blood culture.

Additional Reading: Differential diagnosis of the swollen red eyelid. *Am Fam Physician*. 2015;92(2):106-112.

19. A 16-year-old girl presents with swelling, warmth, and spreading redness at the upper part of her ear. She has recently had her ears pierced. Which one of the following antibiotics is appropriate to prescribe for the next step in her management?

A) Azithromycin
B) Cephalexin
C) Ciprofloxacin
D) Penicillin
E) Tetracycline

The answer is C: The popularity of body piercing at sites other than the earlobe has grown since the mid-1990s. The tongue, lips, nose, eyebrows, nipples, navel, and genitals are frequently used for piercing. Complications include local and systemic infections, poor cosmetic results, and foreign body rejection. Swelling and damage to dentition are common after tongue piercing, and navel, nipple, and genital piercings often have prolonged healing times.

Minor infections, allergic contact dermatitis, keloid formation, and traumatic tearing may occur after piercing of the earlobe. "High" ear piercing through the ear cartilage is associated with more serious infections and disfigurement. Fluoroquinolone antibiotics (eg, ciprofloxacin) are advised for treatment of auricular perichondritis because of their antipseudomonal activity.

Additional Reading: Complications of body piercing. *Am Fam Physician*. 2005;72:2029-2034, 2035-2036.

20. A 3-month-old infant is brought to the office by her mother. She is concerned because for the past 3 to 4 weeks her child has been having mucousy tearing from her left eye. Which one of the following is the most likely diagnosis to account for her presentation?

A) Congenital cataracts
B) *Chlamydia trachomatis* infection
C) Dacryostenosis
D) Glaucoma
E) Viral conjunctivitis

The answer is C: Dacryostenosis (congenital lacrimal duct stenosis) refers to a congenital stenosis of the nasolacrimal duct, which is associated with excessive tearing of the affected eye. The condition is common and affects children from the neonatal period to 2 and 12 months of age. Treatment includes parental massaging of the affected duct two to three times per day. Dacryostenosis typically resolves by 6 to 10 months of age. If the condition persists beyond 12 months of age, the duct may require probing under anesthesia. If copious and persistent purulent discharge is present, treatment with topical antibiotic agents is recommended.

Additional Reading: Congenital nasolacrimal duct obstruction (dacryostenosis) and dacryocystocele. In: *UpToDate*. 2022.

21. Regarding transient cortical blindness, which one of the following statements is true?

A) A consequence is permanent cerebral slowing.
B) It is associated with head trauma.
C) The duration is typically 3 to 5 days.
D) There is associated cerebral edema.

The answer is B: Transient cortical blindness refers to blindness that presents in the absence of other focal neurologic signs and resolves within 24 hours. It is usually caused by mild head trauma, although computed tomography head scans are usually unremarkable and there is little evidence to suggest skull fracture. Electroencephalogram results may initially show some slowing, but this resolves spontaneously as the blindness dissipates.

Additional Reading: Retrochismal disorders. *Nelson Textbook of Pediatrics*. 20th ed. Elsevier/Saunders; 2015.

22. Fluoride helps to reduce the formation of dental caries. What is the goal for fluoride in drinking water, in parts per million (ppm)?

A) 1 ppm
B) 10 ppm
C) 100 ppm
D) 500 ppm
E) 1000 ppm

The answer is A: Fluoride helps to reduce the formation of dental caries and can easily be added to drinking water. The goal for fluoride level in water is 1 ppm. The need for supplementation depends on the amount of fluoride already present in the water and should be considered if fluoride levels are less than 0.6 ppm. Fluoride toothpaste is not sufficient for supplementation. Initiate fluoride supplementation at 6 months of age for infants who are not consuming fluoridated water. Excessive fluoride can cause fluorosis.

Supplemental Fluoride Dosage Schedule

	Milligrams of Fluoride per Day		
Fluoride in Home Drinking Water (ppm)	<0.3	0.3-0.6	>0.6
Birth-6 mo	0	0	0
6 mo-3 y	0.25	0	0
3-6 y	0.50	0.25	0
6-16 y	1.0	0.50	0

Additional Reading: Screening and interventions to prevent dental caries in children younger than 5 years. *Am Fam Physician*. 2022;105(3):online.

The U.S. Preventive Services Task Force recommends that primary care clinicians prescribe oral fluoride supplementation starting at 6 months of age for children whose water supply is deficient in fluoride.

Section III. Neurologic System

Each of the following questions or incomplete statements is followed by suggested answers or completions. Select the ONE BEST ANSWER in each case.

1. You are seeing an 18-month-old boy who had been ill with a fever and then had a seizure. You suspect a febrile seizure. Which one of the following characteristics from this patient's history would indicate the need to perform a lumbar puncture (LP)?

A) He had a generalized seizure.
B) His seizure lasted longer than 10 minutes.
C) He has any signs suggestive of meningitis.
D) He had recently been vaccinated.
E) None of the above—all children with a febrile seizure require an LP.

The answer is C: Most seizures in children <5 years of age are febrile, which refers to any seizure in a child 6 months to 5 years of age, who also has a current or recent fever (at least 38 °C [100.4 °F]). Additionally, they do not have a history of seizure or other neurologic event. Febrile seizures can be simple or complex. Simple febrile seizures are generalized, last less than 15 minutes, and occur only once in a 24-hour period. Complex febrile seizures may have focal features, last longer than 15 minutes, and recur within a 24-hour period.

Viral infections are often present with febrile seizures, often due to human herpes virus 6 and 7, and influenza A and B. There was an increased risk of febrile seizure within 24 hours of receiving diphtheria and tetanus toxoids and whole-cell pertussis vaccines (whole-cell pertussis vaccines are no longer used in the United States) and within 8 to 14 days of receiving an measles-mumps-rubella vaccine.

The risk of recurrence increases in patients who had a first febrile seizure (1) before 15 months of age, (2) with a lower rectal temperature (<40 °C [104 °F]), (3) with shorter duration of fever (<24 hours) beforehand, (4) complex features, and (5) a family history of febrile seizures. The risk of epilepsy development is increased in those who have had simple febrile seizures and is even greater among those who have had one or more complex febrile seizures.

Airway and circulatory support are key components in evaluating a child with a febrile seizure, ideally with noninvasive measures until resolution of the postictal state. A thorough medical history should include past seizures and other neurologic conditions, exposure to medications or toxins, allergies, or trauma. If the seizure duration exceeds 5 minutes, administer benzodiazepines. Antipyretic therapy is not necessary. Conduct mental status and physical examinations after the seizure ends. Obtain a serum blood glucose test and consider electrolytes if considering etiology to be a metabolic abnormality.

Most cases do not require further workup, but in cases in which meningitis is suspected, an LP is indicated. Consider LP in children less than 12 months of age who may not have other evident signs of meningeal infection and in those 12 to 18 months of age who may only demonstrate subtle symptoms of meningitis. Children older than 18 months may present with neck stiffness, positive Kernig or Brudzinski signs, or a clinical picture consistent with intracranial infection.

Neuroimaging only is appropriate in patients at risk of cerebral abscess, increased intracranial pressure, and evidence of trauma and in those with status epilepticus or a history of complex seizure.

After a simple febrile seizure, provide parental education and make plans to follow up and then children can be cared for at home.

Additional Reading: Febrile seizures: risks, evaluation, and prognosis. *Am Fam Physician.* 2019;99(7):445-450.

2. Hyperbilirubinemia is commonly seen in the neonatal period. Which one of the following statements is true regarding hyperbilirubinemia?

A) Complications of kernicterus include hearing loss, seizures, and mental retardation.
B) Coombs testing should not be used in the workup of hyperbilirubinemia.
C) Kernicterus in premature infants occurs with a higher level of bilirubin than does that in term infants.
D) Physiologic jaundice rarely occurs in newborns.
E) Switching from formula to breastfeeding may help decrease bilirubin levels.

The answer is A: Severe neonatal hyperbilirubinemia refers to a total serum or plasma bilirubin >25 mg/dL (428 μmol/L) and is associated with a risk for bilirubin-induced neurologic dysfunction, which occurs once bilirubin crosses the blood-brain barrier and binds to brain tissue. Kernicterus refers to the chronic and permanent sequelae of bilirubin-induced neurologic dysfunction, which develops within the first year of life.

Features include choreoathetoid cerebral palsy, sensorineural hearing loss, gaze abnormalities, and dental enamel dysplasia. Symptoms may include poor feeding, flaccidity, apnea, opisthotonos (spasm of the muscles causing backward arching of the head, neck, and spine), and seizures; in severe cases, death may occur.

Risk factors include jaundice within the first 24 hours of life, having a sibling who required previous phototherapy, cephalohematoma or significant bruising from trauma, prematurity, hemolytic disease resulting from blood incompatibilities, infection, acidosis, and East Asian race.

Physiologic jaundice is the most common form of jaundice, occurring in up to 50% of newborns. Most bilirubin levels peak in 3 to 5 days, resolves within 1 week, and is typically benign. The workup of a child with hyperbilirubinemia includes the following:

- Careful history to detect risk factors and physical examination to rule out petechiae, hepatosplenomegaly, bruising, and signs of infection
- Measurement of bilirubin levels
- Complete blood count, reticulocyte count, and peripheral blood smear
- Coombs test
- Blood typing of mother and infant
- Thyroid function tests

Treatment for hyperbilirubinemia of newborns includes the following:

- Increase formula feedings for the infant to increase gastrointestinal motility and frequency of stools, thereby minimizing the enterohepatic circulation of bilirubin.
- Increasing frequency of breastfeeding. If bilirubin continues to increase, switch from breastfeeding to formula for a few days until bilirubin is <15 mg/dL (the mother should continue with breast pumping during this time).
- Phototherapy to help degrade unconjugated bilirubin.
- Exchange transfusion for severe cases of persistent hyperbilirubinemia (usually >20 mg/dL) or hemolysis with anemia.
- In premature infants, kernicterus may occur with lower bilirubin levels.

Additional Readings:
1. Evaluation and treatment of neonatal hyperbilirubinemia. *Am Fam Physician*. 2014;89(11):873-878.
2. Rebound bilirubin levels after phototherapy in neonates with hyperbilirubinemia. *Am Fam Physician*. 2020;102(9):online

3. A healthy 5-year-old boy is brought to your office by his mother with a concern that he is having recurring staring spells. You consider that he is suffering from absence seizures. Which one of the following is associated with this suspected diagnosis?

A) A marchlike progression of tonic-clonic activity
B) No known genetic transmission
C) Staring episodes that last up to 30 minutes
D) Subnormal intelligence
E) A spike-and-wave (3 per second) electroencephalographic pattern

The answer is E: Absence seizures (formerly called *petit mal seizures*) are characterized by brief 10- to 30-second staring episodes with lack of awareness, followed by resumption of normal activity. During seizure episodes, an electroencephalogram shows a characteristic 3 per second bilateral spike-and-wave pattern. Attacks may occur up to 100 times daily and can be precipitated by hyperventilation.

The seizures usually affect children, and there is some evidence of genetic predisposition. Affected children usually have normal intelligence, and most cases resolve before 20 years of age. Treatment usually involves the use of valproic acid and/or ethosuximide and clonazepam.

Additional Reading: Seizure disorder, absence. In: Domino F, ed. *The 5-Minute Clinical Consult*. Wolters Kluwer; 2022.

4. A 4-year-old boy is brought in urgently by his parents because he has had a high fever and overnight has developed a purplish looking rash. He is lethargic and he does not want to eat or drink. Which one of the following would be the most appropriate step in his care?

A) Admit to the hospital and begin intravenous (IV) antibiotics.
B) Obtain a throat culture and treat if positive for strep.
C) Prescribe oral antibiotics and arrange for next-day follow-up.
D) Prescribe symptomatic measures for this likely viral infection.
E) Send to the laboratory to check Lyme disease titers.

The answer is A: Meningococcemia is a severe infection that is caused by *Neisseria meningitidis*. The mode of transmission is through infected respiratory secretions. Thirty-five percent to 40% of cases occur in children under 5 years of age. The second peak is in adolescence Onset of symptoms is usually abrupt, and the course can be fulminant despite treatment. Symptoms include fever, chills, fatigue, myalgias, and prostration. Mortality rate is between 10% and 15%.

Examination reveals a distinctive petechial or purpuric rash, a purplish discoloration of the skin produced by small bleeding vessels near the surface. Fulminant disease can result in disseminated intravascular coagulopathy and septic shock. Diagnosis can be made with cultures from blood, cerebrospinal fluid, or skin lesions Treatment is high-dose IV penicillin G, central nervous system–penetrating cephalosporins such as ceftriaxone, cefotaxime, meropenem, and chloramphenicol in an intensive care unit setting.

Exposed household, day care, and close school contacts should receive rifampin chemoprophylaxis. Ceftriaxone and ciprofloxacin can also be used for prophylaxis in adults.

Universal meningococcal vaccination against serogroups A, C, W-135, and Y is recommended for children aged 11 to 12 years with a booster dose at 16 years of age.

Additional Reading: Evaluation of purpura in children. In: *UpToDate*. 2022.

5. What is the median age when the anterior fontanel closes?

A) 6 weeks
B) 3 months
C) 18 months
D) 12 months
E) 2 years

The answer is C: An infant has two fontanels at birth, the anterior and posterior fontanels, the largest being the anterior fontanel. On average, the anterior fontanel is about 2 cm in size, and the median time of closure is around 18 months of age. Common causes of a large anterior fontanel or delayed fontanel closure are achondroplasia, hypothyroidism, Down syndrome, increased intracranial pressure, and rickets. A bulging anterior fontanel suggests increased intracranial pressure or intracranial and extracranial tumors. A sunken fontanel suggests dehydration.

The examination with suspected underlying etiology should guide the selection of imaging modality, including plain films, ultrasonography, computed tomography, or magnetic resonance imaging to determine the diagnosis.

Additional Reading: The abnormal fontanel. *Am Fam Physician*. 2003;67(12):2547-2552.

6. Considering the range of normal childhood development, all of the following are normal developmental milestones, except which one?

A) Rolls over at 4 to 5 months
B) Walks at 12 months
C) First words (eg, "mama" and "dada") at 15 months
D) Points to four body parts at 18 months
E) Copies a circle at 3 years

The answer is C: Some important developmental milestones for children include the following:

- *4 to 5 months*: rolls over to supine position.
- *6 months*: sits without support.
- *9 months*: says "mama" and "dada" indiscriminately.
- *9 months*: creeps and crawls, pulls to stand, waves bye-bye.
- *10 months*: says "mama" and "dada" discriminately.
- *12 months*: walks alone.
- *15 months*: creeps upstairs, builds two-block towers, walks independently.
- *18 months*: points to four body parts.
- *24 months*: jumps, kicks ball, removes coat, verbalizes wants.
- *3 years*: copies circle; gives full name, age, and sex; throws ball overhand.
- *4 years*: hops on one foot, dresses with little assistance, puts shoes on the correct feet.
- *5 years*: ties shoes, prints first name, plays competitive games.

Impairments in hearing can relate to delayed development. Therefore, the first step in the evaluation of a child with language delay is hearing assessment.

Additional Readings:
1. Screening for developmental delay. *Am Fam Physician*. 2011;84(5):544-549.
2. CDC's revised developmental milestone checklists. *Am Fam Physician*. 2022;106(4):370-371.

Red flags to consider a developmental delay that warrant a workup to rule out autism or other developmental delays include no babbling or pointing by 12 months; no single word by 16 months; a lack of 2 spontaneous words by 24 months; and any loss of language or social skills at any age.

7. Unfortunately, premature infants are at increased risk for hyperbilirubinemia and the subsequent development of kernicterus. Which one of the following statements regarding premature infants in this situation is true?

A) Decreased bowel motility is common, decreasing enterohepatic bilirubin circulation.
B) Delayed clamping of the umbilical cord is associated with hyperbilirubinemia.
C) Early feedings enhance bilirubin excretion.
D) Enterohepatic circulation begins at 40 weeks' gestation.
E) Feeding does not influence hyperbilirubinemia.

The answer is C: Premature infants develop hyperbilirubinemia more often than do full-term infants. Kernicterus may occur at serum bilirubin levels as low as 10 mg/dL (170 μmol/L) in underweight premature infants. Once bilirubin crosses the blood-brain barrier, it binds to brain tissue and can induce neurologic dysfunction; kernicterus refers to the chronic and permanent sequelae of such effects, which develop within the first year of life.

The higher bilirubin levels in premature infants may be due to inadequately developed hepatic excretion mechanisms, which include deficient bilirubin uptake from the serum, impaired hepatic conjugation of bilirubin, and decreased excretion into the biliary tree. Decreased bowel motility is also a factor because it results in increased enterohepatic circulation of bilirubin, which is present even in premature infants. Enterohepatic circulation refers to the circulation of bilirubin from the liver to the bile, followed by entry into the small intestine, where it is reabsorbed and transported back to the liver. With slower bowel transit time due to decreased motility, more of the bilirubin is reabsorbed, rather than being excreted via the stool.

Early feedings increase bowel motility and thereby reduce bilirubin reabsorption, leading to decreased severity of physiologic jaundice. Delayed umbilical cord clamping is rarely associated with increased risk of hyperbilirubinemia, with large transfusion of red blood cell mass that breaks down and leads to increased production of bilirubin.

Additional Reading: Evaluation and treatment of neonatal hyperbilirubinemia. *Am Fam Physician*. 2014; 89(11):873-878.

8. You are examining a 6-month-old infant for her well-child examination and note that she has flattening of the back of her head. Her examination is otherwise normal, and she appears to be developing as expected. What is the most likely cause of suspected positional head deformity in a child?

A) Child abuse
B) Genetic influences
C) Poorly developed sternocleidomastoid muscle
D) Premature birth
E) Supine positioning

The answer is E: Posterior cranial deformity (occipital plagiocephaly) occurs in infants, who do not have any other risk factors for deformity and have flattening of the back of their head noted on routine examination. The finding is thought to be in relationship to the "Back to Sleep" campaign, which is recommended to reduce the risk for sudden infant death syndrome.

Additional Reading: Diagnosis and management of positional head deformity. *Am Fam Physician*. 2003;67(9):1953-1956.

9. A 5-year-old boy is brought to the office by his mother. Although the boy is generally healthy, the mother is concerned that her son has difficulty interacting with other children at school. The boy's teacher reports that he prefers to quietly play alone, often spending time building elaborate block structures. Based on the suspected diagnosis, which one of the following is least likely to be seen in this patient?

A) Easy to engage in conversation
B) Echolalia
C) Repetitive movements
D) Self-injury behaviors
E) Seizures

The answer is A: Autism spectrum disorder (ASD) is a neurodevelopmental disability characterized by (1) deficits in social and communication functioning and (2) restricted and repetitive behaviors, interests, and activities. The clinical presentation can vary considerably based upon the child/adolescents age, developmental and/or intellectual ability, language skills, and ASD trait intensity.

Echolalia refers to the involuntary repetition of a word or a sentence that was just spoken by another person. This feature is common and may inadvertently enhance the true level of language skill. Individuals with ASD may have deficiencies in symbolic thinking and exhibit stereotypic behaviors (eg, repetitive nonproductive movements of hands and fingers, rocking, and meaningless vocalizations), self-stimulation, and self-injury behaviors. Seizures are also possible. Having an intellectual disability is not a diagnostic criterion, but it is frequently present in the moderate to severe range.

Additional Reading: Autism spectrum disorder: primary care principles. *Am Fam Physician*. 2016;94(12):972-979A.

10. Tick paralysis is associated with all of the following except which one?

A) A neurotoxin produced by the tick's salivary gland
B) A tick that harbors bacteria as a vector for transmission to other species
C) Muscle weakness, anorexia, lack of coordination, and ascending flaccid paralysis
D) Rapid recovery once the tick is removed
E) The bite of *Dermacentor* or *Amblyomma* tick species

The answer is B: Ticks are capable of carrying many diseases. Over 40 species of ticks have been associated with tick paralysis. In North America, most cases are associated with the *Dermacentor variabilis*, the American dog tick, and *Dermacentor andersoni*, the Rocky Mountain wood tick. Manifestations of tick paralysis include muscle weakness fatigue and then an ascending flaccid paralysis. Fever is absent and there is no associated rash, headache or change in mental status. In severe cases, respiratory and bulbar paralysis can occur. The paralysis is likely caused by inoculation of a neurotoxin produced by the tick's salivary gland.

Sensory examination and lumbar puncture are normal. Antibiotics are not indicated for affected patients, as no bacterial infection results. Treatment is simple removal of the tick and symptom support. In severe cases with respiratory compromise, mechanical ventilation may be necessary. Mortality rates can be as high as 10% for those with severe cases who remain untreated. Total recovery typically occurs within a few days of tick removal.

Additional Reading: Tickborne diseases: diagnosis and management. *Am Fam Physician*. 2020;101(9):530-540.

11. All of the following statements are true regarding *N meningitidis*, except which one?

A) In addition to infants, those aged 16 through 23 years have the highest rates of meningococcal disease.
B) Young adults with *N meningitidis* have better outcomes than do other age groups.
C) Meningococcal disease spreads from person to person.
D) Three *N meningitidis* serogroups (B, C, and Y) cause most of the illness seen in the United States.
E) Outbreaks of serogroup B meningococcal disease have been reported from college campuses during the past several years.

The answer is B: *N meningitidis* has an average annual incidence of 1 case per 100,000 in the United States. The disease can cause rapid death or result in severe neurologic and vascular damage, even when antibiotic therapy is administered. Antibiotic chemoprophylaxis with rifampin, ciprofloxacin, or ceftriaxone is recommended for household and other close contacts. The majority of meningococcal cases are sporadic, but outbreaks can occur, and subsequent vaccination of the affected population is required. Adolescents and young adults of 16 to 23 years of age have a higher incidence of disease and a higher fatality rate than do other populations. There are five serogroups ("strains") of *N meningitidis*: A, B, C, W, and Y that cause most disease worldwide. Three of these serogroups (B, C, and Y) cause most of the illness seen in the United States.

There are three types of meningococcal vaccines available in the United States:

1. Meningococcal conjugate vaccines (Menactra, Menveo
2. Meningococcal polysaccharide vaccine (Menomune)
3. Serogroup B meningococcal vaccines (Bexsero and Trumenba)

All 11- to 12-year-olds should be vaccinated with a meningococcal conjugate vaccine (Menactra or Menveo). A booster dose is recommended at age 16 years. Teens and young adults (16- through 23-year-olds) also may be vaccinated with a serogroup B meningococcal vaccine.

Additional Reading: Meningococcal vaccination. https://www.cdc.gov/vaccines/vpd/mening/index.html

12. Syringomyelia present in a child may expand during adolescent years. What is the first neurologic deficit seen when this change occurs?

A) Poor coordination
B) Abnormal lower extremity reflexes
C) Mental confusion
D) Muscle weakness
E) Decreased pain and temperature sensation

The answer is E: Syringomyelia refers to a fluid accumulation that involves the spinal canal and is usually associated with the cervical area; however, it may extend throughout the spinal cord. The lesion may expand during adolescent years and can give rise to various symptoms, with the first being loss of pain and temperature sensation. Other symptoms include loss of sensation in the distal extremities, upper shoulders, and back; spasticity, asymmetric, or absent reflexes; and weakness with muscle wasting. A rapidly progressing scoliosis may be the initial manifestation of syringomyelia.

The congenital abnormality is associated with an Arnold-Chiari malformation, in which differing degrees of cerebellar and brainstem tissues extend into the spinal canal. Diagnosis is confirmed using magnetic resonance imaging of the spine; however, computed tomographic scan and myelography can be used. Treatment requires surgical removal of the fluid pocket.

Additional Reading: Syringomyelia. https://rarediseases.org/rare-diseases/syringomyelia

13. With concern over a case of bacterial meningitis at the local elementary school, you review treatment options. Which of the following patient group vs treatment scenarios is correct in the management of bacterial meningitis?

A) Neonates up to 1 month of age: ampicillin and cefotaxime
B) 1 month to 10 years of age: ampicillin and gentamicin
C) 10 to 18 years of age: cefuroxime and erythromycin
D) Adults: ampicillin and metronidazole

The answer is A: Bacterial meningitis is rare in the United States but can be fatal. The treatment of bacterial meningitis depends on the age of the patient. In neonates, early-onset meningitis (occurring within the first 72 hours of life) is most commonly caused by group B *Streptococcus,* followed by *E coli*. Responsible organisms change as the child ages:

- Term infants to 3 months of age: *E coli*, group B *Streptococcus*, and *Listeria monocytogenes*
- Children < 10 years: *S pneumoniae*, *N meningitidis*, *H influenzae* type B
- Adolescents 10 to 19 years: *N meningitidis*, *S pneumoniae*
- Adults: *S pneumoniae*, *N meningitidis*, *H influenza*, group B *Streptococcus*, *L monocytogenes*

After the neonatal period, it is recommended that infants older than 1 month and children be treated with broad-spectrum empiric antibiotic treatment, which would include ampicillin and ceftriaxone. Recommended treatment for adults 18 to 49 years of age is ceftriaxone and vancomycin intravenously (IV). For adults over 50 years of age and immunocompromised, treatment consists of ceftriaxone, vancomycin, and ampicillin IV.

Dexamethasone may increase survival if given at the time of antibiotic administration for *S pneumoniae* infections.

Family members, nursery school children, and other close contacts of those affected by *N meningitidis* or *H influenzae* meningitis should also receive prophylactic rifampin.

Additional Reading: CDC, Meningitis.

14. You are seeing a 4-year-old boy who has impaired language development, compulsive repetitive behavior, impaired intelligence, and a preoccupation with inanimate objects. What is the most likely diagnosis?

A) A conductive hearing loss
B) Attention-deficit disorder
C) Autism spectrum disorder (ASD)
D) Dyslexia
E) Manic depressive disorder

The answer is C: ASD is a neurodevelopmental disorder characterized by differences in social and communication functioning as well as abnormal behavior patterns that include restricted and fixated interests and restricted and repetitive behaviors. It has a heterogeneous presentation that can make recognition challenging. The condition affects boys more frequently than girls. ASD may be reliably diagnosed at age 14 to 16 months, but the average age of diagnosis is 4 years.

Diagnostic criteria: (A) persistent deficits in social communication and social interaction across multiple contexts as manifest by all 3 of the following: social-emotional reciprocity; nonverbal communicative behaviors used for social interaction; and developing, maintaining, and understanding relationships and (B) restricted and repetitive patterns of behaviors, interests, or activities, as manifested by 2 or more of the following: stereotypic or repetitive mover movements, use of objects, or speech; insistence on sameness, inflexible adherence to routines, highly fixated and restricted interests; hyper- or hyporeactivity to sensory inputs.

Treatment involves targeting the core symptoms of ASD. The modality of behavior therapy with the strongest evidence for improving outcomes is applied behavior analysis (ABA), which is generally administered for 20 to 25 h/wk.

The American Academy of Pediatrics recommends that all children with a diagnosis of ASD have genetic testing consisting of a chromosomal microarray analysis, and to consider fragile X testing.

Additional Reading: Autism spectrum disorder. Primary care principles. *Am Fam Physician*. 2016;94(12):972-979A.

Section IV. Gastrointestinal System

Each of the following questions or incomplete statements is followed by suggested answers or completions. Select the ONE BEST ANSWER in each case.

1. An 8-year-old girl presents for follow-up with recurring episodes of abdominal pain. An evaluation using abdominal ultrasonography revealed the presence of intussusception. The most likely condition that is precipitating this patient's symptoms is which one of the following?

A) A colonic polyp
B) Meckel diverticulum
C) Lymphoma
D) A parasite infection
E) Peyer patch hypertrophy

The answer is C: Intussusception is invagination (telescoping) of intestine onto itself. It has a slight male predominance and can arise from different etiologies that vary with age. In the first 2 years of life, intussusception often arises from reactive hypertrophy of Peyer patches. In older children and adults, the presentation of intussusception warrants further investigation into pathologic etiologies, such as neoplasm. In children older than 6 years, lymphoma is the most common cause. However, in most cases (75%), the cause is not apparent.

Other conditions associated with intussusception include colonic polyps, Meckel diverticulum, lipoma, parasites (*Ascaris lumbricoides*), and foreign bodies. Small intestine intussusception can be triggered by stool bulk mass in the terminal ileum (celiac disease and cystic fibrosis) and hematoma (Henoch-Schönlein purpura). Intermittent small-bowel intussusception is a rare cause of recurrent abdominal pain.

Additional Reading: Gastrointestinal emergencies. *The Harriet Lane Handbook: A Manual for Pediatric House Officers*. 22nd ed. Elsevier/Mosby; 2021.

2. Rotavirus is a major cause of diarrheal disease and is highly contagious. In assessing a child with acute diarrhea, which one of the following findings would make a diagnosis of rotavirus infection *less* likely?

A) An elevated white blood cell (WBC) count
B) A normal WBC count
C) Hypernatremia
D) Metabolic acidosis
E) Watery diarrhea without blood in the stool,

The answer is A: Vomiting is often the first manifestation of rotavirus infection, followed by repeated bouts of watery diarrhea, rarely bloody, within the next 24 hours, sometimes as many as 8 to 20 stools per day. Fever may be as high as 39 °C (102 °F) in up to one-third of patients. Diarrhea usually lasts 3 to 7 days. The WBC count is rarely elevated, and neither WBCs nor red blood cells are found in the stool.

Infection may result in decreased intestinal absorption of sodium, glucose, water and decreased levels of intestinal lactase, alkaline phosphatase, and sucrase activity which may lead to both osmotic and secretory diarrhea. Rotavirus is much more likely to cause dehydration compared to other viral causes of diarrheal illness.

It is critical to replace fluid losses and restore electrolytes, particularly in small infants. Oral rehydration solutions are adequate in most cases. Concurrent probiotic administration, specifically *Lactobacillus rhamnosus* strain GG has also been found to be helpful.

Antidiarrheal medications (eg, loperamide, tincture of opium, and diphenoxylate with atropine) are not effective and can be dangerous.

Although specific identification of rotavirus is not required in every case, especially during outbreak, antigens can be identified in stool.

Prevention of rotavirus is achieved by practicing good hand hygiene and sanitation efforts. Currently, two vaccines are licensed for use in the United States, the pentavalent RotaTeq and the monovalent Rotarix. Both are highly effective (98%-100%) in preventing severe gastroenteritis and reduced diarrhea-related hospitalizations.

Additional Reading: Rotavirus. www.cdc.gov/rotavirus

3. A 6-year-old boy presents to the emergency department with irritability, recurrent episodes of abdominal pain, and bilious emesis. An abdominal radiograph is obtained and shows colonic distension, and a follow-up computed tomographic (CT) scan shows a whirl pattern. What is the most likely diagnosis?

A) Acute appendicitis
B) Intussusception
C) Malrotation
D) Pyloric stenosis
E) Volvulus

The answer is E: Volvulus occurs when an air-filled loop of sigmoid rotates around its mesentery base, which obstructs arterial and venous circulation of the affected segment with rapid distention of the closed loop. The condition is uncommon in children but has been reported in those with abnormal colonic motility and may be the initial presentation in patients with Hirschsprung disease. Symptoms include progressive abdominal pain, nausea, abdominal distension, and constipation. The pain is continuous and can be severe. Children may have an intermittent, atypical presentation due to spontaneous detorsion. Abdominal radiographs can demonstrate a U-shaped, distended sigmoid colon. Diagnostic abdominal CT findings include a whirl pattern caused by the dilated sigmoid colon around its mesocolon and vessels. Nonoperative treatment includes flexible sigmoidoscopy with endoscopic detorsion and placement of a decompression tube. Definitive operative management most commonly consists of sigmoidectomy with primary colorectal anastomosis.

Sigmoid volvulus is a rare problem seen in children and adolescents, but because of the life-threatening nature of its complications, it should be considered in the differential diagnosis of patients with acute and recurrent episodes of abdominal pain or bowel obstruction in children, especially if colonic dilation is seen on radiographs.

Additional Reading: Sigmoid volvulus. In: *UpToDate*. 2022.

4. What is the caloric content/ounce of most regular infant formulas?

A) 1 cal/oz
B) 10 cal/oz
C) 20 cal/oz
D) 50 cal/oz
E) 100 cal/oz

The answer is C: Most regular infant formula preparations provide 20 cal/oz. Formulas can be based on cow's milk, soy, or casein. For a healthy term infant, who is not breastfed or breastfed before 1 year of age, cow's milk–based formula is recommended, because it most closely resembles the nutritional content of human breast milk. Cow's milk–based formula is composed of 20% whey and 80% casein, and it has 50% more protein/dL than breast milk. Additionally, it contains iron, linoleic acid, carnitine, taurine, and nucleotides.

Approximately 32 oz of cow's milk formula meets 100% of the recommended daily allowance for calories, vitamins, and minerals, and is diluted to a standard 20 cal/oz. Infant formulas are typically whey-dominant protein with vegetable oils and lactose. Lactose-free formulas are available. Most standard formula preparations do not contain adequate fluoride; thus, infants who are exclusively formula-fed may require 0.25 mg/d of supplemental fluoride.

Additional Reading: Nutrition and growth. *The Harriet Lane Handbook: A Manual for Pediatric House Officers*. 22nd ed. Elsevier/Mosby; 2021.

Infant formulas can be based on cow's milk, soy, or casein, and most regular preparations provide 20 cal/oz.

5. A 4-year-old boy who attends a day care is brought in by his parents in the middle of June with concern that he has had profuse watery diarrhea. A stool sample is sent for evaluation and shows leukocytes (WBCs), red blood cells (RBCs), and small comma-shaped bacteria that have a corkscrew motion. Which one of the following organisms is most likely responsible for this presentation?

A) *Campylobacter* infection
B) *E coli* infection
C) *Rotavirus* infection
D) *Salmonella* infection
E) *Shigella* infection

The answer is A: *Campylobacter* infection is an important cause of acute diarrhea worldwide; the organism also may produce systemic illness. *Campylobacter* enteritis is typically caused by the bacteria *Campylobacter jejuni* or *Campylobacter coli*. The organism inhabits the intestinal tracts of a wide range of animal hosts, notably poultry; contamination from these sources can lead to foodborne diseases. Young infants who attend day care are particularly prone to infection in the summer months. Contaminated foods include milk, water, poultry, and beef. Although chickens are a classic source of *Campylobacter*, all food sources can harbor the bacteria. Pets can also carry *Campylobacter*.

Symptoms include loose watery stools or bloody and mucus-containing stools. Fever, vomiting, malaise, and abdominal pain are common. Seizures may occur. Children severely affected may show signs of dehydration.

Stool samples contain WBCs, RBCs, and small comma-shaped bacteria that have a characteristic corkscrew motion. Diagnosis is via stool culture, as it is more sensitive than stool microscopy. Since the disease is self-limited, treatment with antibiotics is only used for patients with severe disease or at risk for severe disease. Patients with severe disease include individuals with bloody stools, high fever, extraintestinal infection, worsening or relapsing symptoms, symptoms lasting >1 week. Those at risk for severe disease include immunocompromised individuals, older adults, or pregnant persons.

Preferred treatment is with azithromycin. Fluoroquinolones are an alternative option, but rates of resistance to this class of antibiotics are increasing worldwide.

Additional Reading: Clinical manifestations, diagnosis, and treatment of campylobacter infection. In: *UpToDate*. 2022.

6. You are seeing a 2-month-old child for a well-child check and her mother is wondering at what age she can begin to feed her daughter solid food? She has purchased some iron-fortified cereal and would like to begin giving it to her. You inform the mother that the earliest time to begin such feedings is at what age?

A) 2 to 4 months
B) 4 to 6 months
C) 6 to 8 months
D) 8 to 12 months
E) Only after 1 year

The answer is B: The practice of introducing solid foods and liquids other than breast milk or infant formula during the first year of life has varied over time. The American Academy of Pediatrics and the World Health Organization recommend that foods be introduced around 6 months of age. The infant's ability to tolerate food depends on the infant's needs and readiness.

Neurologic development has progressed sufficiently for tongue and mouth movement to handle solids at approximately 4 months in full-term infants. Before 4 months of age, solid feedings are extremely difficult because the infant's extrusion reflex causes the tongue to push solid food out of the mouth. Current guidelines are that allergenic foods, such as eggs, fish, shellfish, tree nuts, wheat, soy, peanuts, and cow milk–based dairy products, should be introduced between 4 and 6 months of age. It is not necessary to wait several days between each new food introduction.

Avoid easily aspirated food such as large pieces of meat, popcorn, and nuts. Whole milk can replace formula or breast milk at 12 months of age and reduced-fat milk can replace whole milk at 2 years of age. Honey should be avoided in children <1 year of age to reduce the risk of infant botulism.

Additional Reading: Introducing highly allergenic foods to infants and children. In: *UpToDate*. 2022.

7. A 3-year-old boy presents to the office with his father, who thinks the child may have swallowed a small button battery. Chest radiograph and abdominal series confirm the presence of an opacity in the lower esophagus, above the lower esophageal ring. Which one of the following actions is the next appropriate step in his management?

A) Administration of ipecac to induce vomiting
B) Observation and observing his stools for passage
C) Obtaining a barium-swallow study
D) Referral for an endoscopy to remove the battery
E) None of the above

The answer is D: Children younger than 4 years are at risk for the ingestion of foreign bodies. Button batteries, such as those used in wristwatches and cameras, pose a significant risk. If a child ingests a battery, chest and abdominal radiographs can help to localize the position of the battery.

If the battery is lodged in the esophagus, endoscopy should be performed to remove the foreign body because a battery lodged in the esophagus can lead to perforation if left for more than 4 hours. If the battery is distal to the lower esophageal ring, no further therapy is needed; however, if the battery is larger than 1.5 cm, a follow-up radiograph should be performed 48 hours later to make sure the battery has passed through the pylorus.

Additional Reading: Button and cylindrical battery ingestion: clinical features, diagnosis, and initial management. In: *UpToDate*. 2022.

8. You are seeing a child with the acute onset of mid-epigastric pain that radiates to the back, which is worsened by eating, nausea, vomiting, and low-grade fever. Serum amylase and lipase are elevated. You suspect pancreatitis. The most common causes of acute pancreatitis in children include all of the following, except which one?

A) Idiopathic pancreatitis
B) Blunt trauma
C) Gallstones
D) Anatomic anomalies of the pancreas
E) Cystic fibrosis

The answer is C: The incidence of pancreatitis is increasing in children and now approaches that seen in adults. The etiologies of acute pancreatitis differ from those seen in adults, with idiopathic and traumatic causes being the most common among children. Structural and multisystemic cause the remainder of cases. While gallstones can occur in children, they are infrequently a cause of acute pancreatitis.

Additional Reading: Clinical manifestations and diagnosis of chronic and acute recurrent pancreatitis in children. In: *UpToDate*. 2022.

9. Rotavirus causes a viral intestinal infection resulting in a diarrheal syndrome. What age group of children is most commonly affected by rotavirus infection?

A) Infants less than 6 months of age
B) Between 6 months and 2 years of age
C) Between 2 and 7 years of age
D) Adolescents

The answer is B: Rotavirus causes a viral intestinal infection commonly seen in children, often during winter to early spring. Outbreaks can easily occur in day care centers. Most children affected are between 6 months and 2 years of age, but a child of any age could be affected. Symptoms include vomiting, followed by profuse, watery nonbloody diarrhea, mild to moderate fevers, mild abdominal cramping, and occasionally respiratory complaints.

Diagnosis is based on clinical evaluation but can be confirmed by viral antigen detection. Stool will have a normal white blood cell count, which favors diagnosis of a viral infection.

Treatment involves administration of an oral rehydration solution for mild cases and intravenous fluid replacement for moderate to severe dehydration. Lactose-containing foods should be avoided if they appear to exacerbate symptoms. Breastfeeding should be continued during rehydration. A diet consisting of banana, rice, cereal, applesauce, and toast (BRAT diet) is no longer recommended; optimal treatment includes resumption of a normal diet as soon as tolerated.

Additional Reading: *Rotavirus Vaccination*. Centers for Disease Control and Prevention. www.cdc.gov/vaccines/vpd/rotavirus/index.html.

10. Hepatitis B immunization is universally recommended to be administered to children in the United States. Regarding hepatitis B vaccination in healthy infants, which one of the following statements is true?

A) Give the first immunization at birth.
B) Injections should be given in the buttocks to increase immunogenicity-
C) Only infants at risk should receive hepatitis B vaccination.
D) Two doses will provide optimal results.
E) None of the above.

The answer is A: Hepatitis B immunization starting at birth is universally recommended in the United States, with catch-up vaccination for children less than 19 years of age. Adults at risk for hepatitis B virus infection are also recommended to receive vaccinations. Three recombinant vaccines (Recombivax HB, Engerix-B, and Heplisav-B) are used in the United States. Depending on the age of the patient, a three-dose or two-dose schedule is required. Hepatitis B should be initiated during the newborn period, a second dose given 1 to 2 months later, and a third dose given by 6 to 18 months of age. Depending upon the formulation used, children aged 11 to 15 years and adults 19 years of age or older may use a two-dose series.

In infants, administer intramuscularly to the anterolateral thigh muscle. In children over 4 years of age and older through adulthood, administer to the deltoid muscle. Injection in the buttocks or intradermal route may compromise immunogenicity. Most school districts now require hepatitis B immunization before admission to kindergarten or first grade. Evaluation of susceptibility and immunity is not done routinely.

Additional Reading: Hepatitis B. Centers for Disease Control and Prevention. www.cdc.gov/vaccines/vpd/hepb/index.html

➔ **A three-dose schedule is required for adequate hepatitis B vaccination. It is initiated during the newborn period or by 2 months of age, with a second dose given 1 to 2 months later and a third dose given by 6 to 18 months of age.**

11. You receive a call from the mother of a 3-year-old boy who reportedly just swallowed a penny. You have them come into the office and he seems his usual self. His abdominal examination is entirely benign, with no tenderness. You send him to get an abdominal radiograph and the radiologist calls to note that it appears that the coin is in his duodenum. You inform his mother that the next step to address this situation is which one of the following measures?

A) Administer a charcoal suspension.
B) Observe the child for any untoward effects.
C) Prescribe a laxative.
D) Prescribe ipecac syrup.
E) Refer for an endoscopy to remove the coin.

The answer is B: Infants and small children who swallow coins often present asymptomatically to the family physician's office or emergency department. The first step in management includes a radiograph of the chest, neck, and abdominal area to help locate the radiopaque coin. If the coin is localized below the diaphragm (as in this case), the child should be observed until the coin has passed.

If the coin is lodged in the esophagus or if the child exhibits symptoms related to the ingested coin, an endoscopy may be necessary to remove the foreign body. In most cases, sharp objects that have not yet entered the small intestine should be retrieved by endoscopy. Follow-up radiographs of the abdomen can help locate and mark the progress of coins in the intestines. Handheld metal detectors can also aid in localization of the coin's position. The use of ipecac, charcoal, or laxatives is not indicated.

Additional Reading: Foreign bodies of the esophagus and gastrointestinal tract in children. In: *UpToDate*. 2022.

12. A father brings his colicky infant son to the office. Which one of the following situations is true about this condition?

A) Colicky infants are usually small for height and weight.
B) Colic negatively influences maternal mental health.
C) Symptoms begin at birth.
D) Symptoms are more severe in the evening.
E) Symptoms last for approximately 1 year, then resolve.

The answer is D: Infant colic is characterized by paroxysms of crying that has a clear beginning and end, a cry that is qualitatively different from normal crying in that it is louder, higher in pitch and more turbulent. The infant may sound as if they are in pain. Facial flushing, distended abdomen, drawing up of the legs, and clenching of the fists can be seen. During the crying episode, the infant is difficult to console. Episodes tend to cluster in the evening. Up to a third of infant's experience colic within the first few months of life. A presumptive diagnosis of colic can be made in an otherwise healthy infant less than 3 months of age who cries for no apparent reason for more than 3 hours per day for more than 3 days/wk.

The onset of colic typically occurs between the second and sixth weeks of life and remits by 3 months of age. Although colic is typically self-limited, it can overwhelm parents if it persists for many weeks.

Additional Reading: Infantile colic: clinical features and diagnosis. In: *UpToDate*. 2022.

13. You are seeing a 6-month-old infant for his well-child check and his mother reports that he is very "spitty" and regurgitates a lot. You suspect that he has gastroesophageal reflux (GER), as he is otherwise growing well. Which one of the following measures is considered the first step to appropriately manage an infant with GER?

A) Begin an H_2 receptor antagonist.
B) Begin a prokinetic agent.
C) Reduce the number of feedings.
D) Begin a proton pump inhibitor.
E) Thicken the feedings.

The answer is E: GER is common among infants and tends to cause parental anxiety and consequent office visits. GER refers to a physiologic process whereby a healthy infant without underlying systemic abnormalities has regurgitation, or "spitting up," resulting from retrograde passive return of gastric contents into the esophagus. GER prevalence peaks between 1 and 4 months of age and usually resolves by 6 to 12 months of age. There is no gender predilection or definite peak age of onset beyond infancy.

Gastroesophageal reflux disease (GERD) is a more severe, pathologic process in infants manifested by poor weight gain, signs of esophagitis, persistent respiratory symptoms, and changes in behavior. GERD that persists beyond the first year of life tends to be more resistant to complete resolution. Risk factors for GERD include a history of esophageal atresia with repair, neurologic impairment and delay, hiatal hernia, bronchopulmonary dysplasia, asthma, and cystic fibrosis.

Children with GER can be managed with dietary modification. Thickening feedings with dry rice cereal reduces visible regurgitation and fussiness. Recently, concerns have been raised regarding the use of rice cereal as a thickening agent due to elevated levels of inorganic arsenic in all forms of rice. Wherever possible, using organic rice cereal without arsenic is recommended. If thickened feedings do not provide symptom relief after 2 weeks, a trial of cow milk elimination from the mother's diet in breastfed infants or use of an extensively hydrolyzed formula can lead to improvement after 2 weeks in infants who have cow milk protein allergy. Ten percent to 15% of children with cow milk protein allergy will also be allergic to soy.

Medications are generally not indicated for management of uncomplicated GER in infants.

Additional Reading:
1. Pediatric gastroesophageal reflux clinical practice guidelines: joint recommendations of the North American Society for Pediatric Gastroenterology, Hepatology, and Nutrition and the European Society fof Pediatric Gastroenterology, Hepatology, and Nutrition. *JPGN*. 2018;66:516-554.
2. Pharmacologic therapy for gastroesophageal reflux disease in children. *Am Fam Physician*. 2015;92(5):351-352.

14. You have diagnosed a 1-week-old neonate with breast milk jaundice. In addition to monitoring bilirubin levels, which one of the following would be the best advice to give to this infant's mother?

A) Cease breastfeeding and switch to formula feeding.
B) Cease breastfeeding and start phototherapy.
C) Continue breastfeeding and start phototherapy.
D) Initiate breast pumping and start formula feeding.
E) Schedule an exchange transfusion.

The answer is D: Breast milk jaundice is nonpathologic, peaks between days 6 and 14 of life, and occurs in up to one-third of healthy breastfed infants. Total serum bilirubin levels vary from 12 to 20 mg/dL (340 μmol/L). Although the cause is not well understood, it is believed that substances in maternal milk, including β-glucuronidases and nonesterified fatty acids, may inhibit normal bilirubin metabolism. Bilirubin level usually decreases continually after the infant is 2 weeks old but may remain elevated for 1 to 3 months.

If total serum bilirubin level becomes markedly elevated, temporarily discontinuing breastfeeding for the infant is necessary, but the mother should be advised to continue expressing breast milk to maintain production. If formula substitution is implemented, the total serum bilirubin level will decline rapidly over the following 48 hours (at a rate of 3 mg/dL [51 μmol/L]/d), which confirms the diagnosis. Breastfeeding may then be resumed.

Additional Reading:
1. Strategies for breastfeeding success. *Am Fam Physician*. 2008;78(2):225-232.
2. Primary interventions to support breastfeeding. *Am Fam Physician*. 2017;95(8):517-518.

15. You are evaluating an infant in the newborn nursery, who has passed a thickened meconium, and you are concerned that he has meconium ileus. Which one of the following conditions is associated with meconium ileus?

A) Cystic fibrosis
B) Duodenal atresia
C) Hirschsprung disease
D) Malrotation
E) Pyloric stenosis

The answer is A: Meconium ileus is almost always an early sign of cystic fibrosis, in which the infant passes a thickened meconium. In contrast, the meconium plug appears rubbery in meconium plug syndrome. In meconium ileus, the meconium adheres to the bowel mucosa and ultimately causes obstruction at the level of the terminal ileum. Distal to the obstruction, the colon is narrow in diameter and contains dry meconium pellets. The relatively empty colon of small caliber is considered a microcolon. Loops of distended small bowel can sometimes be palpated through the abdominal wall.

Additional Reading: Cystic fibrosis: overview of gastrointestinal disease. In: *UpToDate*. 2022.

16. When are symptoms of pyloric stenosis usually first noticeable?

A) After the first few feedings.
B) Within the first week of life.
C) 4 to 6 weeks after birth.
D) 3 to 4 months of age.
E) Pyloric stenosis is typically asymptomatic.

The answer is C: Pyloric stenosis can cause near-complete gastric outlet obstruction and is seen in male children more often than female children (4:1). Hypertrophy is rare at birth but develops over the initial 4 to 6 weeks of life, when signs of upper intestinal obstruction first appear. The infant presents with forceful projectile nonbilious vomiting of feedings beginning late in the first month of life. Delayed diagnosis may lead to repeated vomiting, dehydration, failure to gain weight, and hypochloremic metabolic alkalosis from continued loss of hydrochloric acid.

Abdominal examination may reveal a discrete, 2- to 3-cm, firm, movable pyloric "olivelike mass" deep in the right side of the epigastrium. Diagnosis is confirmed with identification of the hypertrophied pyloric muscle by abdominal ultrasonography. If diagnosis is uncertain, a barium swallow can be obtained, which will show delayed gastric emptying and the typical "string sign" of a markedly narrowed, elongated pyloric lumen.

Treatment is a longitudinal pyloromyotomy, which leaves the mucosa intact and separates the incised muscle fibers. Postoperatively, the infant usually tolerates feedings within a few days.

Additional Reading: Infantile colic: recognition and treatment. *Am Fam Physician*. 2015;92(7):577-582.

Infant presenting with forceful projectile non-bilious vomiting of feedings late in the first month of life should be evaluated for pyloric stenosis.

17. You are seeing a 7-year-old boy who has been picking at his bottom and his cellophane tape test is positive for pinworms (*Enterobius vermicularis*). You prescribe which one of the following treatments?

A) Mebendazole (Vermox)
B) Metronidazole (Flagyl)
C) Oral vancomycin
D) Permethrin (Elimite)
E) Tetracycline

The answer is A: Pinworm infection is a common pediatric infection caused by the parasite *E vermicularis*. The parasite is a small (1 cm) white worm that lives in the bowel (usually the cecum) and gravid females migrate to the perianal area at night to deposit eggs on the perianal skin, giving rise to severe and intense pruritus. Transmission is per fecal-oral route. Children aged 5 to 10 years are predominantly affected. Young children may report difficulty sleeping. On examination, anal and vulvar inflammation may be evident.

Diagnosis is confirmed with visualization of the worms or by pressing cellophane tape on both sides of the perianal during the night or at the time of waking so that the tape can be evaluated with microscopy the next morning ("Scotch tape test").

Treatment involves two separate doses of mebendazole (Vermox), 2 weeks apart. Albendazole or pyrantel pamoate (over the counter) may be substituted for mebendazole. Bed lines and underclothing should be handled carefully and laundered.

Additional Reading: CDC Enterobiasis.

18. You have diagnosed colic in a 3-month-old infant and the parents are asking about strategies to deal with her colicky periods. Which one of the following would be the most appropriate management of an infant with a colicky episode?

A) Feed the infant sugar water from a bottle.
B) Swaddle the infant.
C) Increase the room temperature.
D) Leave the infant to self-soothe.
E) Place a cold washcloth over the infant's face.

The answer is B: Infant colic is characterized by paroxysms of crying; apparent abdominal pain; and irritability, hypertonicity, and wakefulness that occurs predominately in the evening. Onset of colic typically occurs between the second and sixth weeks of life and remits by 3 months of age. Continued episodes of crying may place significant stress to the family and parents. It is important to reassure parents that the infant's irritability is not because of poor parenting. Treatment of colic involves trying soothing techniques, which can include using a pacifier, taking the infant for a ride in the car or a stroller, rocking, placing the infant in a sling carrier, giving the infant a warm bath, or massaging the infant's abdomen. White noise machines help some infants. *Hip healthy swaddling*, with room for hip and knee flexion and movement of the l can help. If there is suspicion for milk intolerance, a trial feeding with an extensively hydrolyzed formula or avoidance of all dairy in the mother's diet if breastfeeding formula can be tried for 2 weeks to see if there is improvement in the symptoms.

Additional Reading: Colic: management and outcome. In: *UpToDate*. 2022.

19. Which one of the following conditions is the most common malignancy diagnosed in childhood?

A) Acute lymphoblastic leukemia (ALL)
B) Melanoma
C) Osteosarcoma
D) Retinoblastoma
E) Wilms tumor

The answer is A: Leukemia is the most common malignancy diagnosed in childhood, and ALL is the most common type of leukemia in children, accounting for 80% of cases of leukemia. The incidence of ALL is approximately 30 cases per million persons. It is more common in White individuals than with Black individuals, with Hispanic people having the highest risk. Persons with trisomy 21 are at 15 times the risk of developing ALL compared to the general population.

Diagnosis of ALL can be challenging and is often delayed because early symptoms are nonspecific and may resemble viral infections. Children present with generalized malaise, loss of appetite, and low-grade fever. Additional symptoms include pallor, petechiae or ecchymoses, bone pain, and significant weight loss. Examination may only reveal significant lymphadenopathy or hepatosplenomegaly, the latter of which is always an abnormal finding.

For a child with suspicious findings, a complete blood count with a differential smear should be obtained. The presence of blast cells on the peripheral smear is diagnostic of leukemia. Many patients with leukemia only have blast cells in the bone marrow. If there is anemia with reticulocytopenia, or a high mean corpuscular volume, thrombocytopenia, leukopenia, or leukocytosis, a further workup to confirm leukemia is indicated. Diagnoses that can commonly be confused with leukemia include viral suppression, drug-induced cytopenia, immune thrombocytopenic purpura, aplastic anemia, and juvenile idiopathic rheumatoid arthritis, among others.

Additional Readings:
1. Signs and symptoms of childhood cancer: a guide for early recognition. *Am Fam Physician*. 2013;88(3):185-474.
2. Leukemia: an overview for primary care. *Am Fam Physician*. 2014;89(9):731-738.

Section V. Musculoskeletal System

Each of the following questions or incomplete statements is followed by suggested answers or completions. Select the ONE BEST ANSWER in each case.

1. An 11-year-old obese boy presents to your office with persistent bilateral leg pain that occurs only at night. He does not report any pain during the day and his gait is normal. The most likely diagnosis to explain his pain is which one of the following conditions?

A) Benign nocturnal limb pains of childhood
B) Legg-Calvé-Perthes disease
C) Osgood-Schlatter disease
D) Patellofemoral pain syndrome
E) Slipped capital femoral epiphysis

The answer is A: There are several different pathologic concerns for a young male with leg pain, which are important to capture. A diagnosis of benign nocturnal limb pains of childhood (formerly known as "growing pains") requires three criteria: (1) leg pain is bilateral; (2) pain occurs only at night; and (3) there is no limp, pain, or other symptoms during the day. This is a benign, self-limited process that does not require treatment.

Legg-Calvé-Perthes disease presents with limp and hip, knee or thigh pain, and possible joint stiffness.

Osgood-Schlatter disease (tibial apophysitis) presents with pain over the tibial tuberosity, antalgic (pain-avoiding) or straight-legged gait, and aggravation of pain with activity or kneeling.

Patellofemoral pain syndrome presents with anteromedial knee pain that worsens with squatting and other physical activity.

Slipped capital femoral epiphysis would also be considered in an obese child of this age; however, it would present with unilateral hip or knee pain, joint tenderness, and limp.

Additional Reading: Chronic musculoskeletal pain in children: part I. Initial evaluation. *Am Fam Physician*. 2006;74(1):115-122.

A diagnosis of benign nocturnal limb pains of childhood (formerly known as "growing pains") requires three criteria: (1) leg pain is bilateral; (2) pain occurs only at night; and (3) there is no limp, pain, or other symptoms during the day.

2. A 13-year-old boy is brought into your office by his concerned parents. He has had recurring episodes of joint swelling, fever, and rash. On physical examination, there is hepatosplenomegaly and lymphadenopathy. Laboratory evaluation shows anemia, leukocytosis, and thrombocytosis. You suspect juvenile idiopathic arthritis (JIA) and decide to start treatment. Which one of the following medications would be considered as the initial choice for treatment?

A) Acetaminophen
B) Codeine
C) Ibuprofen
D) Methotrexate
E) Prednisone

The answer is C: JIA, formerly known as juvenile rheumatoid arthritis, comprises a diverse group of diseases that is clinically distinct from adult rheumatoid arthritis. Most children with JIA have long remissions without loss of function or significant residual deformity. For a diagnosis of JIA, a patient requires signs of joint inflammation persisting for greater than 6 weeks with the onset before 16 years of age. Although there is no specific laboratory test to aid in diagnosis, an elevated erythrocyte sedimentation rate may suggest polyarticular and systemic types of JIA, and antinuclear antibody may identify patients at an increased risk for uveitis.

Further, it is important to exclude other causes of arthritis, such as reactive arthritis from extra-articular infection, septic arthritis, neoplastic disorders, endocrine disorders (eg, thyroid disease and type 1 diabetes mellitus), degenerative or mechanical disorders, or idiopathic pediatric joint pain.

There are three major subtypes of JIA, with varying clinical presentations and treatment options:

1. Pauciarticular JIA (40%-50%) involves four or fewer large joints in an asymmetrical pattern. Early-onset pauciarticular JIA affects mostly girls younger than 4 years and has a risk of chronic iridocyclitis (30%) and ocular damage (10%). Late-onset pauciarticular JIA affects mostly boys older than 8 years and has later development of spondyloarthropathy and iridocyclitis (10%). Slit-lamp ophthalmic examinations are recommended.
2. Polyarticular JIA (25%-40%) is defined as arthritis in five or more joints and can be positive or negative for rheumatoid factor (RF). Girls 8 years or older are typically RF-positive and have symmetric small-joint arthritis with a worse prognosis compared with those with RF-negative type.
3. Systemic-onset JIA (10%-20%), formerly called Still disease, is characterized by high intermittent fevers (>102 °F), salmon-colored macular rash, hepatosplenomegaly, lymphadenopathy, arthralgias, pericarditis, pleuritis, and growth delay. Laboratory test results may reveal anemia, leukocytosis, and thrombocytosis. Extra-articular symptoms are usually mild and self-limited.

The first line of treatment for mild JIA is to use nonsteroid anti-inflammatory drugs (NSAIDs), such as ibuprofen, and if no response is seen within 4 to 6 weeks, a different NSAID should be tried. If NSAIDs inadequately control symptoms, methotrexate or sulfasalazine is added therapy. Steroids (glucocorticoids) can also be given as intra-articular injections (1-2 joints) or orally (polyarticular, systemic JIA).

Children with JIA often require a great deal of physical and psychological support, in addition to physical and occupational therapy to maintain functionality when children avoid using painful joints.

Additional Reading: Arthritis, juvenile idiopathic. In: Domino F, ed. *The 5-Minute Clinical Consult*. Wolters Kluwer; 2022.

3. A 14-year-old boy presents to your office with his mother. She notes that he has been complaining of pain in his lower left leg for the past few days. You obtain a plain radiograph of the area, and it shows an aneurysmal bone cyst associated with the metaphysis and periosteal elevation of the mid-tibia. The most appropriate management at this time includes which one of the following steps?

A) Apply a leg cast for 6 to 8 weeks.
B) Obtain a technetium bone scan.
C) Prescribe a nonsteroidal anti-inflammatory drug medication along with reassurance.
D) Refer to endocrinology for a growth hormone assessment.
E) Refer to an orthopedic surgeon for possible removal.

The answer is E: Unicameral bone cysts (simple bone cysts) usually affect the metaphysis of long bones in pediatric patients (predominantly femur, humerus). Most are asymptomatic, unless a fracture occurs in the area of the bone cyst. Small cysts tend to heal without difficulty, but larger cysts may require surgery to remove the cyst, with a bone grafting repair. Most patients recover without permanent disability.

An aneurysmal bone cyst can progressively increase in size and expand beyond the metaphyseal cartilage of the long bones. Patients may report pain and swelling in the region of the cyst. Radiographs may show well-circumscribed areas of rarefaction with periosteal elevation, and surgery is required to remove the cyst. Radiation therapy may be used for vertebral lesions that threaten the spinal cord if surgery is contraindicated. Postradiation sarcomas may arise.

Prognosis for both unicameral and aneurysmal bone cysts is excellent after treatment.

Additional Reading: Benign tumors and tumor-like processes of bone. *Nelson Textbook of Pediatrics*. 20th ed. Elsevier/Saunders; 2014.

4. An obese 11-year-old boy presents to your office complaining of gradually increasing hip pain that radiates to his thigh and knee. On examination, pain is elicited with hip abduction and adduction. Radiographs show evidence of acetabular dysplasia. Which one of the following is the most likely diagnosis?

A) Congenital dislocation of the hip
B) Osgood-Schlatter disease
C) Slipped capital femoral epiphysis
D) Sacral insufficiency fracture
E) Transient synovitis of the hip

The answer is C: Slipped capital femoral epiphysis is usually seen in overweight boys between 11 and 14 years of age. The condition occurs when the femoral head slips posteriorly and inferiorly, exposing the anterior and superior aspects of the metaphysis of the femoral neck. If the condition occurs before puberty, an underlying endocrine disorder (hypothyroidism, growth hormone deficiency) should be considered.

Patients typically present with pain and limp with gradual onset, usually involving the hips and possibly referred pain to the thigh or knee. The condition is bilateral in 20% of cases. Frog-leg view radiographs should be obtained and will verify the diagnosis by noting abnormalities and acetabular dysplasia of the femoral head.

A referral to orthopedics is required for surgical treatment using pins to correct the abnormality. If left untreated, complications such as avascular necrosis of the hip and erosion of cartilage may occur.

Additional Reading: Evaluation and management of slipped capital femoral epiphysis (SCFE). In: *UpToDate*. 2022.

5. A 7-year-old boy presents to the office with his father, who reported a worsening limp and progressive left thigh and knee pain for the past 8 days. The patient and his father deny any recent trauma. The boy has previously known delayed bone age. Which of the following is suspected?

A) Legg-Calvé-Perthes disease
B) Morton neuroma
C) Osgood-Schlatter disease
D) Slipped capital femoral epiphysis
E) Transient synovitis of the hip

The answer is A: Children who present with knee pain should be evaluated for an underlying hip pathology. Idiopathic aseptic necrosis of the femoral head can lead to the hip disorder, Legg-Calvé-Perthes disease (LCPD). The disease is often unilateral and found in boys 2 to 12 years of age. Symptoms include hip, groin, and thigh pain, with gradually progressive ambulation difficulty.

Examination findings include an abnormal gait with a painless limp and thigh muscle atrophy. In suspect LCPD, obtain lateral radiographs with frog-leg views. Early in disease, radiographs might be normal, but bone scan will show decreased uptake within the femoral head. Later in disease, radiographs will show a fragmented femoral head with areas of lucency, which may progress to sclerosis and further joint destruction.

Treatment typically involves expectant clinical and radiographic observation; however, severe cases may require abduction casts to contain the femoral head within the acetabulum and surgery.

Additional Reading: Approach to hip pain in childhood. In: *UpToDate*. 2022.

6. In a 5-year-old boy with a limp, which of the following is the most likely cause?

A) Legg-Calvé-Perthes disease
B) Septic joint
C) Slipped capital femoral epiphysis
D) Stress fracture
E) Transient synovitis of the hip

The answer is E: Transient synovitis of the hip is the most common cause of hip pain and limp among children 3 to 8 years of age in the United States and predominately affects boys. The condition usually follows an upper respiratory illness. Despite the frequency of the condition its etiology remains unknown. Physical examination of the affected hip demonstrates limited range of motion, often most severely affecting internal rotation. The hip is usually seen flexed, abducted, and externally rotated.

Complete blood count and erythrocyte sedimentation rate are usually normal. If septic arthritis is suspected, aspiration of the hip may be necessary.

Treatment involves rest and anti-inflammatory drugs. Symptoms usually resolve in 7 to 10 days.

Additional Reading: Approach to hip pain in children. In: *UpToDate*. 2022.

7. You are seeing an obese adolescent boy with his mother and are discussing his recent diagnosis of slipped capital femoral epiphysis (SCFE). You inform them that the most concerning complication of this condition is which one of the following?

A) Avascular necrosis of the hip
B) Intoeing
C) Leg-length discrepancy
D) Osteochondritis dissecans
E) Transient synovitis of the hip

The answer is A: SCFE typically occurs during the adolescent growth spurt and is most frequent in obese children. One or both hips can be affected. Most cases of SCFE are stable and have a good prognosis if diagnosed early.

However, unstable SCFE is associated with a worse prognosis because of the high risk of avascular necrosis. Early radiographic clues include the metaphyseal blanch sign and line of Klein. Treatment is surgical pinning of the displaced femoral head.

Additional Reading: Approach to hip pain in children. In: *UpToDate*. 2022.

8. All of the following statements regarding metatarsus adductus are true, except which one?

A) Boys are more commonly affected than girls.
B) Intoeing is commonly seen with metatarsus adductus.
C) Metatarsus adductus is the most common congenital foot deformity in children.
D) Surgery is rarely needed.
E) Stretching exercises can be effective.

The answer is A: Metatarsus adductus is the most common congenital foot deformity seen in children. Girls are more often affected, and the left side tends to be affected in comparison to the right side. The most likely cause is positioning while in utero.

Examination reveals adduction of the forefoot with a convex lateral border, so that the child appears to have intoeing. The ankle has normal motion. The foot should be assessed for flexibility by holding the heel in neutral position and abducting the forefoot to at least a neutral position. If this cannot be done, then the deformity is rigid (ie, metatarsus varus).

The majority of cases of metatarsus adductus noted at birth resolve without treatment by 1 year of age. Flexible metatarsus adductus is managed by stretching exercises during the first 8 months of life. Parents are instructed to hold the infant's hindfoot in one hand, the forefoot in the other, and stretch the midfoot, opening the "C"-shaped curve and slightly overcorrecting it. Flexible deformities that persist beyond 8 months, and rigid deformities, may need a cast application. Treatment is most effective if started before 8 months of age. If casts are used, they should be changed biweekly and should correct the deformity after three or four casts. Residual adductus causes no long-term disability. Surgery is not typically recommended due to complication risk.

Additional Readings:

1. Managing intoeing in children. *Am Fam Physician*. 2011;84(8):937-944.
2. Lower extremity abnormalities in children. *Am Fam Physician*. 2017;96(4):226-233.

9. Which one of the following statements about osteoid osteoma is true?

A) It is a malignant tumor of long bones.
B) It is more common in girls.
C) It usually presents as a pathologic fracture.
D) Radiographs show radiolucent areas surrounded by sclerosis.
E) Treatment involves systemic chemotherapy.

The answer is D: Osteoid osteoma is a benign tumor that usually involves the long bones of pediatric and adolescent patients. They are found more commonly in boys. Most cases present with bone pain, not fracture. Radiographs show a characteristic radiolucent area surrounded by sclerosis, usually associated with the ends of the tibia or femur. Technetium bone scans are helpful in determining the extent of bone involvement. Treatment for severe refractory cases involves curative surgical resection. Anti-inflammatory drugs are often helpful for mild cases and can relieve the pain.

Additional Reading: Nonmalignant bone lesions in children and adolescents. In: *UpToDate*. 2022.

10. A 12-year-old boy, who recently underwent a growth spurt, presents with his mother because he has been complaining of pain just below his right kneecap for the past week. He denies trauma to the area. On examination, he is tender to palpation over his right tibial tubercle. What is the most likely diagnosis?

A) Legg-Calvé-Perthes disease
B) Osgood-Schlatter disease
C) Osteosarcoma
D) Shin splints
E) Stress fracture

The answer is B: Osgood-Schlatter disease (tibial tubercle apophysitis) is caused by inflammation of the tibial tubercle that usually occurs at the time of a child's growth spurt. It is aggravated by strenuous physical activity such as climbing or running. Boys are more likely to be affected than girls. The condition is usually unilateral, and most patients are between 10 and 15 years of age. Symptoms include pain, swelling, and tenderness over the tibial tubercle. The inflammation results from repeated traction of the inferior patellar tendon on the developing epiphyseal insertion.

Diagnosis is clinical, but radiographs of the knee would show bone fragments at the site of the tibial tubercle. Treatment is rest, refraining from deep knee bending, ice therapy, and anti-inflammatory drugs. If severe, more aggressive therapy, including casting, cortisone injections, and surgery, to remove loose bodies may be necessary.

Additional Reading: Osgood-Schlatter disease (tibial apophysitis). In: Domino F, ed. *The 5-Minute Clinical Consult*. Wolters Kluwer; 2022.

➔ Osgood-Schlatter disease is caused by inflammation of the tibial tubercle that usually occurs at the time of a child's growth spurt.

11. A 3-year-old boy is seen in your office because his parents are concerned about the way he walks. While observing his gait, you notice that the child has toeing in while walking, and on closer examination, you notice that the child exhibits femoral anteversion. The most appropriate treatment at this time is which one of the following?

A) Offer reassurance to the parents.
B) Prescribe a brace to correct internal rotation of the femurs.
C) Refer to an orthopedist for surgery.
D) Refer to a physical therapist for positional stretching.
E) Refer to a podiatrist for corrective shoes.

The answer is A: Femoral anteversion is a common orthopedic finding among young children. The condition results when femoral anteversion leads to excessive internal rotation of the femur. As a result, the child may exhibit "kissing knees," toeing in, and the appearance of incoordination of the lower extremities. Maximal femoral anteversion occurs between 3 and 6 years of age.

Femoral anteversion usually resolves on its own as the child grows, and most cases resolve by age 11 years. Significant abnormalities that persist beyond 8 years of age should be referred to an orthopedist. Severe cases may require osteotomy for rotational correction.

Additional Reading: Approach to the child with intoeing. In: *UpToDate*. 2022.

12. You are performing a well-child check on a 12-year-old student, and his mother is concerned that he has scoliosis because screening performed by the school nurse was thought to indicate the presence of an abnormal spine curvature. You examine his back and inform his mother that which one of the following statements regarding scoliosis is true?

A) A curve greater than 10° may require surgery.
B) Mild cases of scoliosis are treated with bracing.
C) Syringomyelia is often associated with scoliosis.
D) The most common form of scoliosis is congenital.
E) The best way to screen for scoliosis is to perform Adams forward bend test.

The answer is E: Scoliosis is defined as the presence of a lateral spinal curvature of 11° or more. Its prevalence during adolescence is estimated to be between 2% and 3%. Curvatures of more than 100° can contribute to restrictive pulmonary disease; however, deviations of this magnitude are extremely rare.

Scoliosis is classified as idiopathic (80% of cases), congenital (5%), neuromuscular (10%), or miscellaneous (5%). Severe scoliosis is more common in female patients. Idiopathic scoliosis is an inherited autosomal dominant condition that occurs with variable penetrance. Most patients are asymptomatic; however, some may complain of a backache.

The child should be examined with his or her back facing the examiner. The Adams forward bending test is recommended to screen for scoliosis. In performing the test, the patient is asked to flex forward from the waist until the back is horizontal, with feet together and arms hanging and knees in extension. In this position, scapula height is observed. If scoliosis is present, there is asymmetry in scapular height. In most cases, the right shoulder is higher than the left because of a convex curve of the spine to the right in the thoracic area and to the left in the lumbar area. Hip height and symmetry may also be affected.

Consider radiographs when a patient has a curve that might require treatment or could progress to a stage requiring treatment, usually 40° to 100°. Radiographs should include posteroanterior and lateral standing views of the spine. It is recommended that magnetic resonance imaging be obtained in a patient who presents with scoliosis before 8 years of age; rapid curve progression of more than 1° per month; an unusual curve pattern such as left thoracic curve; a neurologic deficit; or significant pain.

Treatment depends on the degree of curvature. The primary goal of treating adolescent idiopathic scoliosis is to minimize progression of the curve. Curves less than 10° to 15° require no active treatment and can be monitored, unless the patient's bones are immature, and progression is likely. Moderate curves between 25° and 45° in patients lacking skeletal maturity have been treated with bracing, but this has never been proven to prevent curve progression and compliance is usually poor. Significant curves (20°-50°) may benefit from bracing, and in severe cases, Milwaukee bracing and/or surgery may be beneficial.

Painful scoliosis may indicate underlying neurologic problems, such as syringomyelia or spinal cord lesion, and is less likely to be idiopathic.

Additional Readings:

1. Adolescent idiopathic scoliosis: diagnosis and management. *Am Fam Physician*. 2014;89(3):193-196.
2. Adolescent idiopathic scoliosis: common questions and answers. *Am Fam Physician*. 2020;101(1):19-23.

13. A young patient is thinking about pregnancy and has questions about Duchenne muscular dystrophy (DMD), as she was told that a family member had suffered from this disease. You inform her that all of the following statements about DMD are true, except which one?

A) Boys are affected more often than girls.
B) Cardiomyopathy can occur.
C) Creatine kinase levels are not affected.
D) Intellectual disability is frequently an associated finding.
E) Proximal muscles are affected before the distal muscles.

The answer is C: DMD is a genetic disorder, often X-linked recessive, affecting the Xp21 locus that interferes with dystrophin production. Dystrophin is found within muscle cell membranes. DMD occurs in 1 in 3600 live male births and often affects boys between 2 and 5 years of age. Becker muscular dystrophy is the same fundamental disease with a genetic defect at the same locus but a milder clinical course. Most patients have no family history of the disorder.

Early manifestations include rapid fatigue on ambulation or running, clumsiness, waddling gait, and a distinctive pattern of climbing up on the legs from a sitting to standing, known as Gowers sign. The proximal muscles are affected before the distal muscles and pseudohypertrophy of the gastrocnemius (seen in 90% of patients), triceps, and vastus lateralis may occur.

Intellectual impairment is seen in all patients, and in advanced cases, cardiomyopathy may also occur. Diagnosis is confirmed by muscle biopsy, which shows degeneration of muscle fibers and proliferation of connective tissue. Electromyographic studies can distinguish between neuropathic and myopathic processes. Laboratory tests show elevated creatine kinase levels.

Mutation analysis of DNA isolated from peripheral blood leukocytes can facilitate identification of defects of the dystrophin gene. Deletions and duplications are present in approximately 65% of patients, and point mutations are present in approximately 25% of patients.

Treatment involves using braces and physical therapy. Prognosis is poor, and most patients die before the second decade because of pneumonia.

Additional Reading: Recognition and management of motor delay and muscle weakness in children. *Am Fam Physician*. 2015;91(1):38-44.

14. A 16-year-old female high school athlete who plays volleyball on the school team presents with complaints of pain in her right lower leg. The pain is dull and achy, and she cannot recall any specific injury, but the pain has slowly worsened over the past couple of months. The pain has recently become more bothersome, particularly at night. What is the most likely diagnosis?

A) Osgood-Schlatter disease
B) Osteosarcoma
C) Shin splints
D) Stress fracture

The answer is B: Patients with osteosarcoma typically present with a progressively worsening dull, aching pain that has persisted for several months and suddenly grew more severe. The increase in pain severity may be related to tumor penetration of cortical bone and periosteal irritation or pathologic fracture. Night pain is common and may awaken the patient from sleep. Patients frequently have a history of a minor injury, sprain, or muscle pull incurred while participating in a sport.

Physical examination may reveal localized tenderness, restricted range of motion of the adjacent joint, limp, or muscle atrophy. Presence of mass, swelling, or deformity may further suggest diagnosis. As children frequently have referred pain, comprehensive examination of the joint above and below the area of complaint and spinal and reflex examinations should be done.

Growing pains are typically bilateral. Shin splints present with pain along the medial tibia caused by repeated trauma and often seen in athletes who run or jump. Osgood-Schlatter disease presents with pain in the front lower part of the knee and presents with intense knee pain during physical activity. Stress fractures result from repetitive trauma with athletics and present with pain with weight-bearing activity.

Additional Reading: Osteosarcoma, pediatric. In: Domino F, ed. *The 5-Minute Clinical Consult*. Wolters Kluwer; 2022.

15. A 16-year-old female dancer presents with pain, swelling, and a sensation that her knee is "giving away." Walking up and down the stairs exacerbates the pain. Physical examination reveals an increased Q angle. What is the most likely diagnosis?

A) Anterior cruciate ligament rupture
B) Iliotibial band syndrome
C) Osgood-Schlatter disease
D) Patellofemoral syndrome
E) Tibial plateau fracture

The answer is D: Patellofemoral syndrome is a common overuse injury associated with the anterior knee and commonly affects young women. In most cases, the syndrome is associated with poor conditioning and the initiation of a new activity, particularly running. Patellofemoral syndrome can also result from other activities including dancing, gymnastics, and figure skating.

Symptoms include pain, swelling, and a "give away" sensation associated with the knee. Ascending or descending slopes or stairs, and repeated squatting or weight bearing on a semiflexed knee, aggravate symptoms. Weakness of the quadriceps muscles, particularly the vastus medialis, contributes to the symptoms.

Patellofemoral syndrome is associated with an increased Q angle (the angle formed from a line down the femur and a line formed by the patellar tendon) and a high-riding patella (patella alta). Sunrise view radiographs of the knees may show patellofemoral malalignment, but imaging is not necessary for diagnosis.

Treatment involves rest, ice, nonsteroidal anti-inflammatory agents, and quadriceps-strengthening exercises. Knee braces have shown no significant benefit toward symptom relief.

Additional Reading: Patellofemoral pain syndrome. *Am Fam Physician*. 2019;99(2):88-94.

16. A 4-year-old boy who recently immigrated to the United States is being evaluated for a septic joint. It is unclear about his prior immunization status. In this situation, the child is most likely infected with which one of the following organisms?

A) *H influenzae*
B) *Mycoplasma pneumoniae*
C) *Neisseria gonorrhea*
D) *P multocida*
E) *S pneumoniae*

The answer is A: Bacterial infections are the most common cause of septic joints. In children between 2 and 5 years of age, osteomyelitis is most likely caused by *S aureus*. Other etiologic agents include *Streptococcus* and gram-negative bacteria. In sexually active teenagers and young adults, *N gonorrhea* is most common. *Staphylococcus*, group A *Streptococcus*, and *S pneumoniae*, viruses, mycobacteria, and fungi are also possible causes.

Before universal vaccination, *H influenzae* type B was the most common etiology and still affects many unimmunized immigrants. *Salmonella* and *S aureus* often cause osteomyelitis in children with sickle cell anemia. Patients with rheumatoid arthritis are at increased risk for septic joints.

In children, the hip and knee are the most commonly affected joints, in contrast to adults who are mostly affected in the knees. A child with a septic joint will have pain with any joint motion, whereas a patient with trauma or toxic synovitis will tolerate some motion of the joint.

Laboratory tests show an elevated white blood cell count and elevated erythrocyte sedimentation rate. Joint fluid should be aspirated and sent for culture and Gram stain. Blood cultures are positive in 30% to 40%.

Treatment, in addition to antibiotic therapy, involves surgical debridement as soon as possible if a bacterial source is suspected.

Additional Reading: Bacterial arthritis: clinical features and diagnosis in infants and children. In: *UpToDate*. 2022.

17. Which of the following sounds is associated with a positive Ortolani sign during the assessment for developmental dysplasia of the hip (DDH)?

A) "Click"
B) "Clunk"
C) "Grinding"
D) "Pop"
E) "Snap"

The answer is B: Although no single physical examination finding is pathognomonic for DDH, a "clunk" indicates a positive Ortolani sign. The neonate should have a reference range of motion of abduction to 75° and adduction to 30°. A physical assessment should include evaluation for asymmetry as well as assessing Ortolani and Barlow signs.

The Ortolani maneuver is performed with the infant supine and the hip and knees flexed to 90° with the physician's index and middle finger along the greater trochanter and the thumb along the inner thigh. The hip is gently abducted to about 45° as gentle pressure is applied to the posterior thigh. A "clunk" (not a high-pitched click) indicates a positive Ortolani sign and occurs as the dislocated femoral head is reduced into the acetabulum.

The Barlow test is the reverse of the Ortolani: the abducted hip is gently adducted, and the femoral head can be felt slipping out of the acetabulum as the knees are brought back together.

With the infant prone, the physician should check for limb-length discrepancy or asymmetric gluteal or thigh folds. In an older infant (about 3 months of age), limited abduction of the hip is a reliable sign of DDH. In infants up to 3 to 4 months of age, a hip ultrasound is the preferred imaging study to diagnosis DDH; after 4 to 6 months a radiograph is indicated.

Physical examination screening for DDH should occur at 2 to 4 days and at each well-child visit (1, 2, 4, 6, 9, and 12 months) until the child is a year old or is reliably able to walk. Treatment involves the use of Pavlik harness, spica cast, and possible surgical reduction.

Additional Reading: Screening for developmental dysplasia of the hip in newborns. *Am Fam Physician*. 2013;87(1):10-11.

Section VI. Respiratory System

Each of the following questions or incomplete statements is followed by suggested answers or completions. Select the ONE BEST ANSWER in each case.

1. In a 7-year-old girl with acute sinusitis, which of the following sinuses is least likely to be infected?

A) Ethmoidal
B) Frontal
C) Maxillary
D) Sphenoidal

The answer is B: Acute bacterial sinusitis refers to infection of the sinuses that lasts for fewer than 30 days and completely resolves. The maxillary and ethmoidal sinuses most commonly involved when mucociliary function and drainage are impaired by an upper respiratory infection or allergic rhinitis. Both the ethmoid and maxillary sinuses are present at birth, having formed in the third to fourth gestational month. The sphenoid sinuses pneumatize as an extension of a posterior ethmoid cell by age 5 years. The frontal sinuses form from an anterior ethmoid cell and appear at around 7 to 8 years. Owing to the chain of sinus development, frontal sinusitis is unusual before age 10 years.

Additional Reading: AAP releases guideline on diagnosis and management of acute bacterial sinusitis in children one to 18 years of age. *Am Fam Physician*. 2014;89(8):676-681.

2. A 17-year-old who has had a sore throat for several days now presents with some trouble swallowing. You suspect that he has a peritonsillar abscess. Which one of the following would be the best test to confirm your diagnosis?

A) Obtain a lateral neck plain film.
B) Obtain an ultrasonography of the area.
C) Obtain a neck computed tomographic (CT) scan.
D) Obtain a neck magnetic resonance imaging evaluation.
E) Perform a needle aspiration.

The answer is E: Peritonsillar abscess is most commonly seen in individuals from 20 to 40 years of age in men and women equally. Although young children are rarely affected unless immunocompromised, the resulting infection can cause significant airway obstruction. Chronic tonsillitis or acute tonsillitis requiring multiple trials of oral antibiotics may predispose the development of a peritonsillar abscess. Presenting symptoms include fever, throat pain, and trismus (reduced opening of the jaws caused by spasm of the muscles of mastication).

Although ultrasonography and CT scanning are useful to confirm a diagnosis, a needle aspiration remains the gold standard. After performing aspiration, appropriate antibiotic therapy (including penicillin, clindamycin, cephalosporin, or metronidazole) must be initiated. In advanced cases, incision and drainage or immediate tonsillectomy may be required. Infectious agents most commonly seen in peritonsillar abscess include aerobic *S pyogenes* (GABHS) and anaerobic *Fusobacterium*. In most cases, a mix of aerobic and anaerobic organisms causes infection.

Additional Reading: Peritonsillar abscess. *Am Fam Physician*. 2017;95(8):501-506.

3. You are seeing a 9-year-old child with asthma in the office. She is short of breath, and you can hear wheezing on auscultation of her lungs. After administering albuterol via a metered-dose inhaler (MDI) with a valved holding chamber ("spacer"), the patient's peak expiratory flow rate (PEFR) is found to be 75%. The next step toward managing this acute asthma exacerbation is to provide which one of the following treatments?

A) Administer epinephrine intramuscularly.
B) Prescribe oral ipratropium.
C) Prescribe oral steroids.
D) Prescribe oral theophylline.
E) Send to the emergency department for intubation/ventilation.

The answer is C: Asthma is characterized by reversible airway obstruction. In treating chronic asthma, attention to the three main aspects of the condition can be targeted for effective treatment: (1) reversible airway obstruction; (2) airway inflammation; and (3) airway hyper-responsiveness to environmental stimuli.

Early treatment of a patient with an acute asthma exacerbation can lessen the likelihood of progression to severe respiratory distress. The first-line treatment is a short-acting inhaled β2-agonist (albuterol), by MDI delivered with the use of a valved holding chamber ("spacer"; two to four puffs, every 20 minutes up to three rounds) or by a nebulizer as a single treatment. Response is adequate if the patient has either sustained symptom relief or improved PEFR to greater than 80% of the child's best measurement. The short-acting β2-agonist treatment can be continued every 3 to 4 hours, for 24 to 48 hours.

If the initial therapy does not result in complete clinical improvement (PEFR between 50% and 80%), continue the β2-agonist every 4 hours and add an oral corticosteroid.

If marked distress or if PEFR persists below 50%, have the patient immediately repeat treatment with β2-agonist and monitor closely.

Additional Reading: Acute asthma exacerbations in children younger than 12 years: overview of home/office management and severity assessment. In: *UpToDate*. 2022.

> **Asthma is characterized by reversible airway obstruction due to underlying inflammation.**

4. Pertussis, also known as whooping cough, is a highly contagious respiratory disease. Which of the following statements regarding pertussis is true?

A) The administration of tetanus toxoids and diphtheria with acellular pertussis (Tdap) vaccine is contraindicated in adolescents.
B) The incidence of pertussis is decreasing.
C) The use of acellular pertussis vaccine is indicated throughout the primary vaccination series.
D) The whole-cell vaccine is safer than acellular vaccine.
E) Vaccination eliminates the risk of contracting pertussis.

The answer is C: Pertussis, also known as whooping cough, is a highly contagious respiratory disease. It is caused by the bacterium *Bordetella pertussis*. Fifty million cases of pertussis are seen each year, leading to about 400,000 deaths, with high-income countries reporting increasing adolescent pertussis rates. The incidence of pertussis among US teens has increased 19-fold since 1996.

Whole-cell vaccines were developed in the 1930s to prevent the illness, yet concerns about adverse effects (eg, convulsions, encephalopathy, hypotonic episodes, fever, and vomiting) encouraged development of an acellular recombinant vaccine, available as diphtheria and tetanus toxoids and acellular pertussis (DTaP) vaccine for children under 7 years of age and Tdap vaccine for children 7 years of age and older. The Centers for Disease Control and Prevention recommends administration of DTaP vaccine at 2, 4, 6, and 15 to 18 months of age, with a booster of the Tdap vaccine between 11 and 18 years of age, and a one-time Tdap booster as an adult.

Acellular and whole-cell vaccines have generally low incidences of adverse effects. Although vaccination decreases the risk of contracting pertussis, it does not eliminate the risk.

Additional Reading: CDC Pink Book: Pertussis.

5. A mother presents with her 4-year-old daughter, who has had a bad cold and was up several times previous night with a very "barky" cough. You suspect croup and her mother is asking if you can prescribe a cough syrup to help with sleep. Which one of the following medications has been shown to be helpful in the treatment of croup?

A) Acyclovir
B) Atropine
C) Dexamethasone
D) Theophylline
E) No medications have been found to be useful

The answer is C: Croup, also known as laryngotracheobronchitis, is a respiratory tract infection caused by various viruses including parainfluenza and influenza viruses. Viral croup is the predominant cause of airway obstruction in children 6 months to 6 years of age. The symptoms are due to inflammation and obstruction of the trachea and larynx which interferes with normal breathing and produces the classic symptoms of a "barking" cough, stridor, and a hoarse voice. Fever and a runny nose are often also present.

For mild croup, symptomatic care and cool mist therapy may be sufficient; however, more severe cases are treated with glucocorticoids, such as dexamethasone. Oral dexamethasone is as effective as intramuscular dexamethasone and show clinical benefit as early as 6 hours after administration.

Additional Reading: Croup: diagnosis and management. *Am Fam Physician*. 2018;97(9):575-580.

6. Cystic fibrosis (CF) is the most common fatal genetic disease in the United States. Which one of the following statements about CF is true?

A) Diagnosis is confirmed with pulmonary function testing.
B) Fertility is never affected.
C) Inheritance is autosomal dominant.
D) Life expectancy is 20 years of age.
E) There is an association with pancreatic insufficiency.

The answer is E: In the United States, CF has an incidence of 1:3500 in whites and 1:17,000 in African Americans. Vertical transmission is autosomal-recessive, and heterozygotes are unaffected. CF comprises a constellation of exocrine, gastrointestinal, and respiratory dysfunction that result from a defect in the cellular chloride channel. Complications include meconium ileus at birth, chronic cough and wheezing with copious mucous production, pancreatic insufficiency with possible development of type 1 diabetes mellitus (up to 8%), retarded growth, infertility, and chronic obstructive pulmonary disease.

Diagnosis is confirmed by evaluation of the sodium and chloride content of sweat (>60 mEq/L), typically accomplished with pilocarpine iontophoresis. Mortality results from pulmonary complications in infection with *S aureus*, *P aeruginosa*, and *H influenzae*. Median survival is 40 years of age.

Additional Reading: Cystic fibrosis. In: Domino F, ed. *The 5-Minute Clinical Consult*. Wolters Kluwer; 2022.

7. You are seeing a previously healthy 17-year-old student with a cough, fever, and malaise. His chest x-ray shows patchy infiltrates, and you diagnose a community-acquired pneumonia. Which one of the following organisms is the most likely cause of a lung infection in the adolescent age group?

A) Adenovirus
B) Chlamydia
C) *H influenzae*
D) *M pneumoniae*
E) *S pneumoniae*

The answer is D: *Mycoplasma* is the most common etiologic agent of lung infections in patients between 5 and 35 years of age. It is transmitted via respiratory droplets among close contacts, school children, military recruits, and family members. It is typically less severe than infections with pneumococcus. Symptoms include malaise, sore throat, coryza, myalgias, and a worsening cough that only becomes productive later in disease with mucopurulent or blood-streaked sputum. A maculopapular rash may be seen. Bullous myringitis can be seen in *Mycoplasma* infections as well.

Chest radiographs of pulmonary *Mycoplasma* show patchy infiltrates in the lower lobes. Rarely, there is lobar consolidation. The white blood cell count is often normal or mildly elevated. Confirmation of diagnosis with acute and convalescent titers is unnecessary.

Treatment is with macrolide antibiotic. Alternatives include fluoroquinolone and tetracycline. Because *Mycoplasma* organism does not have a cell wall, the β-lactam antibiotics are ineffective.

Additional Reading: Pneumonia, mycoplasma. In: Domino F, ed. *The 5-Minute Clinical Consult*. Wolters Kluwer; 2022.

8. You are evaluating a 3-month-old infant whose parents called on New Year's Day with concern that he was wheezing. They note that in addition to audible wheezing, he has had a runny nose, fever, and a cough. The child is attending a day care center where other children have had similar symptoms. On examination, you hear rales and wheezing, and observe intercostal retractions with grunting. The most likely infecting organism to account for his symptoms is which one of the following?

A) Adenovirus
B) Coxsackie virus
C) *H influenzae*
D) Respiratory syncytial virus (RSV)
E) *S pneumoniae*

The answer is D: RSV bronchiolitis affects children between 1 and 6 months of age, with a peak incidence at 2 to 3 months of age. The virus is transmitted by close contacts via fomites and respiratory secretions and tends to occur in outbreaks in places such as day care centers. Infection with RSV often presents in winter, with bronchiolitis and pneumonia.

Symptoms include rhinorrhea, fever, cough, and wheezing. In severe cases, tachypnea, dyspnea, and hypoxia are present. Physical examination shows nasal flaring, rales, and wheezing. Infants may have intercostal retractions with grunting.

Routine laboratory testing is not required but often demonstrates a normal leukocyte count with elevated granulocytes. Chest radiographs are not indicated. Identifying the virus in respiratory secretions with enzyme-linked immunoassay antigen detection or immunofluorescence microscopy is possible but rarely affects management.

Treatment of RSV bronchiolitis is symptomatic by maintaining hydration and monitoring for respiratory distress. Supplemental oxygen is not needed for oxygen saturations greater than 90%. Bronchodilators, corticosteroids, deep suctioning, and chest physiotherapy are not helpful. Respiratory support may be required in severe cases.

Additional Reading: Respiratory syncytial virus bronchiolitis in children. *Am Fam Physician*. 2017;95(2):94-99.

9. You are seeing a 4-year-old child who has been brought in by his mother because of a persistent cough. She notes that her daughter seems to make a whooping sound when she coughs and has occasionally started gagging and vomiting. You diagnose with a pertussis infection. Which one of the following agents is considered to be the first-line treatment for pertussis?

A) Amphotericin B
B) Ciprofloxacin
C) Azithromycin
D) Metronidazole
E) Penicillin G

The answer is C: Pertussis is a highly contagious (gram-negative rod) bacterial disease caused by *B pertussis*. The disease is characterized by a short paroxysmal cough that ends with an inspiratory whoop. The incubation period is usually 7 to 21 days. Transmission occurs via airborne droplets or direct contact. There are three defined stages:

1. Catarrhal stage. This stage is characterized by sneezing, lacrimation, decreased appetite, fatigue, coryza, and a cough that becomes diurnal. This episode lasts 10 to 14 days.
2. Paroxysmal stage. This stage is characterized by whooping cough, possibly vomiting due to persistent cough. This episode lasts up to 4 weeks.
3. Convalescent stage. This stage is characterized by slow improvement of cough and constitutional symptoms. This episode may last up to 3 months.

Polymerase chain reaction rapid tests offer excellent sensitivity if performed on nasopharyngeal specimens taken 0 to 3 weeks after cough onset. Treatment is primarily supportive. If given within 21 days of cough onset, azithromycin will reduce infectivity but not affect the symptoms.

The classic whooping cough may not occur in adults or infants younger than 6 months but consider pertussis in any cough lasting more than 2 weeks. Parapertussis, caused by *Bordetella parapertussis*, causes a similar illness and is clinically similar to pertussis but with a milder course and less subsequent complications.

Additional Reading: Pertussis (whooping cough). Centers for Disease Control and Prevention (CDC). www.cdc.gov/pertussis.

> **Pertussis is a highly contagious bacterial infection caused by *B pertussis*. The disease is characterized by a short paroxysmal cough that ends with an inspiratory whoop.**

10. The Centor score is a useful tool to identify cases of sore throat, which are likely due to streptococcal pharyngitis. Which one of the following is considered a negative predictor for streptococcal pharyngitis?

A) Tender anterior cervical lymphadenopathy
B) A fever (temperature, greater than 38.3 °C [100.9 °F])
C) Pharyngeal or tonsillar exudates on examination
D) A recent cough

The answer is D: The Centor score is used to identify cases of streptococcal pharyngitis, with a point given for each of the following associated findings.

- A fever (temperature greater than 38.3 °C [100.9 °F])
- Tender anterior cervical lymphadenopathy
- Pharyngeal or tonsillar exudates
- Absence of a cough
- Additional variables include adding one point for age less than 15 years, 0 points for age 16 to 44 years, and minus one for age > 45 years. A total score of 4 or 5 provides a 51% to 52% probability of a positive culture for group A β-hemolytic *Streptococcus* infection.

A recent cough is considered a negative predictor for streptococcal pharyngitis, and if it is present, a point would be subtracted from the total.

In patients with a low probability of streptococcal pharyngitis (score of 0-1), no testing is indicated; only follow-up is needed. Those in the intermediate group (score 2-3 points) should be tested further. Patients with a high probability of disease (score of 4 or 5) could be treated empirically with antibiotics, although the current best practice is to obtain a rapid antigen detection test and treat only for a positive result.

Additional Reading: CDC Pharyngitis (Strep throat).

11. An 8-year-old child with cystic fibrosis (CF) presents to the office because of recurrent lung infections and difficulty breathing over the past few years. What is the most likely etiology of his pneumonia?

A) *H influenzae*
B) *M catarrhalis*
C) *M pneumoniae*
D) *P aeruginosa*
E) *S pneumoniae*

The answer is D: *S aureus* is the first organism to colonize and infect young people with CF and is the most common etiology of infection in young children with CF. However, *P aeruginosa* becomes the more predominant organism as children age, with approximately two-thirds of all young adults with CF being colonized with this organism. A mucoid polysaccharide capsule variant of *Pseudomonas* likely contributes to biofilm formation that enables persistent colonization among individuals with CF.

Additional Reading: Cystic fibrosis. In: Domino F, ed. *The 5-Minute Clinical Consult*. Wolters Kluwer; 2022.

12. A 7-year-old girl with a history of mild asthma presents to your office with difficulty breathing. On physical examination, bilateral wheezing is appreciated. The girl is in mild respiratory distress. She has not taken any medications. Which one of the following medications should be prescribed for the management of this patient?

A) Albuterol
B) Cromolyn sodium
C) Inhaled corticosteroids
D) Salmeterol
E) Theophylline

The answer is A: Asthma is a chronic lung disease that is characterized by inflammation and airway reactivity that results in episodes of wheezing and coughing. There are currently 5 million children with asthma in the United States. Asthma can be exacerbated by triggers, including allergens from dust mites or mold spores, animal dander, cockroaches, pollen, indoor and outdoor pollutants, irritants (eg, tobacco smoke, smoke from wood-burning stoves or fireplaces, perfumes, and cleaning agents), pharmacologic triggers (eg, aspirin or other nonsteroidal anti-inflammatory drugs, β-blockers, and sulfites), physical triggers (eg, exercise, hyperventilation, and cold air), and physiologic factors (eg, stress, gastroesophageal reflux, respiratory tract infection [viral, bacterial], and rhinitis).

The four components of asthma management include:

1. regular assessment and monitoring,
2. control of factors that contribute to or aggravate symptoms,
3. pharmacologic therapy, and
4. education of children and their caregivers.

A stepwise approach to pharmacologic treatment should be taken, starting with aggressive therapy to achieve control of symptoms and followed by a "step down" to the minimal therapy that maintains control. Quick relief of symptoms can be achieved preferentially by the use of short-acting β2-agonists (eg, albuterol).

Consider medications for long-term control in children with persistent symptoms. Inhaled corticosteroids are the most potent long-term anti-inflammatory medications. Other options include long-acting β2-agonists (when used in combination with inhaled corticosteroids), cromolyn sodium, antileukotriene agents, and theophylline. These medications each have advantages and disadvantages in individual situations.

Poor compliance is a major problem in pediatric asthma management. Ease of administration challenges compliance; and route, frequency of dosing, side effects, or concern about potential side effects hinders regular use and thus compromises control of asthma. Goals of pharmacologic therapy aim to minimize daytime and nocturnal symptoms, the number of asthma episodes, and the use of short-acting β2-agonists. Adequate management also aims to improve peak exploratory flow to 80% or more of personal best and to allow the child to maintain normal activities without producing adverse medication side effects.

Additional Reading: Asthma in children younger than 12 years: overview of initiating therapy and monitoring control. In: *UpToDate*. 2022.

13. Which of the following is a contraindication to the administration of the seasonal influenza vaccine?

A) Age less than 6 years
B) An allergy to aluminum
C) An allergy to eggs
D) A severe allergic reaction to a prior dose of any influenza vaccine or influenza vaccine component except egg
E) A recent strep infection

The answer is D: Influenza vaccine is optimally given in September but can be given throughout the influenza season. For people 6 months to 64 years of age the Centers for Disease Control and Prevention recommends any available age-appropriate vaccine product. Adults 65 years of age or older are recommended to receive "high"-dose products; however, if none of those vaccines are available, "standard-dose" vaccines can be given.

Children 6 months through 8 years of age should receive 2 doses 4 weeks apart if (1) they are receiving influenza vaccine for the first time, (2) if they have not received a total of at least two doses of the any seasonal influenza vaccine before July 1 of the current year, or (3) if their vaccination history is unknown.

- Some, but not all, available influenza vaccines are prepared by propagation of the virus in embryonated eggs and might contain trace amounts of egg proteins, such as egg albumin. The strain of influenza virus used to make the inactivated and recombinant vaccine is prepared in eggs. Persons with a history of egg allergy who have experienced only hives after exposure to egg should receive the flu vaccine that is appropriate for their age and health status.
- Persons who have had reactions to egg involving symptoms other than hives, such as angioedema, respiratory distress, lightheadedness, or recurrent emesis, or who required epinephrine or another emergency medical intervention, may similarly receive any recommended flu vaccine that is appropriate for their age and health status. However, the vaccine should be administered in an inpatient or outpatient medical setting by a health care provider who is able to recognize and manage severe allergic conditions.
- A previous severe allergic reaction to flu vaccine, regardless of the component suspected of being responsible for the reaction, is a contraindication to future receipt of the vaccine.

Additional Reading: Seasonal influenza vaccine safety: a summary for clinicians. www.cdc.gov/flu/professionals/vaccination/vaccine_safety.htm.

The Centers for Disease Control and Prevention guidelines regarding the administration of the flu vaccine for those with a history of egg allergy who have experienced only hives state that these individuals can receive the flu vaccine, and those with more severe reactions (eg, angioedema, respiratory distress) may similarly receive the flu vaccine. However, the vaccine should be administered in a medical setting by a health care provider who is able to recognize and manage severe allergic reactions.

14. A false-negative purified protein derivative tuberculosis test is most likely seen with which one of the following immunizations?

A) Hepatitis B
B) Influenza
C) Measles-mumps-rubella (MMR)
D) Pneumococcal
E) Tetanus

The answer is C: Some persons may not react to the purified protein derivative skin test even though they are infected with *Mycobacterium tuberculosis*. The reasons for these false-negative reactions may include, but are not limited to, the following:

- Cutaneous anergy (anergy is the inability to react to skin tests because of a weakened immune system)
- Recent tuberculosis infection (within 8-10 weeks of exposure)
- Very old tuberculosis infection (many years)
- Very young age (less than 6 months)
- Recent live virus vaccination (eg, measles and smallpox)
- Overwhelming tuberculosis disease
- Some viral illnesses (eg, measles and chickenpox)
- Incorrect method of skin test administration
- Incorrect interpretation of reaction

Of the vaccines listed, only the MMR is a live virus vaccine.

Additional Reading: Tuberculin skin testing. www.cdc.gov/tb/publications/factsheets/testing/skintesting.htm.

15. Influenza A is prevalent in your community, and you have diagnosed a young adolescent with the flu. Which one of the following medications is *not* approved by the U.S. Food and Drug Administration for the treatment of influenza A in an adolescent?

A) Peramivir
B) Oseltamivir
C) Rimantadine
D) Zanamivir

The answer is C: Several influenza antiviral agents are available in the United States, including amantadine, oseltamivir, rimantadine, zanamivir, and baloxavir marboxil.

Zanamivir, oseltamivir, and peramivir are chemically related antiviral neuraminidase inhibitors that have activity against both influenza A and B viruses. Oral oseltamivir can be used at any age to treat influenza. Inhaled zanamivir is approved to treat persons 7 years or older. Intravenous peramivir can be used in persons 6 months of age and older.

Baloxavir marboxil is a cap-dependent endonuclease inhibitor and can be used in persons 5 years of age and older.

Additional Reading: Antiviral drugs. Centers for Disease Control and Prevention. https://www.cdc.gov/flu/professionals/antivirals.

Section VII. Cardiovascular System

Each of the following questions or incomplete statements is followed by suggested answers or completions. Select the ONE BEST ANSWER in each case.

1. A 12-year-old girl comes to the office with several days of sore throat with fever and acute onset of bilateral knee pain that began yesterday. There is no history of trauma. Laboratory evaluation shows an elevated sedimentation rate. What is the most likely diagnosis?

A) Acute rheumatic fever
B) Juvenile rheumatoid arthritis
C) Lyme disease
D) Osgood-Schlatter disease
E) Patellofemoral syndrome

The answer is A: Rheumatic fever is an acute systemic febrile illness that presents as a complication of group A streptococcal pharyngitis. Associated findings include migratory arthritis involving the large joints, carditis and valvulitis, erythema marginatum rash, subcutaneous nodules, and choreoathetotic movements of Sydenham chorea. Chronic and progressive damage to the cardiac valves leads to significant cardiac dysfunction.

The Modified Jones criteria facilitate the clinical diagnosis of rheumatic fever; without any pathognomonic findings, it can be challenging to identify affected patients. The criteria's major manifestations include carditis, erythema marginatum, polyarthritis, subcutaneous nodules, and Sydenham chorea. Minor manifestations include clinical (eg, arthralgia and fever) and laboratory (eg, elevated C-reactive protein and erythrocyte sedimentation rate, prolonged PR interval on electrocardiogram). Rheumatic fever is diagnosed using the aforementioned criteria with evidence of preceding group A streptococcal infection (positive throat culture or positive rapid streptococcal antigen test, rising or elevated antistreptolysin titer), and *two major* manifestations or *one major and two minor* manifestations.

Arthritis is the most frequent yet least specific manifestation, usually affecting the large joints, often signaling the first sign of illness. The lower extremities generally are affected before the upper extremities. Joint involvement occurs early and more commonly and severely in younger patients. The arthritis may be painful, but it is self-limited, typically resolves without complication, and is treated with nonsteroidal anti-inflammatory drugs and salicylates. Inflammation lasts 2 to 3 days in each joint and 2 to 3 weeks in total.

Carditis is the most often endocarditis but may also present as pericarditis or myocarditis. Endocarditis may be asymptomatic or present with a new heart murmur. Pericarditis presents with chest discomfort, pleuritic chest pain, pericardial friction rub, and distant heart sounds. Myocarditis is rare in isolation and can present with signs and symptoms of heart failure. Cardiac murmurs do not always indicate valvular involvement and may also be transient. If there is valvular disease, it most likely affects the mitral, aortic, tricuspid, or pulmonary valve, with respect to predominance. Electrocardiographic and echocardiographic abnormalities are present in about one-third of patients with carditis.

Rheumatic heart disease is an important long-term consequence of rheumatic fever and is the major cause of acquired valvular disease worldwide. Rheumatic heart disease typically occurs 10 to 20 years after the original rheumatic fever episode. In the event of significant mitral stenosis, surgery is required.

Sydenham chorea is characterized by involuntary movement, muscular weakness, and emotional disturbances and may be more marked on one side of the body or completely unilateral. Emotional symptoms can include crying, restlessness, and, rarely, psychotic features. There is no sensory loss or involvement of the pyramidal tracts. Sydenham chorea is typically self-limited and occurs in <5% of those affected and lasts 2 to 3 months.

Antistreptococcal prophylaxis should be maintained continuously after an attack of acute rheumatic fever or chorea to prevent recurrences.

Additional Reading: Poststreptococcal illness: recognition and management. *Am Fam Physician.* 2018;97(8):517-522.

2. A 3-year-old boy presents with his mother, who is concerned about a high fever that he has had over the past few days. On examination, you note that he has bilateral conjunctivitis, cracked lips, cervical lymphadenopathy, and redness with swelling of his hands and feet. The most likely diagnosis is which one of the following conditions?

A) Infectious mononucleosis
B) Kawasaki disease
C) Lyme disease
D) Rocky Mountain fever
E) Scarlet fever

The answer is B: Kawasaki disease, previously called mucocutaneous lymph node syndrome, is often seen in patients younger than 5 years, with a male predominance. The cause of this disease is unclear, and no specific diagnostic tests exist. Diagnosis is based on having fever for at least 5 days and at least four of the following:

1. Bilateral, painless, nonexudative conjunctivitis
2. Erythema and cracking of the lips, strawberry tongue, and/or erythema of the oral and pharyngeal mucosa
3. Cervical lymphadenopathy (≥1.5 cm in diameter) usually unilateral
4. Rash: maculopapular, diffuse erythroderma, or erythema multiforme–like
5. Erythema and edema of the hands and feet in the acute phase and/or periungual desquamation in the subacute phase

Pathologically Kawasaki disease is characterized by vasculitis of medium sizes, extraparenchymal arteries, with a predilection for the coronary arteries. Coronary artery lesions develop in up to 255% of untreated children and 3% to 5% of children treated with intravenous immunoglobulin (IVIG). Coronary artery lesions can range from mild dilation to giant aneurysms. Echocardiography should be performed at diagnosis to evaluate coronary artery dimensions, myocardial function, valve regurgitation, and pericardial effusion. Repeat echocardiogram is recommended 1 to 2 weeks after diagnosis done 5 to 6 weeks after hospital discharge. Coronary aneurysms regress in size in more than half of the affected segments but endothelial function remains impaired.

The treatment of Kawasaki disease consists of therapy with IVIG and high-dose aspirin. This therapy decreases the incidence of coronary artery dilation and aneurysm formation. Corticosteroids are not recommended.

Additional Readings:
1. Diagnosis and management of Kawasaki disease. *Am Fam Physician*. 2015;91(6):365-371.
2. Kawasaki disease and multisystem inflammatory syndrome in children: an overview and comparison. *Am Fam Physician*. 2021;104(2):244-252.

3. Coarctation of the aorta is associated which one of the following clinical findings?

A) Bounding femoral pulses
B) Blood pressure higher in the legs than in the arms in infants older than 1 year
C) Diastolic murmur heard at the apex, radiating to the axilla
D) Dilation of the thoracic aorta near the ligamentum arteriosus
E) Rib notching on chest radiograph

The answer is E: Coarctation of the aorta is a common congenital heart defect. In most patients, a discrete narrowing of the thoracic aorta near the ligamentum arteriosus is present, although there is a spectrum of aortic narrowing that can occur. The left ventricular outflow is obstructed, leading to proximal hypertension, and left ventricular overload. Other cardiac lesions are common and can include ventricular septal defect, patent ductus arteriosus (PDA), and bicuspid aortic valve. Less severe obstructions are asymptomatic during infancy. However, if congestive heart failure (CHF) occurs, immediate surgical intervention may be required.

Signs of coarctation of the aorta include diminished or absent femoral pulses, blood pressure higher in the arms compared with the legs in infants older than 1 year, a 2 to 3/6 systolic ejection murmur heard over the apex and left upper sternal border, rib notching on chest radiograph (resulting from enlargement of the intercostal arteries), and left ventricular hypertrophy. Diagnosis is based on physical findings and echocardiography or with computed tomography or magnetic resonance imaging angiography.

Treatment depends on the severity of coarctation and the heart's ability to maintain perfusion. In severe cases, prostaglandin E_1 may be used to maintain a PDA until surgery or balloon angioplasty can be performed. In stable patients, β-blockers and afterload-reducing agents can be used to postpone definitive treatment until the child is 3 to 5 years of age, when the treatment can be performed electively. Patients without CHF or a need for surgery tend to have less complications in childhood and adolescence. Those more severely affected are at risk for hypertension, cardiac dysfunction, and subacute infective endocarditis.

Additional Reading: Clinical manifestations and diagnosis of coarctation of the aorta. In: *UpToDate*. 2022.

4. You are examining a young athlete for a preparticipation examination and after hearing an irregular rhythm, an electrocardiogram is obtained. The electrocardiogram demonstrates sinus variation with respiration and a sinus rhythm is maintained throughout. Which of the following would be the most appropriate next step?

A) Obtain a 24-hour Holter monitor.
B) Offer reassurance to the patient and his family.
C) Order an echocardiogram.
D) Prescribe a β-blocker.
E) Request a cardiology consultation.

The answer is B: Sinus arrhythmia is often observed in young, healthy patients and represents no concern for underlying pathology. The variation in heart rate is affected by normal respirations and is associated with the alternating increases and decreases in vagal and sympathetic tone. Patients report no symptoms, and no treatment is required. Other measures would be indicated only if there is suspicion for underlying cardiac pathology.

Additional Reading: Irregular heart rate (arrhythmias) in children. In: *UpToDate*. 2022.

5. What is considered the normal heart rate range of a newborn?

A) 60 to 100 beats per minute
B) 100 to 120 beats per minute
C) 120 to 160 beats per minute
D) 140 to 160 beats per minute

The answer is C: The normal heart rate of a newborn is 120 to 160 beats per minute.

Additional Reading: The pediatric physical examination: General principles and standard measurements. In: *UpToDate*. 2022.

6. Which one of the following congenital heart defects (CHDs) causes cyanosis of the newborn that typically presents within the first few weeks of life?

A) Ventricular septal defect (VSD)
B) Atrial septal defect (ASD)
C) Patent ductus arteriosus (PDA)
D) Coarctation of the aorta
E) Tetralogy of Fallot

The answer is E: CHDs are classified as either cyanotic or acyanotic. Cyanotic heart defects tend to present with signs and symptoms of hypoxia, whereas those of acyanotic nature tend to present with greater heart failure symptoms. Tetralogy of Fallot is a common anatomical abnormality that leads to cyanosis, diaphoresis with feeding, tachypnea, and tachycardia typically within the first 4 to 6 weeks of life. Transposition of the great arteries is another cyanotic heart defect that usually presents with cyanosis within the first few hours of life. This is a rare condition in which the aorta and pulmonary arteries are transposed such that there are two separate circulation systems running in parallel, rather than in sequence.

Tetralogy of Fallot is the most common CHD seen after infancy, requiring surgical repair when the child reaches 3 years of age. Defect comprises (1) a large VSD, (2) right outflow tract obstruction, (3) right ventricular hypertrophy, and (4) an overriding aorta. Classic presentation is characterized by hyperpnea, irritability, cyanosis, and decreased murmur intensity, as pulmonary vascular resistance declines with age. Patient may be seen squatting, which decreases systemic venous return by trapping blood in the legs, breaking the overload-hypoxia cycle. If this maneuver is ineffective, pharmacologic treatment may be necessary. Medical management for Tetralogy of Fallot includes patient and family education on symptom management, prevention of anemia, and prophylaxis for subacute bacterial endocarditis. Surgical palliation consists of shunt placement from the subclavian artery to the ipsilateral pulmonary artery. Total repair is done before 4 years of age and includes VSD repair and widening of the right ventricular outflow tract.

Acyanotic heart defects include VSD, ASD, atrioventricular canal, pulmonary stenosis, PDA, aortic stenosis, and coarctation of the aorta. Infants with acyanotic heart defects are at risk for congestive heart failure (CHF).

VSD: It is the most common CHD that can occur at any point along the septal wall. Severity of the VSD correlates to the size of the defect. Within the first 6 months of life, 30% to 40% of defects spontaneously close; these tend to be of smaller size. CHF can develop as soon as 6 to 8 weeks of age and is managed with diuretics and digoxin (Lanoxin). Surgery is indicated in cases of impaired growth, unresponsive to medical management, and the development of pulmonary hypertension.

ASD: It can occur as one of the three types: sinus venosus, secundum, or primum. Approximately 85% of secundum-type ASDs resolve spontaneously within the first 4 years of life. Primum- and sinus venosus–type ASD with defects >8 mm rarely close spontaneously and tend to require surgery. Most children with an ASD remain asymptomatic, but some develop CHF and require medical management with diuretics and digoxin. Indications for surgical closure are refractory CHF, persistence of the defect beyond 4 years of age, and the presence of other associated defects (VSD, valve anomalies).

Atrioventricular canal: It is characterized by a combination of a primum-type ASD, common atrioventricular valve, and an inlet type of VSD. Hemodynamic disorder arises from the presence of VSD or pulmonary overload that results from mitral regurgitation, left ventricle to right atrium regurgitation, or both. Treatment of CHF with atrioventricular canal can be corrected surgically, before the onset of pulmonary vascular occlusive disease. Palliative pulmonary artery banding could benefit infants with refractory CHF, yet they are still too small for definitive repair.

Pulmonary stenosis: It occurs due to valvular, subvalvular, or supravalvular defects. Clinical manifestations of pulmonary stenosis vary from asymptomatic to frank CHF. Prostaglandin E_1 infusion may help newborns. For valvular-type pulmonary stenosis, use balloon valvuloplasty during cardiac catheterization.

PDA: It is common among premature infants and most defects close spontaneously. Indomethacin can be used for medical closure in premature infants. In term infants, spontaneous closure is unlikely, and indomethacin is not effective. Surgical ligation should be performed as soon as possible. Cardiopulmonary bypass is not necessary. Nonsurgical options for correcting PDA include catheter placement of an embolic device in term infants. Complications of PDA include CHF and recurrent pneumonia. PDA is the only CHD that may be considered surgically curative.

Aortic stenosis: It can arise from valvular, subvalvular, or supravalvular defects. It can be asymptomatic or cause symptoms of CHF. The pressure gradient across the stenotic aorta increases as the child grows and cardiac output increases. Surgical correction is preferred, and timing depends on the patient's cardiopulmonary status, type of procedure (valvulotomy vs valve replacement), and the size of the valve if a graft is needed. Patients who receive a prosthetic valve require lifelong anticoagulation therapy thereafter.

Additional Reading: Common causes of cardiac murmurs in infants and children. In: *UpToDate*. 2022.

PDA is the only CHD that can be surgically corrected to attain relatively normal hemodynamics without long-term sequelae.

7. An infant is found to have a higher blood pressure reading in the upper extremities compared with that of the lower extremities. Pulses are bounding in both arms and diminished in both legs. What is the most likely diagnosis?

A) Aortic stenosis
B) Coarctation of the aorta
C) Tetralogy of Fallot
D) Transposition of the great arteries
E) Ventricular septal defect

The answer is B: Coarctation of the aorta involves narrowing of the aorta, anywhere along its length. Most cases occur just below the origin of the left subclavian artery. Coarctation of the aorta classically presents with the blood pressure and pulse strength findings described in the stem. Treatment involves surgical repair between 2 and 4 years of age. Emergent surgical repair is performed in cases of circulatory shock, cardiomegaly, severe hypertension, or severe congestive heart failure.

Additional Reading: Clinical manifestations and diagnosis of coarctation of the aorta. In: *UpToDate*. 2022.

8. What feature is most likely associated with transposition of the great vessels?

A) A pulmonary vein that empties into the right ventricle
B) A pulmonary artery that arises from the right ventricle
C) An aorta that arises from the left atrium
D) Cyanosis at birth with an intact ventricular septum
E) Cyanosis several weeks after birth with an intact ventricular septum

The answer is D: Transposition of the great vessels is a cause of cyanotic heart disease. Male term infants are more commonly affected than females. Infants of diabetic mothers are also at risk. The condition is associated with an aorta that arises from the right ventricle and a pulmonary artery that arises from the left ventricle. The ventricular septum can have varied involvement and either present intact or with a ventricular septal defect.

Because the systemic blood must mix with the pulmonary circulation, an intact ventricular septum leads to immediate cyanosis and death if untreated. In many cases, the ductus arteriosus remains open for several days, and cyanosis does not develop until it has fully closed, and blood mixing can no longer occur. Congestive heart failure can develop quickly and lead to death. Growth and development delays are common.

Many children have a systolic murmur and some cyanosis at birth. Chest radiographs may be normal or have mild cardiomegaly, an egg-shaped heart, and a narrow superior mediastinum with increased pulmonary vascular markings ("egg on a string"). Cardiac catheterization is used for the diagnosis, and surgery is required to promote normal anatomic circulation or to place an intra-atrial shunt to redirect blood flow.

Additional Reading: Common causes of cardiac murmurs in infants and children. In: *UpToDate*. 2022.

Section VIII. Hematologic/Immune System

Each of the following questions or incomplete statements is followed by suggested answers or completions. Select the ONE BEST ANSWER in each case.

1. Which one of the following statements is true regarding iron deficiency in childhood?

A) It can present with pica.
B) It is relatively common in full-term infants within the first 3 months.
C) It is rarely associated with complications.
D) Ingestion of cow's milk is preventative.
E) Pallor, fatigue, and delayed motor development are typical early signs.

The answer is A: Iron deficiency causes anemia and can adversely affect multiple organ systems. Signs and symptoms vary with the severity of deficiency. Pica can be seen in some patients with iron deficiency anemia. Mild iron deficiency is usually asymptomatic, whereas severe iron deficiency is associated with pallor, fatigue, irritability, and delayed motor development. Consumption of unfortified cow's milk is associated with iron deficiency, and these children may be fat and flabby, with poor muscle tone.

The incidence of iron deficiency in children has decreased substantially because of improved nutrition and the increased availability of iron-fortified infant formulas and cereals. Normal term infants are born with iron stores sufficient to prevent iron deficiency for the first 4 to 5 months of life, and thereafter, adequate iron must be absorbed to maintain the infant's needs during rapid growth. As a result, nutritional iron deficiency most often presents between 6 and 24 months of life. Iron deficiency presenting earlier than 6 months of age may suggest low iron stores at birth, resulting from prematurity, low birth weight, neonatal anemia, or perinatal or subsequent blood loss due to hemorrhage. A child with iron deficiency older than 24 months should be evaluated for blood loss.

Additional Reading: *Anemia. The Harriet Lane Handbook: A Manual for Pediatric House Officers.* 22nd ed. Elsevier/Mosby; 2021.

A child older than 24 months with iron deficiency should be evaluated for blood loss.

2. You are called to see an infant in the newborn nursery, who was delivered at term, 46 hours before your visit. He appears jaundiced but is otherwise healthy and has been breastfeeding without difficulty. You obtain a bilirubin test, and his total serum bilirubin level is 16 mg/dL. Which one of the following actions would be considered the next most appropriate step in his care?

A) Begin phototherapy.
B) Continue observation.
C) Perform a workup for sepsis.
D) Start intravenous hydration.
E) Stop breastfeeding and switch to formula feedings.

The answer is A: Unconjugated hyperbilirubinemia with serum bilirubin 6.5 mg/dL is common in healthy term newborns and rarely indicates serious underlying pathology. The guidelines for at which bilirubin level to initiate phototherapy treatment is stratified by age of the infant in hours, gestational age of the infant, and presence of risk factors (immune hemolytic disease, glucose-6-phosphate dehydrogenase deficiency, asphyxia, significant lethargy, temperature instability, sepsis, acidosis). For term infants without risk factors the bilirubin levels at which to initiate phototherapy are listed below:

- 25 to 48 hours old: level ≥15 mg/dL (257 μmol/L)
- 49 to 72 hours old: level >18 mg/dL (308 μmol/L)
- Older than 72 hours: level >20 mg/dL (342 μmol/L)

Physiologic jaundice peaks on the third or fourth day of life and declines over the first week following birth. Breastfed infants are more likely to develop physiologic jaundice because of the relative caloric deprivation in the first few days of life. If jaundice occurs in breastfed infants, continue assessing for adequacy of milk transfer and milk supply and increase the feeding frequency to more than 10 times/d. Formula supplementation may be necessary.

Jaundice is considered to be pathologic if it occurs within the first 24 hours after birth and total serum bilirubin level increases by >5 mg/dL (86 μmol/L) per 24 hours. The management consists of excluding pathologic causes of hyperbilirubinemia and initiating treatment to prevent harmful neurotoxicity.

Additional Reading: Unconjugated Hyperbilirubinemia in the Newborn. *The Harriet Lane Handbook*. 22nd ed. 2021.

3. An 18-year-old male high school basketball star presents to the office with 6 weeks of difficulty keeping up with his teammates. He reports a swollen lump in his neck, a slight cough, generalized pruritus, and fatigue. Selection for the championship team is next week, and he is disheartened given his current condition. Which one of the following conditions is the most likely diagnosis?

A) Brachial cleft cyst infection
B) Hodgkin lymphoma
C) Infectious mononucleosis
D) Lyme disease
E) *Streptococcus* pharyngitis

The answer is B: The incidence of Hodgkin lymphoma (Hodgkin disease) increases throughout childhood and peaks in the late teens. Traditionally perceived as a malignancy that involves the lymph nodes (LNs), it can originate from primary LN tissues (bone marrow and thymus) and secondary lymphoid tissues (spleen) and nonlymphoid organs (skin, bone, brain, lungs, liver, salivary glands, etc) Although the most common presenting complaint is a painless mass in the neck, other presentations include chest discomfort, superior vena cava syndrome, tachypnea and orthopnea in the case of a large mediastinal mass, abdominal discomfort due to hepatomegaly or splenomegaly or large intra-abdominal mass, headaches and focal neurological signs in cases of central nervous system involvement, and musculoskeletal pain. Pruritus may be present as well.

Constitutional signs include fatigue, anorexia, and so-called B symptoms:

- Fever of at least 100.4 °F (38 °C) for 3 consecutive days, occurring mostly at night in an undulant pattern and progressively becoming worse
- Drenching night sweats
- Weight loss without trying (at least 10% of body weight over 6 months)

Presence of "B" symptoms usually signifies advanced disease and is secondary to inflammatory cytokine release by the tumor.

Factors that have a high predictive value for the nonbenign nature of lymphadenopathy are the following:

- Age > 10 years
- LNs > 2.5 cm
- Supraclavicular site (left side in particular_
- Matting and limited mobility to palpation
- More than 1 noncontiguous LN involved

Recommended investigations include complete blood count, renal and liver function tests, erythrocyte sedimentation rate, C-reactive protein, uric acid, lactate dehydrogenase and alkaline phosphatase levels, chest x-ray, computed tomographic scan of neck, chest and abdomen. Excisional biopsy allows for pathomorphologic evaluation of the tissue and is preferred over fine-needle aspiration or core biopsy.

Additional Reading: Lymphoma: diagnosis and treatment. *Am Fam Physician*. 2020;101(1):34-41.

4. You are seeing a 12-year-old girl with malaise and fever. You suspect infectious mononucleosis. Which one of the following examination findings is seen in patients with infectious mononucleosis?

A) Cobble-stoned appearance of posterior pharynx
B) Palatal petechiae
C) Strawberry tongue
D) Submental lymphadenopathy

The answer is B: Infectious mononucleosis (IM) is caused by an infection of the Epstein-Barr virus (EBV) and is common among patients 10 to 30 years of age who present with sore throat and fatigue. Findings include fever, tender lymphadenopathy (anterior and posterior cervical, auricular, and/or inguinal adenopathy), pharyngitis with palatal petechiae (seen in 33% of patients and not specific to IM), gray-white exudative tonsillitis, hepatosplenomegaly, and sometimes erythematous macular rash.

A complete blood count with differential demonstrates lymphocytosis, with up to 70% of all leukocytes being atypical lymphocytes in peripheral blood. Atypical lymphocytes are not pathognomonic of IM and can be seen in other syndromes. Self-limited, mild neutropenia is seen in 60% to 90% of individuals, Mild thrombocytopenia is present in 50% of patients. Abnormalities of liver function tests are seen in almost 90% of patients. Heterophile antibodies detected by the commonly used "Monospot" test are nonspecific and can provide both false-positive and false-negative results. Specific serologic testing involves testing for EBV-associated antigens, the interpretation of which can determine if the infection is new or recent versus past.

Symptomatic treatment is often sufficient, ensuring adequate hydration, analgesics, antipyretics, and adequate rest. Steroids, antivirals, or antihistamines are not recommended for routine treatment management. However, patients with respiratory compromise or severe pharyngeal edema may benefit from corticosteroids. With infectious mononucleosis, patients should not participate in contact or collision sports for at least 4 weeks after the onset of symptoms. Fatigue, myalgias, and need for sleep may persist for several months after resolution of acute infection.

Additional Reading: Common questions about infectious mononucleosis. *Am Fam Physician*. 2015;91(6):372-376.

5. To prevent hemorrhagic disease of the newborn, which of the following is routinely given at birth?

A) Erythromycin
B) Vitamin C
C) Vitamin K
D) Factor X
E) von Willebrand factor

The answer is C: Newborns are at risk for developing vitamin K deficiency bleeding (VKDB) for several reasons: newborns have low reserves of vitamin K due to minimal plactental transfer during gestation; intestinal flora that synthesize vitamin K are not yet present in the intestinal biome; and breast milk contains low amounts of vitamin K. Following birth, vitamin K–dependent factors II, VII, IX, and X decrease and then gradually return to normal in 7 to 10 days.

At birth, term infants receive 1 mg of vitamin K intramuscularly to prevent hemorrhagic disease of the newborn. Preterm infants are dosed on a mg/kg regimen. Intramuscular (IM) vitamin K administration substantially lowers an infant's risk of developing vitamin K deficiency bleeding. Despite its demonstrated efficacy and safety, parental refusal of IM vitamin K administration is on the rise, as are cases of VKDB.

VKDB can be divided into three types, early, classic, and late.

Early onset occurs in the first 24 hours of life and is seen in mothers who took medications that affected vitamin K metabolism.

Classic VKDB occurs between 1 and 7 days of life and is idiopathic in origin.

Late VKDB occurs between 1 week and 6 months of age, with peak incidence between 2 and 8 weeks of age. It typically occurs in inclusively breastfed infants who did not receive IM vitamin K at birth. It presents with intracranial bleeding in 30% to 60% of cases. Oral, multidose vitamin K regimens have not been shown to be as effective in preventing late-onset VKDB and are not recommended for use.

Additional Reading: *Vitamin K Deficiency Bleeding*. CDC.

6. You are seeing a 9-month-old infant for a well-child check and his mother notes that she has been giving him whole milk for the past few months because she could not afford his formula. Which one of the following is the most likely consequence of providing whole cow's milk to infants younger than 1 year?

A) Hirschsprung disease
B) Iron-deficiency anemia
C) Inflammatory bowel disease
D) Developmental delay
E) None of the above

The answer is B: Providing whole cow's milk to young infants can cause iron-deficiency anemia because cow's milk is low in iron, and this iron is poorly absorbed. Other causes of iron-deficiency anemia among children include having inadequate iron stores at birth due to prematurity, fetal-maternal blood loss, iron-deficient mother, and poor iron intake by the child. The 2022 Bright Futures Guidelines recommend that all children be screened for iron deficiency between at 12 months of age and again thereafter based upon risk factors. Note that in some states screening for iron deficiency anemia is also suggested at 2 and 3 years of age.

Anemia in children between 6 months and 5 years of age is defined as hemoglobin levels <11.0 g/dL (110 g/L). Preventing iron-deficiency anemia among infants can start in the family physician's office with expectant and new parents with a discussion of infant nutrition and encouragement of iron-fortified cereals to accompany breastfeeding or iron-fortified formulas and cereals, as appropriate between the ages of 4 and 6 months.

Additional Reading: Screening for iron deficiency anemia in young children. *Am Fam Physician*. 2015;92(12):1103-1104.

7. Which one of the following statements about immunoglobulin A (IgA) deficiency is true?

A) It is associated with influenza vaccination administration.
B) It is the most common immunodeficiency syndrome.
C) Most individuals do not survive beyond the second decade.
D) Symptoms include night blindness, skin necrosis, and joint pain.
E) Treatment involves scheduled monthly antibiotic administration.

The answer is B: IgA deficiency is the most common immunodeficiency and results in a lack of IgA production in mucosal secretions.

It is the mildest form of immunodeficiency and affects about 1 in 600 individuals. The condition has been associated with phenytoin administration, congenital intrauterine infections, and abnormalities of chromosome 18. Most affected individuals are asymptomatic; however, some may present with decreased immunity and recurrent respiratory tract infections, diarrhea, allergies, and other autoimmune disorders such as systemic lupus erythematous or rheumatoid arthritis.

In most cases of IgA deficiency, no treatment is necessary. In patients with recurrent respiratory infections, frequent antibiotic use may be required. Patients sometimes experience spontaneous remission. Occasionally, patients develop antibodies to IgA, setting the foundation for anaphylaxis during later blood transfusions.

Additional Reading: Evaluation of primary immunodeficiency disease in children. *Am Fam Physician*. 2013;87(11):773-778.

8. A 6-year-old child is brought to the emergency department with nosebleeds that have worsened over the past few days and now his gums started bleeding this morning when he was brushing his teeth. The mother notes that other than a recent cold he has been healthy. On examination, he is looking tired, and you note bruising on his arms and legs. What is the most likely diagnosis to account for this presentation?

A) Hemophilia A
B) Idiopathic thrombocytopenic purpura (ITP)
C) Ingestion of warfarin
D) Meningococcemia
E) Vitamin K deficiency

The answer is B: ITP results from the formation of IgG autoantibodies against the patient's own platelets, resulting in thrombocytopenia. This acute disorder usually affects children between 2 and 6 years of age of both sexes. The condition usually follows a febrile, viral illness (such as varicella-zoster virus, Epstein-Barr virus, or cytomegalovirus) during the winter months. Petechiae, purpura, and bleeding from mucous membranes develop within 3 weeks after the infection.

Thrombocytopenia is seen (platelet counts <20,000 mm^3), and bone marrow shows increased megakaryocytes. Bleeding time is increased, yet prothrombin time and partial thromboplastin time remain normal.

ITP is most common in children ages 2 to 10 years, with a peak incidence between 2 and 4 years of age.

Mild cases do not require treatment. Those with platelet counts between 30,000 and 10,000 have treatment recommendations based upon the presence and severity of associated bleeding symptoms or the risk for bleeding. Treatment is with corticosteroids, intravenous immunoglobulin, or intravenous anti-D immunoglobulin in Rh-positive individuals. .

Approximately 15% to 20% of all pediatric patients with ITP develop moderate or major hemorrhagic problems. Life-threatening bleeding, including intracranial hemorrhage, is rare, with an incidence of 0.1% to 1.0%.

Additional Reading: Thrombocytopenia: evaluation and management. *Am Fam Physician*. 2022;106(3):288-298.

Section IX. Endocrine System

Each of the following questions or incomplete statements is followed by suggested answers or completions. Select the ONE BEST ANSWER in each case.

1. A 4-year-old girl presents with her parents for follow-up on her short stature, and you inform them that her evaluation reveals a delayed bone age. The diagnosis is most likely associated with which one of the following conditions?

A) Constitutional growth delay (CGD)
B) Cartilage growth defects
C) A growth plate disorder
D) Familial short stature (FSS)

The answer is A: Short stature is defined as height that is two or more standard deviations below the mean height for individuals of the same sex and chronologic age in a population. The most common causes of short stature are CGD and FSS. In CGD, children are healthy, but between 3 to 5 years of age, their linear growth and weight track downward to the lower end of the growth chart. Typically, they enter puberty at a later age and have a later growth spurt. A characteristic finding is that their bone age is delayed by 2 or more years. Bone age can be estimated using a radiograph of the left hand and wrist. Delayed or advanced bone age is defined as two standard deviations below or above the mean, respectively.

In FSS, a child consistently grows at a normal rate and has one or both parents who are quite short. Children with FSS tend to enter puberty as a normal age. They generally are within 2 to 3 inches of their target adult height. Target adult height can be calculated by averaging the parental heights, then adding 2.5 inches to that result for boys and subtracting 2.5 inches for girls. Bone age is typically not delayed.

Evaluation of children with short stature serves to identify those children with pathologic etiologies of short stature, including Turner syndrome, underlying systemic disease such as inflammatory bowel disease, Celiac disease, and hormonal abnormalities. In conjunction with history, physical examination, and calculation of height velocity and adult height prediction, a bone age study can be obtained.

Additional Reading: Evaluation of short and tall stature in children. *Am Fam Physician*. 2015;92(1):43-50.

2. A 15-month-old infant is brought in for a well-child check. According to the growth chart, her weight has crossed downward more than 2 major percentiles since 9 months of age after having been stable previously. The next appropriate course of action would be to which of the following?

A) Begin a workup by obtaining a complete blood count, electrolytes, serum glucose levels, and a urinalysis.
B) Consult social services.
C) Prescribe a supplemental calorie beverage.
D) Reassure the family that this is a common finding at this age and that no further workup is necessary at this time.
E) Take a thorough history feeding history and assess for food insecurity in the home.

The answer is E: Growth faltering (formerly termed "failure to thrive") is a symptom of many forms of primary and secondary undernutrition, usually in young children. Childhood growth faltering often derives from the interplay of medical, developmental/behavioral, nutritional, and psychosocial factors resulting in nutritional deficiency. It is defined as attained weight for length or body mass index is below expected on age- and sex-specific growth charts or whose weight on those charts has crossed 2 major percentiles after previously having had stable growth.

Mechanisms of growth faltering can be understood in terms of inadequate energy intake, inadequate absorption, excessive energy expenditure due to an underlying health conditions, or a defective utilization of energy.

The most common cause of growth faltering, inadequate intake, can be due to insufficient supply or consumption of food. Inadequate consumption may occur secondary to feeding difficulties.

History includes the pregnancy and perinatal period, a detailed feeding and nutritional history, a thorough review of systems and a family history for GI disease, atopy, or developmental disorders.

The physical examination should include assessment for tooth decay, tonsillar hypertrophy, skin or neurologic abnormalities, dysmorphisms, cardiac murmur, and organomegaly.

Treatment in most children entails increasing caloric intake using calorically dense foods such as oils, avocados, heavy cream, and peanut butter while avoiding foods with low nutritional value such as sweets and fried foods. Supplemental calorie beverages, if used, should be prescribed with counseling on their ideal use and scheduling so that they are not used in place of food and thus exacerbate feeding difficulties.

Additional Readings:
1. Failure to thrive: a practical guide. *Am Fam Physician*. 2016;94(4):295-299.
2. Nutrition in Toddlers. *Am Fam Physician*. 2018;98(4):227-233.

3. A 13-year-old boy is diagnosed with constitutional growth delay (CGD). The workup including a complete blood count, urinalysis, erythrocyte sedimentation rate, and thyroid studies is unremarkable. Which of the following is the next appropriate step in addressing this child's growth?

A) Monitor his thyroid function tests every 3 months.
B) Offer reassurance to his parents.
C) Prescribe a course of corticosteroids.
D) Prescribe protein supplements.
E) Prescribe vitamin E supplementation.

The answer is B: CGD is a variant of normal growth. Length and weight measurements of affected children are normal at birth, but affected children, generally boys, then experience a slowing of their height velocity in the first 3 to 5 years of age, leading to a falloff in their height percentile. They then resume a normal growth velocity at a lower height percentile. Puberty onset is generally delayed, and there is often a family history of "late bloomers." A hallmark of the condition is a bone age that is delayed.

Reassurance to the parent is the most appropriate management for children who are at Sexual Maturity Rating 2 or 3 and do not have any underlying chronic disease. The parents can be reassured that the child will go through a growth spurt in the near future, and no further testing is warranted. Individuals with CGD undergo complete catch-up growth and achieve an adult height that is within range for their genetic potential.

Additional Reading: Evaluation of short and tall stature in children. *Am Fam Physician*. 2015;92(1):43-50.

4. A 6-year-old boy is brought in for his well-child check. The child's parents are concerned that he is of shorter stature than most of the other children in his class. The child's bone age is consistent with his chronologic age and you observe that his parents are relatively short as well. His height velocity has been normal throughout his life. Which one of the following is the most likely diagnosis to account for this situation?

A) Acromegaly
B) Dwarfism
C) Familial short stature
D) Hypothyroidism
E) Parental neglect

The answer is C: Familial short stature is considered a normal variant, where a child's height is less than 2 standard deviations for his age, but the child is expected to reach the calculated mid-parental height. These children have low normal height velocities, normal laboratory findings, and a bone age that is in agreement with their chronological age.

Additional Reading: Evaluation of short and tall stature in children. *Am Fam Physician*. 2015;92(1):43-50.

5. Type 1 diabetes mellitus (T1DM) is more common in individuals younger than 30 years than adults. Which one of the following statements about T1DM is true?

A) T1DM results from decreased insulin sensitivity.
B) The initial diagnosis is usually made following an episode of nonketotic hyperosmolar coma.
C) Lack of insulin production results from autoimmune destruction of β cells of the islets of Langerhans.
D) Diabetic ketoacidosis is not typically associated with T1DM.

The answer is C: T1DM is the result of an insulin deficiency and appears to be secondary to autoimmune destruction of the β cells of islet of Langerhans. It is more common in individuals younger than 30 years and can run in families. Common symptoms are polyphagia, polyuria, polydipsia, increased thirst, and weight loss despite an increased appetite. Fatigue and blurred vision are also common complaints.

One-third of patients with T1DM present with diabetic ketoacidosis. Signs include severe dehydration, Kussmaul respirations, altered mental status, abdominal pain, enuresis, and fruity breath. Laboratory results show hyperglycemia and glycosuria. This is an acute situation, which requires urgent intravenous fluids and insulin administration.

Treatment of T1DM involves the chronic administration of exogenous insulin. Up to two-thirds of patients experience a period of total or partial remission ("honeymoon period") within a few weeks or months after initiation of insulin therapy. The goal of treatment is to replace insulin, institute a sustainable diet and exercise regimen, and monitor glucose level regularly.

Additional Reading: Epidemiology, presentation, and diagnosis of type 1 diabetes mellitus in children and adolescents. In: *UpToDate*. 2022.

6. A 15-year-old adolescent has decided to follow a strict vegan diet, avoiding all animal products, including eggs and dairy. Adherents to this diet are at risk for which vitamin or mineral deficiency?

A) Calcium
B) Folate
C) Iron
D) Vitamin D
E) Vitamin B_{12}

The answer is E: Vitamin B_{12} is produced exclusively by microorganisms and is found in high concentrations in animal products. Vitamin B_{12} deficiency is a well-known complication of veganism but can also be seen in nonvegans with low consumption of eggs, dairy, fish, or meat or without adequate supplementation. Persons following a vegan diet should be counseled regarding the importance of consuming foods rich in B_{12}, such as some brands of fortified cereals, nutritional yeast, and plant-based milks.

Additional Readings:
1. Nutrition history taking: a practical approach. *Am Fam Physician*. 2022;106(4):427-438.
2. Vitamin B12 deficiency: recognition and management. *Am Fam Physician*. 2017;96(6):384-389.

Section X. Nephrological/Reproductive Systems

Each of the following questions or incomplete statements is followed by suggested answers or completions. Select the ONE BEST ANSWER in each case.

1. You are assessing a 5-year-old boy with nephritic syndrome. Given his age, which one of the following is the most likely cause?

A) Dehydration
B) Nonsteroidal anti-inflammatory drug uses
C) Recent streptococcal infection
D) Trauma
E) Varicella infection

The answer is C: Poststreptococcal glomerulonephritis is the leading cause of acute nephritic syndrome. The condition is most frequently encountered in children between 2 and 6 years of age with a recent history of pharyngitis. It is rare in children younger than 2 years and adults older than 40 years, and the overall incidence of poststreptococcal glomerulonephritis appears to be decreasing. The condition typically develops approximately 10 days after pharyngitis or 2 weeks after skin infection with a nephritogenic strain of group A hemolytic *Streptococcus*.

It has not been determined if antibiotic treatment of the primary skin infection yields protection from the development of poststreptococcal glomerulonephritis. The classic presentation of poststreptococcal glomerulonephritis is a nephritic syndrome with oliguric acute renal failure. Most patients have mild disease and subclinical cases are common. Patients with severe disease experience gross hematuria characterized by red or smoky urine; headache; and generalized symptoms such as anorexia, nausea, vomiting, and malaise. Inflammation of the renal capsule can lead to flank or back pain.

Physical examination may show hypervolemia, edema, or hypertension. Acute poststreptococcal glomerulonephritis is usually diagnosed on clinical and serologic grounds without the need for biopsy, especially in children with a typical history. The overall prognosis in classic poststreptococcal acute proliferative glomerulonephritis is good. Most patients recover spontaneously and return to baseline renal function within 3 to 4 weeks with no long-term complications.

Additional Reading: Poststreptococcal glomerulonephritis. In: *UpToDate*. 2022.

2. A 20-month-old infant is brought to the office by her concerned mother, who reports that over the past few days, her daughter has not been herself, has a low-grade fever, and has not been eating as she normally does. Further clinical evaluation suggests a urinary tract infection (UTI). In addition to administering antibiotics, what additional evaluation should next be completed?

A) Order an intravenous pyelogram.
B) Order a renal and bladder ultrasonography (RBUS).
C) Refer for a cystoscopy.
D) Refer for a voiding cystourethrogram (VCUG).
E) Continue observation with no further testing at this time.

The answer is B: A child between 2 months and 2 years of age, who presents with a first febrile UTI, should have RBUS to evaluate for urinary tract anomalies, including obstruction, renal structural anomalies, nephrolithiasis, or calcification. Older children with recurrent UTIs may also benefit from a RBUS. RBUS cannot detect acute pyelonephritis or vesicoureteral reflux.

Further evaluation with a VCUG is indicated in a child of any age with two or more febrile UTIs; a child with a first febrile UTI and anomaly detected on RBUS; a child with a non–*E coli* pathogen identified; a child with a complex clinical course or known renal scarring.

Additional Reading: Urinary tract infections in young children and infants: common questions and answers. *Am Fam Physician*. 2020;102(5):278-285.

3. You are seeing a 6-year-old boy with glomerulonephritis and suspect that it is a complication of a recent sore throat. In a patient with a suspect poststreptococcal complication, which one of the following blood tests would be the most helpful to confirm that the patient truly had a group A β-hemolytic streptococcal (GABHS) infection?

A) Anti–streptolysin O titer
B) C-reactive protein
C) Complete blood count (CBC)
D) Erythrocyte sedimentation rate

The answer is A: Infections of GABHS pharyngitis, and pyodermic infections such as impetigo can lead to poststreptococcal complications. Once such complication, poststreptococcal glomerulonephritis (PSGN), occurs predominantly among children over 2 years of age, with a peak incidence between 4 and 12 years of age; it is rarely seen in individuals over 18 years of age.

PSGN presents with nephritis 1 to 2 weeks after streptococcal pharyngitis and 3 to 6 weeks after skin infections. Classic signs of nephritis, gross hematuria, edema, and hypertension, may be present; however, more subtle presentations with microscopic hematuria, mildly elevated to normal blood pressure, and no edema can occur and may be never diagnosed.

Evidence of a preceding streptococcal infection can be confirmed by demonstrating an elevated anti–streptolysin O titer, although negative results can occur, especially for preceding skin infections. Assessing other antibody markers, including antihyaluronidase, anti–deoxyribonuclease B (DNase B), and antistreptokinase, has greater specificity but high false-negative rates.

Additional labs to be obtained include C3, CBC, renal function testing, and metabolic panel in addition to the urinalysis with microscopy.

Additional Reading: Poststreptococcal illness: recognition and management. *Am Fam Physician*. 2018;97(8):517-522.

4. In the workup of a child with a recurrent urinary tract infection (UTI), the patient is discovered to have a posterior urethral valve. All of the following statements are true regarding this diagnosis, except which one?

A) The patient is a male child.
B) A prenatal ultrasonography would have shown changes suggestive of the diagnosis.
C) Most cases require surgical correction.
D) There are abnormal valves within the posterior calices of the kidney.
E) Voiding cystourethrogram (VCUG) is used to confirm the diagnosis.

The answer is D: Children with UTIs do not always present with classically associated symptoms such as urinary frequency, dysuria, or flank pain. Infants may present nonspecifically with fever, irritability, or lethargy. Older children may also have nonspecific symptoms, such as abdominal pain or unexplained fever; thus, a urinalysis for any child with unexplained fever or symptoms may suggest the presence of a UTI.

Posterior urethral valves are a common cause of UTIs among young boys. These valves arise secondarily to abnormal folds within the prostatic urethra that enlarge with voiding and ultimately obstruct the urethral lumen. Symptoms include decreased urinary stream, overflow incontinence, and UTIs with dysuria.

Prenatal ultrasonography can facilitate diagnosis by demonstrating the presence of bilateral hydronephrosis, distended bladder, and oligohydramnios if obstruction is severe. In a boy with a UTI and suspected posterior urinary valves, the evaluation is completed with either a VCUG or a perineal ultrasound. Prompt assessment and surgical resection of valves can help reduce the risk of kidney damage.

Additional Reading: Clinical presentation and diagnosis of posterior urethral valves. In: *UpToDate*. 2022.

5. A father presents with his 9-year-old son who continues to wet the bed. He is otherwise healthy but wondering about treatment, as he has not been able to participate in "sleepovers" at his friend's house due to the embarrassment of wetting the bed. Which one of the following statements about enuresis in children is true?

A) It is uncommon for it to occur in families.
B) Enuresis often resolves before 12 years of age.
C) No approved treatment exists.
D) Primary enuresis can occur after a 6-month period of dryness.
E) The diagnosis requires cystoscopy.

The answer is B: Nocturnal enuresis beyond 5 years of age is a relatively common problem. *Primary enuresis* is defined as a patient who has never had an extended period of dryness since birth. *Secondary enuresis* is the onset of bed-wetting after 6 months of dryness. There is a strong hereditary component, and children with a family history of enuresis are more likely to experience enuresis than are their peers.

The patient and family should be reassured that enuresis is common, occurring in 20% of 5-year-old children, with an annual spontaneous resolution rate of 15%. It persists about 1% of late teens. Generally, nocturnal enuresis is not associated with any underlying disorder. The bladder is usually of normal structure and size yet functionally small. Primary nocturnal enuresis is a diagnosis of exclusion, and it is important to consider other causes of bed-wetting.

Secondary enuresis can be caused by neurogenic bladder and associated spinal cord abnormalities, urinary tract infections, urethral stricture, urethral obstruction, posterior urethral valves in boys, or an ectopic ureter in girls. Posterior urethral valves cause significant voiding symptoms such as straining to void and diminished urinary stream. An ectopic ureter causes constant wetting.

Management of primary nocturnal enuresis is primarily observation. Nonpharmacologic treatment includes restricting fluid intake and hour before bedtime, void prior to bedtime, encouraging regular voiding during the day. For children over 8 years of age, enuresis alarm therapy may be used. First-line pharmacologic therapy is DDAVP. Combined therapy with DDAVP and oxybutynin has been shown to be efficacious as well. Imipramine is considered last-line therapy. Most patients outgrow the condition before 12 years of age. Daytime enuresis may indicate underlying pathology or voiding dysfunction and requires further evaluation. Secondary enuresis due to structural abnormality may require surgery.

Additional Reading: Enuresis in children: common questions and answers. *Am Fam Physician*. 2022;106(5):549-556.

Management of primary nocturnal enuresis includes observation, alarm-pad conditioning, or medications (oxybutynin, nasal desmopressin [DDAVP]). Most patients outgrow the condition before 12 years of age.

6. You are seeing a 6-month-old boy for a well-child check and are unable to palpate testis in his scrotum or retracted in the inguinal canal. You diagnose him with cryptorchism and advise his parents that he will likely need to have an orchiopexy at what age?

A) 12 to 24 months.
B) 36 to 48 months.
C) 5 years.
D) 7 years.
E) Orchiopexy is no longer considered necessary surgery.

The answer is A: Either one or both testes may be absent from the scrotum at birth in about one in five premature or low-birth-weight male infants and in 3% to 6% of full-term infants. Cryptorchism is found in 1% to 2% of male children after 1 year of age but can be confused with retractile testes that is associated with a strong cremasteric reflex, which requires no treatment. Cryptorchism should be surgically corrected before 12 to 24 months of age in attempt to reduce the risk of infertility, which occurs in up to 75% of male children with bilateral cryptorchism and in 50% of male children with unilateral cryptorchism.

It is not clear whether such early orchiopexy ultimately improves fertility. Some patients have underlying hypogonadism. Cryptorchism is also associated with testicular carcinoma, which predominantly affects the undescended testicle and with intra-abdominal malposition but can also occur on the unaffected side in up to 10% of cancers.

Additional Reading: Undescended testes (cryptorchidism) in children: clinical features and evaluation. In: *UpToDate*. 2022.

7. A 6-year-old boy presents to your office complaining of scrotal pain and you note swelling of the left testis. Appropriate management at this time should include which one of the following?

A) Elevate the scrotum and apply cold compresses.
B) Observe overnight and reexamine in the morning if unimproved.
C) Obtain a scrotal ultrasonography evaluation with Doppler color flow.
D) Obtain a computed tomographic scan of the pelvis.

The answer is C: Testicular torsion should be suspected in patients, who complain of acute scrotal pain and swelling. Delay in diagnosis may lead to compromised testicular viability and patient fertility. Associated conditions that may resemble testicular torsion yet do not require surgery include torsion of a testicular appendage, epididymitis/orchitis, trauma, incarcerated hernia, varicocele, and idiopathic scrotal edema. Testicular torsion is most common in men younger than 25 years; however, it can occur at any age. A diagnosis of testicular torsion until proven otherwise should be considered in a prepubertal child or a young adult man with acute scrotal pain.

On physical examination, higher testicular lie and absent cremasteric reflex support the diagnosis of testicular torsion. If diagnosis is unclear, proceed with scrotal imaging with ultrasonography evaluation and Doppler color flow. Once the correct diagnosis is established, prompt surgical evaluation should be performed. It is reasonable to perform manual detorsion for immediate noninvasive treatment followed by elective orchiopexy.

Additional Reading: Clinical diagnosis of testicular torsion. *Am Fam Physician*. 2022;106(6):712-713.

8. A 2-year-old girl is found to have symptomatic labial adhesions. Which one of the following is considered the first line of treatment?

A) Application of hydrocortisone cream
B) Application of estrogen cream
C) Application of testosterone cream
D) Gonadotropin-releasing hormone antagonist administration
E) Surgical separation

The answer is B: Labial adhesions are common in prepubertal girls. One possible explanation for the development of labial adhesions is that they arise from the combination of inflammation of the labia and low levels of circulating estrogen seen typically in prepubertal girls. They are usually identified on routine physical examination and may be partial or complete. Most women with partial labial adhesions are asymptomatic, but they can present with difficulty with urination, vulvar pain, vaginal pain or discharge, or recurrent urinary tract infections. Rarely, urinary retention may occur.

Asymptomatic adhesions do not usually require treatment and may resolve as the child develops, and higher levels of circulating estrogen are present. Symptomatic adhesions may be treated with a short course of estrogen cream applied twice daily for up to 4 weeks, which may cause the labia to separate. Beclomethasone cream has also been shown to be effective.

Additional Reading: Overview of vulvovaginal complaints in the prepubertal child. In: *UpToDate*. 2022.

9. An 11-year-old Black girl is in for a well-child check and her mother has a question about puberty. Regarding female sexual development, which one of the following statements is true?

A) Early maturation is associated with greater height.
B) Of the physical changes that occur during sexual maturation, breast development occurs last.
C) Menarche occurs approximately 2.5 years after thelarche (breast budding)
D) Menarche among Black females occurs at a later age compared to Caucasian females.
E) The onset of a height spurt correlates more with development of pubic hair compared with breast development.

The answer is C: Puberty refers to the gonadal activation by pituitary hormones, follicle-stimulating hormones, and luteinizing hormone. Today, normal pubertal development ranges from 10 to 16 years of age, with Black females maturing at a younger age compared with Caucasians. Compared with previous generations, adolescents today are reaching menarche at a younger age.

Early pubertal changes in females are triggered by an increase in the pulsatile secretion of gonadotropin-releasing hormone, signaling the development of breast tissue and skeletal growth often between 8 and 11 years of age. Breast development is often seen before pubic hair growth. The pubertal growth spurt begins with early puberty with peak height velocity being achieved before puberty is complete. Menarche typically occurs 2.5 years after thelarche.

Early pubertal maturation is associated with reaching earlier peak height growth velocity and final attainment of height. Later maturation is typically associated with a greater ultimate height due to a longer period of growth before the spurt. Final height results from a combination of skeletal age of pubertal onset and genetics.

Additional Reading: Physiology of puberty. *Nelson Textbook of Pediatrics*. 20th ed. Elsevier/Saunders; 2014.

10. Which one of the following statements concerning circumcision is true?

A) Circumcision can be performed in the office until 4 months of age.
B) Hypospadias is not a contraindication for circumcision.
C) It is medically indicated for all male children.
D) Male infants with posthitis should not be circumcised.
E) Premature infants should not be circumcised.

The answer is E: Routine circumcision is often performed out of social preference compared with medical necessity. However, urinary tract infections (UTIs) are seen 10 to 15 times more often in uncircumcised infants compared with those who are circumcised. Many recommend circumcision in infants predisposed to UTIs, including those with congenital hydronephrosis or vesicoureteral reflux. Other indications for circumcision include recurrent balanitis (inflammation of the glans), posthitis (inflammation of the foreskin), or paraphimosis (retraction of the prepuce behind the glans that may interfere with blood flow). Because phimosis (tightness of the foreskin so that it cannot be retracted over the glans penis) cannot usually be detected before puberty, it is not an indication for circumcision.

Contraindications for circumcision include prematurity, genital anomalies (including hypospadias or ambiguous genitalia), and bleeding disorders. Circumcision should be performed at least 12 to 24 hours after birth, within 6 weeks of birth, and before discharge from the hospital.

Typical anesthesia includes a dorsal penile nerve block with 1% lidocaine without epinephrine. EMLA cream can also be applied. Beyond 6 weeks of age, circumcision should be postponed until after 1 year of age and be performed with general anesthesia.

Additional Reading: Neonatal circumcision: techniques. In: *UpToDate*. 2022.

11. A young girl is in with her mother for her 10-year-old well-child check, and the mother is asking when she can expect to start menstruating. You inform them that the first sign of sexual development in girls is which one of the following?

A) The development of axillary hair
B) The development of breast buds
C) The development of pubic hair
D) The closure of the epiphyseal growth plates

The answer is B: The development of breast buds (subareolar tissue) is usually the first sign of puberty (8-13 years of age) in females. This is followed shortly thereafter by the development of pubic hair (6-12 months later) and then axillary hair.

Menarche occurs 2.0 to 2.5 years after the development of the breast buds. Peak height velocity occurs predominantly before menarche and then slows. Throughout puberty, the percentage of body fat increases and redistributes, giving rise to adult contours.

Precocious puberty is defined as the presence of breast development or pubic hair before 8 years of age. *Pubertal delay* is defined as the absence of breast development before the age of 13 years or the lack of menstruation 5 years after breast growth.

Additional Reading: Normal puberty. In: *UpToDate*. 2022.

The development of breast buds (subareolar tissue) is usually the first sign of puberty in girls.

12. Changes associated with puberty are relatively predictable. Which one of the following changes would be the first sign of puberty in boys?

A) A skeletal growth spurt
B) Enlargement of the penis
C) Spermarche
D) The development of pubic hair
E) Testicular enlargement

The answer is E: At the onset of puberty, boys undergo testicular enlargement followed by the appearance of pubic hair, enlargement of the penis, and then spermarche (the development of sperm in the testicles). Skeletal and muscle growth are late events in male puberty. The age at which pubertal milestones are attained varies and is influenced by activity level and nutritional status.

Additional Reading: Normal puberty. In: *UpToDate*. 2022.

The first sign of puberty in boys is testicular enlargement.

13. In a boy with delayed sexual development, which one of the following findings would be characteristic?

A) A lack of testicular development by 10 years of age
B) A lack of axillary hair growth by 13 years of age
C) A lapse of five or more years between the initial and completed growth of genitalia
D) A lack of pubic hair growth 1 year after the growth spurt
E) No pubertal-related voice changes before 15 years of age

The answer is C: Definitions of delayed sexual maturation in boys and girls are as follows:

Boys: A lack of testicular development by 14 years of age, pubic hair by 15 years of age, or 5 or more years between the initial and completed growth of the genitalia.

Girls: A lack of breast development by age 13 years, pubic hair before 14 years of age, or absent menstruation within 5 years of the development of breast buds, or if menstruation does not occur by 16 years of age.

Constitutional delay is an inherited delay in maturation that affects the child in a manner similar to that of the parents. Prepubertal growth is normal, but during adolescence, the growth spurt is delayed. Individuals with constitutional delay develop later; however, this development is considered normal. Constitutional delay tends to occur more often in boys than girls. If a girl presents with severe pubertal delay, she should be monitored for primary amenorrhea and a further workup pursued if indicated.

Additional Reading: Normal puberty. In: *UpToDate*. 2022.

14. A young male patient presents with painless swelling of his scrotum. On examination, you palpate a mass which you are able to transilluminate. A follow-up ultrasonography reveals a cystic structure. Which one of the following conditions is the most likely diagnosis for this presentation?

A) A hydrocele
B) A Leydig cell tumor
C) A spermatocele
D) A varicocele
E) Epididymis

The answer is A: A hydrocele is a relatively common condition, resulting from a fluid collection between the tunica vaginalis and the tunica albuginea, surrounding the testicle. It typically presents as a painless, enlarging, cystic structure that transilluminates. Etiology of hydrocele is usually congenital idiopathic but can be associated with injury, infection, and, rarely, tumor. Most cases do not require further treatment, unless the patient is symptomatic or a hernia occurs, at which point surgical consultation is recommended.

Ultrasonographic examination is not usually necessary, unless the diagnosis is uncertain, or the mass does not transilluminate. In these other cases, testicular tumor needs to be ruled out. In some cases, a communicating hydrocele may start out small in the early morning and enlarge throughout the day or may enlarge with Valsalva-type maneuvers (eg, coughing, crying, and changing position). Most hydroceles seen in newborns resolve during the first year, and parents require only reassurance.

A Leydig cell tumor develops from testicular Leydig cells, which are responsible for testosterone production. These are the cells in the testicles that release the male hormone, testosterone. They are most often found in men between 30 and 60 years of age. This tumor is not common in children before puberty, but it may cause early puberty.

A spermatocele is an abnormal cyst that develops in the epididymis. This is benign and generally painless; a spermatocele usually is filled with milky or clear fluid that might contain sperm.

A varicocele is the swelling of the veins inside the scrotum, which are found along the spermatic cord. Most of the time, varicoceles develop slowly. They are more common in men aged 15 to 25 years and are most often seen on the left side of the scrotum.

Epididymitis is inflammation of the epididymis, often caused by the spread of a bacterial infection. Epididymitis is most common in young men aged 19 to 35 years. Infection often begins in the urethra, the prostate, or the bladder. Gonorrhea and chlamydia infections are the most common pathogens in young heterosexual men. In children and older men, it is more commonly caused by *E coli* and similar bacteria.

Additional Reading: Scrotal masses. *Am Fam Physician*. 2022;106(2):184-189.

15. A mother brings her 4-year-old girl in to see you because she has been complaining of vaginal itching. The itching is most bothersome at night, right before going to bed. Considering her symptoms which one of the following organisms is likely causing her symptoms?

A) *A lumbricoides*
B) *Ancylostoma braziliense*
C) *Enterobius*
D) *Pthirus pubis*
E) *Gardnerella vaginalis*

The answer is C: *Enterobius* (pinworms) is the most common parasite among children in the United States, with a prevalence approaching 100% among those institutionalized. Infestation occurs via fomites, surviving for up to 3 weeks. Hand-to-mouth transfer of ova from the perianal area to clothing, bedding, furniture, rugs, and toys can be picked up by a new host, transmitted to the mouth, and swallowed. Although less common, airborne ova may be inhaled and then swallowed. Pinworms mature in the lower GI tract within 2 to 6 weeks, at which point the female worm migrates to the perianal region (usually at night) to deposit ova. Pruritus is caused by movements of the female worm. Most people with pinworm infestation are asymptomatic yet some present with perianal itching that can lead to excoriations from persistent scratching.

Young females presenting with vaginitis may have irritation from pinworm infestation. Diagnosis is confirmed either by microscopic identification of the ova or by finding the female worm, approximately 10 mm long in the perianal region 1 or 2 hours after the child goes to bed at night. In contrast, male worms are 3 mm in length.

The ova can be obtained in the early morning before the child arises by patting the perianal skinfolds with a strip of transparent adhesive tape. This procedure should be repeated on five successive mornings if it is necessary to rule out pinworm infestation.

Treatment, regardless of age, is a single dose of mebendazole, which will eradicate pinworms in about 90% of cases. Pyrantel pamoate can be used, with a repeat treatment after 2 weeks. Treat all symptomatic household members. Extensive hand washing and housekeeping have little effect on the control or treatment of pinworm infestation.

Additional Reading: Pinworms. In: Domino F, ed. *The 5-Minute Clinical Consult*. Wolters Kluwer; 2022.

Section XI. Nonspecific Systems

Each of the following questions or incomplete statements is followed by suggested answers or completions. Select the ONE BEST ANSWER in each case.

1. At what age would you expect children who are developing normally to articulate most words and know basic colors?

A) 3 years
B) 4 years
C) 5 years
D) 6 years
E) 7 years

The answer is B: Motor development during the preschool years results in children running, jumping, and climbing. Children learn to balance on one foot and hop. Vocabulary continues to develop rapidly with the mastery of hundreds of words. Language development proceeds with multiword sentences, the use of pronouns, and the gradual improvement in articulation skills. Children typically master the concept of numbers 1, 2, and 3 by 3.5 years. Four-year-old children should know basic colors and clearly articulate most words.

Additional Readings:
1. Screening for developmental delay. *Am Fam Physician*. 2011;84(5):544-549.
2. CDC's revised developmental milestone checklists. *Am Fam Physician*. 2022;106(4):370-371.

2. A mother is concerned that her 6-year-old son is hyperactive, because he can never seem to sit still for very long. Which one of the following statements is true regarding attention-deficit/hyperactivity disorder (ADHD)?

A) Combining psychosocial and drug therapy is always preferred over drug therapy alone.
B) Specific biologic markers are useful to make the diagnosis.
C) Stimulant medications are rarely beneficial.
D) Symptoms of ADHD typically progress over time.
E) The Conners ADHD Index is useful in identifying children with ADHD.

The answer is E: ADHD is the most common neurobehavioral disorder in childhood. Individuals with the disorder have developmentally inappropriate levels of attention, hyperactivity/impulsivity that result in impairment in areas of academic, social, and emotional functioning. Additionally, individuals with ADHD have a higher rate of comorbid learning, cognitive, language, motor, and behavioral health disorders. Conversely, individuals with developmental disorders, including autism spectrum disorder, have a greater risk of co-occurring ADHD.

Report on prevalence among children aged 3 to 17 years is reportedly 8.9%. Boys are twice as likely to be diagnosed with ADHD as girls. Prevalence increases with increasing age, from 2.1% in children 2 to 5 years of age to 11.9% in 12- to 17-year-olds. There is a strong heritability to the condition.

Core features of ADHD are hyperactivity, impulsivity, and inattention, but the phenotypic expression varies. The diagnosis of ADHD is behaviorally defined and derived from history.

Teacher and parent rating scales are useful to support the diagnosis of ADHD, but they are not diagnostic. They solicit information regarding the 9 core symptoms of both inattentive and hyperactive/impulsive subtypes of ADHD. Commonly used rating scales include the Conners ADHD Index and the Vanderbilt Assessment Scale, which are freely accessible.

First-line pharmacologic management of ADHD is with stimulant medications, which include methylphenidate or amphetamine preparations. Atomoxetine (Strattera) is a selective norepinephrine reuptake inhibitor; a second-tier medication for treatment of ADHD. It can be used as monotherapy or in combination with a stimulant.

Nonpharmacologic treatments such as behavioral modification and intensive contingency-management therapy may improve behavior and academic performance. Although combining drug and psychosocial therapy has not been shown to yield a clear advantage compared with drug therapy alone, it may help augment some of the behavioral components associated with ADHD, such as reducing anxiety and improving social skills.

Long-term follow-up of children with ADHD suggests that those whose symptoms are adequately managed have improved academic outcomes and lower rates of mood disorder, substance abuse, criminal behavior, motor vehicle accidents, injuries, and traumatic brain injuries.

Additional Reading: Attention-deficit/hyperactivity disorder: AAP updates guideline for diagnosis and management. *Am Fam Physician*. 2020;102(1):58-60.

3. Child safety seats have been proven to prevent morbidity and mortality when appropriately utilized. Which one of the following statements is true about the appropriate use of car safety devices?

A) A child no longer needs a forward-facing safety when their shoulders can reach beyond the back of the seat.
B) Low-back booster seats are safe to use in children greater than 40 pounds.
C) Newborn infants always face forward when placed in the backseat.
D) Once a child exceeds 40 pounds, the seat harness should be used.
E) Children can use a standard seat belt when it fits properly, that is, the lap belt is across the upper thighs and the shoulder belt is across the center of the shoulder and chest.

The answer is E: Motor vehicle accidents continue to be the leading cause of death in children 1 to 14 years of age. Although using safety seats can reduce children's morbidity and mortality, they are often misused. Engaging the parents in education regarding proper vehicle safety systems can help protect children in the event of a potentially fatal crash. Children should always sit in the backseat through at least 12 years of age.

Children should use a rear-facing seat from birth to 2-4 years of age.

After outgrowing their rear-facing seat, children should use a forward-facing care seat until 5 years of age. The seat should have a harness and a top tether.

Once a child outgrows their car seat, they should use a booster seat until the seatbelt fits properly as described above.

Additional Reading: Keep Child Passengers Safe on the Road, CDC.

Motor vehicle accidents are the leading cause of death in children 1 to 14 years of age.

4. Early sex education can alleviate the burden of which of the following?

A) Academic difficulties
B) Early sexual activity
C) Increased sexually transmitted diseases
D) Low socioeconomic status
E) Subsequent pregnancies

The answer is B: Early sex education can empower individuals with information that could influence their views on sexual activity from a young age. Engaging patients in early conversations about prevention of pregnancy and infection may reduce early sexual activity in adolescents. Without a proper understanding of safe sex, early sexual activity can lead to unintentional pregnancies and sexually transmitted infections (STIs).

The birth rate among teenagers has been steadily in decline, largely because of the increased use of contraception and more teens abstaining from sexual activity. In 2019, the teen birth rate was 16.7 per 1000 females, a record low. Racial and ethnic disparities exist, with the birth rates for Hispanic teens and non-Hispanic Black teens being more than two times higher than that for non-Hispanic white teens.

Only about 50% of teen mother receive a high school diploma by age 22 years, whereas 90% of women who do not give birth during adolescence graduate from high school.

Of the STI cases reported in the United States, about half occur in adolescents and young adults aged 15 to 24 years.

Additional Reading: About Teen Pregnancy, CDC.

5. All the following statements regarding childhood immunizations are true, except which one?

A) The measles-mumps-rubella (MMR) vaccine does not cause autism.
B) Hepatitis B vaccine is not associated with multiple sclerosis.
C) Children with egg allergies may be given the MMR vaccine.
D) Receiving multiple vaccinations preserved with thimerosal causes mercury poisoning.
E) Children with a prior local reaction to neomycin do not need to avoid the varicella vaccine.

The answer is D: The safety of vaccines has been called into question on multiple fronts, with groups alleging that vaccines can cause autism and lead to serious health issues and that additives, adjuvants, and preservatives in vaccines are unsafe. Currently, there is no credible evidence to support the claims that the MMR vaccine causes autism or that the hepatitis B vaccine causes multiple sclerosis.

Typical side effects to vaccination administration are local reactions of pain, swelling, and redness at the injection site and sometimes fever and irritability. Children with a history of egg allergy may be given MMR vaccine, even though it is derived from chick embryo fibroblast tissue culture. Traces of antibiotics such as neomycin, which is present in varicella (chickenpox), trivalent inactivated poliovirus, and measles-mumps-rubella-varicella vaccines, have been considered as possible causes of adverse reactions. Therefore, a history of anaphylactic reaction to neomycin is a contraindication to future immunization, whereas a local reaction is not.

Thimerosal was eliminated from routine childhood vaccines in 2001 due to concerns that multiple immunizations with vaccines containing this preservative could exceed recommended mercury exposures. All routinely recommended vaccines for US infants are available only as thimerosal-free formulations. The exception is the multidose influenza vaccine used in young children; however, mercury-free formulations are available.

Additional Reading: Counseling parents about vaccine safety. *Am Fam Physician*. 2008;78(11):1248.

6. Which one of the following statements is true regarding immunization for diphtheria and tetanus toxoids and acellular pertussis (DTaP) vaccine?

A) DTaP vaccine is made of inactivated strains of each bacterium.
B) Previous anaphylactic reactions to diphtheria-tetanus-pertussis (DTP) vaccines do not contraindicate future doses within the series.
C) Routine vaccination is recommended at 4, 6, and 12 months, with a booster at 5 years of age.
D) Routine vaccination with DTaP is recommended for all infants.
E) There is less pertussis toxin in DTP vaccine compared with DTaP vaccine.

The answer is D: To protect children from diphtheria, tetanus, and pertussis, DTaP is administered at 2, 4, 6, and 12 to 15 months, and an additional dose at 4 to 6 years. A booster dose of Tdap (tetanus, diphtheria and acellular pertussis) vaccine is recommended at 11 to 12 years of age.

The earliest pertussis vaccines contained the whole cell. While effective, local and systemic reactions to the whole-cell vaccine were common, leading to the development of more purified (acellular) pertussis vaccines. DTaP and TdaP vaccines contain diphtheria toxoid, tetanus toxoid and purified (acellular) pertussis. The Tdap vaccine contains less diphtheria toxoid than the DTaP formulations. DTP vaccines are no longer available in the United States.

DTaP vaccine is available in five combination vaccines that have different age indications and dosing schedules. DTaP vaccine is licensed for use up until 7 years of age; after that, a TdaP formulation should be used, although doing so is off-label for children 7 to 9 years of age.

Adolescents aged 13 to 18 years who did not get the Tdap vaccine or tetanus and diphtheria toxoid booster (11-12 years) should receive a single dose of Tdap vaccine. If the individual was not vaccinated according to a standard schedule, catch-up schedules should be reviewed for timing guidance. Subsequent diphtheria toxoid booster doses every 10 years are recommended for all patients without contraindications.

Contraindications to DTaP and TdaP vaccines include the following:

- Previous anaphylaxis to the vaccine
- Encephalopathy not attributable to another cause occurring within 7 days of vaccination

Precautions to vaccination with DTaP and TdaP vaccines include:

- Moderate or severe acute illness
- Progressive or unstable neurologic disorder
- Uncontrolled seizures
- Progressive encephalopathy
- Guillain-Barre syndrome within 6 weeks after a previous dose of tetanus-containing vaccine
- History of Arthus-type hypersensitivity reactions after a previous dose of diphtheria toxoid or tetanus-toxoid containing vaccine

Additional Reading: Diphtheria. The Pink Book, CDC.

7. All of the following vaccines are recommended for routine vaccination of children, except which one?

A) Diphtheria and tetanus toxoids and acellular pertussis (DTaP)
B) *H influenzae* type B
C) Hepatitis B
D) Live attenuated oral poliovirus vaccine (OPV)
E) Pneumococcal conjugate vaccine (PCV13)

The answer is D: The Sabin vaccine (OPV) for poliomyelitis prevention is an oral, live attenuated, trivalent vaccine that is given at 2, 4, and 18 months, and 5 years of age. Upon ingestion of the OPV, the attenuated polioviruses replicate in the intestinal mucosa and other sites. Vaccine viruses are excreted into the stool of the vaccinated person for up to 6 weeks after a dose and can spread from the vaccine recipient to a contact, leading to vaccine-associated paralytic polio (VAPP). In order to eliminate VAPP, the United States switched to exclusive use of the inactivated poliovirus vaccine (Salk vaccine) in 2000. The OPV vaccine it is still used abroad.

Additional Reading: Poliomyelitis, The Pink Book, CDC.

8. Which one of the following statements is true regarding preterm breast milk?

A) It typically requires fortification with human milk fortifiers.
B) It contains lower concentrations of important electrolytes and immunoglobulins.
C) It contains excessive amounts of calcium.
D) It contains the same components as breast milk produced at term.

The answer is A: The composition of breast milk in mothers of preterm infants does not adequately fulfill the demands of a preterm infant, who requires increased nutrients, compared with a term infant. Preterm breast milk contains higher concentrations of total and bound nitrogen, immunoglobulins, sodium, iron, chloride, and medium-chain fatty acids. However, it may not contain sufficient amounts of phosphorus, calcium, copper, and zinc. Preterm infants are more likely to require fortification with human milk fortifiers to correct these deficiencies. After 4 weeks, the breast milk will satisfy most of the nutritional demands of the infant.

Additional Reading: Enteral nutrition components. In: *The Harriet Lane Handbook. A Manual for Pediatric House Officers*. 22nd ed. Elsevier; 2021.

9. Which one of the following statements about the genetic disorder Down syndrome (trisomy 21) is true?

A) Affected children have an increased risk of leukemia.
B) Infertility is preserved in all cases.
C) Most affected children have normal intelligence quotients (IQs).
D) The average life span is increased compared with the normal population.
E) Younger maternal age is associated with an increased risk.

The answer is A: Down syndrome is genetically characterized by the presence of additional chromosome 21 genetic material (trisomy 21). The condition may result from sporadically occurring meiotic nondisjunction (95% occur in egg), translocation (3%-4%), or mosaicism (1%-2%). Common physical findings include a flattened, hypoplastic midface with a depressed nasal bridge, hypotonicity, small brachycephalic head, epicanthal folds, upward slanting palpebral fissures, small mouth, and ears, Brushfield spots (gray to white spots around the periphery of the iris), excessive skin at the nape of the neck, single transverse palmar crease, short fifth finger clinodactyly, and wide spacing between the first and second toes. The degree of cognitive impairment is variable and may be mild (IQ of 50-70), is usually moderate (IQ of 35-50), and is occasionally severe (IQ of 20-35). Delays in development are common.

Associated medical conditions include congenital heart defects in 50%; gastrointestinal atresia (12%); hearing loss (75%); eye problems (60%-89%); autoimmune disorders, including Hashimoto thyroiditis (13%-39%); and leukemia (1%).

Fifteen percent to 30% of women with trisomy 21 are fertile, and there is an up to a 50% risk that their fetus will also have the condition.

Additional Reading: Role of the family physician in the care of children with Down syndrome. *Am Fam Physician*. 2014;90(12):851-858.

> **Down syndrome is genetically characterized by the presence of additional chromosome 21 material (trisomy 21).**

10. Which one of the following statements is true regarding infectious mononucleosis?

A) Glaucoma can be seen with prolonged cases.
B) Guillain-Barré syndrome is an associated complication.
C) Heterophile agglutination tests are usually positive at the onset of the disease.
D) Rupture of the aorta has been associated with the disease.
E) The disease can result in positive RF formation.

The answer is B: Infections with Epstein-Barr virus (EBV) are extremely common but not always apparent clinically. In low socioeconomic groups, 70% to 90% of children will have EBV seropositivity by 5 years of age. In developed countries, primary infections tend to occur at a later age, that is, adolescence to young adulthood. *Infectious mononucleosis* describes the clinical syndrome caused by the EBV and others, which generally affects individuals between 10 and 35 years of age. Symptoms include fever, sore throat, anorexia, generalized fatigue, lymphadenopathy (especially affecting the posterior cervical chain), splenomegaly, and a maculopapular rash. Hepatitis with hepatomegaly is often seen with occasional jaundice.

Laboratory findings include leukocytosis with many atypical lymphocytes (ie, larger with vacuolated cytoplasm) and a positive heterophile agglutination test (Monospot) before the second week following the onset of illness. The heterophile agglutination test is usually negative in infants and children younger than 4 years. The Centers for Disease Control and Prevention states that Monospot is not recommended for general use, as the antibodies detected by Monospot can be caused by conditions other than infectious mononucleosis. Moreover, studies have shown that Monospot produces both false-positive and false-negative results.

Complications include the development of Guillain-Barré syndrome, myocarditis, and encephalitis. Spleen rupture may occur with trauma; therefore, contact sports should be avoided until the splenomegaly has resolved.

Additional Reading: *About Infectious Mononucleosis; Epstein-Barr Virus and Infectious Mononucleosis*. CDC.

11. A 2-year-old girl is brought in by her mother because she has a low-grade fever and has been less active than usual. On examination, she does not appear to be ill but has an erythematous rash on the face, with a slapped-cheek appearance. The mother reports that the rash has spread to involve her trunk, but it appears that her extremities are spared. Which one of the following conditions is the most likely diagnosis to explain this child's presentation?

A) Congenital syphilis
B) Erythema infectiosum
C) Measles
D) Meningococcemia
E) Rubeola

The answer is B: Erythema infectiosum is referred to as *fifth disease* because it represents the fifth major viral childhood illness (the first four being measles, mumps, rubella, and rubeola). The disease is caused by parvovirus B19 and is characterized by mild constitutional symptoms, such as low-grade fever, malaise, and joint pain (particularly in adult women). The classic rash is an indurated, erythematous maculopapular facial rash that may progress to the trunk and extremities (but spares the palms and soles). The rash is often more pronounced on extensor surfaces. The "slapped-cheek" appearance of the rash is exacerbated with exposure to sunlight, heat, emotional stress, or fever.

The illness usually lasts 5 to 10 days, and only symptomatic treatment is necessary; however, complications can include arthropathies, myocarditis, and a transient aplastic crisis. Fifth disease may occasionally cause fetal death secondary to fetal hydrops. Pregnant women should avoid contact with affected patients.

With the onset of rash, children are no longer infectious, as the rash and arthropathy (if present) are immune-mediated, postinfectious reactions. Isolation from school and day care is not necessary.

Additional Reading: Common skin rashes in children. *Am Fam Physician*. 2015;92(3):211-216.

When children present with the classic "slapped-cheek" rash of erythema infectiosum, also known as *fifth disease*, they are no longer infectious. Isolation from school and/or day care is not necessary.

12. You are seeing a 6-year-old boy with pica and a concern for iron intoxication. You inform his parents that the first-line treatment for iron poisoning is which one of the following?

A) Deferoxamine
B) $CaNa_2EDTA$
C) Penicillamine
D) Plasmapheresis
E) Pralidoxime chloride

The answer is A: For the most part, childhood iron poisonings are unintentional and result in minimal consequences. The most serious ingestions involve prenatal vitamins or ferrous sulfate supplements, which have more elemental iron per tablet (60-65 mg) than other iron preparations. An addition factor is that these are often brightly colored and sugar-coated, with a candylike appearance.

There are five stages associated with iron intoxication:

Stage 1. The patient experiences a hemorrhagic gastroenteritis, which occurs 30 to 60 minutes after ingestion and lasts for 4 to 6 hours. It may result in hematemesis, abdominal pain, irritability, explosive diarrhea, shock, coma, and metabolic acidosis.

Stage 2. This is a symptom-free period, which may last up to 24 hours.

Stage 3. With iron levels >500 mg/dL, there is usually a period of delayed shock. This occurs within the first 48 hours after ingestion. Cerebral dysfunction, fever, seizures, and coma may occur.

Stage 4. Two to 5 days after ingestion, liver damage starts to appear and may lead to hepatic failure. Other manifestations include coagulopathies and hypoglycemia.

Stage 5. Two to 5 weeks after the initial ingestion, gastrointestinal scarring, bowel obstruction, and pyloric stenosis may develop. There may be hyperglycemia and leukocytosis. If serum iron level is >300 mg/dL, an abdominal radiograph may demonstrate the presence of iron particles. Severe poisoning may cause seizures, coma, pulmonary edema, and vascular collapse. Treatment involves induction of vomiting, gastric lavage, and the use of the chelating agent deferoxamine. In severe cases, hemodialysis and exchange transfusion may be necessary.

$CaNa_2EDTA$ is a chelating agent that helps manage poisoning with lead or mercury.

Penicillamine is a copper-chelating agent used to treat Wilson disease.

Pralidoxime chloride treats organophosphate-inactivated acetylcholinesterase poisoning.

Additional Reading: Acute iron poisoning. In: *UpToDate*. 2022.

13. The immunization schedule to follow for premature infants weighing less than 2000 g (except for the administration of hepatitis B vaccine) is which one of the following?

A) Administer immunizations according to their gestational age.
B) Administer immunizations according to their chronologic age.
C) Administer immunizations after 6 months of age, when their immune system is fully developed.
D) Administer immunizations at a younger chronologic age because of their increased susceptibility to vaccine-preventable diseases.
E) Administer immunizations according to the regular schedule but titrate the dosage to adjust for the infant's body weight.

The answer is B: Immunizations should take place at the same chronological ages as for term infants with no adjustments made for premature age. One exception to this recommendation is that hepatitis B vaccination should be delayed in infants who weigh less than 2000 g at birth for 1 month if mothers are negative for hepatitis B surface antigen. Preterm infants weighing less than 2000 g at birth had a decreased response to hepatitis B vaccine; however, by 1-month chronological age, they are as likely to respond as are term infants.

Additional Reading: Immunization in preterm and low birth weight infants. https://redbook.solutions.aap.org/chapter.aspx?sectionid=88187007&bookid=1484. Hepatitis B, The Pink Book, CDC.

14. Children born of teenage mothers are at increased risk for neurodevelopmental disorders. Which one of the following conditions is associated with children of teenage mothers?

A) Cognitive delays
B) Major depression
C) Manic depressive disorder
D) Schizophrenia
E) Suicide

The answer is A: The children of teenage mothers tend to have cognitive delays on intelligence quotient and vocabulary tests. They may also have difficulty with regulating emotion, with displays of rebelliousness, aggressiveness, uncontrollable anger, and impulsiveness. These children are at a greater risk for low birth weight, have a higher chance of experiencing an accident within the home, and are at an increased risk of being hospitalized before 5 years of age. There does not appear to be an association with major affective disorders.

Additional Reading: *Pregnancy in adolescents*. In: *UpToDate*. 2022.

15. Rabies in humans is rare in the United States, but it is recommended that bites from which one of the following animals be treated with rabies postexposure prophylaxis?

A) Fox
B) Gerbil
C) Hamster
D) Rat
E) Squirrel

The answer is A: The Centers for Disease Control and Prevention estimates that up to 40,000 US citizens receive postexposure prophylaxis annually. The risk of infection must be carefully evaluated by the clinician in the management of potential human rabies exposures. More than 90% of reported rabies in animals occurs in wildlife. If bitten by bats, skunks, raccoons, foxes, and most other carnivores, the patient should receive postexposure prophylaxis. Contact with infected bats is the leading cause of human rabies deaths in the United States. Bites from squirrels, hamsters, guinea pigs, gerbils, chipmunks, rats, mice, other small rodents, rabbits, and hares almost never require antirabies postexposure prophylaxis. Administration of postexposure prophylaxis should be done without delay.

Additional Reading: Animals and Rabies. The Centers for Disease Control and Prevention (CDC). https://www.cdc.gov/rabies/index.html.

16. You are seeing a new mother in the postpartum care unit and she is trying to breastfeed. You encourage her efforts and inform her that which one of the following statements about breastfeeding is true?

A) Immediately after delivery, infants should feed at the breast.
B) Colostrum is excreted 7 to 10 days after delivery and contains important antibodies, high calories, and other nutrients.
C) Infants should be weighed before and after each feeding to quantify consumption.
D) Breastfeeding alone provides adequate nutrition for the first 2 to 4 months.
E) Breastfeeding should be based on timed intervals rather than on demand.

The answer is A: Breastfeeding is encouraged for all mothers, and as many as 77% of mothers initiate breastfeeding. The newborn infant should feed at the breast beginning within 1 hour of delivery. Early nursing in the delivery room is associated with an increase in the percentage of mothers who continue breastfeeding at 2 to 4 months post partum compared with initiation 2 hours after birth.

Infants may be sleepy or hungry after birth; less frequent, small feedings are often seen. After 24 hours of age, the infant should feed 8 to 12 feedings in a day. Breastfed infants often require more frequent feedings than bottle-fed infants. Breastfeeding should occur based on the infant's demand as opposed to by scheduled feedings.

Colostrum, a yellowish fluid excreted from the breast immediately after delivery, contains important antibodies, high calories and protein, and nutrients, and helps stimulate the passage of meconium. Delaying breastfeeding, attempting to quantify amount of feeding with weights before and after feedings, and providing infant formula led to decreased breast-feeding among women.

Breastfeeding provides adequate nutrition for up to 6 to 9 months.

Additional Readings:
1. Strategies for breastfeeding success. *Am Fam Physician*. 2008;78(2):225-232.
2. Primary interventions to support breastfeeding. *Am Fam Physician*. 2017;95(8):517-518.

Breastfed infants often require more frequent feedings than bottle-fed infants. Breastfeeding should occur based on the infant's demand as opposed to scheduled feedings.

17. Which one of the following is excreted into breast milk and should be avoided by women who are breastfeeding?

A) Alcohol
B) Amitriptyline
C) Digoxin
D) Heparin
E) Penicillin

The answer is A: Nicotine and alcohol are excreted into breast milk and should be avoided by mothers who are breastfeeding. Breast milk alcohol levels closely parallel maternal blood alcohol levels. The highest alcohol levels in milk occur within 30 minutes of ingestion. Clearance of alcohol from breast milk is related to many factors such as food consumption and the number of drinks consumed.

Nicotine and its metabolites are present in the breast milk of individuals who inhale nicotine or use transdermal delivery patches. Nicotine is thought to be a causative factor in sudden infant death syndrome. It is also associated with decreased breast milk yields.

Amitriptyline, digoxin, and heparin are not excreted into breast milk, and their use is not a contraindication to breastfeeding.

Medication compatibility with breastfeeding is categorized as (1) compatible, (2) use with caution, (3) unknown with concerns, (4) contraindicated, and (5) safety not established. Many references are available to research drug and supplement compatibility with breastfeeding and ideally would be consulted when counseling the breastfeeding parent.

Additional Reading: *Drugs and Lactation Database (LactMed)*. National Library of Medicine, NIH.

18. Breastfeeding has been shown to have many benefits. Which one of the following is associated with early breastfeeding?

A) Fewer apneic spells
B) Higher rates of postpartum depression
C) Improved growth in the first 2 months of life
D) Lower risk of aspiration pneumonia
E) More robust temperature stability

The answer is E: Mothers of newborn infants should initiate breastfeeding as soon as possible after giving birth. When mothers initiate breastfeeding within a half hour of birth, the infant is alert and has a strong suckling reflex, which facilitates feeding. Early breastfeeding is associated with less nighttime feeding problems and better mother-infant bonding. These infants have a higher core temperature and are less prone to temperature instability. The other findings are not associated with early breastfeeding.

Additional Readings:
1. Strategies for breastfeeding success. *Am Fam Physician*. 2008;78(2):225-232.
2. Primary interventions to support breastfeeding. *Am Fam Physician*. 2017;95(8):517-518.

19. Which one of the following foods has been associated with causing botulism in children younger than 1 year?

A) Corn syrup
B) Honey
C) Peanuts
D) Organic cereals
E) Rice cookies

The answer is B: Infant botulism is caused by the ingestion of *botulinum* spores of *Clostridium botulinum*, which produce the toxin in vivo. Honey contains *botulinum* spores and should not be given to children younger than 1 year. Constipation is a common presenting symptom, followed by neuromuscular paralysis of the cranial nerves and progressing to the peripheral and respiratory musculature. Cranial nerve deficits include ptosis, extraocular muscle palsies, weak cry, poor suck, decreased gag reflex, pooling of oral secretions, and an expressionless face. Severity ranges from mild lethargy and slowed feeding to severe hypotonia and respiratory insufficiency. Infants affected are typically between 2 and 3 months of age. Finding *C botulinum* toxin in stool, serum, or food or by culturing botulism neurotoxin-producing species of *Clostridium* from stool confirms the diagnosis.

Treatment is primarily supportive and may involve mechanical ventilation. Administration of an antitoxin may be considered. BabyBIG, Botulism Immune Globulin Intravenous (Human), is available to treat infant botulism types A and B in patients under 15 months of age.

Five kinds of botulism are described: infant botulism, foodborne botulism, wound botulism, iatrogenic botulism, and adult intestinal botulism.

Foodborne botulism is caused by toxin produced by anaerobe *C botulinum*. Symptoms occur within 24 hours after ingestion of contaminated food (usually canned). Symptoms include dry mouth, diplopia, dysarthria, dysphagia, decreased visual acuity, nausea, vomiting, abdominal cramps, and diarrhea. Neurologic disorders include weakness and eventual paralysis, which can lead to respiratory failure and death. Sensory function remains intact. Early treatment with Botulism Antitoxin Heptavalent without waiting for laboratory confirmation if the disease is suspected is warranted.

Additional Reading: Clinical guidelines for the diagnosis and treatment of botulism, 2021. *MMWR*. 2021;70(2):1-30.

20. A 20-month-old girl is brought to the office by her mother, who is concerned about a recent loss of appetite and increasing irritability as well. The child has seemed happy, and she enjoys exploring around the house. The family lives in an old farmhouse in a rural area and drinks well water. You are concerned about lead poisoning. Which of the following statements will be important to discuss with the family regarding this diagnosis?

A) Neurologic deficits are not routinely associated with lead poisoning.
B) Removing lead hazards from the environment before a child is exposed is the most effective way to protect children from the harmful effects of lead exposure.
C) Routine screening for arsenic in well water could have presented the present illness.
D) Symptoms include vomiting, irritability, weight loss, and abdominal pain.
E) Treatment will be with deferoxamine.

The answer is B: Children living in housing built before 1978 and those from low-income households are at highest risk of lead exposure. Children less than 6 years of age are at a higher risk due to frequent hand to mouth activities and greater absorption of lead. Common sources of lead include dust from lead-based paints, paint chips containing lead paint, some water pipes, toys, jewelry, some home remedies, solder, glazed pottery, some candles, some imported spices, and fumes from burning batteries. Lead was banned from paint for residential use in 1978. The use of leaded gasoline was banned in the United States in 1996.

Most children with lead exposure are asymptomatic. In 2021, the Centers for Disease Control and Prevention updated its blood lead reference value (BLRV) from 5.0 μg/dL to 3.5 μg/dL. A BLRV is intended to identify children with higher levels of lead in their blood compared with levels in most children. It is not a health-based standard or a toxicity level but is meant to be used as guide to determine whether medical or environmental follow-up are needed.

Management of confirmed blood levels over 3.5 μg/dL is based upon the blood lead level. Levels 45 μg/dL or higher may cause confusion, irritability, weakness, seizures, coma, nausea, vomiting, and abdominal pain. Presence of such symptoms is an indication to admit the child to the hospital for chelation treatment.

Arsenic can also contaminate well water. Poisoning presents with abdominal pain, rice-water stools, and garlic breath, which this child does not have. An evaluation would be to test a spot urine, with an arsenic level of greater than 1000 μg/L considered diagnostic.

Arsenic poisoning is treated with dimercaptosuccinic acid, penicillamine, or dimercaprol.

Additional Reading: *Childhood Lead Poisoning Prevention Program*. CDC. www.cdc.gov/nceh/lead.

21. A 5-year-old girl is brought to your office by her mother with painful swelling and sores inside her mouth and a vesicular rash that affects her hands and feet. Which one of the following is the most likely etiologic agent to account for this patient's presentation?

A) Adenovirus
B) Coxsackie virus
C) Measles
D) Syphilis
E) Varicella

The answer is B: Coxsackie virus is responsible for various infections that affect the pediatric population. There are differences between the two major types of Coxsackie virus:

Coxsackie virus A

- A16 causes a mild hand, foot, and mouth disease. Findings include stomatitis and a vesicular rash that affects the hands and feet. It is usually mild, affects young children, and may occur in epidemics.
- A2, A4, A5, A6, A7, and A10 cause more severe herpangina. Findings include severe fever that can lead to febrile seizures. Other findings include severe sore throat, vesiculoulcerative lesions of the tonsils, soft palate, and posterior pharynx, headache, myalgias, and emesis.

Coxsackie virus B

- B1, B2, B3, B4, and B5 cause pleurodynia with pain associated with the area of diaphragmatic attachment. Other symptoms include fever, headache, sore throat, malaise, and emesis. Orchitis and pleurisy may be present. Patients with pleurodynia are children or young adults, presenting with severe pleuritic pain, tachypnea, and systemic upset. It is self-limited, and antibiotics are only helpful if there is a secondary bacterial infection. Coxsackie virus B infection is rare in persons older than 60 years; it is more common in children and young adults.

Transmission of the viruses occurs by hand-to-mouth contact and may become widespread. Coxsackie virus has been called "the great pretender" because of various clinical syndromes it can produce. Although most infections are subclinical, more serious conditions include myocarditis, orchitis, myalgia, and pleurodynia.

Additional Reading: COVID-19 Vaccine Safety in Children and Teens | CDC.

22. In a case of school avoidance, what is the most appropriate approach?

A) Allow the child to remain at home until reasons for avoidance are determined.
B) Begin methylphenidate.
C) Begin inpatient psychotherapy.
D) Change teachers or schools.
E) Return the child to school and determine reasons for school avoidance.

The answer is E: School refusal is common and can be accompanied by a variety of physical symptoms which may emulate organic medical problems School avoidance peaks at ages associated with transitions such as entering Kindergarten or middle school. Underlying separation anxiety, generalized anxiety disorder, oppositional defiant disorder, and major depressive disorder may be present. Children may avoid school due to issues with teachers or other adults in the school, bullying, social humiliation, fear of possible failure, or fear of public performance.

Clinicians should use the initial interview to build rapport and trust while taking a holistic approach to data gathering. Organic disease should be ruled out by a thorough history and physical examination coupled with judicious use of laboratory testing.

The parents, clinician, and school personnel must agree upon the shared goal to have the child return to school as soon as possible without waiting upon results of a medical investigation. Specific criteria for school absence, such as presence of an objective fever, need to be discussed and agreed upon.

Treatment may include referral to a mental health professional and is recommended when the child is unresponsive to management; the child has been out of school for more than 2 months; the child has depression, panic attacks, or psychosis; or the family is unable to cooperate with the treatment plan.

Additional Readings:
1. School refusal in children and adolescents. *Am Fam Physician*. 2003;68(8):1555-1561.
2. School absenteeism in children and adolescents. *Am Fam Physician*. 2018;98(12):738-744.

23. You are assessing a newborn and note significant hypotonia on examination. You consider that the infant may have an underlying congenital condition such as Prader-Willi Syndrome (PWS). Which set of the following characteristics would describe a typical patient with PWS?

A) Obese, with hypogonadism and an intellectual disability
B) Short, obese, and precocious puberty
C) Tall, with a long arm span and an increased risk of aortic rupture
D) Thin, with an intellectual disability and precocious puberty

The answer is A: PWS is characterized by decreased fetal movements extreme hypotonia in infancy, growth faltering in infancy, childhood-onset hyperphagia and obesity, intellectual disability. Hypogonadotropic hypogonadism, short stature, small hands and feet, and characteristic facial features are commonly present. Facial characteristics include a narrow bitemporal dimension, almond-shaped eyes, and thin upper lips with downturned corners. Hip dysplasia, scoliosis, and kyphosis may occur. Males should be evaluated for cryptorchidism.

PWS results from the loss of the paternally derived genes from the proximal arm of chromosome 15. There are 3 ways in which this can occur: deletion in the paternally contributed chromosome, maternal uniparental disomy, and an error in the imprinting process.

Deletion of the paternally contributed chromosome is responsible for PWS in over 70% of cases.

In uniparental disomy the individual receives two copies of a chromosome from one parent. In maternal uniparental disomy, active and imprinted paternal genes are not present. Maternal uniparental disomy accounts for about 28% of cases.

Imprinting errors account for less than 2% of PWS cases. In these instances, paternally derived genes are present but not expressed.

Obesity accounts for most cases of morbidity and mortality. Deaths are often the result of cardiorespiratory failure or complications of sleep apnea. Optimal care is best delivered by a multidisciplinary care team.

Additional Reading: Prader-Willi syndrome. In: Domino F, ed. *The 5-Minute Clinical Consult*. Wolters Kluwer; 2022.

PWS is characterized by failure to thrive due to hypotonia and feeding difficulties, which generally improve after 6 to 12 months of age, followed by an uncontrollable appetite with an increase in weight and obesity. The syndrome is caused by two copies of the maternal gene and none of the father's genes on chromosome 15.

24. Varicella-zoster immunoglobulin (VariZIG) postexposure prophylaxis is recommended for which of the following groups?

A) All newborns
B) Hospitalized premature infants older than 28 weeks of gestation, regardless of the mother's history of chickenpox
C) Newborns of mothers with onset of varicella 5 days before delivery
D) Newborns greater than 4500 g regardless of exposure history or mother's exposure history
E) Pregnant women just before delivery who have no history of varicella and were exposed at the time of conception

The answer is C: VariZIG for postexposure prophylaxis is indicated for the prevention of varicella infections in the following groups:

- Neonates whose mothers have varicella around the time of delivery (ie, 5 days before to 2 days after delivery)
- Hospitalized preterm infants born at 28 weeks gestation or later whose mothers do not have evidence of immunity
- Immunocompromised patients without evidence of immunity to varicella
- Pregnant women without evidence of immunity
- Hospitalized premature infants born at 28 weeks gestation or earlier or who weigh 1000 g or less at delivery regardless of maternal history.

VariZIG is given by intramuscular injection. One vial (125 U) is given for each 10 kg of body weight, with a maximum dose of 625 U (five vials). The minimum dose is 62.5 IU (0.5 vial) for patients weighing less than or equal to 2 kg and 125 IU (one vial) for patients weighing 2.1 to 10.0 kg. VariZIG should be given as soon as possible after exposure and within 10 days.

The most common adverse effects of VariZIG are pain at injection site and headache.

Current recommendations include routine vaccination of all children with a single dose of live varicella virus vaccine (Varivax) between 12 and 18 months of age with a second dose between 4 and 6 years of age.

Additional Reading: Updated recommendations for use of VariZIG-United 'states, 2013. *MMWR*. 2013;62(28):574-576.

25. A mother calls you concerned that her child is having "nightmares," as he is waking up in the middle of the night crying and shrieking. Once she settles him down, he goes back to sleep without difficulty. He has otherwise been well and seems to be his usual self the next day. You inform her that it sounds like he is having night terrors. Which one of the following statements about night terrors is true?

A) Adults are more often affected than children.
B) Benzodiazepines should not be prescribed in this situation.
C) They occur during rapid eye movement sleep.
D) They occur during stages of slow-wave sleep
E) Vivid details are often remembered the next morning.

The answer is D: Night terrors occur more frequently in children than in adults. They represent partial awakenings from slow-wave sleep and are characterized by pallor, sweating, pupillary dilation, piloerection, and tachycardia. The child may sit up and scream and appear terrified, and may thrash or run. During a night terror, a child is often unresponsive to parental interventions or soothing. Up to 3% of children will experience the condition, with age of onset at 18 months and resolution by 8 years of age. They do not reflect emotional disturbance but will increase with illness, stress or sleep deprivation Episodes tend to occur in clusters. Most often, the episodes happen in the first third to half of the night.

Parents need to be reassured about the benign nature of these events. In contrast, nightmares occur during rapid eye movement sleep and are frequently remembered in vivid detail.

A short course of diazepam can help patients with severe night terrors, but episodes may recur when the child is weaned or when tolerance develops.

Additional Reading: Common sleep disorders in children. *Am Fam Physician*. 2005;72(7):1322.

26. A woman who is regularly drinking alcohol during her pregnancy is most likely to have a child with which one of the following findings?

A) Hepatitis
B) Low birth weight
C) Palmar erythema
D) Peripheral neuropathy
E) Seizures

The answer is B: Fetal alcohol spectrum disorders (FASD) refer to spectrum of neurobehavioral, physical, and growth abnormalities that occur as a result of prenatal exposure to alcohol. Prenatal alcohol exposure is among the leading causes of developmental disabilities worldwide. Several disorders are contained in the umbrella term of FASD. Fetal alcohol syndrome represents the most severe end of the FASD spectrum and has well-defined clinical diagnostic features. Physical findings of FAS include growth deficiency, smooth philtrum, thin vermillion border, small palpebral fissures, and central nervous system abnormalities that can include microcephaly. Other disorders in the FASD spectrum include partial fetal alcohol syndrome, alcohol-related birth defects, and alcohol-related neurodevelopmental disorder.

There is no defined safe level of alcohol use during pregnancy, and all pregnant women should be advised to abstain from alcohol use throughout pregnancy.

Additional Reading: Fetal alcohol syndrome and fetal alcohol spectrum disorders. *Am Fam Physician*. 2017;96(8):515-522A.

27. Which one of the following is the mostly likely finding to be seen in a patient with Klinefelter syndrome?

A) An extra Y chromosome on karyotyping
B) Precocious puberty
C) Profound intellectual disability
D) Short stature and hirsutism
E) Tall stature with disproportionately long arms and legs

The answer is E: Klinefelter syndrome is a congenital anomaly that occurs in males about 1 to 2.5/1000 and is the result of additional X chromosome of either maternal or paternal origin. Karyotype is 47/XXY in 80% to 90% of cases, but mosaicism can occur. Rarely, men will have more than 2 copies of the X chromosome, for example, XXXY. The phenotype of Klinefelter syndrome is variable and can be correlated with androgen receptor sensitivity, with less sensitivity resulting in a more severe phenotype. Androgen receptor sensitivity is determined by trinucleotide repeats in the noncoding region of the receptor gene.

Infants with Klinefelter syndrome may have micropenis, hypospadias, and cryptorchidism.

Adolescents tend to have delayed puberty onset, scant facial and pubic hair, and absence of testicular enlargement.

Adults with Klinefelter syndrome tend to be tall, with disproportionately long arms and legs. Testes are generally small and firm due to progressive fibrosis and destruction of functional compartments of the testes. Gynecomastia and sexual dysfunction can occur.

Additional Reading: Clinical features, diagnosis and management of klinefelter syndrome. In: *UpToDate*. 2022.

Klinefelter syndrome is associated with the XXY karyotype. Clinical presentation varies, and many men are normal in appearance and intellect, and are typically only detected during a workup for infertility.

28. Measles immunization is accomplished with a vaccine given as part of the measles-mumps-rubella (MMR) vaccine. All of the following statements about measles immunizations are true, except which one?

A) Severe allergies to neomycin are contraindications to the measles vaccine.
B) Those who received a live attenuated measles immunization between 1963 and 1967 should receive a live attenuated booster vaccination.
C) Two doses of MMR are recommended, the first between 12 and 15 months of age and the second between 4 and 6 years of age.
D) Current immunization uses an attenuated line of measles virus.
E) Those born before 1956 are most likely immune.

The answer is B: Measles immunization is accomplished with a live-attenuated virus vaccine given at 12 to 15 months of age as part of the MMR vaccine. A booster dose is given at the preschool physical between 4 and 6 years of age. Infants vaccinated before 12 months of age should receive two additional boosters.

Those vaccinated with the inactivated (killed) measles vaccine in the United States from 1963 to 1967 should be given the live attenuated vaccine, as the inactivated vaccine preparation was ineffective. Those born before 1956 are most likely immune to measles because of natural infection, and they do not require any additional vaccination.

Contraindications for measles vaccination include prior anaphylactic reaction to neomycin.

Additional Reading: Measles, The Pink Book (Centers for Disease Control and Prevention). www.cdc.gov/measles/index.html.

29. Recommendations to ensure successful breastfeeding include all except the following:

A) Help mothers initiate breastfeeding within 1 hour of delivery
B) Practice rooming-in—allow mothers and infants to remain together 24 hours/d
C) Provide lactation support and teaching
D) Offer supplemental formula via bottle routinely

The answer is D: While data are sparse on adverse effects of pacifier use in the newborn period, there is more robust evidence to demonstrate that bottle-feeding formula reduces the prevalence of breastfeeding after discharge. The United Nations Children's Fund/World Health Organization Baby-Friendly Hospital Initiative© UNICEF lists 10 steps to ensure breastfeeding success in the hospital:

Step 1: Have a written breastfeeding policy that is routinely communicated to all health care staff.
Step 2: Train all health care staff in skills necessary to implement this policy.
Step 3: Inform all pregnant women about the benefits and management of breastfeeding.
Step 4: Help mothers initiate breastfeeding within 1 hour of birth.
Step 5: Show mothers how to breastfeed and how to maintain lactation even if they are separated from their infants.
Step 6: Give newborns no food or drink other than human milk, unless medically indicated.
Step 7: Practice rooming-in—allow mothers and infants to remain together—24 hours a day.
Step 8: Encourage breastfeeding on demand.
Step 9: Give no artificial teats or pacifiers to breastfeeding infants.
Step 10: Foster the establishment of breastfeeding support groups and refer mothers to them on discharge from the hospital or clinic.

Available at www.unicef.org/nutrition/index_24806.html

Additional Readings:
1. Strategies for breastfeeding success. *Am Fam Physician*. 2008;78(2):225-232.
2. Primary interventions to support breastfeeding. *Am Fam Physician*. 2017;95(8):517-518.

28. An adolescent comes to the office for an annual examination. Screening for which one of the following should be routinely performed?

A) Anemia
B) Hyperlipidemia
C) Sexually transmitted infections (if sexually active)
D) Tuberculosis
E) Urinary tract infections

The answer is C: Several organizations have developed guidelines for adolescent preventative health services. The Society for Adolescent Health and Medicine's guidelines focus on similarities between the different entities and encourages the following screenings:

- Hypertension.
- Obesity and eating disorders.
- Hyperlipidemia, if indicated (note that Bright Futures recommends universal hyperlipidemia screening once between 17 and 21 years of age).
- Tuberculosis, if at risk.
- Physical, sexual, and emotional abuse.
- Learning or school problems.
- Substance use (both tobacco and alcohol).
- Behaviors or emotions that indicate recurrent or severe depression or risk of suicide.
- Sexual behavior that may result in unintended pregnancy and sexually transmitted diseases, including human immunodeficiency virus (HIV) infection.

- Sexually transmitted diseases, if sexually active.
- HIV infection: The 2006 Centers for Disease Control and Prevention recommendations call for all adolescents seen in health care settings to be tested for HIV infection unless they specifically "opt out."
- Cervical cancer (as indicated).

Additional Reading: Guidelines for adolescent preventative health services: screening. In: *UpToDate*. 2022.

30. Which one of the following conditions is most likely to be seen as a result from the sexual abuse of a child?

A) Cushing syndrome
B) Enuresis
C) Secondary amenorrhea
D) Engaging in sexualized behaviors
E) The early onset of menarche

The answer is D: Sexualized behaviors are suggestive of sexual abuse and can include such behaviors as excessive masturbation; use of adult words associated with sexuality; and simulation of sexual intercourse with another child, doll, or animal.

Behavioral changes can also include aggression, problems in school, sleep disturbances, depression, generalized anxiety, suicidal gestures, and eating disturbances. Sexual abuse may result in vaginal pain, bleeding, vaginal discharge and rectal bleeding, and sexually transmitted infections; however, only a small percentage of sexually abused children will have abnormal findings. In contrast, vaginal discharge in a prepubertal girl is associated with sexual abuse in only 5% to 10% of cases, the most common cause being related to poor hygiene. Approximately 75% of children evaluated for sexual abuse are girls. Ages range from 6 months to 18 years with a median age of 8 years. By the age of 18 years of age, an estimated 12% to 25% of girls and 8% to 10% of boys become victims of sexual abuse. With a high prevalence, it is likely that primary care physicians will encounter child victims of abuse in their practice. Physicians are mandated to report suspected and reported cases of abuse to local child protective services agency. Many communities have access to children's advocacy centers that can provide multidisciplinary assessments of abused children. Providers need to familiarize themselves with services available in their region. Early onset of menarche among females may be associated with an increased risk of sexual abuse; however, it is not a symptom of sexual abuse. Cushing syndrome and secondary amenorrhea are not symptoms of sexual abuse.

Additional Reading: Child abuse: approach and management. *Am Fam Physician*. 2022;105(5):521-528.

31. You are checking in on the parents of a premature neonate, who was admitted to the neonatal intensive care unit. They are asking if you know when their daughter will be discharged. Which one of the following is an acceptable criterion for discharging a premature infant from the neonatal intensive care unit?

A) Her birth weight is maintained.
B) Her body temperature is maintained in an open crib.
C) Her weight gain is at least 5 g/d.
D) Her reaction to external stimuli is appropriate.
E) The tube feeds are tolerated.

The answer is B: Increased survival rate of premature neonates and early discharge from the intensive care units lead to an increasing likelihood that family physicians will provide care to small, premature infants after discharge from the hospital. Most neonatal units have no minimum weight requirement for discharge (although most are at least 1800-2100 g). Medical guidelines for discharge are as follows:

- Body temperature is maintained while the infant is in an open crib, usually at 34 weeks of gestational age or at 2000 g (4 lb, 6 oz) of weight.
- The infant feeds by mouth well enough to have a weight gain of 10 to 30 g/d.
- The infant is not receiving medications that require hospital management.
- No recent major changes in medications or oxygen administration have occurred.
- No recent episodes of apnea or bradycardia have occurred.

During the first 2 years of life, growth is plotted using age corrected for prematurity. Growth charts for the "average" premature infant have been designed for this purpose. After 2 years of age, a standard growth chart for chronologic age may be used. The infant's development during the first 2 years should be plotted from the estimated due date rather than the actual birth date. The Denver Prescreening Developmental Questionnaire, the Denver Developmental Screening Test, and the Gesell Screening Inventory are all accepted tests.

Immunization schedules (except for hepatitis B) are based on chronologic age, not the gestational age. Hepatitis B vaccine should only be given when the infant weighs at least 2000 g.

Additional Reading: Common questions about outpatient care of premature infants. *Am Fam Physician*. 2014; 90(4):244–251.

32. Which etiologic organism is most likely to cause occult bacteremia in unimmunized children 3 to 36 months of age?

A) *N meningitidis*
B) *S pneumoniae*
C) *S aureus*
D) *H influenzae*
E) *Salmonella*

The answer is B: The incidence of occult bacteremia in children fully immunized against *S pneumoniae* (3 doses of PV13) and *H influenzae* (2 or 3 doses depending upon the formulation) is less than 1%. Unimmunized or partially immunized children are at greater risk of occult bacteremia but at rates lower than that seen before the widespread use of the PCV13 and *H influenzae* type B conjugate vaccines due to herd immunity. Prior to the use of the conjugate vaccines, the most common etiologies of bacteremia were *S pneumoniae* (80%) and *H influenzae* (20%). In the post–conjugate vaccine era, the etiology has shifted with *E coli* and *S aureus* now being the predominant organisms. Obtaining an immunization history is essential to assessing the risk of occult bacteremia in young, febrile (fever 39 C or higher) children without a source of infection on examination.

Additional Reading: Fever without a source in children 3 to 36 months of age. In: *UpToDate*. 2022.

33. Many substances including antibiotics are contraindicated in breastfeeding because of the risk they pose to the young, developing infant. Which one of the following substances is permitted for use during breastfeeding?

A) Alcohol
B) Bromocriptine
C) Ciprofloxacin
D) Penicillin
E) Tetracycline

The answer is D: Contraindicated medications during breastfeeding include quinolones, tetracyclines, chloramphenicol, bromocriptine, cyclosporine, cyclophosphamide, doxorubicin, methotrexate, lithium, and ergotamine. Relatively contraindicated medications include metronidazole, sulfonamides, salicylates, phenobarbital, other psychotropic medications, and antihistamines. Large quantities of caffeine should also be avoided. All mothers should be advised to avoid the use of recreational drugs (eg, alcohol, cocaine, and marijuana) while breastfeeding.

Additional Readings:
1. Strategies for breastfeeding success. *Am Fam Physician*. 2008;78(2):225-232.
2. Primary interventions to support breastfeeding. *Am Fam Physician*. 2017;95(8):517-518.

34. Reducing the risk of drowning includes all but which one of the following measures?

A) Install a 4′, 4-sided isolation fence that separates the pool from the house
B) Install self-latching, self-closing gate at the pool access point
C) Prevent unsupervised access to the bathroom, swimming pool or open water
D) Provide infant swimming lessons to "drown-proof" the infant
E) Have children and adolescents wear U.S. Coast Guard–approved life jackets whenever they are in watercraft.

The answer is D: Drowning is the leading cause of injury death in US children, and in 2017, drowning claimed the lives of almost 1000 US children. Children and parents should learn to swim and learn water-safety skills. Not all children will be ready to learn to swim at the same age. Swimming lessons may reduce the risk of drowning, including for those 1 to 4 years of age, but infants younger than 1 year are developmentally unable to learn to swim.

Evidence strongly supports installation of 4′, 4-sided high fencing to isolate a pool from the home with a self-closing, self-latching gate installed. Swim lessons, use of life jackets, and adult supervision are all well-validated interventions that reduce drowning risk.

Additional Reading: Drowning Prevention | CDC.

35. Despite your counseling otherwise, a family requests that their 12-month-old child have their vaccines separated by 1 week per vaccine to minimize the number of injections given in 1 day. They request that the varicella vaccine be given today. Which of the following vaccines cannot be given next week?

A) *H influenzae* vaccine
B) Diphtheria and tetanus toxoids and acellular pertussis vaccine
C) Influenza vaccine
D) Measles-mumps-rubella (MMR) vaccine
E) Pneumococcal vaccine

The answer is D: If any combination of live injected vaccines (MMR, Measles-mumps-rubella-varicella, Varivax) or live attenuated influenza vaccine (FluMist) is not administered at the same time as another live injected vaccine, the vaccine doses should be separated by at least 4 weeks. This interval is intended to reduce or eliminate interference from the vaccine administered first with the vaccine administered later. If any two of these vaccines are administered at an interval of less than 4 weeks, then the vaccine administered second should be repeated in 4 weeks.

Live vaccines administered by the oral route (eg, typhoid Ty21a [Vivotif], rotavirus, and adenovirus vaccines) are not believed to interfere with parenteral or intranasal live vaccines or with each other. Therefore, they may be administered simultaneously with or at any time before or after other live vaccines.

Additional Reading: General Best Practice Guidance for Immunization, The Pink Book, CDC.

36. Which of the following statements regarding inhalant abuse is true?

A) Approximately 5% of children in middle school and high school have experimented with inhaled substances.
B) Drug testing of urine can help aid in the diagnosis of inhalant abuse.
C) Inhalant abuse can become addictive.
D) Reversal of inhalant effects can be achieved with the administration of naloxone (NARCAN).
E) There are no associated fetal abnormalities with inhalant abuse during pregnancy.

The answer is C: Inhalant abuse is a prevalent and common form of substance abuse in teenagers. Study results consistently show that nearly 11% of children in middle school and high school have experimented with inhaled substances. The method of delivery is inhalation of a solvent from its container, sprayed on a heated surface to enhance evaporation. Inhaled from a saturated cloth or spraying into a bag that is then placed over the nose, mouth, or head. Solvents include glue, shoe polish, toluene, gasoline, lighter fluid, spray paint, and nitrous oxide, typically inhaled from a balloon. Inhalant abuse creates a euphoric feeling and can become addictive. Acute side effects primarily are neurologic and can include slurred speech, ataxia, disorientation, headache, hallucinations, agitation, violent behavior, and seizures. Cardiovascular effects such as arrhythmias, myocarditis, and myocardial infarction have been reported. Long-term inhalant abuse can cause heart, kidney, liver, and neurologic damage. Inhalant abuse during pregnancy can cause fetal abnormalities, spontaneous abortions, and premature delivery.

Diagnosis of inhalant abuse is difficult and relies almost entirely on a thorough history and a high index of suspicion. There are currently no specific laboratory tests that could confirm solvent inhalation.

Treatment is generally supportive because there are no reversal agents for inhalant intoxication. Education of young patients and their families is essential to discourage experimentation with potentially harmful inhalants.

Additional Reading: Inhalant misuse in children and adolescents. In: *UpToDate*. 2022.

37. When discussing bicycle safety with patients and their families, it is important to focus on which critically essential component?

A) Ensuring proper bike fitting
B) Looking both ways before crossing an intersection
C) Using proper hand signals
D) Wearing a helmet with every ride
E) Wearing shoes while riding

The answer is D: The peak incidence of bicycle-related injuries and fatalities is in the 9- to 15-year age group, with a male-to-female ratio of 3:1. Important risk factors for bicycle-related injuries include not wearing a helmet, crashes involving motor vehicles, and an unsafe riding environment. In adolescents and young adults, alcohol and substance abuse can be associated with bicycle injury. Most injuries that occur in boys are associated with riding at high speeds. Most serious injuries and fatalities in bike accidents result from collisions with motor vehicles.

Although superficial soft tissue injuries and musculoskeletal trauma are the most common injuries, head injuries lead to the most fatalities and long-term disabilities. Overuse injuries may contribute to various musculoskeletal complaints, compression neuropathies, perineal complaints, and genital complaints. Physicians treating bicycle-riding patients should consider medical factors and suggest adjusting various components of the bicycle, such as the seat height and handlebars. Encouraging bicycle riders to wear helmets is key to preventing injuries. In addition, protective clothing, and equipment along with general safety advice may help the patients further protect themselves.

Additional Reading: Prevention of unintentional childhood injury. *Am Fam Physician*. 2020;102(7):411-417.

Care of the Female Patient (Including Maternity Care)

CHAPTER 3

To help you focus your studying, the questions in this section have been grouped into related categories: Prenatal Care, Labor and Delivery, Contraception, and General Gynecology/Women's Health.

Section I. Prenatal Care

Each of the following questions or incomplete statements below is followed by suggested answers or completions. Select the ONE BEST ANSWER in each case.

1. Gestational diabetes mellitus (GDM) is carbohydrate intolerance that occurs during pregnancy. Which one of the following medications has been used with success in gestational diabetes?

A) Glimepiride (Amaryl)
B) Glipizide (Glucotrol)
C) Glyburide (Micronase, Diabeta)
D) Repaglinide (Prandin)
E) Rosiglitazone (Avandia)

The answer is C: Those affected by GDM are at risk of developing diabetes and related conditions later in life and face a range of complications during pregnancy, including hypertension, preeclampsia, and cesarean delivery. Macrosomia is more common in infants exposed to GDM, which increases the risks of operative delivery, shoulder dystocia, birth trauma, and obesity during childhood.

Women with GDM are often treated initially with diets designed to achieve normal glycemic levels and avoid ketoacidosis. However, an acceptable diet has not been determined, and calorie restriction may increase the chance of ketosis. Several trials have demonstrated reduced risk for fetal macrosomia if the mother is treated with insulin. Although insulin treatment is common in GDM, only 9% to 40% of treated mothers benefit. Treatment aims to achieve postprandial glucose levels of 120 mg/dL and less than 90 mg/dL when fasting.

Oral hypoglycemic agents, with the exception of glyburide, are contraindicated in pregnancy. In one study, glyburide provided outcomes comparable with those achieved with insulin in patients with GDM who had failed to achieve adequate glycemic control with diet alone. Clinical experience and the evidence published thus far also support the safety and efficacy of metformin use in pregnancy with respect to the immediate pregnancy outcomes. However, the long-term impact—positive or negative—of metformin use is still largely unknown (metformin is listed as a category B medication in pregnancy). When glycemic control is satisfactory and no complications occur, mothers with GDM routinely do not require early or operative delivery. Nevertheless, the high incidence of macrosomia and other complications often results in cesarean or other operative delivery.

The most commonly used initial screening test for GDM is the 50-g 1-hour glucose challenge. The accepted optimal limits vary, but at the recommended level of 130 mg/dL (7.2 mmol/L), the screening test has an estimated sensitivity of 79% and a specificity of 87%. The diagnostic test most specific to pregnancy, and with the most supporting data, is the 100-g 3-hour oral glucose tolerance test, which is commonly given to women who have had an abnormal 1-hour glucose challenge test.

Additional Reading:

1. Screening, diagnosis, and management of gestational diabetes mellitus. *Am Fam Physician*. 2015;91(7):460-467.
2. Metformin therapy during pregnancy: good for the goose and good for the gosling too? *Diabetes Care*. 2011;34(10):2329-2330.

2. Pregnancy is accompanied by changes in a woman's hormonal milieu, with associated symptoms that can be problematic. Which one of the following symptoms would present the greatest concern in a pregnant woman?

A) Abnormal cravings
B) Chronic vomiting
C) Heartburn
D) Mild edema
E) Nausea

The answer is B: Symptoms noted in early pregnancy that present concern to the physician include vaginal bleeding or fluid vaginal discharge, severe headaches, visual disturbances, chronic vomiting, fever or chills, dysuria, swelling of the face or hands, and pelvic pain. Abnormal cravings, nausea, mild lower extremity edema, and heartburn are common complaints of pregnancy that are generally of no significant medical concern.

Additional Reading: Nausea and vomiting of pregnancy. *Am Fam Physician*. 2014;89(12):965-970.

3. Several fetal physical parameters are measured with a prenatal ultrasonography. Which one of the following ultrasonography parameters is best used for estimating gestational age during the first trimester?

A) Biparietal diameter
B) Crown-rump length
C) Estimated weight
D) Femur length
E) Head-foot length

The answer is B: An ultrasonography can be used to measure crown-rump length, biparietal diameter, abdominal circumference, and femur length, all of which can be used to confirm dates. The crown-rump length is more accurate during the first trimester, whereas the biparietal diameter and femur length are used more during the second trimester. The ultrasonography is best used in the first trimester for estimating the age of the fetus. As pregnancy progresses, estimation of age is more difficult to assess using ultrasonography examination.

Additional Reading: *Initial prenatal assessment and first trimester prenatal care*. In: *UpToDate*. 2022.

4. In the management of a pregnant patient, medications are classified based on their risk to the fetus. Category C refers to medications that:

A) are associated with teratogenicity in animals.
B) are considered safe during pregnancy.
C) have unknown risk for the fetus.
D) should never be given during pregnancy.
E) should only be given in life-threatening situations.

The answer is C: The following medication classifications are used to determine the risk of their use during pregnancy:

- *Category A*: Controlled studies in women fail to demonstrate the risk to the fetus in the first trimester; considered safe with no harmful effects on the fetus.
- *Category B*: Animal studies do not indicate a risk; however, there are no human studies; considered relatively safe during pregnancy.
- *Category C*: unknown fetal risk with no human studies to support or disprove safety.
- *Category D*: Some risk has been proved for the fetus; these drugs should be used only in life-threatening situations.
- *Category X*: proven harm to the fetus; should not be used in pregnancy.

Additional Reading: Briggs GG, Freeman RK, Yaffe SJ. *Drugs in Pregnancy and Lactation: A Reference Guide to Fetal and Neonatal Risk*. 10th ed. Wolters Kluwer; 2015.

5. Rho(D) immune globulin (RhoGAM) is indicated when:

A) the mother has type AB blood.
B) the father is Rh negative.
C) the mother is Rh positive.
D) the mother is Rh negative.

The answer is D: RhoGAM is indicated when a pregnant patient has a negative Rh antibody test. Rh-negative mothers should be given an immune globulin preparation at 28 weeks' gestation to prevent erythroblastosis fetalis. If the father is also Rh negative, the administration is unnecessary. However, if the Rh status of the father is unknown, RhoGAM should be given; however, extramarital pregnancies should be considered. A dose of RhoGAM should also be given at the time of delivery, depending on the blood type of the infant.

If the infant is Rh positive, the mother's dose can be determined by the *Kleihauer-Betke* test, which measures the amount of fetal erythrocytes in the maternal blood. If the newborn is Rh negative, there is no need for the second immune globulin administration. The immune globulin should also be given to Rh-negative women after elective or spontaneous abortion, placental abruption, ectopic pregnancy, or amniocentesis. Typically, the standard dose is 300 μg, which protects up to 30 mL of Rh-positive fetal whole blood.

Additional Reading: Evidence-based prenatal care: part II. Third-trimester care and prevention of infectious diseases. *Am Fam Physician*. 2005;71:1555-1562.

6. Proper seat belt use decreases the likelihood of maternal injury and mortality after a motor vehicle crash. Which one of the following statements is true regarding seat belt use in pregnancy?

A) The shoulder harness should not be used during pregnancy.
B) The air bag should be disabled.
C) The lap belt should be placed under the gravid uterus and over the thighs with the shoulder harness placed between the breast and over the uterus.
D) The use of correctly positioned seat belts can unfortunately increase the risk of fetal injury in a head-on crash.
E) Seat belt–restrained women who are in motor vehicle crashes have the same fetal mortality rate as women who are not in motor vehicle crashes.

The answer is E: Seat belt–restrained women who are in motor vehicle crashes have the identical fetal mortality rate as women who are not in motor vehicle crashes, but unrestrained women who are in crashes are more than twice as likely to lose their fetuses. Prenatal care should include three-point seat belt instruction. The lap belt should be placed under the gravid abdomen, snugly over the thighs, with the shoulder harness off to the side of the uterus, between the breasts and over the midline of the clavicle. Seat belts placed directly over the uterus can cause fetal injury. Airbags should not be disabled during pregnancy.

Additional Reading: Blunt trauma in pregnancy. *Am Fam Physician*. 2004;70:1303-1310, 1313.

7. A young couple are attending a prenatal visit at 12 weeks' gestation and are asking about the safety of sexual activity. Which one of the following statements about sexual intercourse and uncomplicated pregnancy is true?

A) Intercourse should be avoided during pregnancy because of the risk for placental abruption.
B) Intercourse should be avoided until 36 weeks' gestation because of the risk of premature labor.
C) Intercourse should be avoided the 2 weeks before the estimated date of confinement because of the risk of infection.
D) Intercourse is safe during pregnancy; however, orgasm should be avoided because of the risk of preterm labor.
E) Intercourse is not considered dangerous during normal pregnancy.

The answer is E: Sexual intercourse during pregnancy is generally considered safe as long as the pregnancy has not been complicated by preterm labor, abnormal vaginal bleeding, premature rupture of membranes. Orgasm with uterine contractions does not induce labor; however, milk ejection may occur and is a normal response. Desire for sexual intercourse during pregnancy may be either increased or decreased—both responses are normal. Abstention from sexual intercourse was formerly recommended during the final months of pregnancy; however, it is no longer considered a risk in normal pregnancies.

Additional Reading: Pregnancy myths and practical tips. *Am Fam Physician*. 2020;102(7):420-426.

8. A patient presenting for care in the first trimester of pregnancy requests information on the types of noninvasive testing that are available to detect whether her fetus has Down syndrome. You inform her of which one of the following screening strategies?

A) That it is recommended that all patients should be offered such genetic testing.
B) That only an amniocentesis done in the early second trimester can give her such information.
C) That she should wait until the second trimester to have a maternal quadruple screen and an ultrasonography to look at fetal anatomy.
D) That she will need to meet with a genetic counselor to help decide what testing is right for her.
E) That the combination of a first-trimester ultrasonography and maternal blood testing performed on the same day will help identify if the fetus is at an increased risk for Down syndrome.

The answer is A: The American College of Obstetrics and Gynecology recommends that all pregnant women should be offered aneuploidy (the presence of an abnormal number of chromosomes in a cell) screening before 20 weeks. Currently available screening tests for aneuploidy in the first trimester include an ultrasonography measurement of fetal nuchal translucency as well as a maternal blood screening for levels of β-human chorionic gonadotropin (hCG) and pregnancy-associated plasma protein A.

An increased nuchal translucency is associated with a variety of trisomies, most notably trisomy 21, as well as fetal congenital anomalies such as cardiac defects. Trisomy 21 is also associated with an increased β-hCG level as well as a decreased pregnancy-associated plasma protein S level. Combining the nuchal translucency with first-trimester biochemical markers allows identification of a population of pregnant women at a high risk for aneuploidy early in their pregnancies.

These women should receive genetic counseling and be offered first-trimester chorionic villus sampling (CVS) or second-trimester amniocentesis. If no increased risk is identified with first-trimester screening, this information can be combined later in pregnancy with second-trimester maternal serum screening. This increases the sensitivity of testing for aneuploidy and decreases the false-positive rate of either of these forms of testing done separately. If a fetal anatomical survey done by second-trimester ultrasonography suggests a major congenital anomaly and/or if a high risk for aneuploidy is detected on combined first- and second-trimester screening, the patient should receive genetic counseling and be offered diagnostic fetal chromosomal testing via amniocentesis.

Another option for women is to be offered noninvasive prenatal testing (NIPT) as an alternative to amniocentesis. NIPT allows the isolation of cell-free fetal DNA from the plasma of pregnant women as another detection tool for fetal aneuploidy. Counseling regarding the limitations of NIPT should include a discussion that the screening test provides information regarding only trisomy 21 and trisomy 18 and, in some laboratories, trisomy 13. It does not replace the precision obtained with diagnostic tests such as CVS or amniocentesis and currently does not offer other genetic information.

Additional Reading:

1. Screening for fetal chromosomal abnormalities. ACOG Practice Bulletin no. 77. 2007.
2. Non-invasive screening for fetal aneuploidy. ACOG Practice Bulletin no. 163. 2016. www.acog.org/Resources_And_Publications/Committee_Opinions_List

9. You are caring for a 32-year-old hypertensive woman who is worried that her antihypertensive medication will have a negative effect on her fetus. You note that all of the following medications are used to treat hypertension in pregnancy except which one?

A) Methyldopa
B) Hydralazine
C) Labetalol
D) Nifedipine XL
E) Losartan

The answer is E: During pregnancy, women can suffer from chronic (preexisting) hypertension, which is defined as systolic pressure ≥140 mm Hg and/or diastolic pressure ≥90 mm Hg that antedates pregnancy, is present before the 20th week of pregnancy, or persists longer than 12 weeks post partum. Gestational hypertension refers to elevated blood pressure (BP) first detected after 20 weeks of gestation in the absence of proteinuria or other features of preeclampsia. Over time, some patients will develop proteinuria or end-organ dysfunction characteristic of preeclampsia and be considered preeclamptic, whereas others will be diagnosed with chronic hypertension because of persistent BP elevation post partum.

Most hypertensive women of childbearing age with preexisting hypertension will not have target organ damage, and the risk for short-term cardiovascular consequences during pregnancy is very low. Improved maternal or neonatal outcomes with antihypertensive therapy have not been documented in this group. Therefore, antihypertensive medication might be safely withheld in such patients, provided that BP remains less than 160 mm Hg systolic and 110 diastolic while off medications.

Continuing previous antihypertensive medication is an option; however, angiotensin-converting enzyme inhibitors and angiotensin receptor blockers (eg, losartan) should not be used during pregnancy. Because methyldopa (Aldomet) has the longest track record of safety in pregnancy, it is preferred by many clinicians. Hydralazine, nifedipine, and labetalol are also used.

Additional Reading: Hypertension in pregnancy. ACOG; 2013. http://www.acog.org/Resources_And_Publications/Task_Force_and_Work_Group_Reports/Hypertension_in_Pregnancy

10. Pregnant women should avoid contact with cat litter because of the risk for developing which one of the following infections?

A) Coccidioidomycosis
B) Cryptococcosis
C) Cytomegalovirus infection
D) Erythema infectiosum
E) Toxoplasmosis

The answer is E: Toxoplasmosis is a granulomatous disease caused by the protozoan *Toxoplasma gondii*, which affects the central nervous system. Because the protozoan is found in cat feces, pregnant women should avoid handling cat litter. The disease is extremely common, and affected patients are usually asymptomatic. Symptoms, when present, mimic mononucleosis and include malaise, fever, myalgia, and rashes, with cervical and axillary lymphadenopathy.

Laboratory and physical findings include mild anemia, leukopenia, lymphocytosis, elevated liver function tests, and hypotension. A more severe form may occur in patients with acquired immunodeficiency syndrome or other patients who are immunocompromised; complications include hepatitis, pneumonitis, meningoencephalitis, and myocarditis. Chronic toxoplasmosis can lead to retinochoroiditis, persistent diarrhea, muscular weakness, and headache.

Unfortunately, toxoplasmosis infection during pregnancy can lead to spontaneous abortion or stillbirths. A multitude of congenital defects may also occur, including blindness and severe mental retardation. Diagnosis is usually made by serologic tests with fluorescent antibody techniques. Computed tomographic examination of the brain may show enhancing lesions, and biopsies can be taken to look for the organisms microscopically.

Treatment is reserved for more severe cases and consists of the combined use of pyrimethamine, sulfadiazine, and folinic acid (leucovorin). Immunocompromised patients require maintenance treatment for life.

Additional Reading: Pet-related infections. *Am Fam Physician*. 2016;94(10):794-802.

Toxoplasmosis is a granulomatous disease caused by the protozoan *T gondii*, which is found in cat feces; therefore, pregnant women should avoid handling cat litter.

11. There is interest in early detection and prevention of neural tube defects (eg, spina bifida, meningomyelocele, and anencephaly). Which one of the following statements about neural tube defects is true?

A) Laboratory testing is not useful in the diagnosis of neural tube defects.
B) Nicotinic acid has been shown to help prevent neural tube defects.
C) Elevated α-fetoprotein levels should be further evaluated by obstetric ultrasonography.
D) α-Fetoprotein testing should be done at 24 to 28 weeks' gestation.
E) Elevated α-fetoprotein levels are not associated with normal pregnancies.

The answer is C: Neural tube defects can be screened by performing a serum α-fetoprotein blood test, which is done at 16 to 18 weeks' gestation. Evaluation is based on maternal weight and gestational age. Causes for elevations of maternal α-fetoprotein include inaccurate gestation dates, multiple gestations, abdominal wall defects in the fetus, congenital nephrotic syndrome, fetal demise, and neural tube defects. Low levels of α-fetoprotein are associated with inaccurate gestation dates, chromosome trisomy such as Down syndrome, molar pregnancy, and fetal demise. However, low and high α-fetoprotein levels can also be seen in normal pregnancies; thus it is recommended that an obstetric ultrasonography should be performed if the α-fetoprotein level is abnormal.

Recent studies have shown that the administration of folic acid before pregnancy may help to prevent neural tube defects. The current recommendations are that women who plan to conceive should consume at least 0.4 mg folate per day (which is usually contained in a prenatal vitamin). Preconception counseling should include a discussion of folic acid supplementation.

Additional Reading: Folic acid for the prevention of neural tube defects: recommendation statement. *Am Fam Physician*. 2010;82(12):1526-1527.

12. A 21-year-old woman in her 14th week of pregnancy presents with a painful vesicular rash on her labia. You diagnose genital herpes, and this appears to be her initial outbreak. Which one of the following statements about genital herpes is true?

A) Antiviral medications such as acyclovir are contraindicated in pregnancy.
B) Cesarean section is recommended for delivery, irrespective of whether there are recurrent herpetic lesions at that time or not.
C) Genital herpes is a sexually transmitted disease (STD) that can be treated to prevent future recurrences.
D) Termination of the pregnancy should be considered with an active herpes simplex virus (HSV) infection.
E) The risk for transmission to the neonate is high among women with newly acquired genital HSV near term and lower among those who acquire HSV during the first half of pregnancy.

The answer is E: Genital herpes is a sexually transmitted infection caused by HSV. Unfortunately, this STD is not curable and recurs at a varying rate in all individuals. In pregnancy, the highest risk for neonatal transmission (30%-50%) is among infants of women who experience their first outbreak of genital HSV close to the time of delivery. However, the risk of neonatal transmission is low (<1%) for pregnant women who have a recurrent outbreak near term. However, because recurrent genital HSV is much more common than initial HSV infection in pregnancy, the proportion of neonatal HSV infections acquired from mothers with recurrent herpes is still significant.

Prevention of neonatal HSV infection is best accomplished by preventing the acquisition of new genital HSV infection during late pregnancy, decreasing the recurrence rate of HSV infections near term, and avoiding exposure of the infant to herpetic lesions during delivery. Suppressive antiviral treatment late in pregnancy reduces the frequency of cesarean sections among women who have recurrent genital herpes by diminishing the frequency of recurrences at term.

Women with recurrent HSV infection should be counseled about the use of antiviral therapy such as acyclovir. They should also be informed about the role of cesarean delivery in decreasing vertical transmission, which is typically only offered in the presence of active HSV genital lesions at the time of labor. For women with active lesions after delivery, care should be taken to avoid postpartum transmission to the infant through direct contact.

Additional Reading: *Diseases characterized by genital, anal or perianal ulcers. CDC Sexually Transmitted Disease Treatment Guidelines*. Centers for Disease Control and Prevention; 2021.

13. All of the following conditions are considered risk factors for a group B *Streptococcus* (GBS) infection in the neonate, except which one?

A) Maternal intrapartum fever
B) Maternal GBS anogenital colonization
C) Premature birth (less than 37 weeks' gestation)
D) Prolonged rupture of membranes (more than 18 hours)
E) Twin gestation

The answer is E: GBS infection is responsible for a significant amount of neonatal morbidity and mortality. Up to 30% of women are colonized by GBS. Risk factors for neonatal infection include less than 37 weeks' gestation, prolonged rupture of membranes (>18 hours), and maternal fever.

Multiple organizations recommend that all women be offered GBS screening by vaginal-rectal culture at 35 to 37 weeks' gestation and that colonized women be treated with appropriate intravenous antibiotics at the time of labor or rupture of membranes. GBS bacteriuria indicates heavy maternal urovaginal colonization. Women found to have GBS bacteriuria at any point in their current pregnancy, or a previous infant with GBS infection, should be offered empiric intrapartum antibiotics and therefore do not require vaginal-rectal culture.

Additional Reading:
1. Prevention of perinatal group B streptococcal disease: updated CDC guideline. *Am Fam Physician*. 2012;86(1):59-65.
2. Maternal and neonatal risk factors for early-onset group B streptococcal disease: a case-control study. *Int J Women's Health*. 2013;5:729-735.

14. A 29-year-old pregnant woman at 8 weeks' gestational age is found to have hyperthyroidism. She has been feeling well and appears to be asymptomatic at this time. Which one of the following medications is the drug of choice for the treatment of hyperthyroidism in the first trimester of pregnancy?

A) Levothyroxine
B) Methimazole
C) Propranolol
D) Propylthiouracil (PTU)
E) Radioactive iodine

The answer is D: Hyperthyroidism during pregnancy is usually associated with Graves disease. Other causes include toxic nodular goiter, choriocarcinoma, hydatidiform mole, ovarian teratoma, and iatrogenic thyrotoxicosis. Symptoms may include weight loss, tachycardia, exophthalmos, pretibial myxedema, generalized weakness, and tremor. Laboratory findings include an elevated triiodothyronine and thyroxine, and a low level of sensitive thyroid-stimulating hormone.

Treatment depends on the situation. Antithyroid medications readily cross the placenta and inhibit fetal thyroid function. PTU and methimazole cross the placenta but are used in the treatment of hyperthyroidism during pregnancy. Because of reports of possible teratogenic effects of methimazole, PTU is the drug of choice in the first trimester. Some experts recommend a change to methimazole from PTU at the beginning of the second trimester, because of an association of PTU with liver failure.

β-Blockers can be used to control tremor and tachycardia but should be limited to 2- to 6-week duration if possible to minimize impact on fetal growth. Radioactive iodine ablation of the thyroid is contraindicated during pregnancy. Close monitoring of thyroid hormones is required when administering antithyroid medications during pregnancy. Side effects of the medications include rash, urticaria, arthralgias, and agranulocytosis, which may predispose to maternal infection. Surgery is reserved for severe refractory cases. Untreated hyperthyroidism during pregnancy can lead to premature delivery, neonatal thyrotoxicosis, and spontaneous abortion.

Additional Reading: *Hyperthyroidism during pregnancy: treatment*. In: *UpToDate*. 2022.

15. A gravid woman is being assessed for complaints of right-lower-quadrant abdominal pain and there is a concern for appendicitis. At what month during pregnancy does the mother's appendix move upward to a level above the iliac crest?

A) The third month.
B) The sixth month.
C) The ninth month (with the onset of labor contractions).
D) The appendix does not change location during pregnancy.

The answer is B: As the sixth month of pregnancy approaches, the appendix moves upward, above the iliac crest. Because of the normal changes during pregnancy, such as leukocytosis, nausea, vomiting, anorexia, and abdominal discomfort, the diagnosis of appendicitis may be difficult. The condition occurs with equal frequency during each trimester of pregnancy. The risk for perforation is particularly increased in the third trimester, as is the perinatal risk. Complications of appendectomy include premature labor and wound infection. The differential diagnosis includes placental abruption, round ligament pain, acute pyelonephritis, renal colic, and cholecystitis.

Additional Reading: *Acute appendicitis in pregnancy*. In: *UpToDate*. 2022.

16. An ultrasonography taken for fetal development notes oligohydramnios. In the absence of ruptured membranes, oligohydramnios is correlated with an increased risk for all of the following conditions, except which one?

A) Abnormal fetal heart rate (FHR) tracings
B) Fetal gastrointestinal abnormalities
C) Induction of labor
D) Intrauterine growth restriction
E) Meconium-stained amniotic fluid

The answer is B: *Oligohydramnios* is defined as an amount of amniotic fluid that is less than what is expected (ie, less than fifth percentile) for gestational age. Amniotic fluid is usually quantified with ultrasonography determination, by measuring and adding together four-quadrant vertical fluid pocket measurements to obtain the amniotic fluid index. An amniotic fluid index of <5 at any gestational age is generally accepted as diagnostic of oligohydramnios; however, there is some evidence that using gestational age-specific calculations is more closely associated with perinatal morbidity.

Oligohydramnios seen early in pregnancy is a poor prognostic sign. Fetal gastrointestinal abnormalities that result in the inability of the fetus to swallow amniotic fluid more often result in polyhydramnios, rather than oligohydramnios. Pregnancies that have oligohydramnios from an early gestational age have an increased risk of limb contractures and pulmonary hypoplasia because of restriction in movement of the developing fetus. Oligohydramnios at all gestational ages is associated with underlying renal congenital abnormalities of the fetus that result in a lack of adequate amniotic fluid. Oligohydramnios is more common in postterm pregnancies and also in association with growth-restricted fetuses and is a frequent indication for induction of labor. Meconium-stained fluid and abnormalities of the fetal heart tracing due to either cord compression or uteroplacental insufficiency are also seen more often in patients with oligohydramnios.

Additional Reading: Assessing the optimal definition of oligohydramnios associated with adverse neonatal outcomes. *J Ultrasound Med*. 2011;30(3):303-307.

17. You are providing prenatal counseling to a woman living with human immunodeficiency virus (HIV). Which of the following is true?

A) With adequate antiretroviral therapy (ART), the risk of transmission is essentially zero.
B) She should pursue in vitro fertilization (IVF) as the only safe option for conception.
C) She should stop ART as it is category C for the fetus.
D) She will need a scheduled cesarean delivery.
E) ART is associated with large-for-gestation-age infants.

The answer is A: Women who initiate ART in the prenatal period and maintain a negligible viral load (<50 copies/mL) have a vertical transmission rate that is very close to zero. Depending on viral load, either a vaginal or cesarean delivery will be considered. With an unknown viral load or viral load >1000 copies/mL, cesarean delivery is safest for the infant. IVF may be considered as a means of conception is discordant couples, but if the partner with HIV is on ART with a suppressed viral load, unprotected vaginal intercourse is safe and there is effectively no risk of transmission to the partner. ART has been proven safe and effective in pregnancy, with no increased rates of birth defects. There may be an increase in preterm birth and low for gestational age infants, but these need to be weighed against the risks of unsuppressed viral load in pregnancy and delivery.

Additional Reading: Management of infants born to mothers with HIV infection. *Am Fam Physician*. 2021;104(1):58-62.

18. A 32-year-old woman who is 30 weeks' pregnant is involved in a motor vehicle accident and there is concern for neck trauma. You suggest placing her in which one of the following positions on a backboard for transport to the emergency department?

A) In the left lateral decubitus position
B) In the Trendelenburg position
C) In a prone position
D) In a supine position
E) In a supine position with her right hip elevated

The answer is E: After 20 weeks of gestation, the enlarged uterus may compress the great vessels when a pregnant woman is in a supine position. This compression can cause a decrease of up to 30 mm Hg in maternal systolic BP, a 30% decrease in stroke volume, and a consequent decrease in uterine blood flow. Manual deflection of the uterus laterally or placement of the patient in the lateral decubitus position avoids uterine compression. Because of suspected neck trauma in this patient, placing her supine on a backboard with her right hip elevated 4 to 6 in with towels is the safest position.

Additional Reading: Blunt trauma in pregnancy. *Am Fam Physician*. 2004;70:1303-1310, 1313.

19. A 21-year-old G1P0 woman presents to your office for an initial prenatal visit at 12 weeks' gestation. A urinalysis shows evidence of bacteriuria, and a culture is positive for 100,000 *Escherichia coli*; however, she is completely asymptomatic. Appropriate management includes which one of the following?

A) Discontinue urinalysis at her prenatal visits because of the high rate of false positives.
B) No treatment at this time; repeat urinalysis at her next visit.
C) No antibiotic treatment but encourage the patient to drink more fluids and cranberry juice daily.
D) Reassure the patient that antibiotic administration is not necessary, unless she should develop symptoms.
E) Treat the patient with a 7-day course of amoxicillin.

The answer is E: Asymptomatic bacteriuria is present in 2% to 7% of pregnant women. The condition is defined as more than 100,000 colonies of a single bacterial species per milliliter of urine, which has been cultured from a clean-caught midstream sample. Most women who do not have asymptomatic bacteriuria at their initial prenatal visit will not develop bacteriuria in pregnancy. Accordingly, routine screening for bacteriuria is done at the initial prenatal visit only.

The most common bacterium cultured is *E coli*. Pregnancy does not increase the incidence of asymptomatic bacteriuria. However, pregnancy does increase the incidence of pyelonephritis with asymptomatic bacteriuria. Additionally, pregnant patients with asymptomatic bacteriuria are at higher risk for preterm labor and delivery. Asymptomatic group B *Streptococcus* (GBS) bacteriuria has also been shown to increase the rate of preterm delivery and is associated with genitourinary colonization.

Because of these risks, when asymptomatic bacteriuria is discovered, treatment with an antibiotic is indicated. Treatment options include a 3- to 7-day course of oral amoxicillin, nitrofurantoin (Macrobid), or cephalexin (Keflex). In the case of GBS bacteriuria discovered in a pregnant patient, it is recommended that such patients should be treated at the time of diagnosis and while in labor. The intrapartum antibiotic prophylaxis is used to prevent early GBS infection in newborns.

After the therapy is completed, a urine culture should be repeated to ensure eradication of the infection. This repeat culture also identifies patients with persistent or recurrent bacteriuria. For patients who have persistent or recurrent bacteriuria, consideration should be given to administering suppressive doses of antibiotics.

Additional Reading: *Urinary tract infections and asymptomatic bacteriuria in pregnancy*. In: *UpToDate*. 2022.

20. Prenatal vitamins are important during pregnancy because they help to reduce the incidence of neural tube defects. Which of the following is responsible for this protective effect?

A) Calcium
B) Folic acid
C) Iron
D) Vitamin C
E) Vitamin B_{12}

The answer is B: Prenatal vitamins are recommended for all women of childbearing age who are not actively preventing pregnancy. The following intake is recommended for pregnant women:

- Calcium, 1200 to 1500 mg/d
- Iron, 30 mg/d
- Folic acid, at least 0.4 mg/d

Prenatal vitamins prior to conception provide adequate folic acid, which has been shown to help prevent neural tube defects. An increased dose of 1 mg/d is recommended for women with diabetes mellitus or epilepsy. Excessive vitamin A intake should be avoided due to the risk of birth defects. Furthermore, if the infant is breastfed, the use of prenatal vitamins for the mother is usually encouraged.

Additional Reading: Folic acid for the prevention of neural tube defects. *Am Fam Physician*. 2010;82(12):1533-1534.

21. Which one of the following statements is true regarding bacterial vaginosis (BV) during pregnancy?

A) Oral metronidazole should be avoided in pregnancy because of potential teratogenic effects.
B) Routine screening is recommended for all pregnant patients.
C) Studies have shown that BV is not associated with adverse pregnancy outcomes.
D) Symptomatic women should be treated.
E) Vaginal clindamycin and vaginal metronidazole are recommended choices for treatment of BV in pregnancy.

The answer is D: BV is a condition that is caused by replacement of the normal hydrogen peroxide producing *Lactobacillus* sp in the vagina by an overgrowth of anaerobic bacteria including *Prevotella* sp, *Mobiluncus* sp, *Gardnerella vaginalis*, *Ureaplasma*, and *Mycoplasma*. Treatment is recommended for all pregnancy women with symptomatic BV.

BV in pregnancy is associated with a variety of adverse peripartum outcomes such as preterm rupture of membranes, preterm labor, preterm delivery, intra-amniotic infection, and postpartum endometritis. However, the only proven benefit of treatment is a reduction in signs/symptoms of vaginal infection.

Efforts have been made to assess the benefits of screening for BV in women at high risk for preterm delivery and whether the treatment of asymptomatic BV in pregnancy women who are at low risk for preterm delivery reduces adverse pregnancy events, but neither intervention has consistently been shown to yield improved outcomes. Recommended antibiotic regimens for treating symptomatic pregnant women with BV include the following:

- Metronidazole 500 mg orally bid for 7 days
- Metronidazole 250 mg orally three times a day for 7 days
- Clindamycin 300 mg orally bid for 7 days

Regardless of the antimicrobial agent used to treat pregnant women, oral therapy is preferred because of the possibility of subclinical upper genital tract infection. Providers should also be aware that intravaginal clindamycin cream might be associated with adverse outcomes if used in the latter half of the pregnancy. Multiple studies have shown no documented increase in teratogenic effects in newborns with a history of maternal metronidazole use in pregnancy.

Additional Reading: *Diseases Characterized by Vulvovaginal Itching, Burning, Irritation, Odor or Discharge*. Centers for Disease Control and Prevention; 2021.

22. A triathlete presents for her first prenatal visit and indicates that she wants to stay as active as possible during her pregnancy. You inform her that regular exercise is recommended in pregnancy, but some activities are contraindicated. Which one of the following sports is considered to be contraindicated in pregnancy?

A) Downhill skiing
B) Low-impact aerobics
C) Stationary bicycle
D) Swimming
E) Walking

The answer is A: Concerns have been raised about the safety of some forms of exercise during pregnancy. Because of the body changes associated with pregnancy as well as the hemodynamic response to exercise, some precautions should be observed. Pregnant women should avoid exercise that involves the risk of abdominal trauma, falls, or excessive joint stress, as in contact sports, gymnastics, horseback riding, and skiing.

In the absence of any obstetric or medical complications, the American College of Obstetricians and Gynecologists recommends at least 30 minutes of exercise most or all days of the week during pregnancy. Studies have shown that exercise may contribute to prevention of gestational diabetes in obese women and that exercise can help women with gestational diabetes achieve euglycemia when diet alone is insufficient.

Additional Reading: Exercise during pregnancy. ACOG Committee Opinion no. 267. www.acog.org/Resources_And_Publications/Committee_Opinions_List.

23. Screening for gestational diabetes in patients without significant risk factors should take place during which one of the following prenatal visits?

A) At the first prenatal visit
B) Anytime between 12 and 16 weeks' gestation
C) Anytime between 24 and 28 weeks' gestation
D) Anytime between 30 and 34 weeks' gestation
E) At any random prenatal visit

The answer is C: Gestational diabetes is associated with a number of abnormalities that affect the fetus, including increased risk of spontaneous abortion, congenital anomalies (eg, neural tube defects, cardiac defects, skeletal abnormalities, and malformations of the intestinal and urinary tract), and fetal macrosomia. Risk factors for gestational diabetes include maternal age above 35 years, obesity, family history of diabetes, and prior history of gestational diabetes and/or macrosomia. Women with these risk factors should be screened early in pregnancy.

All other pregnant women (and high-risk women with normal early screening) should be screened for diabetes between weeks 24 and 28 of gestation with a 1 hour 50-g oral glucose tolerance test. If values are >140 mg/dL, a 3-hour glucose tolerance test should be performed. Although most women experience a resolution of diabetes immediately post partum, patients who develop gestational diabetes mellitus are at increased risk of developing type 2 diabetes mellitus later in life and thus should be screened for diabetes 6 weeks post partum and annually thereafter.

Additional Reading: Screening, diagnosis and management of gestational diabetes. *Am Fam Physician*. 2015;91(7):460-467.

24. Many laboratory values are affected during pregnancy because of hormonal changes. Which one of the following laboratory test results would you expect to see with pregnancy?

A) A decreased alkaline phosphatase level
B) A decreased fibrinogen level
C) A decreased lactic dehydrogenase level
D) An increased hemoglobin reading
E) An increased white blood cell count

The answer is E: Many laboratory values are affected during pregnancy. The following are typically increased:

- White blood cell count
- Alkaline phosphatase level
- Fibrinogen levels
- Erythrocyte sedimentation rate
- Lactic dehydrogenase level

- Creatinine phosphokinase level
- Cortisol levels
- Prolactin level
- Thyroxine total levels

Laboratory levels that are usually decreased include the following.

- Hemoglobin/hematocrit
- Albumin level
- Fasting blood glucose
- Calcium (total)

Although mild glycosuria and proteinuria are also common during pregnancy, excessive amounts should prompt for further evaluation to rule out gestational diabetes and preeclampsia.

Additional Reading: *Maternal Physiology. Williams Obstetrics.* 26th ed. McGraw-Hill; 2022.

25. You are counseling a young woman who has been treated for human immunodeficiency virus (HIV). She is concerned that she will transmit HIV to her child. Which one of the following risk factors is considered the most important variable in the transmission of HIV from an infected mother to her newborn?

A) A low maternal CD4 count
B) A preterm delivery (<34 weeks' gestation)
C) IV drug use during pregnancy
D) Low birth weight
E) Prolonged rupture of membranes (>4 hours)

The answer is E: Reported rates of HIV transmission from mother to child have varied; most studies in the United States and Europe have documented transmission rates in untreated women of between 12% and 30%. Perinatal treatment of HIV-infected mothers with antiretroviral drugs has dramatically decreased these rates to less than 2%. All of the listed conditions above increase the rate of vertical HIV transmission, but a prolonged rupture of membranes (>4 hours) is the most important variable that increases that risk.

Cesarean section combined with prenatal, intrapartum, and neonatal zidovudine therapy decreases the transmission rate by 87%. HIV can be transmitted via breast milk and colostrum.

A positive enzyme-linked immunosorbent assay HIV test result should be confirmed with the Western blot test. Antibodies to HIV generally appear in the circulation 2 to 12 weeks after infection. Detection in the newborn is more difficult when the mother is infected with HIV because the child will be positive for the enzyme-linked immunosorbent assay and the Western blot as a result of maternal transmission of the antibody transplacentally. Because of this, the HIV DNA polymerase chain reaction testing is the preferred test in developed countries. Almost 40% of infected newborns have positive tests in the first 2 days of life, with more than 90% testing positive by 2 weeks of age.

Additional Reading: *HIV Among Pregnant Women, Infants, and Children.* Centers for Disease Control and Prevention. www.cdc.gov/hiv/group/gender/pregnantwomen

26. The best time to administer live virus vaccines, such as measles, mumps, and rubella, to unimmunized pregnant women is during which of the following times?

A) At the first prenatal visit following conception
B) During the second trimester
C) During the third trimester
D) After delivery or at least 3 months before conception

The answer is D: Immunizations with live attenuated vaccines, such as measles, mumps, rubella, varicella, and the oral vaccine for polio, are contraindicated in pregnancy and should be given at least 3 months before conception. Immunizations with inactivated virus, such as influenza, *Pneumococcus*, tetanus, pertussis, rabies, and the injectable poliovirus, as well as the hepatitis B recombinant vaccine, are safe to administer.

Additional Reading: *Guidelines for Vaccinating Pregnant Women.* www.cdc.gov/vaccines/pubs/preg-guide.htm

27. Rubella ("German measles") is a highly contagious childhood disease that can affect pregnant mothers. True statements regarding this disease include all of the following statements, except which one?

A) An erythematous morbilliform rash usually develops on the trunk and then spreads to the face.
B) Congenital rubella syndrome includes cataracts, deafness, intellectual disability, and growth retardation.
C) Rubella immunization is safe when breastfeeding.
D) Symptoms of acute infection include fever, cough, and conjunctivitis.
E) Spontaneous abortion occurs more frequently in pregnancies that are complicated by rubella.

The answer is A: Rubella ("German measles") is a highly contagious childhood disease that can affect pregnant mothers. As many as 15% of mothers do not have antibodies to the rubella virus. Symptoms of acute infection include fever, cough, and conjunctivitis. Other symptoms may include headaches, malaise, myalgias, arthralgias, and postauricular and suboccipital lymphadenopathy. An erythematous morbilliform rash usually develops on the face and spreads inferiorly.

Generally, the symptoms of rubella are less severe than those of rubeola, and there is usually no prodrome seen with rubella (unlike with rubeola). Spontaneous abortion occurs two to four times more frequently in pregnancies that are complicated by rubella. Transmission to the fetus occurs by direct infection. If the woman is affected during the first trimester, the risk of birth defects is higher than that if she is affected during the last two trimesters.

Effects of the virus on the fetus (congenital rubella syndrome) include cataracts, glaucoma, blindness, cardiac abnormalities, deafness, intellectual disability, cerebral palsy, growth retardation, hemolytic anemia, and cleft palate. In cases of maternal rubella, therapeutic abortion can be considered if infection occurs in the first two trimesters. All women should receive routine rubella testing during pregnancy. If the test is negative, the patient should be vaccinated during the immediate postpartum period.

There are no contraindications to breastfeeding immediately after receiving the rubella vaccine. Women who are immunized with the live attenuated virus should not become pregnant for 3 months following immunization. The use of immune globulin for pregnant women who are exposed to rubella is not recommended.

Additional Reading: *Guidelines for Vaccinating Pregnant Women.* www.cdc.gov/vaccines/pubs/preg-guide.htm

Congenital rubella syndrome affects the fetus in a number of ways: cataracts, glaucoma, blindness, cardiac abnormalities, deafness, intellectual disability, cerebral palsy, growth retardation, hemolytic anemia, and cleft palate.

28. During pregnancy, it is important to counsel pregnant patients about diet and exercise. Weight gain is expected but varies depending on the patients' prenatal weight. How much weight should an otherwise healthy woman gain during her pregnancy?

A) 5 to 15 lb (2-7 kg)
B) 15 to 25 lb (7-11 kg)
C) 25 to 35 lb (11-16 kg)
D) 35 to 45 lb (16-20 kg)

The answer is C: The amount of healthy weight gain in pregnancy varies. Eating a well-rounded diet and getting at least 30 minutes of exercise per day is recommended for a healthy pregnancy. These are general guidelines:

- If prepregnancy body mass index (BMI) is underweight (<18), the recommended weight gain is 35 to 45 lb (16-20 kg).
- For women with a normal prepregnancy BMI total weight gain is 25 to 35 lb (11-16 kg).
- For women with prepregnancy BMI 25.0-29.9, recommended weight gain is 15 to 20 lbs.
- For women with a prepregnancy BMI > 30, 10 to 20 lb (4-9 kg) weight gain is recommended.

Additional Reading: Pregnancy myths and practical tips. *Am Fam Physician.* 2020;102(7):420-426.

29. Although exercise is recommended during pregnancy, some women with various conditions are advised to restrict activities. In which of the following conditions is aerobic exercise safe?

A) Incompetent cervix
B) Multiple gestations at risk for premature labor
C) Placenta previa after 26 weeks
D) Pregnancy-induced hypertension
E) Preterm labor during a prior pregnancy

The answer is E: There is no reason why women who are in good health should not to engage in exercise while pregnant. However, women with medical or obstetric complications should be encouraged to avoid vigorous physical activity.

Contraindications to exercise during pregnancy include hemodynamically significant cardiac disease, restrictive lung disease, gestational hypertension, preeclampsia, preterm rupture of membranes, preterm labor during the current pregnancy, incompetent cervix or cerclage placement, multiple gestations at risk of preterm labor, persistent second- or third-trimester bleeding, and placenta previa after 26 weeks of gestational age. Preterm labor in a prior pregnancy does not result in exercise restriction in subsequent pregnancies.

Additional Reading: *Physical Activity and Exercise During Pregnancy and the Postpartum Period. ACOG, Number 804.* American Congress of Obstetricians and Gynecologists. 2021.

30. Nonstress tests are used for antenatal well-being studies. Which one of the following statements about the nonstress test is true?

A) An abnormal nonstress test should be followed by a contraction stress test.
B) Late decelerations are usually noted with fetal movements.
C) Nonstress tests should be routinely performed beginning at 38 weeks until delivery.
D) The presence of oligohydramnios is accurately predicted with the results of a nonstress test.
E) Two or more fetal heart rate (FHR) accelerations (at least 15 beats above baseline) that last for 15 seconds in a 20-minute period are reassuring.

The answer is E: Nonstress testing includes the use of a fetal heart monitor and contraction monitor. Testing is usually reserved for complicated pregnancies (eg, intrauterine growth retardation, gestational diabetes, pregnancy-induced hypertension, multiple gestations, and prior stillbirth) or postdate pregnancy. A reassuring nonstress test shows two or more FHR accelerations of at least 15 beats/s above the baseline, which last for at least 15 seconds during a 20-minute period.

If this criterion is not met, a biophysical profile should be performed. Late or variable decelerations are concerning findings. Oligohydramnios is a risk for cord compression but is not well predicted by nonstress testing. Simplistically, the nonstress test is primarily a test of fetal well-being, whereas the contraction stress test is a test of uteroplacental function. In previous practice, a nonreassuring nonstress test required further workup with a contraction stress test, but today a biophysical profile is preferred.

Additional Reading: *Overview of fetal assessment.* In: *UpToDate.* 2022.

31. RhoGAM is given to prevent sensitization of an Rh-negative mother from carrying an Rh-positive fetus; thus, RhoGAM should be given to Rh-negative mothers following which one of the following schedules?

A) At the first prenatal visit and at delivery
B) At 12 and 36 weeks' gestation
C) At 16 weeks' gestation and after delivery, depending on the Rh status of the newborn
D) At 28 weeks' gestation and after delivery, depending on the Rh status of the newborn
E) At 28 and 36 weeks' gestation

The answer is D: The condition of erythroblastosis fetalis is the result of blood incompatibility between the mother and fetus. It results when an Rh-negative woman is impregnated by an Rh-positive man resulting in a fetus with Rh-positive blood type. Red blood cells (RBCs) cross the placenta into the mother's bloodstream throughout pregnancy and during termination or delivery and evoke the production of antibodies in the maternal blood to the fetus' RBCs.

Usually, there are no complications during a woman's first pregnancy. However, in subsequent pregnancies with an Rh-positive partner, the antibodies that were generated in the first pregnancy can cross the placenta and may result in severe, potentially life-threatening anemia. As a reaction to the anemia, the fetal bone marrow releases immature RBCs and erythroblasts (thus the name *erythroblastosis fetalis*). As a result of the antibody destruction of RBCs, there is an increased production of bilirubin that can result in kernicterus, which is characterized by poor feeding, apnea, poor fetal tone, mental retardation, seizures, and death.

Prevention of erythroblastosis fetalis is accomplished by administering RhoGAM, an anti-Rh antibody, to the mother. RhoGAM neutralizes the Rh-positive fetal blood cells when they cross the placenta, before they can involve in the production of maternal antibodies. RhoGAM is administered at 28 weeks' gestation and then again within 72 hours after delivery, if the infant is determined to be Rh positive. Mothers of Rh-negative infants do not need postpartum RhoGAM. It should also be given if abortion or ectopic pregnancy occurs or in any case in which there is fetal-maternal transfer of blood. All mothers should be screened for Rh status at their initial prenatal visit.

Additional Reading: Update on prenatal care. *Am Fam Physician.* 2014;89(3):199-208.

32. A young woman at 10 weeks' gestation presents feeling poorly. She has been coughing and has a runny nose consistent with an upper respiratory tract infection. On examination, her vital signs are normal but her temperature is 38.3 °C (101.0 °F). She is worried about her baby and you inform her that maternal temperature elevations above what temperature can be detrimental to the fetus in the first trimester of pregnancy?

A) 37 °C (98.6 °F).
B) 37.8 °C (100.0 °F).
C) 38.3 °C (101.0 °F).
D) 38.9 °C (102.0 °F).
E) Maternal temperature has no detrimental effects on the fetus.

The answer is D: Some data suggest a teratogenic potential when maternal temperatures increase above 38.9 °C (102 °F), especially in the first trimester. Mothers should be reassured when they have a low-grade temperature and examined to determine the source of a fever and treated appropriately.

Additional Reading: *Intrapartum fever*. In: *UpToDate*. 2022.

33. A gravid patient at 36 weeks' gestation is scheduled for a biophysical profile test. The profile measures all of the following factors in evaluating fetal well-being, except which one?

A) Amniotic fluid volume
B) Body movements
C) Fetal tone
D) Fetal heart rate (FHR)
E) Fetal size

The answer is E: Biophysical profile testing is a more extensive method for evaluating fetal well-being than obtaining a nonstress test. Indications for obtaining a profile include the following:

- Maternal hypertension or diabetes
- Post term pregnancies
- Multiple gestations
- Oligohydramnios
- Intrauterine growth retardation
- Placental abnormalities
- Decreased fetal movement
- Previous intrauterine fetal demise

The test looks at five different aspects of fetal well-being with real-time ultrasonography:

- Fetal breathing
- Body movements
- Fetal tone
- Amniotic fluid volume
- FHR (nonstress test)

Each aspect is given either a score of 0 for abnormal findings or 2 for normal findings. A score of 4 or less is a poor prognostic indicator, whereas a score of 8 or 10 is reassuring for fetal well-being. A score of 6 is suspicious for chronic asphyxia.

Additional Reading: *The fetal biophysical profile*. In: *UpToDate*. 2022.

34. Occasionally, it is necessary to obtain radiographic imaging during pregnancy. However, in utero exposure to ionizing radiation can be teratogenic, carcinogenic, or mutagenic. The maximum acceptable cumulative dose of ionizing radiation during pregnancy is which one of the following doses?

A) 1 rad
B) 5 rad
C) 10 rad
D) 50 rad
E) 100 rad

The answer is B: The accepted cumulative dose of ionizing radiation during pregnancy is 5 rad, and no single diagnostic study exceeds this maximum. The effects are directly related to the level of exposure and stage of fetal development. The fetus is most susceptible to radiation during organogenesis (2-7 weeks after conception) and in the early fetal period (8-15 weeks after conception). Nonurgent radiologic testing should be avoided during this time. Non–cancer-related adverse health effects have not been detected at any stage of gestation after exposure to ionizing radiation of less than 5 rad. However, the risk of childhood cancer (eg, leukemia) is increased regardless of the dose.

Pregnant women should be counseled that radiation exposure from a single diagnostic imaging procedure does not increase the risk of fetal anomalies or pregnancy loss. Spontaneous abortion, growth restriction, and mental retardation may occur at higher exposure levels. Appropriate counseling of patients before radiologic studies are performed is critical. Physicians should carefully weigh the risks and benefits of any radiographic study and include the mother in the decision-making process whenever possible. In utero exposure to *non*ionizing radiation is not associated with significant risks; therefore, ultrasonography is safe to perform during pregnancy.

Additional Reading: Health effects of prenatal radiation exposure. *Am Fam Physician*. 2010;82(5):488-493.

35. You are seeing a G1P0 patient at her 38 weeks' prenatal visit. The nurse notes that her blood pressure (BP) is elevated today and asks about preeclampsia. In addition to elevated BP (systolic BP > 160 or diastolic BP > 110), the diagnosis of preeclampsia requires which one of the following findings?

A) Proteinuria.
B) Proteinuria and edema.
C) Proteinuria, edema, and a seizure.
D) No other findings are required.

The answer is A: The classic preeclampsia triad included elevated BP, proteinuria, and edema; however, an elevated BP is considered sufficient to make the diagnosis. Seizures are the distinguishing component of eclampsia. The criterion for eclampsia includes any one of the following conditions:

- Systolic BP > 160 or diastolic BP > 110 taken 4 hours apart at bed rest
- Proteinuria >300 mg/24 hours
- Platelet count <100,000
- Liver dysfunction
- Progressive renal insufficiency (creatinine >1.1)
- Pulmonary edema
- Cerebral or visual disturbances

Additional Reading: *Hypertension in Pregnancy*. ACOG; 2022. http://www.acog.org/Resources_And_Publications/Task_Force_and_Work_Group_Reports/Hypertension_in_Pregnancy.

36. A young woman who has been receiving treatment for a human immunodeficiency virus (HIV) infection presents now having missed her last menses and is diagnosed with an intrauterine pregnancy. Which one of the following recommendations is correct for such patients?

A) All antiviral medications should be avoided because of their teratogenic potential.
B) Patients receiving efavirenz when the pregnancy is diagnosed should continue to take it.
C) Such patients need only to receive zidovudine at the time of delivery.
D) Zidovudine should be avoided because of its limited effectiveness.
E) Zidovudine should only be prescribed if the CD4+ count is unacceptably low.

The answer is B: Several important changes were made in the July 2012 update of the US Department of Health and Human Services' "Recommendations for Use of Antiretroviral Drugs in Pregnant HIV-1-Infected Women for Maternal Health and Interventions to Reduce Perinatal HIV Transmission in the United States" (see summary and link below), particularly pertaining to zidovudine and efavirenz. Zidovudine (also known as azidothymidine) is no longer a necessary part of a pregnant patient's antiretroviral therapy (ART) regimen. Additionally, azidothymidine is no longer administered intravenously during delivery, so long as the patient is on appropriate therapy with an HIV RNA load of <400 copies/mL near delivery.

Efavirenz (pregnancy category D) can be continued in pregnant women already receiving an effective efavirenz-based regimen who present for antenatal care in the first trimester. Unnecessary antiretroviral drug changes during pregnancy may be associated with loss of viral control and increased risk of perinatal transmission. In addition, the risk of neural tube defects is restricted to the first 5 to 6 weeks of gestation when pregnancy is rarely diagnosed.

There are several ART medications recognized to be generally safe in pregnancy, and all pregnant women should be offered ART. The decision whether to start the regimen in the first trimester or delay until 12 weeks' gestation will depend on CD4 cell count, HIV RNA levels, and maternal conditions such as nausea and vomiting. Earlier initiation of a combination antiretroviral regimen may be more effective in reducing transmission, but benefits must be weighed against potential fetal effects of first-trimester drug exposure.

Additional Reading: Recommendations for use of antiretroviral drugs in pregnant HIV-1-infected women for maternal health and interventions to reduce perinatal HIV transmission in the United States. www.aidsinfo.nih.gov/guidelines/html/3/perinatal-guidelines/0

37. A patient had an abnormal Papanicolaou test and is pregnant; her gynecologist called her to suggest that this should be investigated further with a loop electrosurgical excision procedure (LEEP). She is worried about her pregnancy, and you inform her that laser conization and LEEPs during pregnancy have been associated with which one of the following adverse effects?

A) Higher rates of endometritis during pregnancy
B) Increased peripartum mortality
C) Increased cesarean rates
D) Premature rupture of membranes (PROM)
E) No adverse effects during pregnancy

The answer is D: There is an increased risk of PROM and preterm labor following laser conization or LEEPs during pregnancy. The treatment of high-grade cervical dysplasia is by cervical conization, when a cone-shaped portion of the cervix, including the transformation zone, is excised. Methods to achieve this include using a scalpel, laser, or via an LEEP.

The LEEP provides an intact specimen of a cervical lesion in its entirety; however, the entire lesion is not obtained during pregnancy, and LEEP should not be performed during pregnancy, unless a very strong suspicion of cancer exists, given the concerns for disruption of the endocervical canal and risk for subsequent PROM.

Additional Reading: *Cervical intraepithelial neoplasia: reproductive effects of treatment*. In: *UpToDate*. 2022.

38. A 38-year-old woman presents to your office to discuss concerns over a second pregnancy, as her first child was born with a neural tube defect. Appropriate preconception counseling concerning folic acid intake in this situation would be to recommend that she take a supplement containing which one of the following amounts of folate daily?

A) 1 µg
B) 100 µg
C) 400 µg
D) 1 mg
E) 4 mg

The answer is E: Taking folic acid supplementation before conception reduces the incidence of neural tube defects, including spina bifida and anencephaly. The average woman receives about 100 µg of folic acid per day, mostly from fortified breads and grains. Supplementation should begin at least 1 month before conception and continue through the first 3 months of pregnancy; women should take a daily vitamin supplement containing at least 400 µg of folic acid. Higher dosages are indicated for special-risk groups. A dosage of 1 mg/d is recommended for women with diabetes mellitus or epilepsy. Mothers who have given birth to children with neural tube defects should take 4 mg of folic acid per day for subsequent pregnancies.

Additional Reading: Folic acid for the prevention of neural tube defects. *Am Fam Physician*. 2010;82(12):1533-1534.

39. A 37-year-old G1P0 woman has a history of a prior deep vein thrombosis (DVT). In view of her prior history of DVT, which one of the following would you recommend that she take for DVT prophylaxis during this pregnancy?

A) Aspirin
B) Clopidogrel (Plavix)
C) Heparin
D) Warfarin (Coumadin)
E) No prophylaxis is necessary, unless she has another event.

The answer is C: Women who have a personal or family history of venous thromboembolism should be offered testing for coagulopathy before pregnancy. Women with a prior history of DVT have a 7% to 12% risk of recurrence during pregnancy. Heparin (in regular or low-molecular-weight form) is indicated for prophylaxis and should be started as early in pregnancy as possible. Women receiving warfarin as maintenance therapy for DVT should be switched to heparin before conception, as warfarin has teratogenic properties.

Additional Reading: ACOG Practice Bulletin no. 196. Thromboembolism in pregnancy. *Obstet Gynecol*. 2018.

40. Which one of the following statements regarding varicella during pregnancy is true?

A) A single dose of varicella vaccine is safe during pregnancy.
B) Pregnancy should be delayed 6 months after varicella vaccination.
C) Varicella vaccination should be avoided in breastfeeding women.
D) Susceptible pregnant women who are exposed to varicella are candidates for varicella zoster immune globulin.
E) If a pregnant woman has no history of varicella, and tests negative for antibodies, she should be immunized as soon as possible.

The answer is D: The varicella vaccine is contraindicated in pregnant women because it is a live vaccine. Susceptible pregnant women who are exposed to varicella are candidates for varicella zoster immune globulin. Nonimmune women should be offered postpartum varicella vaccination. The vaccine is considered safe in breastfeeding women.

If varicella testing is performed in the preconception period, women can be offered two doses of varicella vaccine at least 1 month apart. Pregnancy should be delayed 1 month after vaccination. Women found to be nonimmune during pregnancy should be counseled to avoid exposure to chickenpox and to report exposure immediately.

Additional Reading: Evidence-based prenatal care: Part II. Third-trimester care and prevention of infectious diseases. *Am Fam Physician*. 2005;71:1555-1562.

41. A young woman at 34 weeks' gestation presents with fever and chills, and complains of dysuria and flank pain. You diagnose pyelonephritis and decide to treat with which one of the following antibiotics?

A) Ceftriaxone
B) Ciprofloxacin
C) Nitrofurantoin
D) Tetracycline
E) Trimethoprim/sulfamethoxazole

The answer is A: Pyelonephritis is one of the most common serious complications in pregnancy. It occurs in approximately 2% of pregnancies and more frequently in the third trimester. Symptoms include fever, chills, dysuria, flank pain, nausea, vomiting, and malaise. Pregnant women with acute pyelonephritis should be treated initially with a second- or third-generation cephalosporin, such as ceftriaxone 1 g every 12 hours, and then assessed to determine whether further treatment as an outpatient is appropriate. A regimen of ampicillin (2 g intravenously every 6 hours) and gentamicin (1.5 mg/kg every 8 hours) is an acceptable alternative.

Quinolone antibiotics (eg, ciprofloxacin) interfere with fetal cartilage development and should be avoided. Nitrofurantoin is used frequently in pregnancy but can induce hemolysis in patients who are deficient in glucose-6-phosphate dehydrogenase, a condition that affects approximately 2% of African Americans. Sulfonamides (eg, trimethoprim/sulfamethoxazole) are contraindicated in the third trimester of pregnancy because of the risk of kernicterus in newborns. Tetracyclines are contraindicated because they can cause yellowish discoloration in the child's teeth.

Treatment of pyelonephritis is necessary because of the increased risk of premature labor. All pregnant patients with pyelonephritis should be hospitalized, and periodic fetal monitoring should be instituted. Follow-up cultures are indicated to ensure eradication.

Additional Reading:
1. Diagnosis and treatment of acute pyelonephritis in women. *Am Fam Physician*. 2011;84(5):519-526.
2. Urinary tract infections and asymptomatic bacteriuria in pregnancy. In: *UpToDate*. 2022.

42. A previously healthy young mother presents for her first prenatal visit. She reports that her last menstrual period was about 10 weeks ago. In addition to a pelvic examination, which one of the following laboratory tests is indicated at this time?

A) α-Fetoprotein
B) Antibody test (indirect Coombs test)
C) Free T4
D) Glucose tolerance test
E) Quantitative β-human chorionic gonadotropin

The answer is B: Prenatal testing is usually performed at the initial prenatal visit. Tests include Papanicolaou test (if due based on age-appropriate screening intervals), complete blood count, urinalysis with culture, ABO blood type, Rh status, antibody test (indirect Coombs test), rubella antibody titer, syphilis, human immunodeficiency virus, and hepatitis B surface antigen testing. Other tests may include urine or cervical testing for chlamydia and gonorrhea, tuberculosis skin test, sickle cell prep, hepatitis C antibody, varicella antibody, and thyroid-stimulating hormone.

α-Fetoprotein testing is usually done with the maternal serum screening at 15 to 18 weeks' gestation. A 1-hour glucose challenge test (Glucola) is done at 24 to 28 weeks' gestation and hematocrit and Rh antibody screening at 28 weeks' gestation. Patients at high risk for sexually transmitted diseases (STDs) may need repeated STD screening later in pregnancy. Vaginal-rectal swab for group B *Streptococcus* (GBS) should be obtained from all pregnant women 35- to 37-week gestational age except those already known to have had GBS bacteriuria.

Additional Reading: Update on prenatal care. *Am Fam Physician*. 2014;89(3):199-208.

43. When a pregnant patient in the first trimester experiences vaginal bleeding, which one of the following tests should be obtained to evaluate fetal viability?

A) Qualitative β-human chorionic gonadotropin (β-hCG) determination
B) Serial quantitative β-hCG measurements
C) Transvaginal ultrasonography
D) Serum progesterone levels

The answer is C: Approximately 25% of pregnant women experience vaginal spotting or heavier bleeding during the first trimester of pregnancy, and 25% to 50% of these pregnant women experience spontaneous abortion. Genetic anomalies are the most common cause of spontaneous abortion in the first trimester.

Qualitative hCG determination is consistent with a diagnosis of pregnancy because the positive test reflects the presence of hCG, usually at a level of >25 mIU/mL. However, it does not give any information regarding the viability or location of an actual pregnancy. When first-trimester bleeding is present, potential viability of the pregnancy can be determined with serial quantitative β-hCG determinations, which are repeated 3 to 5 days after a baseline level is determined. The β-hCG level should double every 48 hours, when a normal pregnancy is present, but does not definitively diagnose an intrauterine viable pregnancy until confirmed by ultrasonography.

A fetus should be seen with vaginal ultrasonography by the 33rd to 35th day after the last menstrual period, or when the β-hCG level has reached 1500 to 2000 mIU/mL. If the β-hCG level exceeds 1500 to 2000 mIU/mL and no intrauterine pregnancy is found with vaginal ultrasonography, an ectopic pregnancy should be suspected, especially if an adnexal mass is palpated on physical examination or the patient experiences lower abdominal pain.

Progesterone levels of less than 5 ng/dL usually indicate a nonviable pregnancy, but progesterone measurements are not generally used for diagnosis of viability.

Additional Reading: First trimester bleeding. *Am Fam Physician*. 2009;79(11):985-992.

44. You have been caring for a 25-year-old woman since she was child and helping to manage her well-controlled seizure disorder. She would like to get pregnant and have a child and is asking for advice about the use of her anticonvulsant medications (ACMs) during pregnancy. Which one of the following statements is true concerning the use of ACMs during pregnancy?

A) Most ACMs are considered safe (category B).
B) Seizure activity in mothers has no impact on fetal outcomes.
C) Single ACM agents are preferred to multiple medications.
D) Multiple ACMs are preferred to maintain low doses of each medication.
E) ACM should be discontinued and the patient cautioned not to drive at the time pregnancy is confirmed.

The answer is C: Children of mothers with epilepsy have a 4% to 8% risk of congenital anomalies, which may be caused by ACM or may be related to an increased genetic risk. These children also have an increased risk of developing epilepsy. Preconception counseling should include optimizing seizure control, prescribing folic acid supplements of 1 to 4 mg/d, and offering referral to a genetic counselor.

Tonic-clonic seizures in pregnancy can lead to hypoxia in the fetus, and pregnant women with any type of seizure are also at risk for trauma (eg, falls), which can also adversely impact the fetus. The therapeutic goal for women with seizure disorders who are pregnant is to prevent seizures while minimizing teratogenic damage to the fetus.

If possible, use of multiple anticonvulsants should be discouraged. It is advisable to use the best single agent for the seizure type at the lowest protective level. A committee assembled by the American Academy of Neurology reassessed the evidence related to the care of women with epilepsy during pregnancy, including ACM teratogenicity. Some of the conclusions published by this committee related to specific medication concerns are as follows:

- First-trimester valproate (VPA) exposure has higher risk of major congenital malformations compared with carbamazepine, and possibly compared with phenytoin and lamotrigine.
- ACM polytherapy likely contributes to the development of major congenital malformations and reduced cognitive outcomes compared with monotherapy. VPA monotherapy probably reduces cognitive outcomes.
- If possible, avoidance of VPA and ACM polytherapy during the first trimester of pregnancy should be considered to decrease the risk of major congenital malformations. If possible, avoidance of VPA and ACM polytherapy throughout pregnancy should be considered to prevent reduced cognitive outcomes.
- If the patient has been seizure-free for 2 years or longer, drug discontinuation with a long taper period (3 months) may be successful.

Additional Reading: Management issues for women with epilepsy-focus on pregnancy. *Epilepsia*. 2009;50(5):1237-1246.

45. You are seeing a 22-year-old woman who is interested in getting pregnant. She reports that she smokes a pack of cigarettes per day and wants to know about the risks of smoking during her pregnancy. Which one of the following statements is true regarding smoking during pregnancy?

A) Bupropion (Zyban) is contraindicated during pregnancy.
B) Nicotine patches are a safe alternative during pregnancy.
C) Smoking increases the risk of attention-deficit disorder in the child.
D) Infants born to mothers with a smoking history, regardless of when the mother stopped smoking, are at risk for neonatal complications.
E) When compared with total abstinence, reducing the number of cigarettes smoked has no effect on fetal outcomes.

The answer is C: Smoking increases the risk of miscarriage, low birth weight, perinatal mortality, and subsequent attention-deficit disorder in the child. If the mother smokes less than 1 pack of cigarettes per day, the risk of a low-birth-weight infant increases by 50%; with more than 1 pack per day, the risk increases by 130%. However, if the mother quits smoking by 16 weeks of pregnancy, the risk to the fetus is similar to that of a nonsmoker.

Behavioral techniques, support groups, and family assistance may be beneficial. Nicotine patches or gum may be helpful before conception, but most authorities recommend avoiding them during pregnancy. Bupropion may be used during pregnancy after a discussion of risks and benefits. If the patient cannot stop smoking, the physician should help her establish a goal to decrease her number of cigarettes to fewer than 7 to 10 per day, as many of the adverse effects are dose related.

Additional Reading: Smoking cessation in pregnancy (2013). ACOG Committee Opinion Paper no. 471. 2013. www.acog.org/Resources_And_Publications/Committee_Opinions_List

46. Your 23-year-old patient with an anxiety disorder is being treated with clonazepam by her psychiatrist. She wants to get pregnant and have a child and is asking if it is OK to continue to use her medication during her pregnancy. You inform her that the use of benzodiazepines during pregnancy has been associated with which one of the following conditions?

A) Cleft lip
B) Developmental delay
C) Growth retardation
D) Polydactyly
E) Spina bifida

The answer is A: Maternal use of benzodiazepines during pregnancy has been associated with anomalies such as cleft lip and palate, as well as a withdrawal syndrome in the newborn.

Additional Reading: ACOG guidelines on psychiatric medication use during pregnancy and lactation. *Am Fam Physician*. 2008;78(6):772-778.

47. An obese patient (body mass index [BMI] 32) presents to discuss pregnancy. She has always been overweight and wants to know if her weight will cause any problems during her pregnancy or for her infant. You inform here that all of the following conditions are associated with maternal obesity during pregnancy, except which one?

A) Maternal diabetes
B) Maternal hypertension
C) Neonatal hydrocephalus
D) Neonatal macrosomia
E) Preeclampsia

The answer is C: Obesity increases the risks of maternal hypertension, preeclampsia, diabetes, and macrosomia (which is, in itself, related to birth complications such as shoulder dystocia). Women who are obese (BMI > 30) should attempt to lose weight and reduce their caloric intake to 1800 cal/d prior to conception. Additionally, overweight women should only gain 10 to 20 lb (4-9 kg) during pregnancy.

Additional Reading: Obesity in pregnancy. ACOG Committee Opinion no. 549. 2013. http://www.acog.org/Resources_And_Publications/Committee_Opinions_List

48. A 25-year-old primigravida presents to your office with a concern over itchy skin lesions that have developed on her abdomen. The rash is composed of reddened spots. Her face, palms, and soles are spared. She is pregnant with a twin gestation and is in her third trimester. The most likely diagnosis for such a presentation is which one of the following conditions?

A) Herpes zoster
B) Hyperbilirubinemia
C) Pruritic urticarial papules and plaques of pregnancy (PUPPP)
D) Scabies infection
E) Varicella infection

The answer is C: PUPPP, also known as *polymorphic eruption of pregnancy*, is the most common dermatologic complaint of pregnancy. The etiology is not well understood. The condition occurs in up to 1 in 160 pregnancies, with an increased incidence in multiple gestations. It usually occurs in primigravidae in the third trimester, and recurrence in subsequent pregnancies is unusual.

The rash may first appear postpartum. PUPPP typically presents with a marked pruritic component, the onset of which coincides with the skin lesions. The rash typically begins over the abdomen, commonly involving the striae gravidarum, and may spread to the breasts, upper thighs, and arms. The face, palms, soles, and mucosal surfaces are usually spared. The lesions typically consist of polymorphous, erythematous, nonfollicular papules, plaques, and sometimes vesicles. The lesions can be painful.

The rash usually resolves near term or in the early postpartum period. Topical moisturizers and moderately potent steroids in combination with oral antihistamines can provide symptomatic relief.

Additional Reading: The skin disorders of pregnancy: a family physician's guide. *J Fam Pract*. 2010;59(2):89-96.

Section II. Labor and Delivery

Each of the following questions or incomplete statements below is followed by suggested answers or completions. Select the ONE BEST ANSWER in each case.

1. A young woman presents with regular contractions at 34 weeks and has yet to attend her prenatal "birthing" classes. She is asking if the baby will be OK as she thought her due date is 2 months away. You inform her that she is in "preterm" labor, which is defined as regular contractions with cervical change before which one of the following weeks of gestation?

A) 39 weeks' gestation
B) 38 weeks' gestation
C) 37 weeks' gestation
D) 36 weeks' gestation
E) 35 weeks' gestation

The answer is C: According to the American College of Obstetricians and Gynecologists, *preterm labor* is defined as regular contractions associated with cervical change before 37 weeks' gestation.

Additional Reading: American College of Obstetricians and Gynecologists. Assessment of risk factors for preterm birth. ACOG Practice Bulletin no. 31. www.acog.org/Resources_And_Publications/Committee_Opinions_List

2. External cephalic version is a technique used to turn a fetus that is in the breech or transverse position. Which one of the following is a contraindication for using this technique?

A) Maternal age of 35 years
B) Maternal diabetes
C) Maternal obesity
D) 36 weeks' gestation
E) Polyhydramnios

The answer is D: External cephalic version can be attempted on fetuses that are found to be mispositioned (ie, breech or transverse lie) before the onset of labor and after 37 weeks' gestation. A tocolytic is delivered, and abdominal manipulation is performed under ultrasonography guidance. Version before 37 weeks is not recommended because of the risk that the fetus may revert to a breech presentation before delivery and the risk of delivery of a premature infant. The success rate is approximately 75%.

The procedure should be performed in the hospital so that cesarean section can be done if complications arise. The most common complications are placental abruption and cord compression. Contraindications for external cephalic version include uteroplacental insufficiency, hypertension, intrauterine growth retardation, oligohydramnios, or a history of prior uterine surgery.

Additional Reading: *External cephalic version*. In: *UpToDate*. 2022.

3. A young patient at 32 weeks' gestation is experiencing preterm labor. Which one of the following is not considered appropriate to use for up to 48 hours of tocolysis in this situation?

A) Ceftriaxone
B) Indomethacin
C) Magnesium sulfate
D) Nifedipine
E) Ritodrine

The answer is A: Evidence supports the use of tocolytic treatment with a variety of agents including magnesium sulfate, β-adrenergic agonist (eg, ritodrine), calcium channel blockers (CCBs) (eg, nifedipine), or nonsteroidal anti-inflammatory drugs (NSAIDs) (eg, indomethacin).

Tocolytics are recommended for short-term prolongation of pregnancy (up to 48 hours) to allow for the administration of antenatal steroids. Corticosteroids are recommended for all pregnant women between 24 and 34 weeks of gestation who are at risk of preterm delivery within 7 days. Antibiotics (eg, ceftriaxone) should not be used to prolong gestation or improve neonatal outcomes in women with preterm labor and intact membranes.

There is accumulated evidence that magnesium sulfate ($MgSO_4$) reduces the severity and risk of cerebral palsy in surviving infants if administered when birth is anticipated before 32 weeks' gestational age. Hospitals that elect to use $MgSO_4$ are expected to develop specific guidelines for this indication. Maintenance therapy with tocolytics (ie, beyond 48 hours of use) is ineffective for preventing preterm birth and improving neonatal outcomes and is not recommended for this purpose.

Additional Reading:

1. Management of preterm labor. ACOG Practice Bulletin no. 127. 2012. www.acog.org/Resources_And_Publications/Committee_Opinions_List
2. Preterm labor: prevention and management. *Am Family Physician*. 2017;95(6):366-372.

4. Several bacterial infections have been associated with preterm labor. Which one of the following bacterial infections is *not* generally associated with preterm labor?

A) *Bacteroides* species.
B) *G vaginalis*.
C) *Mycoplasma hominis*.
D) *Ureaplasma urealyticum*.
E) All are associated with preterm labor.

The answer is E: Several bacterial infections have been associated with preterm labor, including *U urealyticum*, *M hominis*, *G vaginalis*, and *Peptostreptococcus* and *Bacteroides* species. These organisms are usually of low virulence, and it is unclear whether they are etiologic or associated with an acute inflammatory response of another etiology.

Additional Reading: American College of Obstetricians and Gynecologists. Assessment of risk factors for preterm birth. ACOG Practice Bulletin no. 31. www.acog.org/Resources_And_Publications/Committee_Opinions_List

5. A young woman presents with contractions at 36 weeks' gestation. Which one of the following tests best predicts the likelihood of preterm birth in women presenting with symptomatic preterm uterine contractions and can be used to guide pharmacologic management of preterm labor?

A) Screening for genitourinary infections
B) Measurement of salivary estriol
C) Cervical length measurement
D) Fetal fibronectin screening
E) Both C and D

The answer is E: A positive fetal fibronectin test, in conjunction with a shortened cervical length, is a useful predictor of preterm delivery in a patient presenting with symptoms of preterm labor. These screening tests have been shown to have a high sensitivity and high positive predictive value, as well as a high negative predictive value. Therefore, they are useful in guiding decisions regarding steroid and tocolytic administration in women who have positive results and allow avoidance of these therapies in women with negative results.

Additional Reading:

1. Improving the screening accuracy for preterm labor: is the combination of fetal fibronectin and cervical length in symptomatic patients a useful predictor of preterm birth? *Am J Obstet Gynecol*. 2013;208(3):233.
2. Preterm labor: prevention and management. *Am Family Physician*. 2017;95(6):366-372.

6. You are monitoring a 27-year-old G2P1 mother in active labor. Overall, the labor has been going smoothly and the fetal heart tracing shows repeated late decelerations. This type of tracing is consistent with which one of the following conditions?

A) Abnormal presentation
B) Head engagement
C) Rapid descent of the fetus
D) Uteroplacental insufficiency
E) Normal progression of labor

The answer is D: Repetitive late decelerations of the fetal heart rate (FHR) may signal uteroplacental insufficiency and require evaluation of the patient and interventions aimed at improving placental blood flow and fetal oxygenation.

Early decelerations may be caused by head compression and are usually of little concern. Late deceleration patterns look similar to early decelerations but begin well after the contraction begins and return to baseline after the contraction ends.

Variable decelerations do not have the uniform appearance of early or late decelerations and may occur without a contraction. Assessing the associated FHR is important; it is concerning if the rate repeatedly drops to less than 70 beats per minute and persists at a low rate for at least 60 seconds before returning to baseline. Variable decelerations can be caused by cord compression.

Additional Reading: Intrapartum fetal monitoring. *Am Fam Physician*. 2009;80(12):1388-1396.

7. Which one of the following is an absolute contraindication to tocolysis for a patient experiencing preterm labor?

A) A biophysical profile score of 8
B) Chorioamnionitis
C) Four centimeters of cervical dilation
D) Hyperthyroidism
E) Oligohydramnios

The answer is B: Absolute contraindications to the use of tocolytics include the following:

- Severe abruptio placentae
- Infection (chorioamnionitis)
- Severe bleeding
- Severe pregnancy-induced hypertension
- Fetal anomalies that are incompatible with life
- Fetal death
- Severe growth retardation
- Fetal distress

Relative contraindications include the following:

- Hyperthyroidism
- Uncontrolled diabetes
- Maternal heart disease
- Hypertension
- Mild abruptio placentae
- Stable placenta previa
- Fetal distress
- Mild growth retardation
- Cervical dilation greater than 5 to 6 cm

Additional Reading: Preterm labor: prevention and management. *Am Family Physician*. 2017;95(6):366-372.

8. Intrauterine fetal demise in the third trimester is not only a disastrous consequence for parents but can also cause adverse health effects for the mother. The most appropriate management for intrauterine fetal demise in the third trimester includes which one of the following?

A) Administration of intravenous (IV) oxytocin (Pitocin) after serial misoprostol 25 to 50 μg every 4 hours until the cervix ripened
B) High-dose misoprostol (200-400 μg) every 4 hours
C) Heparin plus antibiotic prophylaxis and observation
D) Immediate cesarean section
E) Observation for up to 4 weeks until the mother goes into labor

The answer is A: The risk of disseminated intravascular coagulation is increased if a nonviable fetus has been retained in utero for more than 4 weeks. Therefore, it is practical to provide expectant management for patients with in utero fetal demise for up to 1 to 3 weeks. However, because many patients experience significant psychological stress from carrying a nonviable fetus, patients who have experienced a fetal demise should be offered hospital admission and induction of labor.

Induction is most effective if vaginal prostaglandins such as misoprostol are given first to provide cervical ripening followed by IV Pitocin. Doses of misoprostol for cervical ripening in the third trimester of pregnancy are typically 25 to 50 μg through vagina every 4 hours, whereas higher doses (200-400 μg every 4 hours) can be used to achieve uterine evacuation for second-trimester intrauterine fetal demise.

Additional Reading: *Diagnosis and management of stillbirth*. In: *UpToDate*. 2022.

9. A 26-year-old primiparous woman pushed effectively during a 2-hour second stage with subsequent delivery of the infant's head followed by a "turtle sign." She was unable to deliver the infant's shoulders with the normal amount of downward traction and maternal expulsive efforts. You diagnose a shoulder dystocia. In addition to asking the patient to stop pushing, the next appropriate step is which one of the following interventions?

A) Apply fundal pressure.
B) Place the mother in the left lateral position.
C) Perform McRoberts maneuver.
D) Perform a cesarean section.
E) Use a rotational maneuver, either the Rubin II or Wood corkscrew maneuver.

The answer is C: The "turtle sign" is when the fetal head retracts back against the mother's perineum after it emerges from the vagina. The retraction of the fetal head is caused by the baby's anterior shoulder catching on the back of the maternal pubic bone, preventing delivery of the remainder of the baby. The recommended sequence for reducing shoulder dystocia begins with calling for help and asking the mother to stop her pushing efforts.

The first step is the McRoberts maneuver, in which assistants hyperflex the mother's hips against her abdomen, thereby rotating the symphysis pubis anteriorly and decreasing the forces needed to deliver the fetal shoulders. A retrospective study found this maneuver to be the safest and most successful technique for relieving shoulder dystocia. An assistant can add gentle posterolateral suprapubic pressure while the physician continues moderate posterior traction on the fetal head. Fundal pressure should be avoided, because it tends to increase the impaction.

Rotational maneuvers may be tried next, beginning with the Rubin II maneuver, which is done by inserting the fingers of one hand vaginally behind the posterior aspect of the anterior shoulder of the fetus and rotating the shoulder toward the fetal chest. This will adduct the fetal shoulder girdle, reducing its diameter. If the Rubin II maneuver is unsuccessful, the Wood corkscrew maneuver may be attempted. Two fingers are placed on the anterior aspect of the fetal posterior shoulder, applying gentle upward pressure around the circumference of the arc in the same direction as with the Rubin II maneuver.

The Rubin II and Wood corkscrew maneuvers may be combined to increase forces by using two fingers behind the fetal anterior shoulder and two fingers in front of the fetal posterior shoulder. If these efforts are unsuccessful, clavicular fracture may be attempted, followed by maternal symphysiotomy, and finally Zavanelli maneuver (involves pushing the fetal head back inside the uterus to perform a cesarean section).

Additional Reading: Shoulder dystocia. *Am Fam Physician*. 2004;69(7):1707-1714.

10. A patient who is at 38 weeks' gestation calls panicked that she is experiencing some vaginal bleeding—but is not having any pain or contractions. This scenario is most likely due to which one of the following conditions?

A) Bloody show
B) Cervical ripening
C) Placenta accreta
D) Placenta previa
E) Vaso previa

The answer is D: Painless hemorrhage is the hallmark sign of placenta previa. Although spotting may occur during the first and second trimesters of pregnancy with placenta previa, the first episode of hemorrhage usually begins at some point after the 28th week and is characteristically described as being sudden, painless, and profuse. However, blood loss is not usually extensive, seldom produces shock, and is almost never fatal. In about 10% of cases, there is some initial pain because of coexisting placental abruption, and spontaneous labor may be expected over the next few days in 25% of patients. In rare cases, bleeding is less dramatic or does not begin until after spontaneous rupture of membranes or the onset of labor. Occasionally, nulliparous patients can reach term without bleeding, possibly because the placenta has been protected by an intact cervix.

Additional Reading: *Clinical features, diagnosis, and course of placenta previa*. In: *UpToDate*. 2022.

11. The normal amount of blood loss for a vaginal delivery is which one of the following?

A) 250 mL
B) 500 mL
C) 1000 mL
D) 1500 mL
E) 2000 mL

The answer is B: The average pregnant patient typically loses 500 mL of blood at the time of vaginal delivery and 1000 mL during a cesarean delivery. Appreciably more blood can be lost without clinical evidence of a volume deficit as a result of the

40% expansion in blood volume that occurs by the 30th week of pregnancy.

Additional Reading: *Overview of postpartum hemorrhage*. In: *UpToDate*. 2022.

12. A young patient expecting her first child is asking about the use of epidural anesthesia for her labor. Which one of the following statements about epidural anesthesia is true?

A) Anesthesia is only provided for lumbar and sacral nerve roots.
B) Epidural anesthesia should only be used for multigravida women.
C) Epidurals are safe for use in hemophiliacs.
D) Hypotension can be an associated side effect.
E) The epidural catheter should be placed at the L2-L3 level.

The answer is D: Epidural anesthesia is used as a regional block during childbirth. The procedure is performed by inserting a needle between L3 and L4, and threading a catheter into the epidural space. The catheter is then aspirated to check for the presence of cerebrospinal fluid. If this occurs, the catheter must be repositioned. A test dose is then administered to reconfirm the position. When the position is confirmed, a full dose of anesthetic is administered through the catheter. Analgesia is usually established with fentanyl plus a small dose of bupivacaine. Fentanyl works better for the visceral pain that is associated with labor, whereas bupivacaine is more effective for somatic pain. The dose may need to be repeated to maintain anesthesia during delivery. In most cases, a full dose provides anesthesia of nerve roots T10-S5.

Risks that are involved with epidural anesthesia include drug reaction, hypotension, and rare neurologic complications. If the dura is penetrated, a spinal headache eventually develops in many patients. Contraindications to epidural anesthesia include adverse effects to anesthesia, bleeding tendency (eg, hemophilia), infection of the lumbar area, or underlying neurologic defects.

Some studies have reported that epidural anesthesia may prolong labor, but it seems that this is a possible outcome only if the epidural is given prior to active labor; but if given after active labor has begun, cesarean delivery rates are the same as someone who received intravenous analgesia.

Additional Reading:
1. Labor analgesia. *Am Fam Physician*. 2012:85(5):447-454.
2. Analgesia and cesarean delivery rates. ACOG Committee Opinion Number 339. American Congress of Obstetricians and Gynecologists; 2016.

13. Tocolysis is the process of stopping preterm labor contractions with medications. All of the following medications are used for tocolysis, except which one?

A) Magnesium sulfate
B) Nifedipine
C) Propranolol
D) Ritodrine
E) Terbutaline

The answer is C: Medications that are used for tocolysis include β-sympathomimetics (ritodrine, terbutaline), magnesium sulfate, prostaglandin synthetase inhibitors (indomethacin), and calcium channel blockers (nifedipine). Tocolysis is usually not successful if the cervix has dilated to greater than 4 cm. Contraindications to tocolysis include fetal distress, fetal anomalies, significant risk to the mother, abruptio placentae, or placenta previa with heavy bleeding.

Additional Reading: Preterm labor: prevention and management. *Am Family Physician*. 2017;95(6):366-372.

14. Your patient is in the early stages of labor and you have diagnosed her with preeclampsia as her blood pressures are elevated. The drug of choice for controlling eclamptic seizures is which one of the following?

A) Diazepam
B) Hydralazine
C) Magnesium sulfate
D) Phenobarbital
E) Phenytoin

The answer is C: Magnesium sulfate is considered the drug of choice for controlling eclamptic seizures. Fewer intubations are required in the neonates of eclamptic women who are treated with magnesium sulfate. In addition, fewer newborns require placement in neonatal intensive care units.

In the treatment of eclampsia and preeclampsia, magnesium sulfate is often given according to established protocols. If serum magnesium levels exceed 10 mEq/L (5 mmol/L), respiratory depression can occur. This problem may be counteracted by the rapid intravenous infusion of 10% calcium gluconate. Magnesium sulfate should be used with caution in patients with impaired renal or cardiac status, and it should not be used in patients with myasthenia gravis.

Additional Reading: *Magnesium sulfate use in obstetrics. ACOG Committee Opinion Number 652*. American Congress of Obstetricians and Gynecologists; 2016.

15. You are discussing a vaginal delivery after cesarean with a young mother, who is pregnant with her second child. She had a cesarean section for her first childbirth. You inform her that which one of the following would be considered an absolute contraindication for a trial of labor after cesarean (TOLAC) section?

A) A twin gestation
B) A previous vertical uterine cesarean section
C) An unknown type of previous cesarean section
D) Two prior low cervical transverse cesarean sections

The answer is B: All pregnant women who have had prior lower cervical transverse cesarean section should be counseled regarding the availability of a TOLAC section and the benefits of successful vaginal delivery after cesarean. These benefits include decreased maternal morbidity as well as a decreased risk of complications in future pregnancies.

The risks of a TOLAC section with a focus on the risk of uterine rupture during labor need to be reviewed, and this risk is related to the type of uterine incision that women have had in their prior cesarean sections. Women who have had a previous cesarean section via a vertical (classic) incision should undergo repeat cesarean section for delivery because of the increased risk of uterine rupture.

Preferably, candidates for a TOLAC section have documentation of one prior lower cervical transverse cesarean. However, women who have unknown uterine scars can be allowed to attempt a TOLAC section if it is not thought to be high risk of a previous classical incision, on the basis of the history obtained from the patient regarding the circumstances of her previous cesarean. There are limited data on TOLAC sections in women who have had two prior cesarean sections; however, these women can be allowed a TOLAC section after appropriate counseling regarding risks and benefits.

Women who attempt a TOLAC section after adequate antepartum counseling are quite successful (approximately 60%-80%) in vaginal deliveries with subsequent births. Women who are unsuccessful during a trial of labor and require repeat cesarean section at that time have higher complication rates than women who undergo elective repeat cesareans. Women with previous cesarean sections (low transverse incision) can also receive oxytocin during labor, but the contractions and the fetus should be closely monitored. Misoprostol as a cervical ripening agent in the third trimester is contraindicated in women with prior cesarean section because of the increased risk for uterine rupture.

Additional Reading: Vaginal birth after previous cesarean delivery. ACOG Practice Bulletin no. 115. 2013. www.acog.org/Resources_And_Publications/Committee_Opinions_List

16. You have just assisted in the delivery of a full-term newborn. The labor was uneventful, but now the mother is continuing with postpartum bleeding. The most common reason to explain this scenario is which one of the following conditions?

A) Coagulopathy
B) HELLP syndrome
C) Retained placenta
D) Uterine atony
E) Vaginal laceration

The answer is D: Hemorrhage after placental delivery should prompt vigorous fundal massage while the patient is rapidly given oxytocin in their intravenous fluid. If the fundus does not become firm, uterine atony is the presumed (and most common) diagnosis. While fundal massage continues, the patient may be given methylergonovine (Methergine) intramuscularly, with the dose repeated at 2- to 4-hour intervals if necessary. Methylergonovine may cause cramping, headache, and dizziness. The use of this drug is contraindicated in patients with hypertension.

Alternatively, carboprost (Hemabate), 15-methyl prostaglandin F_{2a}, may be administered intramuscularly or intramyometrially every 15 to 90 minutes, up to a maximum dosage. As many as 68% of patients respond to a single carboprost injection, with 86% responding by the second dose. Another prostaglandin that is increasingly used in the treatment of postpartum hemorrhage is misoprostol, which is most commonly administered rectally as an 800- to 1000-μg dose; however, it can also be administered buccally or vaginally.

Additional Reading:
1. *Obstetrical* Hemorrhage. *Williams Obstetrics*. 26th ed. McGraw-Hill; 2022.
2. Postpartum hemorrhage: prevention and treatment. *Am Fam Physician*. 2017;95(7):442-449.

17. A 19-year-old G1P0 female patient is in the second stage of labor. She begins to complain of abdominal pain between uterine contractions. You suspect which one of the following conditions?

A) A breech presentation
B) A posterior presentation
C) A vasa previa
D) An abruptio placentae
E) Uterine atony

The answer is D: The patient in labor who develops abdominal pain between uterine contractions or who has a tender uterus must be presumed to have abruptio placentae. Ultrasonography examination has a high false-negative rate in diagnosing placental abruption and, as a result, this complication is diagnosed clinically. In one prospective study, 78% of patients with abruptio placentae presented with vaginal bleeding, 66% with uterine or back pain, 60% with fetal distress, and only 17% with uterine contractions or hypertonus.

The management of abruptio placentae is primarily supportive and entails both aggressive hydration and monitoring of maternal and fetal well-being. Coagulation studies should be performed, and fibrinogen and D-dimers or fibrin degradation products should be measured to screen for disseminated intravascular coagulation. Packed red blood cells should be typed and held. If the fetus appears viable but compromised, urgent cesarean delivery should be considered.

Additional Reading: *Placental Abruption. Williams Obstetrics*. 25th ed. McGraw-Hill; 2018.

18. Oxytocin is a natural hormone released into the bloodstream during labor and therefore used as a medication to facilitate childbirth. All of the following statements are true regarding the administration of oxytocin when used for this indication, except which one?

A) Oxytocin must be given through a controlled infusion device.
B) Oxytocin must be administered as a continuous infusion or in "pulsed" doses.
C) Oxytocin can have a diuretic effect with high doses.
D) Oxytocin can result in uterine hyperstimulation.

The answer is C: Oxytocin is mixed for use by placing 10 U in 1 L of isotonic intravenous (IV) solution to achieve a concentration of 10 mU/mL. Because severe hypotension can occur, especially during rapid IV administration, and because the drug is infused into the main IV line, a controlled infusion device must be used to determine its rate. However, it can be administered as a continuous infusion or in "pulsed" doses.

Effect of oxytocin is noted within 3 to 5 minutes, and a steady state is achieved within 15 to 30 minutes. Studies show a wide range of effective dosages—no regimen has been shown to be clearly superior. Oxytocin has many advantages: the medication is potent and easy to titrate, has a short half-life (1-5 minutes), and is generally well tolerated. Dose-related adverse effects can occur.

Because oxytocin is close to vasopressin in structure, it has an antidiuretic effect when given in high dosages (40 mU/min); thus, water intoxication is a possibility in prolonged inductions. Uterine hyperstimulation and uterine rupture can also occur. When the resting uterine tone remains above 20 mm Hg, uteroplacental insufficiency and fetal hypoxia can result.

Additional Reading: Oxytocin augmentation during labor with epidural analgesia. *Am Fam Physician*. 2013;87(11):760-761.

19. A young woman is contracting in premature labor. In assessing the extent of lung development for her fetus, which one of the following laboratory results would be consistent with lung maturity in a fetus?

A) A lecithin-sphingomyelin (L/S) ratio of 1.5
B) An L/S ratio less than 1.0
C) A lamellar body count (LBC) of >10,000
D) Undetectable levels of phosphatidylglycerol (PG)
E) An L/S ratio of 2.2 with a positive PG level

The answer is E: Premature birth can result in severe lung-related problems (ie, respiratory distress syndrome [RDS]) secondary to inadequate lung development. Tests for lung maturity include the

LBC, L/S ratio, and detection of PG. The levels are measured by obtaining amniotic fluid via amniocentesis.

The LBC provides a direct measurement of surfactant production by the fetal lungs, and testing for these is less labor-intensive and therefore faster than the L/S ratio, which is often done simultaneously with PG testing. LBCs that are less than 30,000/mL are considered to represent underlying fetal lung immaturity, whereas LBCs greater than 50,000/mL are associated with positive fetal lung maturity.

LBCs in the range of 30,000 to 50,000/mL are inconclusive; therefore, some centers do LBCs as an initial screen. If results are very high or very low, a diagnosis of fetal lung maturity or immaturity is made, and if the LBC is indeterminate because of decrease in the middle range, the lengthier L/S and PG testing is then done.

RDS is rare if the L/S ratio is >2 and PG is present. If the L/S ratio is <2 but PG is present, RDS develops in <5% of infants.

A variety of medications have been used to improve lung maturation. The use of antenatal corticosteroids reduces mortality and the incidence of RDS and intraventricular hemorrhage in new preterm infants. Treatment is typically administered between 24 and 34 weeks. The benefits usually peak at 24 hours and continue for 7 days. Treatment consists of betamethasone given in two intramuscular doses 24 hours apart. Antenatal steroids should be administered, unless immediate delivery is anticipated.

Additional Reading: *Assessment of fetal lung maturity*. In: *UpToDate*. 2022.

20. A 27-year-old primipara has had prolonged, difficult labor, and a decision is made to proceed with a cesarean section as the fetal heart rate tracing has shown signs of fetal compromise. The nurse is asking if you want to prescribe an antibiotic. Which one of the following would be indicated in this situation?

A) Administer preoperative antibiotics within 1 hour of starting surgery.
B) No antibiotics are indicated because of the risk of resistant neonatal infection.
C) Administer antibiotics only if the surgery is prolonged (>1.5 hours).
D) No antibiotics are necessary in low-risk patients.
E) Administer antibiotics only if an infection is suspected.

The answer is A: According to the American College of Obstetricians and Gynecologists, all patients undergoing cesarean delivery should receive prophylaxis with narrow-spectrum antibiotics such as a first-generation cephalosporin within the hour prior to surgical skin incision. Infection is the most common complication of cesarean delivery and can occur in 10% to 40% of women who have a cesarean compared with 1% to 3% of women who deliver vaginally.

In previous practice, antibiotics were given to patients requiring cesarean sections at the time when the umbilical cord is clamped. This practice was based on the concern that any antibiotic entering the baby's bloodstream via transfer from the mother would interfere with newborn laboratory tests or could lead to antibiotic-resistant infections. However, studies have shown that prophylactic antibiotics given before initiation of cesarean section significantly reduce maternal infection and do not cause harm to newborns.

Additional Reading: Antimicrobial prophylaxis for cesarean delivery: timing of administration. ACOG Committee Opinion no. 465. www.acog.org/Resources_And_Publications/Committee_Opinions_List

21. A woman with a favorable cervix is a good predictor of the likelihood of vaginal delivery when labor is induced, but induction will most likely fail even at term with a cervix that is unfavorable (firm, posterior, neither dilated nor effaced). Therefore, if the cervix is unfavorable, a ripening process is generally required. Which one of the following medications can be safely used for cervical ripening in term pregnancies?

A) Bromocriptine
B) Methotrexate
C) Misoprostol
D) Terbutaline
E) Thalidomide

The answer is C: Cervical ripening is a process that results in softening and distension of the cervix, leading to effacement and dilatation. These changes are naturally induced by hormones (estrogen, progesterone, relaxin), as well as cytokines and prostaglandins. The two major techniques for inducing cervical ripening are physical interventions, such as insertion of catheters or cervical dilators, or medical application of cervical ripening agents.

Misoprostol (Cytotec) is a synthetic prostaglandin E1 analogue that has been approved by the U.S. Food and Drug Administration (FDA) for gastric protection. Although it is not approved for use in labor induction, this drug has been extensively investigated for use in cervical ripening. Low-dose (25 μg) intravaginal misoprostol appears to be safe and effective for cervical ripening in term pregnancy for patients without a history of cesarean section. Because of a potential increased risk of uterine rupture, the use of misoprostol for labor induction in women with a previous cesarean section is relatively contraindicated.

Compared with other cervical ripening methods, misoprostol has an increased rate of vaginal delivery within 24 hours without significant differences in cesarean section rates or fetal outcomes. A 50-μg dose of intravaginal misoprostol causes increased rates of uterine hyperstimulation and may be associated with an increased cesarean section rate.

Additional Reading: *Techniques for ripening the unfavorable cervix prior to induction*. In: *UpToDate*. 2022.

22. You are seeing a patient pregnant with her first child at 38 weeks' gestation. She is asking about the option for having epidural anesthesia during her labor. In discussing the risks of placing an epidural during labor, you inform your patient of which one of the following?

A) Early epidural anesthesia increases the risk of cesarean section.
B) Epidural anesthesia may increase the rate of vacuum extraction.
C) Epidural anesthesia has no effect on the length of the second stage of labor.
D) Epidural anesthesia is of little help with pain management in early labor.
E) Epidural anesthesia use in nulliparous women is not recommended until cervical dilation has reached 4 to 5 cm.

The answer is B: Epidural analgesia during labor is an effective pain reliever for labor, which is commonly used. Despite wide acceptance of this use, the timing of epidural placement remains controversial, with conflicting reports on the risk for subsequent cesarean deliveries and the length of the latent phase of labor. There are data from several studies suggesting that epidural anesthesia does lengthen the duration of the second stage of labor and may increase the rate of instrumented vaginal deliveries, such as the need for vacuum extraction.

The American College of Obstetricians and Gynecologists had recommended using other forms of analgesia in nulliparous women until they reach dilatation of 4 to 5 cm. However, a follow-up report recommends that maternal request is a sufficient indication for epidural analgesia during labor and that it should not be denied on the basis of cervical dilatation.

Additional Reading: Management of spontaneous vaginal delivery. *Am Fam Physician*. 2015;92(3):202-208.

23. A 21-year-old primipara is experiencing fatigue and struggling with effective pushing. The decision is made to assist using a vacuum extractor. When attempting such a delivery, it is recommended that the procedure be abandoned for which of the following situations?

A) After 20 minutes of trying to deliver the infant
B) If three consecutive pulls do not produce any progress
C) If three consecutive pulls do not result in the delivery of the infant
D) If there have been three disengagements, also known as "pop-offs," of the vacuum device
E) Any of the above

The answer is E: The use of a vacuum device should be halted when there are three disengagements of the vacuum (or "pop-offs"), more than 20 minutes have elapsed, or three consecutive pulls result in no progress or delivery.

Additional Reading: Instruments for assisted vaginal delivery. *Am Fam Physician*. 2011;84(1):26-27.

24. When deciding to use a vacuum extractor to assist in a delivery, it is important to ensure proper placement of the extractor to avoid injury to the mother and infant. Which one of the following is suggested as to the correct location for placing the center of the cup?

A) Cover the posterior fontanel.
B) Place over the sagittal suture extending to the posterior fontanel.
C) Place over the sagittal suture and 3 cm in front of the posterior fontanel.
D) Place anywhere on exposed cranium.
E) Place it as far anteriorly as possible.

The answer is C: When the vacuum extractor is placed on the fetal scalp, the center of the cup should be over the sagittal suture and about 3 cm (1.2 in.) in front of the posterior fontanel. As a general guide, the cup is placed as far posteriorly as possible. This cup placement maintains flexion of the fetal head and avoids traction over the anterior fontanel. In positioning the cup, the physician should be careful to avoid trapping maternal soft tissue (eg, labia) between the cup and the fetal head.

Additional Reading: Vacuum-assisted vaginal delivery. *Am Fam Physician*. 2008;78(8):953-960.

25. Shoulder dystocia occurs in 1 of 300 deliveries. Which one of the following is considered a major risk factor for shoulder dystocia?

A) Gestational diabetes
B) Precipitous delivery
C) Preterm delivery
D) Thin body habitus
E) Young maternal age

The answer is A: Risk factors include diabetes, postterm pregnancy, obesity, previous shoulder dystocia, prolonged second stage of labor, advanced maternal age, and multiparity.

Risk of shoulder dystocia is related to the size of the fetus:

- Less than 3000 g = 0%
- 3001 to 3500 g = 0.3%
- 3501 to 4000 g = 1.0%
- 4001 to 4500 g = 5.4%
- Greater than 4500 g = 19%

Warning signs for shoulder dystocia include a prolonged second stage of labor and retraction of the fetal head tightly against the vaginal introitus after delivery of the head. Complications include a fractured clavicle or humerus, brachial plexus injuries, anoxic brain injuries, and even death of the fetus.

Additional Reading: Shoulder dystocia. *Am Fam Physician*. 2020;102(2):84-90.

26. Antibiotic treatment is indicated for women in labor who are colonized with group B *Streptococcus* (GBS) to decrease the risk of infection in the newborn. Which one of the following antibiotics is the drug of choice in this situation?

A) Oral amoxicillin
B) Oral ciprofloxacin
C) Intramuscular ceftriaxone
D) Intravenous (IV) penicillin G
E) IV vancomycin

The answer is D: IV penicillin G is the preferred antibiotic for the prevention of GBS infection in newborns, with ampicillin as an alternative. Penicillin G should be administered at least 4 hours before delivery for maximum effectiveness. Cefazolin is recommended in women allergic to penicillin who are at low risk of anaphylaxis. Clindamycin and erythromycin are options for women at high risk for anaphylaxis if testing shows that their GBS isolates are sensitive to these agents. Vancomycin should be used in women allergic to penicillin and whose cultures indicate resistance to clindamycin and erythromycin or when susceptibility is unknown.

Additional Reading: Prevention of perinatal group B streptococcal disease. *ACOG Practice Bulletin 797*. 2022.

27. You have just assisted in the delivery of a 10-lb 4-oz boy and the mother developed a perineal laceration with her final push. When considering the repair of her perineal laceration, which one of the following statements is true?

A) Interrupted transcutaneous sutures are superior to running subcuticular sutures.
B) Repair with skin sutures leads to better outcomes.
C) Skin sutures may increase the incidence of perineal pain.
D) Skin sutures are required for adequate skin approximation.
E) Sutures should begin at the anterior point of the skin laceration.

The answer is C: When the perineal muscles are repaired anatomically, the overlying skin is usually well approximated, and skin sutures are generally not required. Skin sutures have been shown to increase the incidence of perineal pain at 3 months after delivery. If the skin requires suturing, running subcuticular sutures have been shown to be superior to interrupted transcutaneous sutures. Synthetic rapidly absorbable sutures are preferable to catgut, standard absorbable sutures, and these sutures should start at the posterior apex of the skin laceration and should be placed approximately 3 mm from the edge of the skin.

Additional Reading: Absorbable suture materials for primary repair of episiotomy and second degree tears. *Cochrane Database Syst Rev*. 2010;6:CD000006.

28. The obstetrical nurses are monitoring a patient in active labor and call with concerns over a category III fetal heart rate (FHR) tracing. Which one of the following measures is the appropriate response to such a finding?

A) Attempt fetal scalp stimulation, and if an increase in FHR is not observed, continue to watch the patient closely and reattempt scalp stimulation in 30 minutes.
B) Begin in utero resuscitation and proceed to cesarean section within 30 minutes if FHR tracing does not improve.
C) Increase Pitocin to induce a more rapid vaginal delivery.
D) Prepare for expectant management.
E) Proceed to cesarean section immediately.

The answer is B: Because of high interobserver variability in the interpretation of FHR tracings, the American College of Obstetricians and Gynecologists, the Society for Maternal-Fetal Medicine, and the US National Institute of Child Health and Human Development convened a workshop in 2008 to standardize definitions and interpretation of electronic fetal monitoring, propose management guidelines, and develop research questions. The workshop created standard guidelines for FHR interpretation and a three-tier system (categories I, II, and III) for the categorization of intrapartum electronic fetal monitoring. A category III tracing is defined by either of the following criteria:

1. Absent baseline FHR variability and (any of the following):
   a. Recurrent late decelerations
   b. Recurrent variable decelerations
   c. Bradycardia

or

2. A sinusoidal pattern

Category III tracings are abnormal and associated with an increased risk of fetal hypoxic acidemia. Patients with category III tracings should be prepared for delivery while initiating resuscitative measures, such as intravenous fluid bolus, oxygen administration, left-sided positioning, discontinuation of uterotonics, consideration of tocolytics, and request for anesthesia to administer α-adrenergic agonist if the patient has recently received an epidural. If these measures and scalp stimulation do not result in FHR acceleration, delivery should be accomplished expeditiously, ideally within 30 minutes (usually via cesarean section) of beginning the category III tracing.

Additional Reading: American College of Obstetricians and Gynecologists. ACOG Practice Bulletin no. 106: Intrapartum fetal heart rate monitoring – nomenclature, interpretation, and general management principles. *Obstet Gynecol*. 2009;114:192.

29. You have been called to the newborn nursery to assess a febrile neonate. In considering the diagnosis of sepsis, you would determine whether any of the following situations were present, as they are known risk factors for early-onset neonatal sepsis, except which one?

A) Low socioeconomic status
B) Macrosomia
C) Maternal group B *Streptococcus* (GBS) colonization
D) Preterm birth
E) Prolonged rupture of membranes (>18 hours)

The answer is B: The major risk factors for early-onset neonatal sepsis are preterm birth, maternal GBS colonization, prolonged rupture of membranes (>18 hours), and maternal intra-amniotic infection. Other variables include low socioeconomic status, male sex, and low Apgar scores. African American women are at higher risk for GBS colonization as well.

Preterm birth and low birth weight are the risk factors most closely associated with early-onset sepsis. Infant birth weight is inversely related to risk of early-onset sepsis; therefore, macrosomia is not of concern.

In the United States, the most common pathogens responsible for early-onset neonatal sepsis are GBS and *Escherichia coli*. Initial therapy for the treatment of these pathogens, as well as *Listeria monocytogenes*, usually includes ampicillin and an aminoglycoside (eg, gentamicin). Third-generation cephalosporins (eg, cefotaxime) provide a reasonable alternative to an aminoglycoside. However, several studies have reported rapid development of resistance when cefotaxime has been used routinely for the treatment of early-onset neonatal sepsis.

Because of its excellent cerebrospinal fluid penetration, empirical or therapeutic use of cefotaxime should be restricted for use in infants with meningitis attributable to gram-negative organisms. Ceftriaxone is contraindicated in neonates because it is highly protein-bound and may displace bilirubin, leading to an increased risk of kernicterus.

Additional Reading: Management of neonates with suspected or proven early-onset bacterial sepsis. *Pediatrics*. 2012;129(5):1006-1015.

30. A patient had excessive postpartum bleeding with severe hypotension; there is concern that she suffered an infarction of her pituitary gland, as she has been unable to breastfeed because of a lack of milk production. This complication of severe postpartum hemorrhage is known as which one of the following syndromes?

A) Asherman syndrome
B) Cushing syndrome
C) Nelson syndrome
D) Sheehan syndrome
E) Stein-Leventhal syndrome

The answer is D: Sheehan syndrome is a complication of childbirth that results from shock and excessive peripartum bleeding. During pregnancy, the pituitary gland usually enlarges and is vulnerable to infarction if excessive bleeding compromises blood flow. Necrosis of the pituitary can occur with varying loss of pituitary function. Symptoms of Sheehan syndrome include lack of postpartum milk production as a result of low prolactin levels, breast atrophy, loss of pubic or axillary hair, amenorrhea, depressed mental status, low blood pressure, loss of libido, and lack of sweating.

Laboratory findings include evidence of hypothyroidism, adrenal insufficiency, and decreased gonadotropin hormone secretion. Treatment involves the replacement of inadequate hormones, including thyroxine, glucocorticoids, and sex hormones.

Asherman syndrome is the development of adhesions, also known as "uterine synechiae," within the endometrial cavity, most commonly as a result of instrumentation such as dilatation and curettage post partum or from intrauterine infection.

Cushing disease is a condition that is caused by excess corticosteroids, especially cortisol, usually from adrenal or pituitary hyperfunction, and is characterized by obesity, hypertension, muscular weakness, and easy bruising.

Nelson syndrome refers to a spectrum of symptoms and signs arising from an adrenocorticotropin-secreting pituitary macroadenoma after a therapeutic bilateral adrenalectomy.

Stein-Leventhal syndrome is an older term for polycystic ovary syndrome characterized by anovulation, oligorrhea or amenorrhea, excess androgens, obesity, insulin resistance, and infertility.

Additional Reading: *Overview of postpartum hemorrhage*. In: *UpToDate*. 2022.

Sheehan syndrome is a complication of childbirth that results from shock and excessive peripartum bleeding, with subsequent infarction of the pituitary gland. Symptoms can include lack of postpartum milk production as a result of low prolactin levels.

31. You are caring for an Rh-negative mother, who has delivered an Rh-positive infant. A standard dose of Rh immune globulin (300 μg) is administered after birth. This standard amount of immune globulin prevents sensitization from fetomaternal hemorrhage of up to how many milliliters of whole blood?

A) 15 mL
B) 30 mL
C) 60 mL
D) 100 mL
E) Any amount of whole blood

The answer is B: 300 μg of Rh immune globulin is sufficient to prevent sensitization of up to 30 mL of whole blood or 15 mL of packed red blood cells. The risk of developing alloimmunization for an RhD-negative woman carrying an RhD-positive fetus is approximately 1.5%. This risk can be reduced to 0.2% with Rho(D) immune globulin (RhoGAM). Testing for ABO blood group and RhD antibodies should be performed early in pregnancy. Rho(D) immune globulin, 300 μg, is recommended for nonsensitized women at 28 weeks' gestation and again within 72 hours of delivery if the infant has RhD-positive blood.

Rho(D) immune globulin should also be administered if the risk of fetal-to-maternal transfusion is increased (eg, with chorionic villus sampling [CVS], amniocentesis, external cephalic version, abdominal trauma, or bleeding in the second or third trimester). Although alloimmunization is uncommon before 12 weeks' gestation, women with a threatened early spontaneous abortion may be offered Rho(D) immune globulin, 50 μg. Rh immune globulin must be administered to an Rh-negative mother immediately after termination of pregnancy or delivery (live or stillborn).

It is necessary to identify women with fetomaternal hemorrhage to calculate the doses needed to prevent sensitization via a screening rosette test, which, if positive, is followed by a quantitative test (eg, *Kleihauer-Betke*). RhoGAM does not need to be given if the infant is Rho(D) and Du negative, the mother's serum already contains anti-Rho(D), or the mother refuses to take it.

Additional Reading: Evidence-based prenatal care: part II. Third-trimester care and prevention of infectious diseases. *Am Fam Physician*. 2005;71:1555-1562.

Section III. Contraception

Each of the following questions or incomplete statements below is followed by suggested answers or completions. Select the ONE BEST ANSWER in each case.

1. A young patient is asking about the use of a diaphragm for contraception. You inform her that all of the following statements about diaphragm contraception are true, except which one?

A) The diaphragm should be left in place for 8 hours after intercourse.
B) The diaphragm should not be used with contraceptive jelly because of the risk of slippage.
C) The diaphragm is associated with an increase in vaginal and urinary infections.
D) The diaphragm is prescribed after a customized "fitting" in the office.
E) The diaphragm is not associated with an increased risk of cervical cancer.

The answer is B: The diaphragm is a contraceptive device. It is a round, dome-shaped piece of rubber that has a spring incorporated on the outer edge. The device is placed in the vagina and positioned so that it covers the cervix. The diaphragm should be placed in the vagina before intercourse and left in place for 8 hours after intercourse. Contraceptive foam or jelly should always be used with the diaphragm to improve its effectiveness.

When used properly, pregnancy rates are approximately 3% but can be as high as 15% with improper use. The diaphragm is associated with an increased risk of vaginal and urinary tract infections. Patients who desire to use a diaphragm should have it fitted by a physician, and they should demonstrate proper diaphragm positioning to the physician before leaving the office to ensure proper use.

Additional Reading: Diaphragm fitting. *Am Fam Physician*. 2004;69(1):97-100.

2. You see a 16-year-old female patient for contraception counseling. Which of the following is true regarding long-acting reversible contraception (LARC) in this age group?

A) Intrauterine devices (IUDs) should be avoided in this age group due to risk of sexually transmitted infections (STIs) and pelvic inflammatory disease (PID).
B) IUDs should be encouraged because placement of IUDs leads to lower rates of teen pregnancy, birth, and abortion.
C) IUDs should be avoided as they are painful and difficult to place.
D) Implantable contraceptive devices should be avoided due to concerns over future fertility.
E) Implantable contraceptive devices should be encouraged because they can treat acne as well.

The answer is B: IUD placement in teens leads to a drastic decrease in pregnancy, birth, and abortion. When given free IUDs, teens experienced a pregnancy rate of 34 per 1000 (compared to 158.5 in a comparable sexually experienced teen cohort), a birth rate of 9.7 per 1000 (compared to 94.0 per 1000), and an abortion rate of 9.7 per 1000 (compared to 41.5 per 1000). Teens should be counseled that LARC methods do nothing to prevent STIs, including human immunodeficiency virus infection, so condoms are recommended. However, rates of PID and infection are not higher in teenagers with IUDs. While IUD placement can be challenging and painful, that is not a reason to avoid engaging in shared decision-making with teenage patients. It is certainly not a contraindication to placement. Patients can premedicate with nonsteroidal anti-inflammatory drugs and a para cervical block can be used. Neither implants nor IUDs impact fertility. Progesterone-only methods of contraception, such as implants, may actually worsen acne.

Additional reading: Adolescents and long-acting reversible contraception: implants and intrauterine devices. ACOG Committee Opinion No. 735. American College of Obstetricians and Gynecologists. *Obstet Gynecol*. 2018;131:e130-e139.

3. You care for a 22-year-old patient, assigned female sex at birth, who has decided to pursue gender-affirming care. He has changed his pronouns to "he/him" and has decided to pursue testosterone therapy along with gender-affirming surgery in the future. All of the following are true except:

A) He should have age-appropriate cancer screening that aligns with his assigned sex at birth.
B) He should have a mammogram prior to surgery despite his age.
C) He should be counselled on contraceptive options if he is engaging in sexual activity that can result in pregnancy.
D) The use of testosterone means that he will not need osteoporosis screening in the future.
E) Counselling on future fertility plans is an important part of holistic care.

The answer is D: Testosterone therapy does not negate the need for osteoporosis screening starting at age 65 (or earlier with risk factors) for people assigned female sex at birth. Knowing the sex assignment at birth is an important consideration in providing appropriate preventive care. This includes pap smear, if a cervix is still present, done in a sensitive manner at the same screening intervals as cisgender women. Prior to mastectomy, mammograms are recommended for all transgender patients. If they choose not to undergo mastectomy, mammograms should be done per the U.S. Preventive Services Task Force guidelines.

Understanding that sexual identity and preference are separate from gender identity is important. Determining the types of sexual activity a patient engages in will inform discussions about sexually transmitted infections and pregnancy prevention. Similarly, discussing future fertility plans prior to initiating therapy is an important step in whole person care. While it is not necessary to harvest eggs prior to testosterone therapy, it can be distressing and confusing to interrupt testosterone therapy in the future to allow ovaries to recover enough to release eggs. For this reason, some patients wish to consider egg retrieval or in vitro fertilization prior to starting hormone therapy.

Additional Reading: Center of Excellence for Transgender Health, University of California, San Francisco, Department of Family and Community Medicine. Primary and Gender-Affirming Care of Transgender and Gender Nonbinary People. https://prevention.ucsf.edu/transhealth

4. Oral contraceptives are associated with a variety of effects; which one of the following conditions is associated with oral contraceptive use?

A) A decreased risk of cervical cancer
B) A decreased risk of liver cancer
C) A decreased risk for ectopic pregnancy
D) An increased risk of endometrial cancer
E) An increased risk of ovarian cancer

The answer is C: The neoplastic effects of oral contraceptives have been extensively studied, and a meta-analysis indicates that there is a reduction in the risk of endometrial and ovarian cancer, a possible small increase in the risk for breast and cervical cancer, and an increased risk of liver cancer. Benefits include reduction in menstrual-related symptoms, fewer ectopic pregnancies, a possible increase in bone density, and possible protection against pelvic inflammatory disease.

Additional Reading: *Risks and side effects associated with estrogen-progestin contraceptives*. In: *UpToDate*. 2022.

5. A 27-year-old woman presents to your office with questions regarding an intrauterine device (IUD) for birth control. Which one of the following statements is true about this contraceptive method?

A) IUD use has been decreasing in the United States.
B) IUD failure rates can be as high as 10%.
C) IUDs currently available in the United States pose little risk for pelvic inflammatory disease (PID).
D) IUD placement may affect future fertility.
E) IUDs containing copper or levonorgestrel produce similar bleeding patterns in users.

The answer is C: An IUD is a contraceptive method that involves placing a foreign body through the cervical os and into the uterus. Interest in IUDs started in the 1960s, and their use in the United States increased in the 1970s. However, a 1974 study linked the Dalkon Shield, an early IUD, to maternal death and found it to have a disproportionately higher rate of infection than any other IUD. The cause of infection was the multifilament string (or tail), which was a modification of the monofilament tails used by other IUDs. This multifilament tail provided a pathway for bacteria, enabling them to bypass the immunologic barrier provided by the endocervix. This design flaw caused a fivefold increase in PID and an increase in septic abortion.

The Dalkon Shield was removed from the market, but the use of IUDs declined in the United States. However, there are currently three IUDs on the market in the United States, all of which have an improved design, which has shown them to be a safe and efficacious form of birth control. The availability of these IUDs and their improved safety record have led to increased use of IUDs in the United States over the past 20 years.

The "ParaGard" copper T308A is a type of IUD that can be used for up to 10 years and can also be used as emergency contraception. A common side effect of the copper IUD is menorrhagia, which necessitates its removal in some women.

The "Mirena" levonorgestrel-secreting IUD is effective for at least 5 years, and some sources suggest that it may effectively prevent pregnancy for up to 7 years. Recently, a physically smaller IUD called the Skyla that releases a lower dose of levonorgestrel was approved for use up to 3 years. The levonorgestrel exerts a direct effect on the uterus, which diminishes menstrual bleeding.

Combined failure rates of both types of IUDs are less than 1% to 1.9% over 10 years, which is comparable to female sterilization. Contraindications for the use of IUDs include current cervical or uterine infections and pregnancy. Multiple studies conclude that the IUD poses little or no increased risk of PID. Multiple studies have shown no increased risk for cervical or uterine malignancies in IUD users.

Additional Reading:

1. Long-acting reversible contraception: implants and intrauterine devices. ACOG Practice Bulletin no. 1. 2011. www.acog.org/Resources_And_Publications/Committee_Opinions_List
2. Intrauterine devices: an update. *Am Fam Physician*. 2014;89(6):445-450.

6. A 37-year-old mother of two is requesting to go back on "the Pill." Noting that she is 37 years of age, you ensure that she has no contraindications to being prescribed an oral contraceptive pill (OCP). All of the following are considered absolute contraindications to using oral contraceptives in women above 35 years of age, except which one?

A) A family history of stroke
B) Hypertension (systolic >160 and diastolic >99)
C) Previous DVT
D) Diabetes with neuropathy
E) Smoker (1 pack per day)

The answer is A: Risks associated with combination OCPs may limit their use in women older than 35 years. Before the use of OCPs is initiated, a thorough medical history should be obtained and blood pressure (BP) should be measured.

Although the use of OCPs increases the risk of venous thromboembolism, the absolute risk of venous thromboembolism is very low (1 case per 10,000 OCP users per year). The risk of myocardial infarction may be increased in women using OCPs, especially if smoking (>10 cigarettes per day) or other cardiovascular risk factors are present, such as diabetes with neuropathy. The association between OCP use and ischemic stroke is not clear, although increased risk has been demonstrated in OCP users who have migraines.

Absolute contraindications to prescribing OCPs for women older than 35 years:

- Pregnancy
- Less than 6 weeks post partum and breastfeeding
- Age more than 35 years and heavy smoker (>15 cigarettes per day)
- Systolic BP > 160 mm Hg, diastolic BP > 99 mm Hg
- Hypertension with vascular disease
- Diabetes with neuropathy, retinopathy, nephropathy, or vascular disease
- History of deep vein thrombosis or pulmonary embolism
- Major surgery with prolonged immobilization
- History of ischemic heart disease
- History of stroke
- Complicated valvular disease (with atrial fibrillation, pulmonary hypertension, bacterial endocarditis)
- Severe headaches with focal neurologic symptoms
- Current breast cancer
- Active viral hepatitis, severe cirrhosis, benign or malignant liver tumors

The best OCP in women above 35 years of age is the one with the lowest effective estrogen dose. Follow-up should include annual BP measurements, lipid profiles in patients with a baseline abnormality, and a review of symptoms that could signify an important adverse effect.

Additional Reading: *United States Medical Eligibility Criteria for Contraceptive Use*. vol. 65. No. 3. Centers for Disease Control and Prevention, 2016.

7. A young woman is requesting to use depot medroxyprogesterone acetate (DMPA) as her form of contraception because her friend recommended it to her as a convenient method. You inform her that DMPA does not protect against sexually transmitted infections and is associated with which one of the following adverse effects?

A) An increased risk of endometrial cancer
B) An increased pregnancy risk
C) Increased risk of teratogenicity in future pregnancies
D) Migraines
E) Reversible bone loss

The answer is E: DMPA (brand name Depo-Provera) is associated with a decrease in bone mineral density (BMD) that is usually temporary and reversible. Data suggest that the loss in BMD is rapid within the first 2 years of use but slows dramatically after those first 2 years. Although women have a decrease in BMD while using DMPA, studies have consistently demonstrated that BMD returned to baseline levels when DMPA is discontinued. There have been no randomized trials on DMPA use and fracture risk.

The benefits of excellent protection against pregnancy that DMPA provides are felt to outweigh the risks of bone loss in most healthy women. However, long-term DMPA use is inadvisable in women with conditions that place them at high risk for osteoporosis and fracture, such as long-term corticosteroid use, disorders of bone metabolism, and a strong family history of anorexia nervosa.

Additional Reading: CDC updates recommendations for contraceptive use. *Am Fam Physician*. 2017;95(2):125-126.

8. A variety of side effects are associated with oral contraceptive use, including an increase in blood pressure (BP). Which one of the following statements is true regarding this situation?

A) An increase in BP is rarely a problem in patients with underlying hypertension.
B) An increase in BP is more common in women with a positive family history for hypertension.
C) An increase in BP is not associated with increased age of the patient.
D) An increase in BP is related to a permanent increase in BP despite discontinuation of the contraceptive.
E) An increase in BP is an indication to begin antihypertensive therapy.

The answer is B: A slight increase in BP (5-6 mm systolic/1-2 mm diastolic) is expected in some women who take oral contraceptives. In fact, hypertension is five to six times more likely to develop in women who use oral contraceptives than in those who do not use them. Women who are older, have a positive family history for hypertension, or have been using oral contraceptives for longer durations are at an increased risk.

BP increases may occur within weeks; however, it may not be noted for months or even years after starting medication. Discontinuation of oral contraceptives in most patients allows the BP to decrease to normal levels, and most patients will not require antihypertensive therapy. Patients should be seen for a BP check within 3 months after the initiation of the contraceptive. If significant increases occur, oral contraception medication should be discontinued. Underlying preexisting hypertension is a relative contraindication for oral contraceptive use.

Additional Reading: Contraception choices in women with underlying medical conditions. *Am Fam Physician*. 2010;82(6):621-628.

9. Although oral contraceptive pills (OCPs) have numerous benefits, there are also concerns with their use as well. Which one of the following statements concerning OCP use is true?

A) OCP use increases the risk of cholelithiasis.
B) OCP use increases the risk for an ectopic pregnancy.
C) OCP use increases the risk for pelvic inflammatory disease (PID).
D) OCP use increases the risk for endometrial carcinoma.
E) OCP use may decrease the risk of cervical cancer.

The answer is A: The use of oral contraceptives for birth control is widely accepted and prescribed. Properly used, the pill approaches 100% effectiveness in preventing pregnancy. Its mechanism of action involves the prevention of ovulation by the regulation of hormones (suppression of follicle-stimulating hormone and luteinizing hormone) during the menstrual cycle, induction of atrophic changes to the endometrium that are not conducive to implantation, and the alteration of cervical mucus.

There are two types of OCPs: combination pills that include both estrogen and progestin components and pills that contain only progestin. Pills that contain only progestin are best suited for women older than 35 years, smokers, or those who cannot tolerate estrogen. Additionally, OCPs are divided into monophasic (a fixed combination of estrogen and progestin component) and multiphasic (a varying amount of progestin during each of the 3 weeks of medication with a fixed amount of estrogen). Overall, the multiphasic oral contraceptives are highly effective and may provide a lower dose of estrogen and progestin.

Complications associated with OCP use include an increased risk of cholelithiasis, increased blood pressure, midcycle bleeding between periods, headaches, weight gain, hirsutism, acne, melasma, increased risk for myocardial infarction in smokers older than 35 years, and, rarely, benign hepatic lipomas.

Women who use oral contraceptives are at decreased risk for ovarian cancer, endometrial cancer, PID, and ectopic pregnancy. No consistent association has been found between breast cancer and oral contraceptive use, except for the possibility of a slightly elevated risk in users of OCPs for more than 3 years before 25 years of age.

Additional Reading: CDC updates recommendations for contraceptive use. *Am Fam Physician*. 2017;95(2):125-126.

10. A young woman calls asking for advice regarding emergency contraception after having unprotected intercourse. You inform her that which one of the following statements is true regarding the use of such treatments?

A) Birth defects often occur if the method is unsuccessful.
B) Emergency contraception is 95% effective.
C) Emergency contraception is most effective if administered within 72 hours.
D) Ulipristal (Ella) is less effective than levonorgestrel taken as a single 1.5-mg pill (Plan B One-Step).

The answer is C: Women should be offered the option to use emergency contraception to prevent pregnancy after known or suspected failure of birth control or after unprotected intercourse. Emergency contraception is about 75% to 85% effective. It is most effective when initiated within 72 hours after unprotected intercourse. Despite the large number of women who have received emergency contraception, there have been no reports of major adverse outcomes. If a woman becomes pregnant after using emergency contraception, she may be reassured about the lack of negative effects that emergency contraception has on fetal development.

Products contain levonorgestrel (Plan B, Next Choice, etc) or ulipristal (Ella). Plan B One-Step simplified the original Plan B two-tablet regimen to administer a single 1.5 mg dose of levonorgestrel, which was shown to be equally effective emergency contraception without causing an increase in side effects. A third approved method of emergency contraception is the insertion of a copper-containing intrauterine device.

The mechanism of action may vary, depending on the day of the menstrual cycle on which treatment is started. Ulipristal is a selective progesterone receptor modulator and, when taken as a single 30 mg dose, is a safe and effective emergency contraceptive that can be used from the first day and up to 5 days following unprotected intercourse. During clinical development, ulipristal acetate has been shown to be more effective than levonorgestrel in delaying or inhibiting ovulation.

Additional Reading: Emergency contraception: safety and effectiveness. *Am Fam Physician*. 2020;101(11):651-652.

➔ Emergency contraception is 75% to 85% effective. It is most effective when initiated within 72 hours after unprotected intercourse.

11. Intrauterine devices (IUDs) are increasingly being used for contraception. All of the following statements are true regarding IUDs, except which one?

A) The risk of unintended pregnancy in the first year of IUD use is less than 1%.
B) One-year continuation rates for IUD use are near 60%.
C) IUDs can be placed at any time during the menstrual cycle, as long as pregnancy can be reasonably excluded.
D) The copper IUD is an effective method of emergency contraception when inserted within 5 days of unprotected intercourse.
E) Women with mucopurulent cervical discharge or known gonorrhea or chlamydial infection should be treated before placement of an IUD.

The answer is B: The 1-year continuation rate for the copper IUD is 78% and that for the levonorgestrel-containing IUD is 80%, and both types of IUDs have 1-year pregnancy rates of <1%. IUDs may be inserted anytime during the menstrual cycle. Insertion may be performed during menstruation to provide additional reassurance that the woman is not pregnant; however, documentation of a negative pregnancy test, preferably at least 2 weeks after the last unprotected intercourse, is also recommended.

The copper IUD is a more effective method of emergency contraception than oral emergency contraceptives and reduces the chance of pregnancy by 99% when taken within 5 days of unprotected intercourse. The effectiveness of levonorgestrel-containing IUD for emergency contraception has not been studied and is not recommended.

The IUD should not be placed in a patient with documented chlamydial, gonococcal, or nonspecific mucopurulent cervicitis until treatment has been given. Routine screening for sexually transmitted infections is recommended before IUD placement in high-risk women but not in low-risk women. Screening may be performed on the same day of the IUD placement.

Additional Reading: Intrauterine devices: an update. *Am Fam Physician*. 2014;89(6):445-450.

12. You are seeing an adolescent girl who is complaining of facial acne. She is asking if an oral contraceptive pill (OCP) would help. You note that which one of the following OCPs is U.S. Food and Drug Administration (FDA)–approved for the treatment of acne vulgaris in women and adolescent girls?

A) Ethinyl estradiol-desogestrel (Desogen)
B) Ethinyl estradiol-levonorgestrel (Preven)
C) Ethinyl estradiol-norgestimate (Ortho Tri-Cyclen)
D) Ethinyl estradiol-norelgestromin (Ortho Evra patch)
E) Norethindrone (Micronor)

The answer is C: OCPs may be a useful adjunctive therapy for all types of acne in women and adolescent girls. Sebum production is controlled by androgens, and oral contraceptives are known to decrease androgen levels by increasing sex hormone–binding globulin levels, thus reducing the availability of biologically active free testosterone. The third-generation progestin norgestimate has lower intrinsic androgenicity than other progestins and is effective in treating moderate inflammatory acne. Ortho Tri-Cyclen is a triphasic combination of norgestimate and ethinyl estradiol that has been labeled by the FDA for the treatment of acne vulgaris in women and adolescent girls.

Other contraceptive agents that contain norgestimate (Ortho-Cyclen) or desogestrel (Desogen) are also reasonable choices but are not FDA-approved for this indication. Two other FDA-approved OCPs for use in acne treatment are ethinyl estradiol-norethindrone (Estrostep) and drospirenone-ethinyl estradiol (YAZ). Two to 4 months of therapy may be required before improvement is noted, and relapses are common if medication is stopped.

Additional Reading: Diagnosis and treatment of acne. *Am Fam Physician*. 2012;86(8):734-740.

13. An 18-year-old woman has recently been regularly taking oral contraceptives and is in the office for a follow-up visit. She reports that she is feeling fine but notes some darkened areas have appeared on her face. The most likely diagnosis is to explain this finding is which one of the following conditions?

A) Acne
B) Lupus pernio
C) Malignant melanoma
D) Melasma
E) Sebaceous hyperplasia

The answer is D: Melasma occurs in some women taking oral contraceptives and often also occurs in pregnancy. The condition is characterized by areas of darkened pigmentation that may affect the face. There is a genetic predisposition to melasma, with at least one-third of patients reporting other family members to be affected, and it is more common in African Americans and Latinas, and is worse with sun exposure. The cause of melasma is unknown. The pigmentation is due to overproduction of melanin by the melanocytes, which is taken up by the keratinocytes (epidermal melanosis) and/or deposited in the dermis (dermal melanosis). Usually, the areas fade when pregnancy is complete or oral contraceptives are discontinued.

Lupus pernio is a chronic, raised, indurated lesion of the skin, often purplish in color, and associated with underlying sarcoidosis. Melanoma lesions are typically dark black and are not associated with oral contraceptive use.

Sebaceous hyperplasia is a disorder of the sebaceous glands in which they become enlarged, sometimes in response to the hormones of pregnancy, producing yellow shiny bumps on the face, but do not alter the pigmentation of the skin. Oral contraceptives can both predispose patients to acne and improve it. However, acne lesions do typically appear as dark areas, except in cases of postacne scar formation.

Additional Reading: Common skin conditions during pregnancy. *Am Fam Physician*. 2007;75(2):211-218.

14. A 23-year-old patient has been using the vaginal ring for contraception and is confused about how long it can be left in place. You inform her that the ring can be left in place for what time period?

A) 3 days
B) 1 week
C) 4 weeks
D) 3 months
E) 1 year

The answer is C: With typical use, after 3 weeks, the contraceptive vaginal ring is removed for 1 week, after which a new ring is inserted. It is possible to use a single ring for 4 weeks with the same efficacy and skip the withdrawal bleed. Withdrawal bleeding occurs during the ring-free week. If the ring is removed from the vagina for more than 3 hours, an additional backup contraception should be used for 7 days until the ring has been back in place.

Additional Reading: *Contraceptive vaginal ring*. In: *UpToDate*. 2022.

15. A 32-year-old woman with well-controlled hypertension on enalapril is requesting an oral contraceptive pill (OCP). Which one of the following OCPs should be used cautiously with enalapril, as it can lead to hyperkalemia?

A) Ethinyl estradiol-drospirenone
B) Ethinyl estradiol-levonorgestrel
C) Ethinyl estradiol-norgestimate
D) Ethinyl estradiol-norelgestromin
E) Norethindrone

The answer is A: Drospirenone has antimineralocorticoid activity and has been shown to decrease the water retention, mood changes, and appetite changes that are commonly associated with a woman's menstrual cycle. Serum potassium levels should be monitored when using this OCP in conjunction with other medicines that also raise potassium levels, because of the risk of developing hyperkalemia from antimineralocorticoid actions.

Additional Reading: Contraception choices in women with underlying medical conditions. *Am Fam Physician*. 2010;82(6):621-628.

14. The oral contraceptive pill (OCP) levonorgestrel-ethinyl estradiol (Seasonale) is different from 28-day oral contraceptives due to having which one of the following characteristics?

A) Higher adherence to correct usage
B) Increased effectiveness
C) More days of active pills and fewer days of nonhormonal pills
D) Once-a-month dosing

The answer is C: The extended-cycle levonorgestrel-ethinyl estradiol OCP regimen consists of 84 days of active pills and 7 days of nonhormonal pills, prescribed as a 91-day extended-cycle pack (eg, Seasonale, Seasonique, and LoSeasonique). These OCPs may be especially desirable for women who do not want monthly periods, as this regimen results in only four menses per year. Fewer withdrawal bleeds per year, with fewer hormone-free intervals may benefit women with estrogen withdrawal symptoms, dysmenorrhea, or endometriosis.

No differences in effectiveness, safety, and adherence have been shown between extended cycle vs 28-day cycle. Lybrel is a continuous-cycle levonorgestrel-ethinyl estradiol pill taken daily throughout the year with no hormone-free interval to induce a scheduled withdrawal bleed. Women on Lybrel often have initial unscheduled spotting, then ultimately amenorrhea.

Additional Reading: The new extended-cycle levonorgestrel-ethinyl estradiol oral contraceptives. *Clin Med Insights: Reprod Health*. 2011;549-554.

Section IV. General Gynecology/Women's Health

Each of the following questions or incomplete statements below is followed by suggested answers or completions. Select the ONE BEST ANSWER in each case.

1. A 27-year-old patient is being seen with complaints of menstrual cramping. She has lower abdominal pain, which starts a day before she is expected to start her menses and will continue for a day or two after she starts bleeding. She is asking you to prescribe something to help with the cramps. Which one of the following medication classes is considered to be the first-line therapy for primary dysmenorrhea?

A) Antiestrogens
B) A calcium channel blocker
C) Nonsteroidal anti-inflammatory drugs (NSAIDs)
D) Selective serotonin reuptake inhibitors
E) Tricyclic antidepressants

The answer is C: Primary dysmenorrhea is defined as cramping pain in the lower abdomen occurring just before and/or during menstruation. There are no concerns for other pelvic pathology such as endometriosis. The initial presentation of primary dysmenorrhea typically occurs in adolescence, and prevalence rates are as high as 90% in menstruating women. The condition is associated with increased production of endometrial prostaglandin, resulting in increased uterine tone and stronger, more frequent uterine contractions. A diagnostic evaluation is unnecessary in women with typical symptoms and in the absence of risk factors for secondary causes.

NSAIDs are the most effective treatment, with the addition of oral contraceptive pills when necessary. About 10% of affected women do not respond to these measures. In these cases, it is important to consider secondary causes of dysmenorrhea in affected women.

Additional Reading: Dysmenorrhea. *Am Fam Physician*. 2021;104(2):164-170.

2. A 37-year-old woman presents to your office to discuss irregular menses. You do an in-office pregnancy test, which is positive. This is an unintended and undesired pregnancy and the patient wishes to terminate. Gestational age was found to be 8 weeks 2 days. Which of the following is true?

A) She should be referred for surgical termination as she is beyond 6 weeks.
B) She should be referred for ultrasound for cardiac activity to be certain she wishes to terminate.
C) If she is Rh negative, she will need RhoGAM.
D) Medication abortion with a combination of mifepristone and misoprostol has a greater than 95% success rate.
E) Significant hemorrhage occurs in 3% of patients treated with medication abortion.

The answer is D: Medication abortion is a safe and effective outpatient procedure for women up to 70 days' gestation. Data show that telehealth and in-office visits have similar efficacy, safety, and complications rates. There is no benefit to ultrasound for dating if last menstrual period, exam, and human chorionic gonadotropin (hCG) levels convincingly place the pregnancy at less than 11 weeks. Significant bleeding occurs in roughly 0.1% of all patients. The World Health Organization states that determination of Rh status is not considered a prerequisite for early medical abortion <12 weeks' gestation. The decision to administer RhoGAM in an early termination is done through shared decision-making and is not mandatory.

The regimen for medication abortion includes mifepristone 200 mg followed by misoprostol 800 μg 24 to 48 hours later. Follow-up in the office or by phone is recommended to monitor bleeding (either too much or not enough, signaling incomplete abortion), signs of infection, and downtrending hCG levels.

Additional Reading: Macnaughton H, Nothnagle M, Early J. Mifepristone and misoprostol for early pregnancy loss and medication abortion. *Am Fam Physician*. 2021;103(8):473-480.

3. A 22-year-old previously healthy patient presents to your office complaining of abnormal vaginal bleeding. Your first consideration in the differential diagnosis is which one of the following?

A) Coagulopathy
B) Foreign body
C) Infection
D) Pregnancy
E) Trauma

The answer is D: Pregnancy is the first consideration in women of childbearing age who present with abnormal uterine bleeding.

Additional Reading: Abnormal uterine bleeding in premenopausal women. *Am Fam Physician*. 2019;99(7):435-443.

4. A young couple is in to discuss conception. They report regular intercourse in an attempt to conceive but have been unsuccessful for the last year. They are worried that something is wrong and request a workup. You advise them that which one of the following investigations would be considered the first step in an evaluation of infertility?

A) An evaluation of the woman's hormone levels
B) A hysterosalpingogram
C) A postcoital test of the woman
D) A semen analysis of the man
E) An endometrial biopsy

The answer is D: Infertility affects as many as 10% to 15% of couples in the United States and appears to be increasing in incidence. The definition of infertility is the lack of conception after 1 year of unprotected intercourse for women under age 35. For women 35 years and older, the time is shortened to 6 months.

As much as 26% to 30% of infertility is the result of male factors, such as inadequate sperm production, abnormal sperm motility, or abnormally formed sperm. Female factors include previous pelvic infections with fallopian tube damage, anovulation, low progesterone levels, hypothyroidism, hyperprolactinemia, or the presence of antisperm antibodies.

In the evaluation of infertility, evaluation of the man occurs first, because the female evaluation may be more extensive and invasive. If the sperm is found to be adequate, evaluation of the woman proceeds with hormonal evaluations, endometrial sampling, and a hysterosalpingogram (which can determine the patency of the fallopian tubes). Markers of ovulation, including monitoring basal body temperatures, cervical mucus, and home ovulation tests are also recommended.

Additional Reading: Evaluation and treatment of infertility. *Am Fam Physician*. 2015;91(5):308-314.

4. A 28-year-old woman presents for an office visit with complaints of hirsutism and difficulty with conception. Her body mass index is

31, and her menses occur every 5 to 6 months. Based on her likely diagnosis, she is at increased risk for which of the following malignancies?

A) Breast cancer
B) Colon cancer
C) Endometrial carcinoma
D) Ovarian carcinoma
E) Pancreatic cancer

The answer is C: Polycystic ovary syndrome is the most common endocrine abnormality in women of reproductive age. The syndrome is associated with chronic anovulation, oligomenorrhea, and infertility. Chronic anovulation predisposes women to endometrial hyperplasia and carcinoma. Macrovascular diseases such as type 2 diabetes mellitus, hypertension, and atherosclerotic heart disease are also more likely in women with PCOS.

Symptoms that prompt women to seek attention include irregular menses, hirsutism, or infertility. The earliest manifestations of PCOS are noted around the time of puberty. Adolescent girls affected with PCOS often have early puberty and show hyperandrogenism and insulin resistance. In the early reproductive period, chronic anovulation results in difficulty with fertility. If pregnancy is achieved, first-trimester spontaneous abortion is common, or the pregnancy is complicated by gestational diabetes.

More than 50% of those affected are obese. Abnormal androgen production declines as menopause approaches (as it does in women without PCOS), and menstrual patterns may normalize. PCOS appears to follow a familial distribution. Luteinizing hormone (LH) and follicle-stimulating hormone (FSH) levels are often elevated in PCOS, with the LH to FSH ratio greater than 3 to 1.

Individualized therapy should incorporate steroid hormones, antiandrogens, and insulin-sensitizing agents such as metformin. Metformin increases ovulation rates in some women with PCOS and also may reduce fasting insulin concentrations, lower blood pressure, and reduce low-density lipoprotein cholesterol. Weight loss by way of reduced carbohydrate intake and exercise is the most important intervention; this step alone can restore menstrual regularity and fertility, and provide long-term prevention against diabetes and heart disease.

Additional Reading: *Clinical manifestations of polycystic ovary syndrome in adults*. In: *UpToDate*. 2022.

5. Infertility may be a result of antisperm antibodies. Which one of the following classes of medications may help reduce such antibodies?

A) Corticosteroids
B) Gonadotropin-releasing hormone agonists
C) Estrogen-containing oral contraceptive pills
D) Progesterone-containing contraceptives (medroxyprogesterone)
E) None of the above

The answer is A: Immunologic infertility can occur in women as a result of the development of local and circulating antisperm antibodies. In men, there may also be circulating antibodies that prevent conception. Men with previous vasectomies have an increased risk of antisperm antibodies.

Immunologic tests are now available for the detection of these antibodies. In some cases, spontaneous remission of antibodies has occurred. In cases in which they persist, steroids may be useful in lowering the levels of antibodies, thus allowing pregnancy.

Additional Reading: *Evaluation of male infertility*. In: *UpToDate*. 2022.

6. You are assessing a young woman with abdominal pain and a positive urinary pregnancy test. Which one of the following evaluations is the test of choice for the detection of an ectopic pregnancy?

A) A quantitative β-human chorionic gonadotropin (β-hCG) level
B) Computed tomographic scan of the pelvis
C) Diagnostic laparoscopy
D) Magnetic resonance imaging of the pelvis
E) Transvaginal pelvic ultrasonography

The answer is E: Ectopic pregnancy occurs in 1.5% to 2% of pregnancies and is potentially life-threatening. Although there has been decreased mortality associated with this condition because of early detection and treatment before rupture, ectopic pregnancy still accounts for 0.5 deaths per 1000 pregnancies, which represents 6% of all maternal deaths. Risk factors for ectopic pregnancy include prior pelvic inflammatory disease, tubal surgery, and previous ectopic pregnancy. If a pregnancy occurs in the presence of an intrauterine device, there is a higher risk that it will be ectopic.

When diagnosed early, ectopic pregnancy may be treated medically rather than surgically. Therefore, ectopic pregnancy should be considered and quickly ruled out in all women of reproductive age who present with abdominal pain or vaginal bleeding. Transvaginal ultrasonography used in conjunction with serial quantitative β-hCG levels is the best method for diagnosis of ectopic pregnancy.

Additional Reading: Ectopic pregnancy: diagnosis and management. *Am Fam Physician*. 2020;101(10):599-606.

7. Which one of the following statements about molar pregnancy is true?

A) Further pregnancies are discouraged after a molar pregnancy.
B) Hyperemesis gravidarum is usually an associated sign.
C) Serial α-fetoprotein levels are useful to monitor for malignant transformation.
D) Those with a history of a molar pregnancy are not at an increased risk for a subsequent molar pregnancy.
E) The majority of molar pregnancies result in malignant transformation.

The answer is B: A molar pregnancy (hydatidiform mole) occurs when the placenta undergoes trophoblastic transformation and results in a placental neoplasm. The abnormal placenta is usually swollen, edematous, and vesicular, resembling a cluster of grapes. The condition usually affects women younger than 20 years and older than 40 years. Those with a prior history of hydatidiform mole are at increased risk for subsequent molar pregnancies. Hydatidiform moles are usually associated with hyperemesis gravidarum and preeclampsia that occurs before the third trimester. Other associated conditions include vaginal bleeding, signs and symptoms of hyperthyroidism, trophoblastic embolization that may cause cough, tachypnea, and cyanosis; enlarged uterus associated with gestation; and theca lutein cysts resulting in ovarian enlargement.

In 80% of patients, the molar pregnancy resolves after dilation and curettage without complications. However, in 20%, there is a malignant transformation of the tissue. Therefore, serum human chorionic gonadotropin determination (which is usually significantly elevated at the time of diagnosis) should be monitored every 2 weeks after evacuation of the uterus until the value drops to a nonpregnant level, then every 1 to 2 months for 1 year. The lungs are the most common sites for metastasis; therefore, a chest x-ray should be performed at the time of evacuation and 4 to 8 weeks after evacuation to check for metastasis.

Repeated pelvic examinations should be performed on a monthly basis after a molar pregnancy for the first year. Patients should avoid pregnancy for at least 1 year after the development of a molar pregnancy. Those who have had recurrent molar pregnancies are at an increased risk for malignant transformation. Malignant transformation is usually treated with methotrexate.

Additional Reading: *Gestational Trophoblastic Neoplasia. Williams Obstetrics*. 26th ed. McGraw-Hill; 2022.

8. A 44-year-old woman presents with irregular vaginal bleeding. Appropriate initial management includes which one of the following?

A) Endometrial biopsy
B) A trial of oral contraceptives
C) Medroxyprogesterone injection
D) Pelvic ultrasonography
E) Referral for diagnostic laparoscopy

The answer is A: Women who are reproductively mature (older than 40 years) and experience irregular vaginal bleeding should be evaluated with an endometrial biopsy to rule out endometrial hyperplasia or carcinoma. In addition, tests to rule out thyroid dysfunction and bleeding disorders should be considered. Adolescents with abnormal vaginal bleeding can be regulated with oral contraceptive medications once pregnancy and infection have been ruled out. Vaginal bleeding before the age of 9 years and after the age of 52 years in the absence of hormone replacement is a cause for concern and requires more aggressive investigation.

Additional Reading: Abnormal uterine bleeding in premenopausal women. *Am Fam Physician*. 2019;99(7):435-443.

9. Early diagnosis of an ectopic pregnancy allows for the possibility of utilizing a medical, rather than surgical treatment. Which one of the following medications has been shown to be comparable to laparoscopic excision in the treatment of small ectopic pregnancies that have not ruptured?

A) Bromocriptine
B) Methotrexate
C) Misoprostol
D) Oxytocin
E) Thalidomide

The answer is B: In recent years, intramuscular methotrexate has been suggested as an alternative to salpingostomy for management of ectopic pregnancy. In addition, there is interest in using serum human chorionic gonadotropin (hCG) or progesterone levels to monitor resolution of ectopic pregnancy after intervention. A single dose of intramuscular methotrexate appears comparable to laparoscopic salpingostomy for the treatment of a small, unruptured ectopic pregnancy. The fact that serum progesterone levels resolved faster than serum hCG levels suggests that serum progesterone may be a better marker for monitoring resolution of ectopic pregnancy.

Guidelines have been developed to choose appropriate candidates for medical treatment of ectopic vs surgical. A good candidate for methotrexate must be hemodynamically stable, with no evidence of pending or current rupture, preferably with an hCG level of less than 5000K, an ectopic mass size less than 3 to 4 cm, and an ability to comply with follow-up. Patients with abnormal renal or hepatic function at baseline or certain gastric or hematologic disorders are not generally candidates for this therapy.

Additional Reading: *Ectopic pregnancy: choosing a treatment and methotrexate therapy*. In: *UpToDate*. 2022.

A single dose of intramuscular methotrexate appears comparable to laparoscopic salpingostomy for the treatment of a small, unruptured ectopic pregnancy.

10. Which one of the following statements about uterine adenomyosis is true?

A) It is associated with the invasion of myometrial tissue into the peritoneal cavity.
B) It commonly causes intense pelvic pain, dysuria, and dyspareunia.
C) It is associated with an increased risk of endometrial cancer.
D) It is considered benign and usually causes no associated symptoms.
E) It results from uterine atony after delivery.

The answer is D: Uterine adenomyosis is defined as the invasion of endometrial tissue into the myometrium. This common disorder is benign and usually causes no symptoms. Those who do have symptoms complain of menorrhagia, irregular vaginal bleeding, pelvic pain, and bladder or rectal discomfort. Uterine adenomyosis is more likely to cause secondary dysmenorrhea than fibroids, endometrial polyps, cervical papillomas, or polycystic ovary disease.

Pelvic examination may reveal an enlarged uterus that feels softer in consistency. Associated fibroid tumors may also be present on examination. Hysterectomy may be indicated for those beyond their childbearing years if symptoms are severe. Oral contraceptives and gonadotropin-releasing hormone agonists have not been found to be very effective treatments.

Additional Reading: Adenomyosis. In: Domino F, ed. *The 5-Minute Clinical Consult*. Wolters Kluwer; 2022.

11. A 23-year-old woman is seen in the emergency department with complaints of a high fever, nausea, vomiting, myalgias, and lethargy. On examination, she is found to have hypotension and a generalized erythematous rash with desquamation of the hands and feet. Laboratory test results show an increased white blood cell count, blood urea nitrogen, and serum creatinine. She has decreased urine output. The most likely diagnosis is which one of the following conditions?

A) Gonorrhea
B) Lyme disease
C) Pelvic inflammatory disease (PID)
D) Tertiary syphilis
E) Toxic shock syndrome

The answer is E: Toxic shock syndrome is a condition that is characterized by high fever, nausea and vomiting, myalgias, mental status changes, and an erythematous, sandpaper-like skin rash with the development of severe hypotension, and vascular collapse. Desquamation of the hands and feet is also common. Complications include multisystem failure, adult respiratory distress syndrome, and even death in severe cases.

First recognized in 1978, the condition tends to affect young menstruating women and is associated with the use of vaginal tampons. The syndrome is a result of staphylococcal or streptococcal infection that produces an exotoxin. Occasionally, the syndrome is associated with postoperative infections, diaphragm use, contraceptive sponges, septic abortions, insect bites, and other infections that involve staphylococcal and streptococcal organisms.

Laboratory studies often reveal an elevated white blood cell count, increased blood urea nitrogen, serum creatinine with decreased urine output, and thrombocytopenia followed by thrombocytosis. Mortality may be as high as 5% to 15%.

Treatment with a β-lactamase-resistant penicillin or cephalosporin is recommended because it is supportive treatment to replace fluid loss and electrolytes. Steroids may be indicated for severe cases. Patients with toxic shock syndrome should be encouraged not to use high-absorbency tampons or diaphragms. Oral contraceptives may help to reduce the number of recurrent cases.

Disseminated gonococcal infections typically present with scattered papular skin lesions that can progress to bullae, petechiae, and necrotic lesions with or without associated synovitis.

Acute Lyme disease is a summer "flulike" illness with symptoms including low-grade fever, myalgias, joint pain, swollen lymph nodes, and headaches. The characteristic rash of early Lyme disease is flat and circular with a "bull's eye" appearance with reddened outer margins and a pale central portion.

PID can present with fever, usually with prominent pelvic pain and rarely with sepsis, but has no associated rash.

A rash on the palms and soles is more commonly seen with secondary syphilis rather than tertiary syphilis; the manifestations of tertiary syphilis include aortic aneurysms; valve disease; central nervous system disorders; and infiltrative tumors of skin, bones, or liver.

Additional Reading: Staphylococcal toxic shock syndrome. In: Domino F, ed. *The 5-Minute Clinical Consult*. Wolters Kluwer; 2022.

12. A 32-year-old woman presents to your office complaining of an itchy yellowish-white vaginal discharge. Microscopic examination shows evidence of pseudohyphae. The most appropriate treatment is to prescribe which one of the following agents?

A) Doxycycline capsules
B) Metronidazole (Flagyl) tablets
C) Penicillin G injection
D) Terconazole (Terazol) vaginal cream
E) Topical acyclovir ointment

The answer is D: Yeast vaginitis (monilial vaginitis) is caused by *Candida albicans*. Predisposing factors include the recent use of wide-spectrum antibiotics, the use of oral contraceptives, pregnancy, menstruation, diabetes mellitus, constrictive undergarments, the use of immunosuppressive drugs (eg, steroids), or immunodeficient states (eg, diabetes). Twenty percent of women harbor *C albicans* as part of their natural vaginal flora and are asymptomatic.

Symptoms include intense vulvar irritation, pruritus, and vaginal discomfort. Erythema that affects the vulvar area, vaginal lining, and cervix is usually present. A copious, white, vaginal discharge, which many women describe as "cottage cheese–like," also generally occurs.

Diagnosis is made by microscopic examination of vaginal secretions following the application of potassium hydroxide to a glass slide. Characteristic budding yeastlike cells are noted with projections of pseudohyphae. Vaginal pH is less than 4.5.

Treatment consists of local antifungal vaginal cream (eg, terconazole, miconazole, and others) applied nightly for 3 to 7 days. Oral antifungals (Diflucan) are also effective. Incorrect diagnosis and administration of antibiotics such as penicillin, doxycycline, and metronidazole can allow further overgrowth of yeast in the vagina and increase symptoms. Acyclovir, given either topically or orally, is a usual treatment for symptomatic genital herpes simplex infections.

Additional Reading: Vaginitis: diagnosis and treatment. *Am Fam Physician*. 2018;97(5):321-329.

13. You are evaluating a young woman with complaints of dysmenorrhea, dyspareunia, and pelvic pain. You believe that endometriosis is the most likely cause of her symptoms. The diagnosis of endometriosis is generally made by which one of the following?

A) Measurement of premenstrual estrogen levels
B) Obtaining a pelvic ultrasonography
C) Ordering a pelvic computed tomographic scan
D) Performing an endometrial biopsy
E) Laparoscopy

The answer is E: Endometriosis is the presence of endometrial tissue outside the uterus, in locations such as the ovaries, fallopian tubes, uterosacral ligaments, peritoneal cul-de-sac, and uterovesical peritoneum. Rarely, endometrial tissue can be found in the nasal mucosa and lungs. The gold standard for diagnosis is laparoscopy. Theories for the development of endometriosis are abundant and include the migration of endometrial tissue through the fallopian tubes and into the peritoneal cavity, or the transformation of existing epithelium into endometrial-type tissue.

Symptoms include dysmenorrhea, dyspareunia, infertility, dysuria, irregular vaginal bleeding, and pelvic pain. As many as 33% of affected individuals have no symptoms. Risk factors include nulliparity and a positive family history. Most patients have normal examination results. However, some have a tender retroverted uterus or adnexal masses that are tender with palpation.

Treatment of mild disease involves the use of analgesics, progesterone, and oral contraceptives to regulate a patient's menstrual cycle. More advanced disease can be treated with danazol (Danocrine), an anabolic steroid that has androgen activity. Side effects of danazol therapy include weight gain, fluid retention, fatigue, acne, chloasma, irregular vaginal bleeding, cholestatic jaundice with prolonged use, and hepatic dysfunction in patients who receive high doses. Gonadotropin-releasing hormone agonists are also used for treatment. Severe cases may require surgery.

Additional Reading: Endometriosis: evaluation and treatment. *Am Fam Physician*. 2022;106(4):397-404.

14. You are seeing a young woman with painful menses. Which one of the following statements about primary dysmenorrhea is true?

A) Endometriosis is a common cause.
B) Oral contraceptives usually aggravate the condition.
C) Symptoms typically present after 30 years of age.
D) The cramping and pain are associated with excessive prostaglandin activity.
E) The condition is related to adenomyosis.

The answer is D: Primary dysmenorrhea is defined as pain that occurs during menstruation in the absence of pelvic pathology. The onset is usually before 20 years of age, and it affects women during the first day or two after the onset of menstruation. The cause is thought to be secondary to excessive prostaglandin activity, which leads to uterine contractions and ischemia, giving rise to pelvic discomfort. Other symptoms include headache, nausea and occasionally vomiting, constipation, diarrhea, and urinary frequency.

Premenstrual symptoms, including water retention, irritability, nervousness, and depression, may also persist during the early period of menstruation.

Treatment usually involves reassurance, nonsteroidal anti-inflammatory agents, and heating pads to the lower abdomen. A trial of oral contraceptives may be beneficial. In women who do not desire hormonal contraception, there is some evidence of benefit with the use of the Japanese herbal remedy toki-shakuyaku-san; thiamine, vitamin E, and fish oil supplements; a low-fat vegetarian diet; and acupressure.

In secondary dysmenorrhea, patients report the same symptoms as those of primary dysmenorrhea, except there is evidence of pelvic pathology (ie, endometriosis, fibroids, chronic pelvic inflammatory disease, intrauterine device use, cervical stenosis, or adenomyosis). The age of onset is usually older than 20 years, and the course can be progressive. The treatment is correction of the underlying cause.

Additional Reading: Dysmenorrhea. *Am Fam Physician*. 2021;104(2):164-170.

15. A 34-year-old woman who is 2 weeks post partum presents to your office with her newborn for a well-child check; her infant is doing well and has regained his birth weight. At the visit, the mother asks about her health and wants to know more about her gestational diabetes that developed during the first trimester. You inform her that women who develop gestational diabetes should:

A) have no further monitoring, unless she develops symptoms of diabetes.
B) have no different risk of developing type 2 diabetes in the future than anyone else.
C) be screened for diabetes with either fasting blood glucose measurements or a 2-hour glucose tolerance test 6 weeks post partum and yearly thereafter.
D) be tested for diabetes 6 months after delivery via fasting blood glucose measurements on two occasions or a 2-hour oral 75-g glucose tolerance test.

The answer is C: Women with gestational diabetes are at sevenfold increased risk for developing type 2 diabetes in the future and should be tested for diabetes 6 weeks after delivery. Diagnostic tests include fasting blood glucose measurements on two occasions or a 2-hour oral 75-g glucose tolerance test. Normal values for a 2-hour glucose tolerance test are less than 140 mg/dL. Values between 140 and 200 mg/dL (11.1 mmol/L) represent impaired glucose tolerance, and values greater than 200 mg/dL are diagnostic of diabetes. Screening for diabetes should be repeated annually thereafter, especially in patients who had elevated fasting blood glucose levels during pregnancy.

Additional Reading: Screening, diagnosis, and management of gestational diabetes mellitus. *Am Fam Physician*. 2015;91(7):460-467.

16. You are evaluating a young woman whom you suspect is suffering from nongonococcal urethritis. Which one of the following infectious agents is most commonly associated with this condition?

A) *Chlamydia*
B) Herpes simplex virus (HSV)
C) *Ureaplasma*
D) *Treponema pallidum*
E) *Trichomonas*

The answer is A: Nongonococcal urethritis is diagnosed when examination or microscopy findings indicate inflammation without the presence of the gram-negative intracellular diplococci that cause gonorrhea. This condition is commonly caused by chlamydial infections (documented in 15%-40% of cases). Chlamydia is currently the most common sexually transmitted infection in the United States. Other causes include *Trichomonas vaginalis*, HSV, *Mycoplasma genitalium*, and adenovirus.

Women are often completely asymptomatic. Symptoms, when they are present, include vaginal discharge, dysuria, frequency, pelvic pain, and dyspareunia. The incubation period is between 7 and 28 days.

Nucleic acid amplification tests are the preferred method for diagnosing chlamydial infection because of their sensitivity, ability to detect chlamydia in urine samples, and ease of testing concurrently for chlamydia and gonorrhea from the same sample. Rapid and accurate diagnosis is essential because of need for partner notification and referral to treatment.

Chlamydial infection in women can result in PID and infertility, whereas infection in men can result in epididymitis and Reiter syndrome. Chlamydia is adequately treated either with single-dose azithromycin 1 g or doxycycline 100 mg bid for 7 days. Single-dose azithromycin, especially with witnessed dosing in medical clinics, is associated with high treatment success rates.

Additional Reading: Chlamydia – CDC fact sheet. Centers for Disease Control and Prevention. 2022. www.cdc.gov/std/chlamydia/stdfact-chlamydia.htm

17. A woman presents with complaints of irregular menstrual bleeding. You suspect dysfunctional uterine bleeding. In which setting is this most likely to occur?

A) After sexual intercourse
B) At the time of menopause
C) During pregnancy
D) In premenarche
E) With the development of pelvic inflammatory disease

The answer is B: If the patient is young and otherwise healthy, and the bleeding is not profuse, medical treatment can be initiated with high-dose oral estrogens every 6 hours, which usually stops the bleeding within the first 24 hours. After the cessation of bleeding, the patient should continue with daily estrogen for the rest of the month, followed by the administration of progesterone during the final 10 days of the month. After the addition of progesterone, withdrawal bleeding should occur within a few days, and the patient can then begin oral contraceptive pills to regulate menstrual cycles. If bleeding continues, further evaluation with an endometrial biopsy or dilation and curettage may be necessary.

Older women in the perimenopausal state may initially need endometrial biopsy and possible dilation and curettage to rule out endometrial hyperplasia or endometrial cancer.

Additional Reading: Abnormal uterine bleeding in premenopausal women. *Am Fam Physician*. 2019;99(7):435-443.

18. You are evaluating a young triathlete, who is worried that she has stopped having her menses. Which one of the following statements about exercise-induced amenorrhea is true?

A) It usually affects women who have gained more than 10% to 15% in muscle mass.
B) It can be associated with osteoporosis.
C) It is usually associated with prolactinomas.
D) Hormone therapy is contraindicated in those affected.
E) The condition is rarely reversible with weight gain.

The answer is B: Exercise-induced amenorrhea is a condition that is noted in competitive female athletes. The cause appears to be a relative energy deficit due to a high caloric output and insufficient caloric intake. Menstrual irregularities or amenorrhea are most likely to develop in women who weigh less than 115 lb or those who have lost more than 10% to 15% of their normal weight while training.

The basis of amenorrhea is unknown but may be associated with hypothalamic dysfunction. In most cases, weight gain reverses the condition. However, many women are unwilling to gain the additional weight. This was previously called "female athlete triad," but is now called "RED-S," which stands for relative energy deficiency in sport. It is defined as the combination of inadequate caloric intake, amenorrhea, and low bone mineral density (BMD). The consequences of lost BMD can be devastating for the female athlete. Stress fractures and premature osteoporotic fractures can occur, and lost BMD may never be regained. Athletes with prolonged oligomenorrhea (infrequent menses) or amenorrhea lasting for at least 6 months should undergo bone density evaluation with a dual-energy x-ray absorptiometry scan. Dual-energy x-ray absorptiometry screening should also be performed on female athletes who have normal menstrual cycles but have experienced two or more stress fractures.

Early recognition can be accomplished by the family physician through risk factor assessment and screening questions. Instituting an appropriate diet and moderating the frequency of exercise may result in the natural return of menses. Hormone therapy should be considered early to prevent the loss of bone density.

Additional Reading: Care of the active female. *Am Fam Physician*. 2022;106(1):52-60.

19. The Amsel criteria present a standard approach to diagnosing bacterial vaginosis (BV). The criteria include all of the following findings except which one?

A) A positive "whiff" test
B) The presence of a milky, homogeneous, adherent discharge
C) The presence of clue cells on light microscopy
D) Vaginal pH greater than 4.5
E) Vaginal itching

The answer is E: The Amsel criteria are a standard diagnostic approach to BV. The criteria include the following: milky, homogeneous, adherent discharge; vaginal pH > 4.5; positive whiff test (the discharge typically has a fishy smell); and presence of clue cells in the vaginal fluid on light microscopy. If three of the four criteria are met, there is a 90% likelihood of a BV infection.

Additional Reading: Vaginitis: diagnosis and treatment. *Am Fam Physician*. 2018;97(5):321-329.

20. Which of the following screening tests has been shown to reduce breast cancer-related mortality in average-risk women?

A) Breast self-examination
B) Mammogram
C) Mammogram with clinical breast examination
D) Magnetic resonance imaging (MRI)
E) Screening for *BRCA* mutation

The answer is B: Breast cancer is the most common nonskin cancer and the second leading cause of cancer death in North American women. Mammography is the only screening test shown to reduce breast cancer–related mortality. There is general agreement that screening should be offered at least biennially to women 50 to 74 years of age. For women 40 to 49 years of age, the risks and benefits of screening should be discussed, and the decision to perform screening should take into consideration the individual patient risk, values, and comfort level of the patient and physician.

Information is lacking about the effectiveness of screening in women 75 years and older. The decision to screen women in this age group should be individualized, keeping the patient's life expectancy, functional status, and goals of care in mind.

For women with an estimated lifetime breast cancer risk of more than 20% or who have a *BRCA* mutation, screening should begin at 25 years of age or at the age that is 5 to 10 years younger than the earliest age that breast cancer was diagnosed in the family.

Screening with MRI may be considered in high-risk women, but its impact on breast cancer mortality is uncertain. Clinical breast examination plus mammography seems to be no more effective than mammography alone at reducing breast cancer mortality. Teaching breast self-examination does not improve mortality and is not recommended; however, women should be aware of any changes in their breasts and report them promptly.

Additional Reading: Breast cancer screening: common questions and answers. *Am Fam Physician*. 2021;103(1):33-41.

The U.S. Preventive Services Task Force recommends biennial screening mammography for women aged 50 to 74 years.

21. A 26-year-old woman presents with pelvic pain, fever, vaginal discharge, and nausea with vomiting. She reports recent intercourse with a new sexual partner and is worried that she has "caught something." On pelvic examination, you detect significant cervical motion tenderness. The most likely diagnosis to account for the scenario is which one of the following conditions?

A) Bacterial vaginosis
B) Ectopic pregnancy
C) Pyelonephritis
D) Pelvic inflammatory disease (PID)
E) Yeast vaginitis

The answer is D: PID is an infection of the fallopian tubes, cervix, endometrium, or ovaries. It is usually seen in women younger than 30 years who are sexually active. The use of condoms lowers the risk of PID. The use of intrauterine devices and multiple sex partners increase the risk.

Causative agents include *Chlamydia*, *N gonorrhoeae*, and multiple organisms found in the normal vaginal flora. Many cases involve polymicrobial infections. Acute symptoms include pelvic pain, fever, vaginal discharge, dyspareunia, nausea, and vomiting; however, some cases of PID present with more mild or subtle symptoms.

Physical examination reveals adnexal, uterine, and cervical motion tenderness (positive Chandelier sign). Laboratory findings include elevations of white blood counts, elevated erythrocyte sedimentation rate, and elevated C-reactive protein. Increased white blood cells on microscopy of cervical secretions as well as positive testing for chlamydia and/or gonorrhea in the lower genital tract is often present; however, negative gonorrhea or chlamydia testing does not rule out PID.

The differential diagnosis includes appendicitis, ectopic pregnancy, urinary tract infection, and peritonitis from other causes. Complications of PID include chronic PID, tubo-ovarian abscesses, infertility, and ectopic pregnancy. Outpatient therapy with oral antibiotics can be used in the majority of patients with PID and includes a single dose of ceftriaxone 250 mg intramuscularly and oral doxycycline 100 mg bid for 14 days with or without metronidazole 500 mg bid for 14 days. Parenteral treatment for a patient who is unable to tolerate oral medications consists of cefotetan or cefoxitin plus doxycycline. Follow-up care must be available within 72 hours to evaluate the response to treatment.

Additional Reading: Pelvic inflammatory disease: diagnosis, management, and prevention. *Am Fam Physician*. 2019;100(6):357-364.

22. A 63-year-old woman presents with complaints of painful intercourse for the last few months. You suspect atrophic vaginitis. Which one of the following findings is a characteristic of this condition?

A) Endometrial cells noted on wet-mount microscopic examination
B) Increased vaginal rugae noted on pelvic examination
C) Milky discharge noted on underwear
D) Odorous vaginal discharge noted on pelvic examination
E) Vaginal pH of 5 to 7 measured on pelvic examination

The answer is E: The decline in estrogen levels during perimenopause and after menopause can cause vaginal atrophy and resulting atrophic vaginitis. Physiologic changes include thinning of the vaginal epithelium and the loss of subcutaneous glycogen, which leads to changes in the vaginal pH and flora. Many women with these vaginal changes are minimally symptomatic and require only explanation and reassurance. In women with more severe changes, vaginal irritation, dyspareunia, and fragility may become problems.

Atrophy is diagnosed by the presence of a thin, clear, or bloody discharge; a vaginal pH of 5 to 7; loss of vaginal rugae; and the finding of parabasal epithelial cells on microscopic examination of a wet-mount preparation.

Additional Reading: *Clinical manifestations and diagnosis of vaginal atrophy*. In: *UpToDate*. 2022.

23. A middle-aged woman is in the office with vaginal itching and discharge. You diagnose candidal vulvovaginitis, her fourth episode in a year. Appropriate management for this patient should include which of the following approaches?

A) Continue observation and treatment only if symptomatic.
B) Order laboratory testing to rule out hypothyroidism.
C) Order laboratory testing to look for the presence of diabetes or human immunodeficiency virus infection.
D) Prescribe prophylactic therapy with weekly metronidazole.
E) Refer for a hysterosalpingogram to rule out pelvic structural abnormalities.

The answer is C: Recurrent vulvovaginal candidiasis is defined as four or more yeast infections in 1 year. The possibility of uncontrolled diabetes mellitus or immunodeficiency should be considered in women with recurrent vulvovaginal candidiasis. Only after it has been determined that no reversible causes are present (eg, antibiotic therapy and diabetes) and initial therapy has been completed, maintenance therapy may be appropriate. Selected long-term regimens include the use of clotrimazole and fluconazole. The role of boric acid and *Lactobacillus* therapy remains in question.

Additional Reading: Treatment of recurrent vulvovaginal candidiasis. *Am Fam Physician*. 2011;83(12):1482-1484.

24. A 20-year-old woman presents to your office complaining of pelvic pain, dysuria, and a purulent yellowish-green vaginal discharge. The laboratory reports that a Gram stain of the cervical secretions shows gram-negative diplococci. The most appropriate antibiotic treatment regimen for this situation is which one of the following combinations?

A) Ceftriaxone + azithromycin
B) Cefuroxime + tetracycline
C) Cefoxitin + doxycycline
D) Metronidazole + doxycycline
E) Penicillin G + azithromycin

The answer is A: Gonorrhea is caused by the gram-negative diplococcus *Neisseria gonorrhoeae*. Symptoms include purulent, yellowish-green vaginal or rectal discharge, urethritis, genital irritation, and discomfort. Other symptoms can include abdominal or pelvic pain and pharyngeal discomfort if the patient also has an oral infection. Some patients, especially women, are completely asymptomatic.

Disseminated gonococcal infection can give rise to polyarthralgias; tenosynovitis; and a hemorrhagic papular or pustular skin rash that affects the genitalia, hands, feet, and other areas of the body. The disease is spread by sexual contact. Incubation is 2 to 14 days for men and 7 to 21 days for women. Diagnosis is accomplished with Gram stains that show leukocytes with intracellular gram-negative diplococci and, more accurately, with cultures made on Thayer-Martin chocolate agar media. Urogenital *N gonorrhoeae* infections can also be diagnosed with nonculture (eg, the nucleic acid amplification test) techniques that can simultaneously test for chlamydial infection.

For patients with uncomplicated genital, rectal, and pharyngeal gonorrhea, the Centers for Disease Control and Prevention (CDC) currently recommends combination therapy with ceftriaxone 250 mg as a single intramuscular dose, plus either azithromycin 1 g orally in a single dose *or* doxycycline 100 mg orally twice daily for 7 days. In instances where ceftriaxone is not available, the CDC recommends cefixime 400 mg orally, plus either azithromycin 1 g orally *or* doxycycline 100 mg orally twice daily for 7 days. For patients with a severe allergy to cephalosporins, the CDC recommends a single 2 g dose of azithromycin orally. In both of these circumstances, the CDC recommends a test of cure for these patients 1 week after treatment, and partners should also be located and treated.

Other sexually transmitted diseases (eg, syphilis, acquired immunodeficiency syndrome, and hepatitis) may also coexist and need appropriate diagnosis and treatment; however, chlamydial infection will be adequately covered by these suggested regimens.

Additional Reading: *Gonorrhea Treatment and Care*. Centers for Disease Control and Prevention. www.cdc.gov/std/gonorrhea/treatment.htm

Gonorrhea bacteria have developed resistance to nearly every antibiotic traditionally used for treatment. Therefore, the CDC recommends dual therapy to treat gonorrhea.

25. You performed a Papanicolaou test on a premenopausal 49-year-old patient, who was otherwise feeling well and having normal monthly menses with no other vaginal bleeding. The Papanicolaou test comes back as negative for cervical pathology, but the report notes the presence of benign appearing endometrial cells. Appropriate management in this situation would be to pursue which one of the following tests?

A) Colposcopy
B) Dilation and curettage
C) Endometrial biopsy
D) Ultrasonography examination of the uterus
E) No further testing at this time

The answer is E: The presence of endometrial cells on a Papanicolaou test is reported for all women above 40 years of age. If a woman is still menstruating, the presence of endometrial cells is rarely associated with any significant underlying pathology, and such women do not need additional evaluation. However, in postmenopausal women, current evidence supports further evaluation if benign endometrial cells are observed on a Papanicolaou test. This evaluation may include transvaginal ultrasonography, office endometrial biopsy, or both.

Hormone replacement therapy may increase the rate of benign endometrial shedding, but postmenopausal women on hormone replacement therapy still require evaluation for this finding. The presence of any atypical endometrial cells on a Papanicolaou test requires additional evaluation, regardless of age or menopausal status of the woman.

Additional Reading: Endometrial biopsy: tips and pitfalls. *Am Fam Physician*. 2020;101(9):551-556.

26. A 57-year-old woman presents for her well-woman examination. She has been seen yearly for the last 10 years and has always been found to have normal cytology on routine annual Papanicolaou tests. She is otherwise healthy. She has not had any sexually transmitted diseases and has been in a monogamous relationship with her husband for 30 years. She has never had testing for the presence of high-risk human papillomavirus (HPV) infection. She inquires about her annual Papanicolaou test and you reply with which one of the following?

A) An annual Papanicolaou test is necessary in her age group because of the risk of cervical cancer.
B) An appropriate interval for her to have a repeat Papanicolaou test is 5 years.
C) An appropriate interval for her to have a repeat Papanicolaou test is 3 years.
D) Papanicolaou tests are no longer required for women in her age group.
E) She does not need to repeat a Papanicolaou test but needs HPV screening.

The answer is C: For women aged 30 to 65 years, the U.S. Preventive Services Task Force (USPSTF) recommends screening every 3 years with cervical cytology alone, or every 5 years with high-risk human papillomavirus (hrHPV) testing alone, or every 5 years with hrHPV testing in combination with cytology (cotesting). USPSTF cervical cancer screening recommendations are categorized by the age of the patient:

1. Adolescents should not have screening; rather, cervical cancer prevention efforts should be focused on universal HPV vaccination.
2. Women aged 21 to 29 years should be screened every 3 years with Papanicolaou cytology alone. Routine cotesting for oncogenic (high-risk) HPV is not recommended.
3. Women aged 30 to 65 years should have cytology screening every 3 years or cytology plus hrHPV testing every 5 years.
4. Women above age 65 years and those who have undergone removal of the cervix with hysterectomy and have no history of cervical intraepithelial neoplasia II or greater or cervical cancer do not need Pap screening.

This patient has had negative annual Papanicolaou testing via cytology alone and can wait for a repeat Papanicolaou cytology examination in 3 years. The USPSTF is working on updating its recommendations, with planned publication in 2023.

Additional Reading: *Recommendation: Cervical Cancer – Screening | United States Preventive Services Taskforce* (uspreventiveservicestaskforce.org).

27. A 17-year-old woman who is yet to have a menstrual period presents to your office with her mother, and they are concerned. On examination, she is found to be obese, has evidence of excessive facial hair, and her mother reports that she had similar problems. Laboratory testing shows normal estrogen levels but increased luteinizing hormone (LH), low follicle-stimulating hormone (FSH), elevated testosterone level, and elevated urinary 17-ketosteroids. The most likely diagnosis to account for this presentation is which one of the following conditions?

A) Acromegaly
B) Adrenal adenoma
C) Cushing disease
D) Pregnancy
E) Stein-Leventhal syndrome

The answer is E: Polycystic ovary syndrome (PCOS; or Stein-Leventhal syndrome) is an inherited condition characterized by cystic ovaries, hirsutism, amenorrhea, and obesity. It is the most common cause of anovulation and hirsutism. Although some patients present with primary amenorrhea, others may present with abnormal or irregular periods. In some cases, periods may be normal.

Laboratory studies show normal or increased levels of estrogen, increased LH, normal or decreased FSH, normal or increased testosterone, and increased urinary 17-ketosteroids. Glucose intolerance with increased insulin levels may also be present. Pelvic ultrasonography can also aid in the diagnosis by demonstrating bilateral enlargement of the ovaries.

Administration of progesterone usually results in withdrawal bleeding for patients with amenorrhea. Treatment for PCOS depends on symptoms and pregnancy goals. First-line agents for hirsutism and menstrual irregularities include antiandrogens (spironolactone [Aldactone], flutamide [Eulexin], cyproterone [Cyprostat]), as well as combined oral contraceptives and metformin.

Spironolactone, in a dosage of 25 to 100 mg administered bid, is the most commonly used antiandrogen because of its safety, availability, and low cost. However, spironolactone is pregnancy risk category C; thus, these agents are contraindicated in pregnant women or women who wish to become pregnant. Flutamide is usually given in a dosage of 250 mg bid, and cyproterone is given in a dosage of 25 to 50 mg/d for 10 days each month. If a woman with PCOS desires pregnancy, first-line agents include clomiphene (a selective estrogen receptor modulator) and metformin.

Gonadotropin-releasing hormone (GnRH) analogues such as leuprolide (Lupron) should be reserved for use in women who do not respond to combination hormonal therapy or cannot tolerate oral contraceptive pills. GnRH analogues should be used cautiously, with particular attention given to long-term consequences (eg, hot flashes, bone demineralization, and atrophic vaginitis) that can occur secondary to hypoestrogenemia induced by these agents. Surgery (wedge resection of the ovary) has also been shown to restore ovulatory periods and fertility.

Cushing disease is a condition that is caused by excess corticosteroids, especially cortisol, usually from adrenal or pituitary hyperfunction, and is characterized by obesity, hypertension, muscular weakness, and easy bruising.

Many adrenal adenomas do not produce any symptoms of hormonal excess; however, when “active” or “functioning,” they can lead to Cushing disease or primary aldosteronism.

Acromegaly is abnormal growth of the hands, feet, and face, caused by overproduction of growth hormone by the pituitary gland.

Additional Reading: Diagnosis and treatment of polycystic ovary syndrome. *Am Fam Physician*. 2016;94(2):106-113.

28. A 48-year-old otherwise healthy woman has undergone a hysterectomy secondary to abnormal vaginal bleeding. Pathology results confirm no evidence of malignancy. She asks you how often she should have a Papanicolaou test. The appropriate response is which one of the following?

A) Yearly Papanicolaou tests for an additional 3 years are recommended.
B) Papanicolaou tests should be reinstituted if she develops atrophic vaginitis.
C) Papanicolaou tests should be repeated every 3 years.
D) Papanicolaou tests should be performed every 5 years.
E) No further Papanicolaou tests are necessary if the cervix was removed in the hysterectomy.

The answer is E: Multiple studies have concluded that vaginal cuff smear testing is not necessary in women who have undergone hysterectomy with removal of the cervix for benign conditions.

Additional Reading: Cervical cancer screening among women by hysterectomy status and among women aged >65. *MMWR Morb Mortal Wkly Rep*. 2013;61(51):1043-1047.

29. You had performed a routine Papanicolaou test on a 25-year-old woman, and the results have returned with atypical squamous cells of undetermined significance (ASC-US). Human papilloma virus (HPV) typing is negative for high-risk HPV. Appropriate management at this time would be to recommend which one of the following?

A) Perform a colposcopy.
B) Refer for a loop electrosurgical excision procedure.
C) A repeat Papanicolaou test in 3 years.
D) A repeat Papanicolaou test in 6 months.
E) A repeat Papanicolaou test in 1 year with high-risk HPV testing.

The answer is C: Because of the very low cervical cancer risk observed in women with atypical squamous cells of undetermined significance (ASC-US) cytology, accompanied by a negative high-risk HPV test, such patients should continue with routine screening per age-specific guidelines. Data from published studies have shown that the risk of precancerous lesions following an HPV-negative, ASC-US cytology result is very low, and not qualitatively different from a negative cotest. In the case of a 21- to 29-year-old woman, a 3-year interval for cytology-only screening is appropriate.

Additional Reading: ACS, ASCCP, ASC screening guidelines for the prevention and early detection of cervical cancer. *J Low Genit Tract Dis*. 2012;16(3):1-29.

30. A 43-year-old patient presents noting bilateral milky nipple discharge. You diagnose galactorrhea and state that the most common cause of this condition is which one of the following?

A) Hypothyroidism
B) Nipple stimulation
C) Prolactinoma
D) Psychotropic medication use
E) Sexual intercourse

The answer is C: Galactorrhea is defined as the presence of lactation in the absence of pregnancy. Therefore, pregnancy testing should occur before any further workup. For nonpregnant patients, galactorrhea is most commonly caused by hyperprolactinemia, especially when associated with amenorrhea. The most common cause for hyperprolactinemia is a prolactinoma in the pituitary gland or other sellar or suprasellar lesions. Other causes include psychotropic medications, opioids, antihypertensive drugs (α-methyldopa), hypogonadism, nipple stimulation, bronchogenic carcinomas, herpes zoster, hypothyroidism, renal insufficiency, and trauma.

After pathologic nipple discharge is ruled out by cytology, patients with galactorrhea should be evaluated by measurement of their prolactin level. The result can range from slightly elevated (>23-25 ng/mL) to a thousand times the upper limit of normal, and those with hyperprolactinemia should also have their thyroid and renal function assessed. In general, adenomas are more common when prolactin levels are greater than 200 ng/mL.

Elevated prolactin levels should prompt computed tomographic or magnetic resonance imaging scans of the sella turcica to exclude pituitary adenomas. Visual field defects may also be present if tumors impinge on the optic chiasm.

Patients with prolactinomas are usually treated with dopamine agonists (bromocriptine or cabergoline); surgery or radiation therapy is rarely required. Medications causing hyperprolactinemia should be discontinued or replaced with a medication from a similar class with lower potential for causing hyperprolactinemia. Patients with normal prolactin levels are suffering from idiopathic galactorrhea and can be reassured and do not need treatment. However, those with bothersome galactorrhea usually respond to a short course of a low-dose dopamine agonist.

Additional Reading: Evaluation and management of galactorrhea. *Am Fam Physician*. 2012;85(11):1073-1080.

31. A Papanicolaou test result for a 23-year-old female patient comes back with atypical cells of undetermined significance, and the report cannot exclude high-grade intraepithelial lesion. Appropriate management at this time would be to recommend which one of the following interventions?

A) A repeat Papanicolaou test in 1 year.
B) A repeat Papanicolaou test in 6 months.
C) Perform a colposcopy.
D) Refer for cervical cryotherapy.
E) Refer for a loop electrosurgical excision procedure.

The answer is C: Although high-grade intraepithelial lesion is less common than atypical squamous cells of undetermined significance, the risk of underlying cervical intraepithelial neoplasia (CIN) II or III is higher and colposcopy is recommended. Women aged 21 to 24 years with no CIN II or III identified at the time of colposcopy should be observed with colposcopy and cytology every 6 months up to 2 years, until two consecutive negative Papanicolaou tests are reported and no high-grade colposcopy abnormality is observed.

Additional Reading: Cervical colposcopy: indications and risk assessment. *Am Fam Physician*. 2020;102(1):39-48.

32. A 40-year-old woman's Papanicolaou test result comes back as having atypical glandular cells (AGCs). Appropriate management at this time would be to recommend which one of the following?

A) A repeat Papanicolaou test in 1 year
B) A repeat Papanicolaou test at 6 months
C) A colposcopy
D) A colposcopy with endocervical and endometrial sampling
E) Human papilloma virus (HPV) testing and colposcopy only if high-risk HPV identified

The answer is D: For women older than 35 years, with AGCs (except atypical endometrial cells), colposcopy with endocervical sampling is recommended regardless of the HPV result. Accordingly, triage by reflex HPV testing or repeat cervical cytology is not recommended.

Endometrial sampling is also recommended for women younger than 35 years, with clinical indications suggesting they may be at risk for endometrial neoplasia. These include unexplained vaginal bleeding or conditions suggesting chronic anovulation.

For women with atypical endometrial cells, initial evaluation limited to endometrial and endocervical sampling is preferred, with colposcopy acceptable either at the initial evaluation or deferred until the results of endometrial and endocervical sampling are known; if colposcopy is deferred and no endometrial pathology is identified, colposcopy is then recommended.

Additional Reading: Cervical colposcopy: indications and risk assessment. *Am Fam Physician.* 2020;102(1):39-48.

33. A 54-year-old postmenopausal woman presents noting that she has had some vaginal bleeding over the past couple of months. You are concerned about endometrial cancer. The most sensitive method to diagnose this cancer is with which one of the following tests?

A) Computed tomography of the pelvis
B) Endometrial biopsy
C) Fractionated endometrial curettage
D) Papanicolaou test
E) Ultrasonography

The answer is C: Adenocarcinoma of the endometrium usually occurs in postmenopausal women between 50 and 60 years of age and arises from the columnar cells of the endometrial lining. Associated conditions that constitute risk factors include adenomatous hyperplasia; unopposed estrogen use; delayed menopause; infertility; polycystic ovary syndrome; previous breast, colon, or ovarian cancer; diabetes; long-term tamoxifen use; hypertension; and obesity.

The hallmark symptom is unexplained, irregular vaginal bleeding, particularly in postmenopausal women. The diagnosis can be made with Papanicolaou tests in 40% of patients. However, because of the relatively high rate of false-negative results, diagnosis is better made with endometrial biopsy, ultrasonography, or the gold standard fractionated endometrial curettage. Using this technique, each section of the uterus is examined and curetted to obtain specimens of the endometrium from all parts of the organ.

Treatment involves surgical excision with total abdominal hysterectomy and bilateral oophorectomy followed by lymph node sampling. Chemotherapy using cytotoxic drugs, as well as progesterone and radiation, is also used in the treatment of endometrial cancer. Prognosis depends on the stage and differentiation of the cancer. Well-differentiated, well-localized tumors have a 5-year survival rate of close to 95%, whereas poorly differentiated tumors with metastasis have less than a 20% 5-year survival rate.

Additional Reading: Endometrial cancer and uterine sarcoma. In: Domino F, ed. *The 5-Minute Clinical Consult.* Wolters Kluwer; 2022.

Adenocarcinoma of the endometrium usually occurs in postmenopausal women between 50 and 60 years of age. The hallmark symptom is unexplained, irregular vaginal bleeding, and the diagnosis is made with endometrial biopsy, ultrasonography, or the gold standard fractionated endometrial curettage.

34. A young mother is complaining of postpartum breast engorgement. Which one of the following therapies should you recommend?

A) Bromocriptine orally prn
B) Cabbage leaf compresses
C) Firm binding of breast with a comfortable wrap
D) Initiation of oral contraceptives
E) Topical vitamin E ointment

The answer is C: One of the best ways to prevent postpartum breast engorgement is to bind the breasts firmly with a comfortable wrap. Other suggestions include cold packs, analgesics, mechanical expression of some breast milk, and the avoidance of direct warm water during showering. The use of cooled cabbage leaves is common in some cultures but has not been shown to have clear benefit over placebo. A Cochrane review noted that although some interventions may be promising for the treatment of breast engorgement, such as cabbage leaves, cold gel packs, herbal compresses, and massage, the certainty of evidence is low and they could not draw robust conclusions about their true effects.

The use of bromocriptine (a dopamine agonist) to stop lactation is associated with rebound lactation after discontinuation of the medication, hypotension, hypertension, seizures, and stroke; it is no longer approved by the U.S. Food and Drug Administration for this use. Other medications, such as estrogen and testosterone combinations, are not recommended because of their increased risk for thromboembolism and hair growth, respectively. In most cases, breast engorgement resolves within 72 hours.

Additional Reading: ACOG Committee on Obstetric Practice: Breast Feeding Challenges. *Obstet Gynecol*. 2021;137(2).

35. A 38-year-old woman has a Papanicolaou test result of "AGC—favor neoplasia." She undergoes colposcopy and no invasive disease is found. The appropriate management at this time would be to recommend which one of the following tests?

A) A loop electrosurgical excision procedure (LEEP)
B) Cold-knife conization procedure
C) Repeat Papanicolaou test in 1 year
D) Repeat Papanicolaou test in 6 months
E) Repeat colposcopy in 6 months

The answer is B: The category of atypical glandular cells (AGC) is divided into "not otherwise specified" and "favor neoplasia" or adenocarcinoma in situ. For women with AGC "favor neoplasia" or endocervical adenocarcinoma in situ cytology, a diagnostic excisional procedure is recommended even if invasive disease is not identified during the initial colposcopic examination. It is recommended that the type of diagnostic excisional procedure used in this setting provides an intact specimen with interpretable margins, such as a cold-knife cone procedure. Excision via an LEEP may affect interpretation of specimen margins;therefore, it is not the preferred procedure. Endocervical sampling after excision is preferred.

Additional Reading: 2012 updated consensus guidelines for the management of abnormal cervical cancer screening tests and cancer precursors. *J Low Genit Tract Dis.* 2013;17(5):S1–S27.

36. Endometrial cancer is the most common gynecologic malignancy and the fourth most common cancer in women worldwide. Risk factors include infertility and obesity. In addition to unopposed estrogens, which one of the following medications is also associated with an increased risk of endometrial carcinoma?

A) Alendronate (Fosamax)
B) Bromocriptine (Parlodel)
C) Oral contraceptives
D) Progesterone
E) Tamoxifen (Nolvadex)

The answer is E: Risk factors for endometrial cancer include unopposed estrogens and tamoxifen use. A number of other factors have also been identified, including the following:

- Early menarche/late menopause
- Nulliparity
- Personal or family history of colon or reproductive system cancer
- Obesity
- Diabetes mellitus
- Hypertension
- Polycystic ovary syndrome
- Estrogen-secreting tumor
- Endometrial hyperplasia
- Increasing age

Additional Reading: Endometrial cancer and uterine sarcoma. In: Domino F, ed. *The 5-Minute Clinical Consult*. Wolters Kluwer; 2022.

37. A 17-year-old woman presents to your office complaining of irregular menstrual periods for the past few months. She is otherwise well and denies pregnancy. Appropriate management in this situation consists of which one of the following?

A) Obtain an endometrial biopsy.
B) Order a pelvic ultrasonography.
C) Obtain an endometrial biopsy and order a pelvic ultrasonography.
D) Perform a dilation and curettage.
E) Prescribe an oral contraceptive and follow-up.

The answer is E: Dysfunctional uterine bleeding is defined as abnormal uterine bleeding in the absence of inflammation, pregnancy, or tumors. It is most commonly associated with anovulation. Endometrial cancer is rare in 15- to 18-year-old women. Therefore, most adolescents with dysfunctional uterine bleeding can be treated safely with hormone therapy and observation, without diagnostic testing.

Additional Reading: Abnormal uterine bleeding in premenopausal women. *Am Fam Physician*. 2019;99(7):435-443.

38. Pubic lice are readily transmitted sexually and individuals with such an infection should be evaluated for other sexually transmitted infections. Which one of the following medications should only be used for failed therapy attempts in the treatment of pediculosis because of concerns regarding potential toxicity?

A) Ivermectin
B) Lindane
C) Malathion
D) Permethrin
E) Pyrethrins/piperonyl butoxide

The answer is B: Pubic lice are readily transmitted sexually. There is some evidence that occasionally they may be transmitted through contaminated clothing or towels; however, this is controversial. The presence of pubic lice should prompt an evaluation for other common sexually transmitted diseases, such as chlamydial infection and gonorrhea. Treatment is the same as that for head lice.

Recommended treatments include permethrin 1% or pyrethrins 0.3%/piperonyl butoxide 4% as first-line agents, and alternative regimens of malathion 0.5% lotion or oral ivermectin at 250 µg/kg, repeated in 2 weeks. Lindane is not recommended as first-line therapy because of potential neurotoxicity. It should not be used in children, elderly patients, or patients weighing <110 lb. It should only be used as an alternative if the patient cannot tolerate other therapies or if other therapies have failed. The mainstay of treatment for body lice is laundering clothing and bedding in hot water and regular bathing. Sexual contacts also should be treated if infested.

Additional Reading: Lice and scabies: treatment update. *Am Fam Physician*. 2019;99(10):635-642.

39. Fibroid tumors are frequently diagnosed in women. These tumors are associated with which one of the following conditions?

A) Amenorrhea
B) An increased risk of ovarian carcinoma
C) An increased risk for endometrial hyperplasia
D) Postpartum hemorrhage
E) Renal lithiasis

The answer is B: Fibroid tumors are irregular enlargements of the uterus. They are the most common benign tumors of the female genital tract, with as many as 20% of 40-year-old women affected. The tumors are composed of smooth muscle and connective tissue. In most cases, the condition is asymptomatic; however, it can cause dysmenorrhea with heavy menstrual blood loss leading to anemia and irregular periods along with difficult pregnancies with dystocia and excessive postpartum hemorrhage. Other complications include urinary frequency or difficulty in defecating if the tumors press on the bladder or colon. Occasionally, the fibroids degenerate, giving rise to intense pelvic pain and the development of pelvic infections. In some cases, infertility can occur when a fibroma blocks the fallopian tube.

Diagnosis is usually made with ultrasonography, computed tomographic scan, magnetic resonance imaging, or hysteroscopy. Treatment involves gonadotropin-releasing hormone analogues (leuprolide), which may decrease the size of the fibroid. However, regrowth often occurs after the medication is discontinued. For severe cases, surgery, including myomectomy or hysterectomy, may be indicated. Treatment with estrogen can produce growth of the tumors and worsening of symptoms.

Additional Reading: Uterine myomas. In: Domino F, ed. *The 5-Minute Clinical Consult*. Wolters Kluwer; 2022.

40. A 50-year-old previously healthy woman who only takes a daily multivitamin presents noting a lack of menses for the past few months and inquires if she has gone through menopause. She has had an occasional "hot flashes," but they have been very mild. Which one of the following findings would support the diagnosis of menopause in this situation?

A) A vaginal pH greater than 4.5
B) A follicle-stimulating hormone (FSH) level less than 10 mIU/mL
C) Finding endometrial cells on her Papanicolaou test
D) A thyroid-stimulating hormone level greater than 5.6
E) A progesterone level greater than 100 pg/dL

The answer is A: A vaginal pH greater than 4.5 indicates menopause in women who are not receiving estrogen therapy and do not have acute vaginitis. Studies have shown that vaginal pH is similar in accuracy to FSH levels in establishing the diagnosis of low estrogen levels or menopause. A vaginal pH of 4.5 or less can be used to monitor adequate response to estrogen replacement therapy. Bacterial vaginosis can also cause a vaginal pH to be >4.5 and thus should be ruled out. FSH levels greater than 40 mIU/mL typically indicate a menopausal state. Low progesterone levels (<100 pg/mL) are often seen in menopause; however, low progesterone levels can also be seen in women taking oral contraceptives.

Additional Reading: Vaginal pH for diagnosing status of menopause. *Am Fam Physician*. 2005;71(5):979.

41. You are seeing a postmenopausal woman who is concerned about osteoporosis as her mother had fallen and broken her hip. Which one of the following statements is true regarding these conditions?

A) About 50% of hip fractures are caused by falling.
B) Bone mineral density (BMD) testing is recommended in all women aged 65 years and older, regardless of risk factors.
C) BMD testing should be performed only in postmenopausal women younger than 65 years if they have two or more risk factors for osteoporosis (in addition to menopausal status).
D) Impaired eyesight is not a factor to consider in the decision to start medication.
E) Weight-bearing exercise should be avoided in postmenopausal women.

The answer is B: Each year, about 300,000 elderly are hospitalized for hip fractures and more than 95% of hip fractures are caused by falling (usually falling sideways). BMD testing is recommended for all women aged 65 years and older, regardless of risk factors. All women should be counseled about the risk factors for osteoporosis. Risk factors for osteoporotic fracture include personal history of fracture as an adult, history of pathologic fracture in a first-degree relative, White race, advanced age, female sex, dementia, poor health/frailty, cigarette smoking, low body weight (<127 lb [58 kg]), estrogen deficiency, lifelong low calcium intake, alcoholism, impaired eyesight despite adequate correction (which leads to increased falls), recurrent falls, and inadequate physical activity.

BMD testing should be considered in women aged below 65 years who have one or more additional risk factors for osteoporosis (in addition to menopause). All postmenopausal women with a fracture should be evaluated for osteoporosis using BMD testing to determine if the woman has osteoporosis and to determine disease severity. Bone mineral tests provide a T score expressed in standard deviations; the more negative the number, the greater the risk of fracture. Each standard deviation represents a 10% to 12% bone loss, and a T score of −2.5 indicates osteoporosis. A measurement of the hip is the best predictor of hip fractures, and hip measurement can predict fractures at other sites as well.

Additional recommendations for all women to reduce risks for osteoporosis and falls include the following:

- Consume an adequate intake of dietary calcium (1200 mg/d, including supplements if necessary) and vitamin D (400-800 IU/d for persons at risk of deficiency).
- Avoid smoking.
- Limit alcohol intake to moderate levels.
- Participate in regular weight-bearing and muscle-strengthening exercises.

Additional Reading: Recommendation: Osteoporosis to Prevent Fractures – Screening | United States Preventive Services Taskforce (uspreventiveservicestaskforce.org)

U.S. Preventive Services Task Force guidelines recommend BMD testing for all women aged 65 years and older, regardless of risk factors (grade A recommendation). This recommendation has a planned update for 2023.

42. A young patient has been complaining of vaginal irritation, with a gray, foul-smelling discharge. You diagnose bacterial vaginosis (BV) and prescribe which one of the following regimens as the treatment of choice for BV?

A) Ceftriaxone
B) Doxycycline
C) Metronidazole
D) Nystatin vaginal tablets
E) Vinegar douche

The answer is C: BV is a condition that is caused by replacement of the normal hydrogen peroxide–producing *Lactobacillus* sp. in the vagina by an overgrowth of anaerobic bacteria including *Prevotella* sp, *Mobiluncus* sp, *G vaginalis*, *Ureaplasma*, and *Mycoplasma*. BV is associated with having multiple male or female partners, a new sex partner, douching, lack of condom use, and lack of vaginal lactobacilli. However, women who have never been sexually active can also be affected. The cause of the microbial alteration that characterizes BV is not fully understood, nor is whether BV results from acquisition of a sexually transmitted pathogen.

The condition accounts for as many as 50% of all cases of vaginitis. Patients often report vaginal irritation and a gray, foul-smelling vaginal discharge; however, a majority of patients with BV are asymptomatic. When 10% to 20% potassium hydroxide is applied, the discharge gives off a characteristic aminelike fishy odor. Microscopic examination of the discharge shows "clue cells" (epithelial cells that are covered with coccobacilli on the cell walls). The vaginal secretion pH is greater than 4.5.

The treatment of choice is oral or vaginal metronidazole. Topical 2% clindamycin cream can also be used. Cultures are not helpful because *Gardnerella* may be a normal inhabitant of the vagina. Women with BV are at increased risk for the acquisition of other sexuallt transmitted infections (eg, human immunodeficiency virus, *N gonorrhoeae*, *Chlamydia trachomatis*, and HSV-2), complications after gynecologic surgery, pregnancy complications, and recurrence of BV. Treatment of male sex partners has not been beneficial in preventing the recurrence of BV.

Additional Reading: Bacterial Vaginosis - STI Treatment Guidelines (cdc.gov). 2021.

43. A 15-year-old girl presents to the office with her mother over a concern that she has not had a period in the past 3 months. The young girl emphatically states that there is no way that she could be pregnant, and her mother assures you she is not pregnant, as well. The most appropriate initial test would be which one of the following?

A) Progesterone challenge test
B) Serum prolactin level
C) Serum cortisol level
D) Thyroid function test
E) Urine pregnancy test

The answer is E: Abnormal menses are normal in the immediate pubertal period. Lack of menses for 3 to 4 months presents no concern if there is no possibility that the girl is pregnant. However, the first step in the evaluation of amenorrhea is to ensure that the patient is not pregnant. Other tests for the workup of amenorrhea include a serum prolactin level and sensitive thyroid-stimulating hormone.

If these tests are normal and the pregnancy test is negative, a progesterone challenge test can be performed. In this test, medroxyprogesterone acetate is given for 7 to 10 days, and withdrawal bleeding is usually induced after administration. If withdrawal bleeding occurs (positive test), the diagnosis of anovulation can be made. If no withdrawal bleeding occurs (negative test), the differential diagnosis includes polycystic ovary syndrome or an adrenal enzyme deficiency that leads to an excess of progesterone.

If amenorrhea continues on a regular basis and the patient is diagnosed with anovulation, a daily dose of medroxyprogesterone can be prescribed for the first 10 days of alternative months. Pathologic amenorrhea is divided into primary amenorrhea (absence of menses before the age of 16) and secondary amenorrhea (absence of menses for 3 months or more in patients who have had previous periods).

Additional Reading: Amenorrhea: a systematic approach to diagnosis and management. *Am Fam Physician*. 2019;100(1):39-48.

44. You are assessing a young mother who has not been feeling well and diagnose postpartum depression. Which one of the following statements about this condition is true?

A) Postpartum depression usually occurs 9 to 12 months after delivery.
B) Social support has little impact on the development of postpartum depression.
C) Those with obstetric complications are at increased risk.
D) Those affected are at increased risk for postpartum depression with subsequent pregnancies.
E) Patients who have postpartum depression have no higher risk of developing depression in later years when compared with the general population.

The answer is D: Mild postpartum depression (also referred to as the "baby blues") is usually seen within the first few days after delivery. The incidence ranges up to 25%, and those with poor social support are more commonly affected. There appears to be no relationship with obstetric complications. Symptoms vary but are usually mild and self-limited. In most cases, reassurance that these feelings are common is all that is needed.

In more severe cases, in which the mother's symptoms last for extended periods or if the mother shows a lack of interest in the newborn, has suicidal or homicidal thoughts or gestures, or shows psychotic behavior, further therapy (including medication and psychotherapy) may be needed.

Women who are affected with severe postpartum depression are at the risk for development of further depressive episodes and recurrent postpartum depression with subsequent pregnancies.

Additional Reading: Cognitive behavior therapy for postpartum depression. *Am Fam Physician*. 2019;100(4):244-245.

45. A 66-year-old woman presents to your office concerned about her uterine prolapse. During her pelvic examination, the cervix is visible outside the vaginal introitus, although the uterus itself is not visible. Based on your findings, you classify this finding as which one of the following conditions?

A) A first-degree uterine prolapse
B) A second-degree uterine prolapse
C) A third-degree uterine prolapse
D) An impending uterine prolapse

The answer is B: Uterine prolapse is classified by degree. In first-degree uterine prolapse, the cervix is visible when the perineum is depressed. In second-degree prolapse, the cervix is visible outside the vaginal introitus whereas the uterine fundus remains inside. In third-degree prolapse, or *procidentia*, the entire uterus is outside the vaginal introitus. Uterine prolapse is associated with urinary incontinence, vaginitis, cystitis, and, possibly, uterine malignancy. Although pessaries may be used for mild, symptomatic prolapse, surgical repair or hysterectomy is indicated for more severe prolapse.

Additional Reading: Pelvic organ prolapse. *Am Fam Physician*. 2017;96(3):179-185.

46. A young woman is distraught after having a miscarriage at 10 weeks' gestation and is asking about what may have caused this to happen. You inform her that the most common cause of a first-trimester spontaneous abortion is which one of the following conditions?

A) An older maternal age
B) Cervical incompetence
C) Chromosomal abnormalities
D) Inadequate progesterone production during the luteal phase
E) The presence of a lupus anticoagulant

The answer is C: Up to 15% of recognized pregnancies end in miscarriage, and as many as 80% of miscarriages occur in the first trimester, with chromosomal abnormalities (usually autosomal trisomies that are incompatible with life) as the leading cause. Other factors that may contribute to spontaneous abortion include maternal smoking, increased maternal age, maternal illness, incompetent cervix, lupus anticoagulant, and inadequate levels of progesterone during the luteal phase of the menstrual cycle.

In general, no interventions have been proven to prevent miscarriage. Occasionally, women can modify their risk factors or receive treatment for relevant medical conditions. Patients with miscarriage usually report vaginal bleeding and uterine cramps. Unless products of conception are seen during pelvic examination, the diagnosis of miscarriage is made with ultrasonography or by measuring serial β-human chorionic gonadotropin levels.

Management options for early pregnancy loss include expectant management, medical management with misoprostol, and uterine aspiration with a manual vacuum device. Misoprostol in a dose of 800 μg administered vaginally is effective and well tolerated. Compared with dilation and curettage in the operating room, uterine aspiration is the preferred procedure for early pregnancy loss; aspiration is equally safe, quicker to perform, more cost-effective, and amenable to use in the primary care setting. All management options are equally safe; thus, patient preference should guide treatment choice.

Additional Reading: Common treatments for miscarriage. *Am Fam Physician*. 2011;84(1):85-86.

47. A young woman complains of dysuria and her urine dipstick is positive for leukocyte esterase, yet her subsequent urine culture is negative. The presence of sterile pyuria in a sexually active individual such as this is most commonly associated with which one of the following infectious agents?

A) *Chlamydia*
B) *N gonorrhoeae*
C) Herpes simplex
D) HPV
E) *T pallidum*

The answer is A: Pyuria is defined as the presence of 10 or more white cells per cubic millimeter in a urine specimen or a urinary dipstick test that is positive for leukocyte esterase. Sterile pyuria refers to finding white cells in the urine in the absence of bacteria (ie, no growth on subsequent culture). The presence of sterile pyuria in a sexually active individual should raise the suspicion of chlamydia. Chlamydia is a sexually transmitted disease that is caused by *C trachomatis*. Approximately 50% of nongonococcal urethritis, and most cases of cervicitis, are caused by chlamydia. Men usually report discomfort associated with the urethra, dysuria, or a clear to mucopurulent discharge that occurs 1 to 3 weeks after exposure, but most women are asymptomatic; however, they may report dysuria, pelvic discomfort with dyspareunia, and vaginal discharge that may have a clear to yellow mucopurulent appearance.

Diagnosis is made with immunologic studies performed on urine, vaginal or cervical secretions, or culture. The presence of gonorrhea must be ruled out, and patients should be treated for gonorrhea if chlamydia is found and vice versa. Single-dose therapy with azithromycin 1 g orally is as effective as a 7-day course of doxycycline, and both are first-line regimens for treatment of chlamydial infection. Erythromycin and quinolones, including levofloxacin or ofloxacin, are alternative regiments used to treat *C trachomatis*. Erythromycin is less efficacious than azithromycin and doxycycline, and its adverse gastrointestinal effects may decrease patient compliance. Ofloxacin and levofloxacin are as effective as the recommended regimens but offer no dosing or cost advantages. Doxycycline and fluoroquinolones are contraindicated in pregnant women.

Additional Reading: Sterile pyuria. *N Engl J Med*. 2015;372: 1048-1054.

48. Vaginismus is a condition that is characterized by involuntary spasm of the lower vaginal muscles, resulting in an unconscious effort to prevent penetration. Treatment for vaginismus includes which one of the following therapies?

A) Desensitization therapy with continued regular intercourse
B) Psychotherapy
C) Kegel exercises
D) Transcutaneous electrical nerve stimulation treatment
E) Treatment with muscle relaxants

The answer is B: Causes of vaginismus include psychiatric factors, local trauma, infection, or mechanical factors, including vaginal stenosis or dryness. Women with vaginismus frequently have a history of sexual abuse or other sexual trauma in their past. Women report extreme discomfort with attempts at penetration. Treatment involves correction of reversible causes, psychological and sexual counseling, and gradual and repeated attempts at vaginal dilation with vaginal probes. Treatment can be continued by the patient at home in a private environment after the appropriate technique has been learned. Intercourse can be attempted once the patient is able to tolerate larger dilators without discomfort. Communication with the patient's partner often is helpful in overcoming the patient's fears.

Additional Reading: Dyspareunia in women. *Am Fam Physician*. 2011;84(1):85-86.

49. Which of the following is *not* useful in treating premenstrual syndrome (PMS)?

A) Vitamin B_6 supplements
B) Selective serotonin reuptake inhibitors
C) Calcium and vitamin D supplementation
D) Decreased intake of caffeine, salt, and refined sugar

The answer is D: PMS is defined as recurrent, moderate psychological and physical symptoms that occur during the luteal phase of menses and resolve with menstruation. It affects 20% to 32% of premenopausal women. Women with premenstrual dysphoric disorder (PMDD) experience affective or somatic symptoms that cause severe dysfunction in social or occupational realms. The disorder affects 3% to 8% of premenopausal women. Proposed etiologies include increased sensitivity to normal cycling levels of estrogen and progesterone, increased aldosterone and plasma renin activity, and neurotransmitter abnormalities, particularly serotonin.

The *Daily Record of Severity of Problems* is one tool with which women may self-report the presence and severity of premenstrual symptoms that correlate with the criteria for PMDD. Symptom relief is the goal for treatment of PMS and PMDD.

Serotonergic antidepressants (such as citalopram, escitalopram, fluoxetine, sertraline, and venlafaxine) are first-line pharmacologic therapy for PMDD and can be used daily, with consideration for an increased dose during the luteal phase. There is some evidence to support the use of chasteberry, calcium, vitamin D, and vitamin B_6 supplementation, and insufficient evidence to support cognitive behavior therapy or other oral supplements such as *Ginkgo biloba*, saffron, St. John's wort, soy, or vitamin E. Although some women may benefit from a decreased intake of caffeine, salt, and refined sugar, there is no evidence to support effectiveness in treating premenstrual disorders.

Additional Reading: Premenstrual syndrome and premenstrual dysphoric disorder. *Am Fam Physician*. 2016;94(3):236-240.

Serotonergic antidepressants (such as citalopram, escitalopram, fluoxetine, sertraline, and venlafaxine) are first-line pharmacologic therapy for PMDD and can be used daily, with consideration for an increased dose during the luteal phase.

50. A 22-year-old woman is diagnosed with primary syphilis. She has no allergies and is otherwise healthy. The drug of choice is which one of the following?

A) Oral azithromycin
B) Oral ciprofloxacin
C) Oral penicillin
D) Intramuscular ceftriaxone
E) Intramuscular penicillin G

The answer is E: Syphilis is a systemic disease caused by the sexual transmission of *T pallidum*. It can occur as primary, secondary, tertiary disease, or latent. Primary disease presents with one or more painless ulcers, or chancres, at the inoculation site. Secondary disease manifestations include rash and adenopathy. Cardiac, neurologic, ophthalmic, auditory, or gummatous lesions characterize tertiary infections. Latent disease may be detected by serologic testing, without the presence of signs and symptoms. Early latent disease is defined as disease acquired within the preceding year. All other cases of latent syphilis are considered late latent disease or disease of unknown duration.

Penicillin G, administered parenterally, is the preferred drug for treating all stages of syphilis. The preparation used (ie, benzathine, aqueous procaine, or aqueous crystalline), the dosage, and the length of treatment depend on the stage and clinical manifestations of the disease. For primary, secondary, and early latent syphilis, benzathine penicillin G 2.4 million units intramuscularly in a single dose is the treatment of choice.

Selection of the appropriate penicillin preparation is important because *T pallidum* can reside in sequestered sites (eg, the central nervous system and aqueous humor) that are poorly accessed by some forms of penicillin. Combinations of benzathine penicillin, procaine penicillin, and oral penicillin preparations are not considered appropriate for the treatment of syphilis. Pregnant patients with syphilis who are allergic to penicillin should be desensitized and treated with penicillin as well. Alternatives to penicillin G in nonpregnant patients with a penicillin allergy include doxycycline, tetracycline, and ceftriaxone (for neurosyphilis).

Additional Reading: Syphilis - STD information from CDC.

51. Vulvar cancer is relatively uncommon but must be considered in older women who present with vaginal complaints. The most frequently reported symptom in women with vulvar cancer is which one of the following?

A) Bleeding
B) Dyspareunia
C) Itching
D) Vaginal dryness
E) Vaginal discharge

The answer is A: The most frequently reported symptom of vulvar cancer is vaginal bleeding. Other common presenting symptoms include vulvar itching, discharge, dysuria, and pain. The most common presenting sign of vulvar cancer is a vulvar lump or mass. Rarely, patients present with a large, fungating mass. Any suspicious lesions should be biopsied. Vulvar cancer is most commonly diagnosed in older women. Risks include exposure to human papilloma virus and smoking. An early diagnosis reduces the likelihood that extensive treatment will be needed.

Additional Reading: Vulvar malignancy. In: Domino F, ed. *The 5-Minute Clinical Consult*. Wolters Kluwer; 2022.

52. A 69-year-old woman presents with severe vulvar itching of several months' duration and recently she has been unable to have intercourse due to discomfort. On examination, the vulvar skin appears thin and whitened, with attenuation of the labia minora and narrowing of the introitus. A vulvar punch biopsy shows lichen sclerosus. Appropriate treatment at this point includes which one of the following?

A) 1% hydrocortisone cream
B) High-potency corticosteroid ointment
C) Oral estrogen replacement therapy
D) Testosterone cream
E) Topical estrogen cream

The answer is B: Lichen sclerosus is a type of vulvar nonneoplastic epithelial disorder that is characterized by intense vulvar itching and can affect women of all ages; however, it manifests most commonly in postmenopausal women. Initially, the skin may appear white, thickened, and excoriated, with edema and resorption of the labia minora. As the disease progresses, the skin loses pigmentation and becomes very thin and wrinkled, classically referred to as a "cigarette paper" appearance. With further progression, anatomic features may become severely distorted as the clitoris becomes buried under the clitoral hood, the labia minora disappear, and the introitus narrows. This architectural distortion can be partly responsible for dyspareunia and dysuria.

Definitive diagnosis of lichen sclerosus depends on the histology of biopsied tissue. Moreover, it is important to identify and biopsy any thickened areas of epithelium in patients with lichen sclerosus because such acanthotic epidermal areas can be suggestive of squamous cell hyperplasia. Patients with lichen sclerosus—especially those with squamous cell hyperplasia—have an increased risk of vulvar malignancy and should be monitored accordingly. The increased risk of developing squamous cell carcinoma is approximately 5% in patients with lichen sclerosus.

Lichen sclerosus is treated with potent topical steroids to alleviate symptoms, prevent architectural damage, and reverse histologic changes. The recommended regimen for lichen sclerosus begins with a high-potency corticosteroid (eg, clobetasol propionate 0.05% ointment) used daily until all active lesions have resolved (usually in 2-3 months), then tapered to once or twice per week. Clobetasol is more effective than testosterone, and 2% testosterone is no more effective than petrolatum ointment.

Additional Reading: Common benign chronic vulvar disorders. *Am Fam Physician*. 2020;102(9):550-557.

53. You are caring for a 51-year-old woman who was treated for ovarian cancer with an oophorectomy 3 months ago. Which one of the following tumor markers can be used to follow the effectiveness of ovarian cancer treatment?

A) α-Fetoprotein
B) β-Human chorionic gonadotropin
C) Carcinoembryonic antigen
D) Cancer antigen (CA) 125
E) None of the above

The answer is D: Ovarian carcinoma usually affects women in their 50s. It is the fifth most common cancer that affects women, and approximately 25,000 new cases are diagnosed yearly in the United States. Because of the difficulty in diagnosis, most cases have metastasized outside the pelvis at the time of diagnosis; therefore, prognosis is usually poor. The blood test CA 125 can be used to follow up patients for recurrence of tumor after surgery or the response to chemotherapy but is not a suitable screening test.

Risk factors for ovarian cancer include a positive family history, *BRCA1* gene mutation, white race, high-fat diet, asbestos or talc exposure, and low or nulliparity. The use of oral contraceptives may be protective. Any ovarian mass in any woman greater than 5 cm deserves careful follow-up. Postmenopausal women usually have atrophic ovaries that are not palpable; thus, any palpable ovary in a postmenopausal woman deserves further investigation. The types of tumors are divided histologically into those that arise from the ovarian epithelium:

- Serous cystadenocarcinomas (most common)
- Clear cell carcinomas
- Mucinous cystadenocarcinomas
- Endometrioid tumors
- Celioblastomas (Brenner tumors)

In addition, tumors arise from germ cells and stroma, such as the following:

- Sertoli-Leydig cell tumors
- Malignant teratomas
- Dysgerminomas
- Granulosa-theca cell tumors

Patients may report lower abdominal fullness or discomfort, gastrointestinal complaints, abnormal vaginal bleeding, or pelvic pain. Diagnosis is usually aided with ultrasonography or computed tomographic examination. Treatment of ovarian carcinoma depends on the staging and cell type but involves surgical excision and, in some cases, chemotherapy or radiation. Metastasis is usually to lung or bone.

> **Additional Reading:** Serum biomarkers for evaluation of an adnexal mass for epithelial carcinoma of the ovary, fallopian tube, or peritoneum. In: *UpToDate*. 2022.

54. A 61-year-old woman is noted to have fullness in her right adnexa on a routine pelvic examination. A follow-up ultrasonography reveals a 2.5-cm unilocular ovarian cyst and cancer antigen (CA) 125 level is in the normal range. Appropriate management at this time would be which one of the following?

A) Order a cone radiation ablation.
B) Periodically repeat the ultrasonography and CA 125 levels.
C) Refer for laparoscopic surgical removal.
D) Refer for a hysteroscopic biopsy.

The answer is B: In postmenopausal women, most ovarian cysts <5 cm in diameter are benign and can be managed safely by regular monitoring of cyst size and serum CA 125 level.

> **Additional Reading:** *Serum biomarkers for evaluation of an adnexal mass for epithelial carcinoma of the ovary, fallopian tube, or peritoneum*. In: *UpToDate*. 2022.

55. A young mother is being seen for a postpartum visit and is worried about her stretch marks. Which one of the following statements about stretch marks is true?

A) Stretch marks rarely fade after pregnancy.
B) Stretch marks usually respond to topical corticosteroids.
C) Stretch marks are secondary to excessive weight gain (>40 lb) during pregnancy.
D) Stretch marks are the result of excessive corticosteroids produced during pregnancy.
E) None of the above.

The answer is D: Stretch marks, also called striae distensae or gravidarum, are abnormal skin findings that are noted with varying degree during pregnancy. They affect up to 50% of pregnant women. They can occur in different areas but are usually found associated with the abdomen, breast, or hips. The cause of stretch marks was once believed to be excessive stretching of the skin. Today, it is believed that the development of stretch marks is likely multifactorial and a result of excessive corticosteroids produced endogenously during pregnancy, combined with the body changes that occur with pregnancy. Although stretching of the skin may occur during excessive weight gain, excessive weight gain itself is not the reason for stria development. Unfortunately, there is no effective treatment for stretch marks. They usually fade after pregnancy and are barely noticeable.

> **Additional Reading:** Common skin conditions during pregnancy. *Am Fam Physician*. 2007;75(2):211-218.

56. Which one of the following conditions is considered an independent risk factor for the development of vulvar cancer?

A) Chlamydial infection
B) Diabetes mellitus
C) Human papilloma virus (HPV) infection
D) Hypertension
E) Obesity

The answer is C: Vulvar intraepithelial neoplasia is a premalignant finding and is associated with HPV infection (subtypes 16 and 18). Hypertension, diabetes mellitus, and obesity have been found to coexist in up to 25% of patients, although they are not considered independent risk factors.

> **Additional Reading:** Vulvar malignancy. In: Domino F, ed. *The 5-Minute Clinical Consult*. Wolters Kluwer; 2022.

57. Human papilloma virus (HPV) is associated with the development of cervical and other anogenital cancers. Which one of the following HPV subtypes is associated with the development of these cancers?

A) Types 7 and 9
B) Types 16 and 18
C) Types 24 and 28
D) Types 33 and 40
E) Types 43 and 54

The answer is B: A preponderance of evidence suggests a causal link between HPV infection and cervical neoplasia. Low-risk HPV subtypes 6 and 11 cause the majority of genital warts. Virtually, all cervical cancers are caused by HPV, with subtypes 16 and 18 responsible for about 70% of all cases. HPV 16 is responsible for approximately 85% of anal cancers, and HPV types 16 and 18 have been found to cause close to half of vulvar, vaginal, and penile cancers.

A quadrivalent recombinant HPV vaccine (Gardasil) is offered to women between the ages of 10 and 25 years and protects against HPV subtypes 6, 11, 16, and 18.

> **Additional Reading:** Human papillomavirus: screening, testing, and prevention. *Am Fam Physician*. 2021;104(2):152-159.

58. Female children of women who are exposed to diethylstilbestrol during their pregnancy are at increased risk for which of the following?

A) Congenital limb defects
B) Developmental disabilities
C) Ovarian carcinoma
D) Precocious puberty
E) Vaginal clear cell carcinoma

The answer is E: Diethylstilbestrol was widely used from the 1940s to the early 1970s to help prevent spontaneous abortion in diabetic pregnant women. Approximately 2 to 3 million fetuses were exposed to the medication. Unfortunately, later studies showed that girls who were born to mothers who took the medication while they were pregnant were at increased risk of developing clear cell carcinoma of the vagina as well as cervical and vaginal intraepithelial neoplasia. These patients are also at risk for vaginal adenosis (the most common anomaly associated with exposure), septated vagina, cervical collar, hypoplasia of the cervix, and uterine abnormalities. In addition to lower genital tract anomalies, upper genital tract anomalies occur in 50% of patients. The most common is a T-shaped uterus and small uterine cavity.

Daughters of women who took this drug may have difficulty in conceiving, higher rates of ectopic pregnancy, spontaneous abortion, and premature births as well as a slightly increased risk for breast cancer. All exposed women are encouraged to undergo thorough vaginal examinations, including colposcopy, starting at menarche or age 14, whichever comes first. Male children of women who took the medication may show testicular or epididymal abnormalities and low sperm counts.

Additional Reading: Diethylstilbestrol exposure. *Am Fam Physician*. 2004;69(10):2395-2400.

59. A 45-year-old woman presents with concern that her hair is thinning, and she is finding more hair in her comb after brushing. Which one of the following is the most common cause of hair loss in women?

A) Alopecia areata
B) Androgenetic alopecia
C) Cicatricial alopecia
D) Telogen effluvium
E) Traumatic alopecia

The answer is B: Androgenetic alopecia is the most common cause of hair loss in women and men. In men, this condition is also known as male pattern baldness, with hair loss beginning above both temples with the hairline receding to form a characteristic "M" pattern. Hair also thins at the crown (near the top of the head), often progressing to partial or complete baldness. In women, androgenetic alopecia rarely leads to total baldness, the hair becomes thinner over the head, and the hairline does not recede. Alopecia areata results in smooth hairless patches, which often spontaneously resolve. Cicatricial alopecia causes permanent hair loss from destruction of the hair follicles by inflammatory or autoimmune diseases. Telogen effluvium is a sudden loss of hair, which usually regrows once the precipitating cause is addressed. Traumatic alopecia results from a variety of local mechanical insults.

Additional Reading: Hair loss: common causes and treatment. *Am Fam Physician*. 2017;96(6):371-378.

CHAPTER 4

Mental Health/ Community Health

The questions in this chapter have been grouped in sections to help with your review and allow you to focus and read about a particular condition in one setting. The sections include (1) Substance Use Disorders, (2) Pediatric Behavioral Health, (3) Population Health, and (4) Mental Health.

Section I. Substance Use Disorders

Each of the following questions or incomplete statements is followed by suggested answers or completions. Select the ONE BEST ANSWER in each case.

1. Understanding factors related to beginning to smoke is useful in designing prevention programs. Risk factors for smoking initiation include all of the following situations except which one?

A) Availability of flavored tobacco products
B) Identifying as a cisgender, heterosexual male
C) Presence of a smoker in the family
D) Poor academic performance
E) Single parent at home

The answer is B: Risk factors for smoking include exposure to secondhand smoke, presence of a smoker in the household, comorbid psychiatric disorders, strained relationship with parent and/or single parent at home, low level of expressed self-esteem and self-worth, poor academic performance, increased adolescent perception of parental approval of smoking, affiliation with smoking peers, and availability of cigarettes.

An additional risk factor includes sexual and gender minority adolescents who are more likely than their heterosexual and cisgender peers to smoke cigarettes.

Additional Reading: *Prevention of smoking and vaping initiation in children and adolescents*. In: *UpToDate*. 2022.

2. Smoking is associated with a wide range of diseases, including many types of cancer, chronic obstructive pulmonary disease, coronary heart disease, stroke, peripheral vascular disease, and peptic ulcer disease. In addition, smoking is associated with an increased risk of various women's health concerns, including all of the following conditions except which one?

A) Ectopic pregnancy
B) Infertility
C) Multiple gestations
D) Premature menopause
E) Spontaneous abortion

The answer is C: Smoking is associated with an increased risk of various women's health concerns, including infertility, spontaneous abortion, ectopic pregnancy, and premature menopause. Although a positive family history is a risk factor for multiple gestations, smoking is not.

Additional Reading: *Overview of smoking cessation management in adults*. In: *UpToDate*. 2022.

3. A number of medications are used to assist with smoking cessation. Which one of the following antidepressants has been shown to be beneficial?

A) Bupropion
B) Doxepin
C) Fluoxetine
D) Sertraline
E) Venlafaxine

The answer is A: Bupropion (also marketed as Wellbutrin) has been available for use as an antidepressant in the United States since 1989 and is thought to act by enhancing central nervous system noradrenergic and dopaminergic function. Bupropion can lower the seizure threshold. A sustained-release formulation of the drug (Zyban) is licensed as an aid to smoking cessation. Varenicline (Chantix) has also shown to be beneficial in smoking cessation.

Additional Reading: Promoting smoking cessation. *Am Fam Physician*. 2012;85(6):591-598.

4. The U.S. Preventive Services Task Force recommends that physicians should address smoking cessation with all patients who use tobacco. The 5 As framework has been developed to guide counseling efforts. The "5 As" include all of the following except which one?

A) Ask
B) Advise
C) Assess
D) Argue
E) Assist

The answer is D: Although intensive group and individual psychologic counseling are effective in helping smokers achieve abstinence, many smokers are not interested in participating in such interventions. The 5 As framework (ask, advise, assess, assist, and arrange) has been developed to assist physicians to incorporate smoking cessation counseling into a patient encounter.

Additional Reading: Interventions for tobacco smoking cessation in adults, including pregnant persons: recommendation statement. *Am Fam Physician*. 2021;103(12).

5. Xander, a 19-year-old queer-identifying youth, presents to your office for their routine physical examination. They admit to using smoking flavored e-cigarettes and want to use them as a way to stop smoking regular cigarettes. What would be the best response to this situation?

A) Flavored e-cigarettes are not likely to become addictive.
B) Behavioral support and quit dates are not shown to be effective when trying to quit smoking.
C) Explain that although e-cigarettes are likely less harmful than cigarettes, they are not US Food and Drug Administration–approved cessation devices and safety in their use is largely unknown.
D) The only chemical to worry about in e-cigarettes is the highly addictive nicotine.

Additional Reading: Electronic cigarettes: common questions and answers. *Am Fam Physician*. 2019;100(4) 227-235.

6. Unfortunately, patients with severe alcohol use disorders tend to relapse despite successful cessation efforts. Which one of the following statements is *false* with regard to the risk of relapse?

A) Higher level of alcohol consumption predicts higher likelihood of later relapse.
B) Younger men are more likely to relapse than older men after recovery.
C) Attempts at controlled drinking recovery techniques result in more relapses than abstinence techniques.
D) There is no evidence supporting the effectiveness of Alcoholics Anonymous (AA) in preventing relapse.
E) Women are more likely to relapse than men.

The answer is E: Alcohol dependence is a chronic illness; therefore, with all treatment approaches, relapse is fairly common. Factors associated with higher rates of relapse include male sex, younger age, fewer social supports, greater alcohol consumption before treatment, and poor compliance with drug therapy. Physicians, who continue to be supportive, encourage counseling, and treat comorbid anxiety or depression, may help reduce the incidence of relapse.

Abstinence represents the most stable form of remission for most recovering alcoholics. However, although abstinence is the best outcome, not every individual achieves this end, and controlled drinking for some individuals is an achievable aim, which reduces risk to patients. Common interventions for alcohol-related disorders include motivational enhancement therapy, psychotherapy, cognitive behavior techniques, and referral to 12-step recovery programs, such as AA and Narcotics Anonymous.

AA is the best-known peer support program for substance use disorders. It is an international organization of recovering alcoholics, which offers emotional support and a model of abstinence for people recovering from alcohol dependence using a 12-step approach. Abstinence is encouraged on a "one day at a time" basis. Members attend meetings (either open to all or restricted to participants with alcoholism) in which experiences related to drinking and recovery are shared, and the steps in the Twelve Steps to Recovery are discussed.

The Twelve Steps to Recovery program entails acknowledgment that alcohol has led to loss of control and that recovery is a spiritual journey through belief in a higher power, personal exploration, and acceptance. Despite the long history and popularity of AA, no experimental studies unequivocally demonstrated the effectiveness of AA or 12-step programs for reducing alcohol dependence or problems.

Additional Reading: Screening and behavioral counseling interventions in primary care to reduce alcohol misuse. *Am Fam Physician*. 2014;89(12):971-972.

6. Club drugs are substances commonly used at nightclubs, music festivals, raves, and dance parties to enhance social intimacy and sensory stimulation. Many are associated with adverse health effects. Which one of the following drugs is linked with hyperthermia and can be life threatening?

A) 3,4-Methylenedioxymethamphetamine (MDMA)
B) Cocaine
C) Flunitrazepam (Rohypnol)
D) γ-Hydroxybutyrate (GHB)
E) Ketamine (Ketalar)

The answer is A: The most widely used club drugs are MDMA (also known as ecstasy), GHB, flunitrazepam, and ketamine. These drugs are popular because they are inexpensive and are conveniently dispensed as small pills, powders, or liquids. Club drugs usually are taken orally and may be taken in combination with each other, with alcohol, or with other drugs.

Adverse effects of MDMA ingestion result from sympathetic overload and include tachycardia, mydriasis, diaphoresis, tremor, hypertension, arrhythmias, parkinsonism, esophoria (tendency for eyes to turn inward), and urinary retention. However, the most dangerous potential outcome of MDMA ingestion is hyperthermia and the associated "serotonin syndrome." Serotonin syndrome is manifested by grossly elevated core body temperature, rigidity, myoclonus, and autonomic instability; it can result in end-organ damage, rhabdomyolysis and acute renal failure, hepatic failure, adult respiratory distress syndrome, and coagulopathy.

GHB produces euphoria, progressing with higher doses to dizziness, hypersalivation, hypotonia, and amnesia. Overdose may result in Cheyne-Stokes respirations, seizures, coma, and death. Coma may be interrupted by agitation, with flailing activity described as similar to a drowning swimmer fighting for air. Bradycardia and hypothermia are present in about one-third of patients admitted to a hospital for using GHB and appear to be correlated with a decreased level of consciousness. The long-term use of GHB may produce dependence and a withdrawal syndrome that includes anxiety, insomnia, tremor, and in severe cases, treatment-resistant psychoses.

In the United States, imported Rohypnol came to prominence in the 1990s as an inexpensive recreational sedative and is known as the "date rape" drug. Effects of Rohypnol occur about 30 minutes after ingestion, peak at 2 hours, and may last up to 8 to 12 hours. The effects are much greater with the concurrent ingestion of alcohol or other sedating drugs. Some users experience hypotension, dizziness, confusion, visual disturbances, urinary retention, or aggressive behavior.

Ketamine is difficult to develop; therefore, most of the illegal supply is obtained from human and veterinary anesthesia products. Ketamine is distributed in a liquid form that can be ingested or injected. In clubs, it is usually smoked in a powder mixture of marijuana or tobacco, or is taken intranasally. A typical method uses a nasal inhaler, called a "bullet" or "bumper"; an inhalation is called a "bump." Ketamine is often taken in "trail mixes" of methamphetamine, cocaine, sildenafil citrate (Viagra), or heroin.

Effects of ketamine ingestion appear rapidly and last about 30 to 45 minutes, with sensations of floating outside the body, visual hallucinations, and a dreamlike state. Along with these "desired" effects, users also commonly experience confusion, anterograde amnesia, and delirium. They also may experience tachycardia, palpitations, hypertension, and respiratory depression with apnea. "Flashbacks" or visual disturbances can be experienced days or weeks after ingestion. Some long-term users become addicted and exhibit severe withdrawal symptoms that require detoxification.

Additional Reading: Club drugs: MDMA, gamma-hydroxybutyrate (GHB), rohypnol, and ketamine. *Am Fam Physician*. 2004;69:2619-2627.

7. Diagnosis of inhalant abuse is difficult and relies almost entirely on a thorough history and a high index of suspicion. Which one of the following statements is true regarding inhalant abuse?

A) A comprehensive drug screen can help identify the inhalant used.
B) Inhalant use is not addictive.
C) Hepatic damage is not associated with inhalant abuse because of the lack of enterohepatic circulation of the substance.
D) Reversing agents can assist with recovery from an inhalant toxicity.
E) Twenty percent of children in middle school and high school have experimented with inhalants.

The answer is E: Inhalant abuse is prevalent in adolescents. Studies show that roughly 20% of children in middle school and high school have experimented with inhalants. The method of delivery is inhalation of a solvent from its container, a soaked rag, or a bag. Solvents include household cleaning agents or propellants, paint thinners, glue, and lighter fluid.

Inhalant abuse typically can cause a euphoric feeling and can become addictive. Acute effects include sudden sniffing death syndrome, asphyxia, and serious injuries (eg, falls, burns, and frostbite). The long-term inhalant abuse can cause cardiac, renal, hepatic, and neurologic damage. Inhalant abuse during pregnancy can lead to fetal abnormalities.

No specific laboratory tests confirm solvent inhalation. There are no reversal agents for inhalant intoxication.

Additional Reading: Inhalant abuse. *Pediatrics*. 2007;119(5).

8. Chronic alcohol abuse is associated with which one of the following laboratory abnormalities?

A) An alanine aminotransferase (ALT)/aspartate aminotransferase (AST) ratio of 2:1
B) Hyperuricemia
C) Decreased mean corpuscular volume
D) Decreased γ-glutamyl transferase
E) Decreased triglycerides

The answer is B: Alcohol use disorder is a problematic pattern of alcohol use leading to clinically significant impairment or distress. Complications include gastritis, peptic ulcer disease, cirrhosis, sexual dysfunction, nutritional deficiencies, neuropathy, and pancreatitis. Laboratory findings may include mild elevations of liver function tests. Most causes of liver cell injury are associated with an AST level that is lower than the ALT level. However, an AST/ALT ratio of 2:1 or greater is suggestive of alcoholic liver disease, particularly in the setting of an elevated γ-glutamyl transferase.

Hypertriglyceridemia, hyperuricemia, and elevations in γ-glutamyl transferase are also seen. Hyperuricemia can lead to gout flares; therefore, patients with gout should be counseled about alcohol intake. A macrocytosis with an elevated mean corpuscular volume is usually the result of folate deficiency.

Treatment has historically been aimed at abstinence of alcohol and participation in rehabilitation programs such as Alcoholics Anonymous. However, harm reduction models of treatment to reduce the negative consequences of alcohol use and focus on safety are more common and just as relevant in primary care settings. Close monitoring, including hospitalization, may be necessary if withdrawal symptoms are anticipated.

Additional Reading: Alcohol abuse and dependence. In: Domino F, ed. *The 5-Minute Clinical Consult*. Wolters Kluwer; 2022.

> **Although most causes of liver cell injury are associated with an ALT level higher than the AST level, an AST/ALT ratio of 2:1 or greater is suggestive of alcoholic liver disease, particularly in the setting of an elevated γ-glutamyl transferase level.**

9. A patient with a long history of drinking has decided to stop on his own, and his wife calls because he appears ill and you are concerned that he is having withdrawal symptoms. Which one of the following medications is preferred in the treatment of alcohol withdrawal syndrome?

A) Carbamazepine
B) Haloperidol
C) Lorazepam
D) Phenytoin
E) Phenobarbital

The answer is C: Pharmacologic treatment of alcohol withdrawal syndrome involves the use of medications that are cross-tolerant with alcohol. Benzodiazepines have been shown to be safe and effective, particularly for preventing or treating seizures and delirium, and are the preferred agents for treating the symptoms of alcohol withdrawal syndrome.

Additional Reading: Outpatient management of alcohol withdrawal syndrome. *Am Fam Physician*. 2013;88(9):589-595.

10. Ethanol (ethyl alcohol) is the principal type of alcohol found in alcoholic beverages. Ethanol acts through effects on which one of the following neurotransmitters?

A) Acetylcholine
B) Dopamine
C) γ-Aminobutyric acid (GABA)
D) Norepinephrine
E) None of the above

The answer is C: Alcohol enhances the effect of GABA on GABA-A neuroreceptors, resulting in decreased overall brain excitability. Long-term exposure to alcohol results in a compensatory decrease of GABA-A neuroreceptor response to GABA, evidenced by increasing tolerance of the effects of alcohol.

Additional Reading: Medications for alcohol use disorder. *Am Fam Physician*. 2016;93(6):457-465.

11. A 53-year-old professor with a history of alcohol use disorder and associated liver disease presents to your office and is asking for medication to help stop drinking. To prevent alcohol withdrawal, you select which of the following medications?

A) Buspirone
B) Clonazepam
C) Diazepam
D) Flurazepam
E) Lorazepam

The answer is E: An evidence-based guideline from the American Society of Addiction Medicine recommends benzodiazepines as a first-line agent for the treatment of alcohol withdrawal. The guideline notes that although agents with a longer duration of action may provide fewer breakthrough symptoms, those with a shorter duration of action, such as lorazepam, may be preferred when there is concern about prolonged sedation (eg, in patients with significant comorbidities or liver disease).

Additional Reading: Medications for alcohol use disorder. *Am Fam Physician*. 2016;93(6):457-465.

12. You have placed a middle-aged man on disulfiram (Antabuse) to help with his attempt to stop drinking alcohol abuse. Which one of the following laboratory test results should be monitored while he is being treated with this medication?

A) Alkaline phosphatase
B) Alanine aminotransferase (ALT)
C) Ammonia level
D) Amylase
E) Creatinine

The answer is B: Disulfiram, acamprosate (Campral), and naltrexone (Revia) are approved for the treatment of alcohol dependence. Although disulfiram is reported to be effective as an aversive drug, placebo-controlled clinical trials have been inconclusive. Disulfiram inhibits the metabolism of anticoagulant drugs, phenytoin, and isoniazid. It should be used cautiously in patients with liver disease and is contraindicated during pregnancy and in patients with ischemic heart disease. Disulfiram can cause hepatitis, and therefore monitoring of liver function studies (ALT) is essential.

Acamprosate works by its effect on the GABA system. Side effects include diarrhea, insomnia, anxiety, depression, pruritus, and dizziness. The other drug approved for use in the treatment of alcohol dependence is the opioid antagonist naltrexone. Naltrexone is believed to reduce consumption of alcohol and increase abstinence by reducing the craving for alcohol. The rate of relapse is highest within the first 90 days of abstinence, and it is during this time that naltrexone may be beneficial. Daily dosages may range from 25 to 100 mg. Side effects include nausea, headache, anxiety, and sedation. Naltrexone can be hepatotoxic at higher dosages and should be used with caution in patients with chronic liver disease.

Selective serotonin reuptake inhibitors (SSRIs), including fluoxetine and sertraline, have been found to decrease alcohol intake in heavy drinkers without a history of depression. However, in some trials, SSRIs were found to be no more effective than a placebo. Any drug therapy should be combined with psychotherapy or group therapy to help address the social and psychologic aspects of alcohol dependence.

Additional Reading: Outpatient management of alcohol withdrawal syndrome. *Am Fam Physician*. 2013;88(9):589-595.

13. A 23-year-old woman is brought to the emergency department after suffering a seizure. She is febrile, tachycardic, and hypertensive. Physical examination reveals her to be in a postictal state and she has a perforated nasal septum. Electrocardiogram (ECG) findings suggest an acute myocardial infarction (MI). Her friends report that she has been using cocaine. Which of the following drugs is indicated?

A) Dexfenfluramine
B) Diazepam
C) Flumazenil
D) Propranolol
E) Phenytoin

The answer is B: Cocaine is a strong narcotic stimulant that is often abused. Its mechanism of action involves the release of norepinephrine and the blockage of its reuptake. Effects of cocaine begin within 3 to 5 minutes (within 8-10 seconds with smoking "crack" cocaine), and peak effects occur at 10 to 20 minutes. The effects rarely last more than 1 hour. Cocaine toxicity is characterized by seizures, hyperpyrexia, tachycardia, mental status changes including paranoid behavior, hypertension, stroke, MI, and rhabdomyolysis. Nasal septum perforation may also occur.

In most cases, treatment involves the use of diazepam to treat agitation, hypertension, and tachycardia. Nitroprusside or calcium channel blockers can be used for hypertensive crisis. β-Blockers should be avoided given the risk of coronary vasoconstriction and paradoxical hypertension. Other complications, such as cerebrovascular accidents, rhabdomyolysis, and MIs, should be managed in a conventional manner. Fortunately, cocaine has a short half-life and symptoms are usually self-limited. Individuals who use cocaine may become rapidly addicted.

Additional Reading: Cocaine poisoning, emergency medicine. In: Domino F, ed. *The 5-Minute Clinical Consult*. Wolters Kluwer; 2022.

14. A 51-year-old trans woman with alcohol use disorder presents reporting that she is not feeling well since she stopped drinking 2 days ago. She also feels nauseated and anxious. On examination you note that she is diaphoretic, tachycardic, and hypertensive. The most appropriate management at this time is which one of the following approaches?

A) Administer disulfiram and diazepam and follow up with the patient in 1 week.
B) Hospitalize the patient, administer diazepam, and closely observe.
C) Prescribe diazepam and refer the patient to a drug treatment program.
D) Reassure the patient, compliment her decision to stop drinking, and explain that her symptoms are to be expected.
E) Refer the patient to psychiatry.

The answer is B: Symptoms of alcohol withdrawal usually occur 6 to 48 hours after the last alcoholic drink. These symptoms include sweating, anxiety, tremor, weakness, gastrointestinal (GI) discomfort, hypertension, tachycardia, fever, and hyperreflexia. Other symptoms include hallucinations and, in severe cases, delirium tremens that are characterized by disorientation with hallucinations, drenching sweats, severe tremors, and electrolyte disturbances that can lead to seizures.

Treatment involves hospitalization and close observation when the patient has significant symptoms as in this case. Antianxiety medications, including chlordiazepoxide, lorazepam, diazepam, midazolam, and oxazepam, are used for treatment and are slowly tapered to prevent withdrawal-related symptoms. Oral multivitamin supplementation with thiamine, folate, and pyridoxine is also recommended.

Additional Reading: Outpatient management of alcohol withdrawal syndrome. *Am Fam Physician*. 2013;88(9):589-595.

15. A 37-year-old man is hoping to quit smoking on his birthday next week and is asking if a medication will help. You inform him that the most effective therapy for tobacco cessation is which one of the following?

A) Bupropion
B) Clonidine
C) Nicotine transdermal patch
D) Nicotine polacrilex gum
E) Varenicline

The answer is E: Tobacco dependence is a chronic disease that often requires pharmacologic therapy, but counseling improves the effectiveness of any treatment for this indication. The greater the number of office visits and the longer the counseling time, the higher the smoking cessation rates.

The most effective drugs available for treatment of tobacco dependence are bupropion (Zyban and others) and varenicline (Chantix). Varenicline appears to be the most effective single drug for treatment of tobacco dependence, but bupropion has been available much longer and is also well tolerated.

Bupropion is a dopamine-norepinephrine reuptake inhibitor used mainly for treatment of depression, but it also has some nicotine receptor–blocking activity. A partial agonist that binds selectively to $\alpha4/\beta2$ nicotinic acetylcholine receptors stimulates receptor-mediated activity, relieving cravings and withdrawal symptoms during abstinence.

Varenicline binds to the $\alpha4/\beta2$ receptor with greater affinity than does nicotine and it also acts as an antagonist to nicotine delivery from active cigarette use, thus reducing the reward of smoking. Although varenicline is more effective, bupropion offers the benefit of mitigating the weight gain that often accompanies smoking cessation.

All nicotine replacement therapies (NRTs) deliver nicotine, which acts as an agonist at the nicotinic acetylcholine receptor, to the central nervous system in a lower dose and at a substantially slower rate than tobacco cigarettes. All of these products roughly double smoking cessation rates. Nicotine is subject to first-pass metabolism, limiting the effectiveness of oral pill formulations. Nicotine gum, lozenges, and patches are available without a prescription; these products appear to be as effective as those that require a prescription (the oral inhaler and nasal spray).

All of the NRTs appear to be about equally effective, but results may be better with the combination of a patch and a rapid-onset nicotine medication. NRTs should be started 1 to 4 weeks before the target quit date. The optimum duration of treatment is not clear, 3 to 6 months is probably the minimum, and some patients may need even longer treatment to remain abstinent.

All patients who smoke should be encouraged to stop. The physician should always ask about smoking; if the patient does smoke, there should be an attempt by the physician to motivate the patient to stop. Setting a stop date may be helpful, and follow-up is necessary to provide support and reinforce the patient's commitment to stop.

Additional Reading: Promoting smoking cessation. *Am Fam Physician*. 2012;85(6):591-598.

16. A 22-year-old woman has been struggling with opioid dependence since she was in high school. She is asking about medication to help her avoid the use of opioids. The drug of choice for addressing this condition is which one of the following?

A) Bupropion
B) Diazepam
C) Disulfiram
D) Methadone
E) Naloxone

The answer is D: Opioid dependence is a chronic, often relapsing, disorder that can be challenging to treat. Between 500,000 and 1,000,000 Americans are believed to be opioid dependent at any point in time. Opioid-related disorders are more prevalent in men than in women by a ratio of up to 4:1. Opioid dependency is often linked to a history of drug-related criminal activity, antisocial personality disorder, and coexisting mood disorders, especially depression.

Methadone and buprenorphine seem equally effective at stabilizing opioid use. Methadone has the longest track record and is effective in reducing illicit narcotic use, retaining patients in treatment, and decreasing illegal drug use. Ongoing methadone maintenance decreases the risk of contracting and transmitting human immunodeficiency virus (HIV), hepatitis B virus, and hepatitis B virus and is considered a cost-effective intervention.

Long-term maintenance is more successful in averting relapse than shorter-term treatment. The goals of early treatment are to decrease withdrawal symptoms, diminish opioid craving, and arrive at a tolerance threshold, while preventing euphoria and sedation from overmedication. Detoxification is indicated when a patient demonstrates consistent, long-term abstinence and possesses adequate supportive resources (eg, productive use of time and a stable home life). Patient acceptance of community resources for opiate addicts such as Narcotics Anonymous is a good prognostic sign.

Additional Reading: Opioid use disorder. *Am Fam Physician*. 2019;100(7):416-425.

17. The management of those taking chronic opioids for non–cancer-related pain can be challenging, and appropriate patient monitoring is recommended. Which of the following is recommended in the management of those taking chronic opioids?

A) Opioid contracts
B) Random pill counts
C) Urine drug screens
D) State-sponsored prescription monitoring records
E) All of the above

The answer is E: Physicians should explain the process of monitoring for those taking chronic opioids for non–cancer-related pain and should have the patient sign an opioid contract that outlines the process. Various methods should be used in the monitoring process on the basis of the level of risk associated with abuse. Methods include urine drug screens, random pill counts, and state-sponsored physician prescribing records that are available in some states.

Additional Reading: Weighing the risks and benefits of chronic opioid therapy. *Am Fam Physician*. 2016;93(12):982-990.

18. The following statements are true in regard to using buprenorphine as form medication for opioid use disorder except.

A) Behavioral treatment does not directly affect other substance use, and should be addressed in this context.
B) A medical setting is needed for induction.
C) Buprenorphine is prescribed as long as it continues to benefit the patient.
D) Buprenorphine should not be withheld from patients taking benzodiazepines.
E) Relapse indicates that the patient needs additional support and resources rather than cessation from buprenorphine treatment.

Additional Reading: Opioid use disorder: medical treatment options. *Am Fam Physician*. 2019;100(7):416-425.

Opioid use disorder should be treated as a chronic condition with team-based, patient-centered care. Similar to hypertension and type 2 diabetes, opioid use disorder has genetic, environmental, and behavioral causes; the disorder responds best to long-term treatment with medication supplemented by behavior therapies.

Section II. Pediatric Behavioral Health

Each of the following questions or incomplete statements is followed by suggested answers or completions. Select the ONE BEST ANSWER in each case.

1. An 18-year-old man is brought in by his parents because they note that his behaviors are changing. They have observed that he has an inflated self-esteem about his abilities, yet is distracted when asked to work on a project. Additionally, he seems to have lots of energy despite sleeping for only a few hours nightly. The most likely diagnosis for this presentation is which one of the following?

A) Antisocial personality
B) Borderline personality
C) Depression
D) Hypothymia
E) Mania

The answer is E: The diagnosis of mania consists of a distinct period of abnormally and persistently elevated, expansive or irritable mood and abnormally and persistently increased goal-directed activity or energy, lasting at least 1 week and present most of the day, nearly every day. During the period of mood disturbance and increased energy or activity, three or more of the following are present in sufficient degree and represent a noticeable change from usual behavior:

1. Inflated self-esteem or grandiosity
2. Decreased need for sleep (eg, feels rested after only 3 hours of sleep)
3. More talkative than usual or pressure to keep talking
4. Flight of ideas or subjective experience that thoughts are racing
5. Distractibility (ie, attention too easily drawn to unimportant or irrelevant external stimuli)
6. Increase in goal-directed activity (either socially, at work or school, or sexually) or psychomotor agitation
7. Excessive involvement in pleasurable activities that have a high potential for painful consequences (eg, engaging in unrestrained buying sprees, sexual indiscretions, and foolish business investments)

Additional Reading: American Psychiatric Association. *Diagnostic and Statistical Manual of Mental Disorders*. 5th ed. American Psychiatric Publishing; 2013.

2. A 19-year-old college student presents to her dentist. Her vital signs are normal. Her weight is within normal limits. On examination, extensive upper dental erosion is noted. Which one of the following is the most likely diagnosis?

A) Anorexia nervosa
B) Behcet disease
C) Bulimia nervosa
D) Crohn disease
E) Dental enamel dysplasia

The answer is C: The core features of bulimia nervosa are binge eating (ie, eating an amount of food that is definitely larger than most people would eat under similar circumstances), inappropriate compensatory behavior to prevent weight gain, and excessive concern about body weight and shape. The prototypic sequence of behavior in bulimia nervosa consists of caloric restriction, followed by binge eating, and then self-induced vomiting. Other manifestations of compensatory behaviors include excessive exercise and the misuse of diuretics, laxatives, or enemas.

Common physical signs in bulimia nervosa include hypotension, tachycardia, and dry skin. In addition, menstrual irregularities are seen in approximately one-third to one-half of female patients. Regular vomiting can cause dehydration, hypokalemia, hypochloremia, metabolic alkalosis, and dental enamel erosion (particularly the upper dentition; the lower dentition is protected by the tongue during vomiting), as well as hypertrophy of the parotid glands and "puffy" cheeks. Severe cases may also result in gastric dilation, esophagitis, electrolyte abnormalities, aspiration, or pancreatitis.

Although the cause of this disorder is unknown, genetic and neurochemical factors have been implicated. Bulimia nervosa is more common in women than men by a ratio of 3:1, and the median age of onset is 20 years. The condition usually becomes symptomatic between the ages of 13 and 20 years, and it has a chronic, sometimes episodic, course. Unlike anorexia nervosa, those affected with bulimia are usually within 15% of their appropriate weight.

Treatment involves psychotherapy with behavior modification and the use of antidepressants (selective serotonin reuptake inhibitors, especially fluoxetine). Many patients relapse and require long-term therapy.

Additional Reading: Initial evaluation, diagnosis, and treatment of anorexia nervosa and bulimia nervosa. *Am Fam Physician*. 2015;91(1):46-52.

3. Children who exhibit symptoms of school avoidance with nausea, vomiting, and abdominal pain are suffering from separation anxiety and may benefit from which one of the following treatments?

A) Antidepressant medication
B) Benzodiazepines
C) Methylphenidate
D) Mood stabilizers
E) Psychotherapy

The answer is E: Separation anxiety disorder affects children below the age of 18 years and consists of developmentally inappropriate and excessive anxiety concerning separation from home or a major attachment figure that lasts for at least 4 weeks. Periods of exacerbations and remissions are typical. These children (in many cases, school-aged children with school avoidance) often have no siblings and come from an extremely close family. Boys and girls are equally affected.

It is a normal developmental response for children to cry when their parents leave the room beginning at approximately 8 months of age and continuing up to 2 years of age. The response varies with each child. Many first-time parents overreact and fear that the child is emotionally harmed by the separation.

Reassuring the parents that this is a normal response is appropriate for treatment. However, occasionally, a child exhibits symptoms of nausea, vomiting, and abdominal pain, with separation from a major attachment figure, which signals an abnormal response. Psychotherapy (family therapy) may be necessary for these children. Medication is not recommended.

Additional Reading: Anxiety disorders in children and adolescents: epidemiology, pathogenesis, clinical manifestations, and course. In: *UpToDate*. 2022.

4. After anxiety and depression, which unfortunately has been on the rise during the COVID-19 pandemic, which of these problems rates highest among US teens as a top concern?

A) Bullying
B) Pressure to have sex
C) Pressure to drink alcohol
D) Pressure to do drugs
E) Racism

The answer is A: Childhood bullying has been viewed as an inevitable part of growing up. Survey data show that American youth and parents are concerned about bullying especially online and through social media.

Additional Reading: Childhood bullying: implications for physicians. *Am Fam Physician*. 2018;97(3):187-192.

5. An 18-year-old girl is brought to your office by her parents. They report that she has been having hallucinations over the past year and recently experienced an episode of psychotic behaviors that lasted for several days. She has been out of school for 3 years and has not been able to hold even a part-time job. Her mother reports that the girl often remains in her room. The most likely diagnosis to explain this situation is which one of the following conditions?

A) Agoraphobia
B) Major depression
C) Panic attacks
D) Schizophrenia
E) School avoidance

The answer is D: Schizophrenia is a common psychiatric disorder and there is often a family history for the disorder. Typically, patients are in the late teens or early 20s when the condition is identified. The definition describes a condition in which there is chronic impairment of functioning that involves disturbances of thinking, feeling, and behavior, with continuous signs of the symptoms for at least 6 months. Specific criteria involve two or more of the following and at least one of these must be positive symptoms (1, 2, or 3):

1. Delusions
2. Hallucinations
3. Disorganized speech
4. Grossly disorganized or catatonic behavior
5. Negative symptoms (diminished emotional expression or avolition)

Signs must be present for a significant portion of time during a 1-month period and must impair level of functioning. Often, patients experience social isolation, difficulties with social functioning or job requirements, peculiar behavior, impaired hygiene, abnormal thought processes, inappropriate affect, and lack of energy or interest.

Additional Reading: Schizophrenia. *Am Fam Physician*. 2022;106(4):388-396.

6. A 7-year-old boy is brought to your office. The parents report that the child has had problems in school for the past 6 months. His teacher reports lack of concentration and excessive fidgeting. The child typically interrupts others and often loses objects. After further assessment and a diagnosis of attention-deficit/hyperactivity disorder (ADHD), the most appropriate treatment is which one of the following?

A) Antidepressant medication
B) Disciplinary behavioral plan
C) Reassurance
D) Short-acting benzodiazepines
E) Stimulant medication

The answer is E: ADHD is a condition characterized by a persistent pattern of inattention and/or hyperactivity-impulsivity that interferes with functioning or development and is characterized by (1) a short attention span and/or (2) distractibility that persists for longer than 6 months.

Other symptoms include failure to attend to details, making careless mistakes, not listening when spoken to, inability to follow through on tasks, difficulty with organization, loses things often, forgetful in daily activities, fidgeting or squirming in one's seat, restlessness, inability to remain seated when required to do so, difficulty in awaiting one's turn, excessive talking, blurting out answers to questions before they are completed, interrupting others, and engaging in dangerous activities without consideration of the consequences.

Boys are more commonly affected, and the onset typically occurs before 7 years of age but must be present by the age of 12 years. Symptoms must occur in two or more settings. The clinical history is usually all that is needed to determine the diagnosis; however, psychologic and educational testing may help to support the diagnosis.

Treatment is often accomplished with stimulants, such as methylphenidate and dextroamphetamine, which have a paradoxical calming effect on young patients with ADHD. Atomoxetine (Strattera) is a selective norepinephrine reuptake inhibitor that is approved for use in children above age 6 years. Most children show improvement with medication; drug holidays (at least 2 wk/y) are important during long-term therapy to see if further medication is necessary. Behavior modification for the child and family counseling may also be helpful.

Additional Reading: Diagnosis and management of ADHD in children. *Am Fam Physician*. 2014;90(7):456-464.

ADHD is characterized by a persistent pattern of inattention and/or hyperactivity-impulsivity that interferes with functioning or developments and is characterized by a short attention span and/or distractibility that persists for longer than 6 months.

7. An effective method for disciplining infants and toddlers would be which one of the following strategies?

A) Bargaining
B) Dependency
C) Inconsistency
D) Redirecting
E) Variability

The answer is D: Discipline plays an important role in the social and emotional development of children. Physicians should discuss safe, effective methods of discipline with parents during well-child examinations. Discipline should be instructive and age-appropriate and should include positive reinforcement for good behavior and redirecting undesirable behavior.

Commonly, children misbehave when they are tired, bored, or hungry. Children may also misbehave when they are deprived of adult attention, and when misbehavior elicits adult attention, which can unintentionally reinforce the undesired behavior. Parental attention is a powerful form of positive reinforcement, and parents should attempt to use attention and other positive reinforcers when they are pleased with their child's behavior.

Consistent, reliable standards and expectations are all helpful parenting practices as well. One good method for infants and toddlers is *redirecting*. When one redirects a child, one replaces an unwanted (bad) behavior with an acceptable (good) behavior. For example, if throwing a ball inside the house is not allowed, a parent can take the child outside to throw the ball.

Time-out is a commonly practiced parenting technique to try to eliminate unacceptable behavior and can be effective when implemented correctly. Time-out involves removing the child from the problem situation to a neutral, boring, nonfrightening, and safe setting for a specified and brief period of time. Time-out works well for children from 18 months up to 5 or 6 years of age.

Additional Reading: Childhood discipline: challenges for clinicians and parents. *Am Fam Physician*. 2002;66(8):1447-1453.

8. Which one of the following is true regarding ADHD?

A) ADHD is more common in females than males.
B) ADHD symptoms tend to increase over time.
C) ADHD is best diagnosed using rating scales from parents and teachers and the *Diagnostic and Statistical Manual of Mental Disorders*, 5th edition (*DSM 5*) criteria.
D) Other psychiatric comorbidities are rare with ADHD.
E) Treating ADHD by combining psychosocial therapy with medication has proven to be superior to medication alone.

The answer is C: ADHD presents as some combination of inappropriate hyperactivity, impulsivity, and inattention. ADHD cannot be easily diagnosed by a specific test or biologic marker. Based on study results, the pooled prevalence of ADHD is between 6.8% and 10.3%, with boys having a threefold higher rate. Psychiatric comorbidities, including oppositional defiant disorder, conduct disorder, depressive disorder, and anxiety disorders, are common.

There are several ADHD-specific checklists with high sensitivity for identification of children with the disorder when several checklists are completed by multiple adults with knowledge of the child's behavior in different settings (eg, Vanderbilt Rating Scales and Conners ADHD Index and symptom scales).

Reviews of the pharmacologic management of ADHD with methylphenidate hydrochloride, dextroamphetamine sulfate, and pemoline show these drugs to be effective. Nonpharmacologic treatments that have some beneficial effect on behavior and academic performance are behavioral modification and intensive contingency management therapy. Combining drug therapy with psychosocial therapy shows no clear advantage when compared with drug therapy alone. However, the addition of behavioral therapies to medication may have some benefit, including reduction of anxiety and improvement in social skills. Other psychiatric comorbidities are common and should be identified and properly managed. The symptoms of ADHD tend to decrease over the long term but may continue into adolescence and adulthood. The most common treatment is stimulant medication.

Additional Reading: Diagnosis and management of ADHD in children. *Am Fam Physician*. 2014;90(7):456-464.

9. An adolescent boy is brought in by his mother. He has been diagnosed with Tourette syndrome (TS) and she is asking if there is a medication that can help control his tics. Which one of the following medications would be the drug of first choice for the treatment of moderate to severe TS?

A) Carbamazepine
B) Clonidine
C) Phenobarbital
D) Lorazepam
E) Phenytoin

The answer is B: TS is a genetically transmitted disorder that begins in childhood as a simple tic, progressing to multiple tics as the patient ages. Tics may begin as grunts or barks and progress to involuntary compulsive utterances called *coprolalia*. These outbursts may become severe and significantly disable the patient from a physical or social standpoint.

Tics tend to be more complex than myoclonus but less flowing than choreic movements, from which they must be differentiated. The patient may be able to voluntarily suppress them for seconds or minutes.

For simple and complex tics, alpha-2 adrenergic agonists such as clonidine or guanfacine are first-line treatment choices and are effective in some patients; however, its limiting adverse effect is hypotension. For more severe cases, antipsychotics, such as haloperidol, olanzapine, or risperidone, may be required. Side effects of dysphoria, parkinsonism, akathisia, and tardive dyskinesia may limit their use. Antipsychotics should be started cautiously, and patients should be told about potential adverse outcomes.

Additional Reading: Tourette syndrome. In: Domino F, ed. *The 5-Minute Clinical Consult*. Wolters Kluwer; 2022.

10. Tourette syndrome (TS) is a complex tic disorder. Which one of the following statements is true regarding TS?

A) Girls are more frequently affected by TS than boys.
B) Patients with TS rarely have other associated psychological conditions.
C) TS is a familial disorder.
D) Tricyclic antidepressants are the treatment of choice for TS.
E) The long-term prognosis for treating TS is poor.

The answer is C: TS is a movement disorder most commonly seen in school-age children. The prevalence is about 1% in boys and 0.25% in girls. TS is a chronic familial disorder with a fluctuating course; the long-term outcome is generally favorable. Although the exact underlying pathology has yet to be determined, evidence indicates a disorder localized to the frontal-subcortical neural pathways.

TS is associated with ADHD, obsessive-compulsive disorder, behavior problems, and learning disabilities. These associated conditions can make the management of TS more difficult. The use of antipsychotic medications (risperidone, pimozide, olanzapine, and haloperidol) and clonidine can be effective but may be associated with significant side effects, and stimulant use for comorbid ADHD can worsen tic symptoms.

Additional Reading: Tourette syndrome. In: Domino F, ed. *The 5-Minute Clinical Consult*. Wolters Kluwer; 2022.

11. During an infant's 2 month well-child check, the patient's mother screens a score of 10 on the Edinburgh Postnatal Depression Scale. The patient has no history of psychosis or bipolar disorder but did have anxiety and depression in college but never used a medication before. Using informed decision-making, you and the patient decide to proceed with an antidepressant. Which of the following medications would be the best first choice?

A) Bupropion
B) Sertraline
C) Mirtazapine
D) Citalopram
E) Fluoxetine

The answer is B: Sertraline (Zoloft), paroxetine (Paxil), and fluvoxamine were found to be first-choice medications for breastfeeding mother. Sertraline has the lowest degree of translactal passage and fewest reported adverse effects compared to other antidepressants In general, if an antidepressant has helped, it is best to continue it during lactation.

Additional Reading: Antidepressant use during pregnancy. *Am Fam Physician*. 2011;90(10)1211-1215.

12. A 7-year-old child is brought into the office by his parents, because of problems at school. His teachers report that although he has no problems following instructions and seems able to understand normal conversation, he is having problems reading. The issue appears to involve single-word decoding. The father reports that he had similar problems when he was in school. The most likely diagnosis to account for this situation is which one of the following?

A) Attention-deficit disorder
B) Autism
C) Congenital hearing loss
D) Dyslexia
E) Intellectual disability

The answer is D: Dyslexia is a specific learning disability that is neurological in origin. It is characterized by difficulties with accurate and/or fluent word recognition and by poor spelling and decoding abilities. These difficulties typically result from a deficit in the phonologic component of language that is often unexpected in relation to other cognitive abilities and the provision of effective classroom instruction. Secondary consequences may include problems in reading comprehension and reduced reading experience that can impede the growth of vocabulary and background knowledge.

According to the *DSM 5*, dyslexia fits within the category of a specific learning disorder with impairment in reading and is one of the most common manifestations of a specific learning disorder. The inability to learn derivational rules of printed language is often considered part of dyslexia. Affected children may have difficulty in determining root words or word stems and determining which letters in words follow others and in forming specific sound-symbol associations, such as vowel patterns, affixes, syllables, and word endings.

The cause of dyslexia is unknown, but a strong genetic link has been established. Cerebrovascular accidents, prematurity, and intrauterine complications have been linked to dyslexia. Most experts agree that dyslexia is left hemisphere-related and is associated with deficiencies or dysfunctions in the areas of the brain that are responsible for language association (Wernicke area) and sound and speech production (Broca area) and in the interconnection of these areas.

Most dyslexics are not identified until kindergarten or first grade, when symbolic learning is taught. However, dyslexia in preschool children may manifest itself as delayed language production, speech articulation problems, and difficulties in remembering the names of letters, numbers, and colors, particularly in children with a family history of reading or learning problems. Many dyslexics confuse letters and words with similar configurations or have difficulty in visually selecting or identifying letter patterns and clusters (sound-symbol association) in words.

Reversals or visual confusions tend to be seen frequently during the early school years. Most reading and writing reversals occur because dyslexics forget or confuse the names of letters and words that have similar structures; subsequently, *d* becomes *b*, *m* becomes *w*, *h* becomes *n*, *was* becomes *saw*, and *on* becomes *no*, for example.

Students with a history of delayed language acquisition use or who are not accelerating in word learning by the middle or end of first grade, or who are not reading at the level expected for their verbal or intellectual abilities at any grade level, should be evaluated.

Many dyslexics develop functional reading skills with direct instruction, although dyslexia is a lifelong problem, and many dyslexics never reach full literacy. Compensatory approaches, such as taped texts, readers, and scribes, are used to assist the dyslexic with higher-order learning.

Additional Reading: Learning disabilities, pediatric. In: Domino F, ed. *The 5-Minute Clinical Consult*. Wolters Kluwer; 2022.

13. When initiating antidepressants in children and adolescents, it must be remembered that the risk of suicide is highest during which one of the following time periods?

A) The first hours of medication administration
B) The first few weeks of medication administration
C) The first few months of medication administration
D) Usually a year or more after starting therapy
E) The risk of suicide is not increased in this age group

The answer is B: The US Food and Drug Administration advisory panel concluded there is a small, but real, increased risk of suicidal thoughts or behavior in children taking antidepressants compared with placebo. The risk appears to be greatest in the first few weeks after initiation of therapy. Careful monitoring of symptoms can be helpful when the benefits of pharmacotherapy for depression in children and adolescents outweigh the risks.

Additional Reading: Are some antidepressants safer than others regarding suicide risk? *Am Fam Physician*. 2015;92(1):52a–54.

14. Divorce is associated with significant stress for the divorcing parties but often children are involved as well. Children whose parents are divorcing are at increased risk for which one of the following issues?

A) School problems
B) Externalizing behaviors and acting out
C) Relationship difficulties
D) Somatic symptoms and complaints
E) All of the above

The answer is E: Exposure to high levels of parental conflict is predictive of poor emotional adjustment by the child regardless of the parents' marital status. Still, up to half of children show a symptomatic response during the first year after their parents' divorce. Risk factors for continuing childhood difficulty include ongoing parental discord, maternal depression, psychiatric disorders in either parent, or poverty.

The clinical manifestations of divorce in children depend on many variables, including the child's age; the predivorce level of the family's psychosocial functioning; the parents' ability in the midst of their own anger, loss, and discomfort to focus on their child's feelings and needs; and the child's temperament and temperamental fit of parents with their children. At all ages, children frequently have psychosomatic symptoms as a response to anger, loss, grief, feeling unloved, and other stressors.

Infants and children younger than 3 years may reflect their caregivers' distress, grief, and preoccupation; they often show irritability, increased crying, fearfulness, separation anxiety, sleep and gastrointestinal problems, aggression, and developmental regression.

Children 4 to 5 years of age often blame themselves for the breakup and parental unhappiness, becoming clingier, with externalizing behavior (acting out), misperceive the events of the divorce situation, fear that they will be abandoned, and have more nightmares and fantasies.

School-aged children may be moody or preoccupied; show more aggression, temper, and acting-out behavior; seem uncomfortable with gender identity; and feel rejected and deceived by the absent parent. School performance may decrease, and they may agonize about their divided loyalties and feel that they should be punished.

Adolescents may feel decreased self-esteem and may develop premature emotional autonomy to deal with negative feelings about the divorce and their deidealization of each parent. Their anger and confusion often lead to relationship problems, substance abuse, decreased school performance, inappropriate sexual behavior, depression, and aggressive and delinquent behavior.

Factors that lead to better outcomes include positive child temperament and an optimistic view of the future, consistent parental discipline, parental acceptance and warmth, and maintenance of as normal a routine as possible. Some children have long-lasting emotional and adjustment problems associated with their parents' divorce; however, most adjust and function well over time, particularly those who have supportive relationships and a positive temperament and receive professional counseling.

Additional Reading: Is divorce bad for children? *Scientific American*. 2013.

15. A number of medications are useful in treating attention-deficit/hyperactivity disorder (ADHD). All of listed medications are recommended as first-line agents except which one?

A) Amphetamines (Adderall)
B) Clonidine (Kapvay)
C) Dextroamphetamine (Dexedrine)
D) Methylphenidate (Ritalin)

The answer is B: Stimulant medications (amphetamines, methylphenidate) are often prescribed as the first-line agents to treat children, adolescents, or adults diagnosed with ADHD. Although these medicines are stimulants, in children and adults with ADHD they have a calming effect. In most systematic reviews, methylphenidate, dexmethylphenidate, and amphetamines appear to be equally effective and to have similar adverse effect profiles. The preferences of the patient and family must be taken into consideration when choosing among these agents.

α2-Adrenergic agonists (clonidine) are usually used when children respond poorly to a trial of stimulants or atomoxetine, have unacceptable side effects, or have significant coexisting conditions.

ADHD is the most common pediatric psychiatric disorder. Diagnosis of ADHD requires a detailed history from the family and the use of rating scales to collect observations from two or more settings. Effective treatment, including behavior management, appropriate educational placement, and stimulant medication, improves academic performance and behavior in most patients. Children, for whom initial management fails or for whom the diagnosis is unclear or complicated, should be referred to appropriate mental health professionals.

Additional Reading: Diagnosis and management of ADHD in children. *Am Fam Physician*. 2014;90(7):456-464.

16. An 18-year-old nonbinary high school student presents with her mother to your office. The mother is concerned because their teenager is binge eating and then purging to lose weight. You suspect bulimia. Of the medications listed, which would be best indicated in treatment of the condition?

A) Bupropion (Wellbutrin)
B) Fluoxetine (Prozac)
C) Paroxetine (Paxil)
D) Sertraline (Zoloft)
E) Venlafaxine (Effexor)

The answer is B: Persons affected by bulimia nervosa are often normal weight and are not easily detected by physiologic and medical markers. This disorder is characterized by these key features: binge eating; compensatory behaviors to prevent weight gain (eg, purging); excessive concern about body weight and shape; as well as self-evaluation being unduly influenced by body weight and shape. Bulimia is most common in late adolescent girls. Associations with other psychiatric disorders are also common.

Pharmacotherapy is efficacious for bulimia nervosa and may be used alone or added to other first-line treatments, which consist of nutritional rehabilitation plus psychotherapy. Nutritional rehabilitation aims to restore a structured and consistent meal pattern, typically three meals and two snacks per day. Cognitive behavioral therapy and interpersonal psychotherapy can effectively facilitate nutritional rehabilitation.

Interestingly, disturbances in serotonergic systems have been suggested as contributing to bulimia and the selective serotonin reuptake inhibitor fluoxetine has been approved by the US Food and Drug Administration for the treatment of bulimia. Fluoxetine is the first-line treatment because of its efficacy for the behavioral and cognitive symptoms of bulimia nervosa, as well as its tolerability. Fluoxetine has been more widely studied for bulimia nervosa than any other medication with evidence of decreased bingeing and purging episodes as well as improved dietary restraint, food preoccupation, and excessive concern and dissatisfaction with body weight and shape. The target dosage for fluoxetine in bulimia nervosa is 60 mg/d, which is higher than the standard dosage for major depression.

Most bulimics purge by vomiting; however, abuse of laxatives or diuretics can also occur. The number of times a bulimic patient purges can vary widely, from as seldom as once or twice weekly to as often as 10 times per day. (At least once a week for 3 months is required for *DSM 5* diagnosis.) Repeatedly induced vomiting can lead to the loss of dental enamel, increased dental caries, swollen salivary glands, Mallory-Weiss esophageal tears, and gastroesophageal reflux. Laxative abusers can develop constipation on withdrawal of laxatives.

The typical electrolyte abnormalities associated with bulimia are hypokalemia and metabolic acidosis. Although severe hypokalemia in an otherwise healthy young woman suggests bulimia, most patients who purge do not develop electrolyte abnormalities. As a result, screening for hypokalemia or other electrolyte disturbances is not a sensitive means for detecting bulimia.

Treatment of the complications associated with bulimia is usually possible, but the underlying disorder can be challenging to treat. Fluoridated mouthwash and toothpaste can help prevent dental caries, and the use of sour candies may decrease salivary gland swelling. Antacid medications help reduce gastroesophageal reflux symptoms, and nonstimulant laxatives may be used to decrease constipation in those with stimulant laxative abuse. Oral replacement of potassium is typically accomplished with 40 to 80 mEq/d of supplementary potassium, until a normal serum potassium level is achieved. Patients with severe hypokalemia and metabolic alkalosis need volume repletion with intravenous normal saline to allow normalization of potassium levels.

Additional Reading: Initial evaluation, diagnosis, and treatment of anorexia nervosa and bulimia nervosa. *Am Fam Physician*. 2015;91(1):46-52.

17. Anorexia nervosa in adolescent girls can affect growth and development and is associated with a number of adverse effects. Which one of the following findings is not associated with this condition?

A) Bradycardia
B) Hypotension
C) Low bone density
D) Low estradiol levels
E) Precocious puberty

The answer is E: Adolescent girls with anorexia nervosa have an increased risk for hematologic, metabolic (low estradiol levels), hemodynamic, and skeletal abnormalities (low bone density), including bradycardia, hypotension, and pubertal delay, compared with healthy girls.

Additional Reading: Eating disorders in primary care: diagnosis and management. *Am Fam Physician*. 2021;103(1):22-32.

18. You are seeing a 22-year-old man with a history of persistent depression. He reports having difficulty completing assignments at community college along with trouble falling asleep, some unintentional weight loss, and loss of interest in hobbies. He has tried antidepressants including, bupropion, fluoxetine, and citalopram. He reports that there was a week or so when his mood felt much more normal. He needed only 2-3 hours of sleep each night that week. He admits that he was somewhat impulsive, had an increased sex drive, and experienced racing thoughts at that time. He has a family history of suicide in both his brother and mother, who also abused substances. He denies any alcohol, tobacco, or illicit drug use. Which of the following medications is most likely to help this patient?

A) Escitalopram
B) Mirtazapine
C) Trazodone
D) Aripiprazole
E) Lithium

The answer is D: Patients with bipolar II disorder, such as this patient, may have a hypomanic episode that goes unrecognized, and the patient may present with persistent depression. There are many options to treat bipolar disorder and typically lithium can be used but is often reserved for bipolar type I without mixed features. The best choice would be Abilify or other atypical antipsychotics like lamotrigine, lurasidone, or quetiapine.

Additional Reading: Bipolar disorders: evaluation and treatment. *Am Fam Physician*. 2021;103(4):227-239.

Section III. Population Health

Each of the following questions or incomplete statements is followed by suggested answers or completions. Select the ONE BEST ANSWER in each case.

1. Recent concerns have been raised over the use of psychotropic agents in nursing homes. Which one of the following statements regarding this situation is true?

A) Phenobarbital does not require monitoring.
B) Sedative-hypnotics should be reserved to sedate patients who are at risk for falls.
C) Periodic dose reductions of psychotropic agents should be performed.
D) The physician is ultimately responsible for monitoring drug utilization.
E) Tranquilizers, regardless of their effectiveness in patients before admission to the nursing home, should not be used.

The answer is C: All psychotropic drugs (antidepressants, anxiolytics, sedative-hypnotics, and antipsychotics) are subject to the "unnecessary drug" regulation of the Omnibus Budget Reconciliation Act (OBRA). According to the federal government guidelines, "nursing home residents must be free of unnecessary drugs," which are defined as those that are duplicative, excessive in dose or duration, or used in the presence of adverse effects or without adequate monitoring or indication.

Medical, environmental, and psychosocial causes of behavioral problems must be ruled out, and nonpharmacologic management must be attempted before psychotropic drugs are prescribed to nursing home residents. Because treatment with psychotropic medications is indicated only to maintain or improve functional status, diagnoses and specific target symptoms or behaviors must be documented and the effectiveness of drug therapy must be monitored. Specific dosage limits must be observed, and periodic dosage reductions or drug discontinuations must be undertaken. Side effects (of antipsychotics in particular) must be monitored.

Barbiturates and certain other older tranquilizers may not be prescribed unless they were being used successfully before a patient was admitted to a long-term care facility. Phenobarbital can be used only to control seizures. OBRA restricts the use of antipsychotic drugs only in patients with dementia. None of the OBRA dosage restrictions or monitoring requirements apply in patients with psychotic disorders (eg, schizophrenia).

According to the OBRA strategy, the long-term care facility, rather than the prescribing physician, is accountable for monitoring drug use. Each nursing home is surveyed annually. Because facilities that do not meet the federal government's requirements may be denied Medicare reimbursement, physicians who prescribe medications for nursing home residents must document the medical necessity of noncompliance with regulations (eg, drug prescriptions in excess of OBRA-mandated dosages). In most cases, a local consultant pharmacist reviews all charts monthly and assists with compliance.

Regardless of where final responsibility lies, physicians need to be aware of the federal government's interpretive guidelines for the fulfillment of OBRA requirements.

Additional Reading:
1. Nursing home care: part I. Principles and pitfalls of practice. Am Fam Physician. 2010;81(10):1219-1227.
2. Nursing home care: part II. Clinical aspects. Am Fam Physician. 2010;81(10):1229-1237.

2. Preventive measures are classified into three levels. Which one of the following is an example of tertiary prevention?

A) Administration of neonatal erythromycin eye drops
B) Hepatitis A vaccination for travelers
C) Pneumococcal vaccination
D) Purified protein derivative determination in a patient who is affected with tuberculosis
E) Smoking cessation counseling in a patient with chronic obstructive pulmonary disease

The answer is E: The following are three types of prevention:

Primary prevention: These types of treatments are administered to prevent the development of disease. Examples include vaccinations (eg, tetanus, influenza, and pneumococcal and intraocular administration of erythromycin to prevent neonatal chlamydia or gonorrhea).

Secondary prevention: These are steps taken to detect disease early in the course of the illness, to help identify those who are affected. Examples include purified protein derivative determination in patients affected with tuberculosis or Venereal Disease Research Laboratory determination in those with syphilis.

Tertiary prevention: These are steps that are taken after the development of a condition to help treat the patient and decrease the incidence of disease complications. Examples include counseling a patient with emphysema or chronic bronchitis to stop smoking.

Additional Reading: Definitions of prevention. In: Rakel, ed. *Textbook of Family Medicine*. 9th ed. Saunders/Elsevier; 2016.

3. Intimate partner violence (IPV) is unfortunately more common than recognized, and various factors have been identified that appear to be related to an increased risk of abuse. Which one of the following factors may contribute to an increased risk of IPV?

A) A power differential in the relationship
B) More than three children in the home
C) One partner with depression
D) One spouse undergoing schooling
E) Prior divorce

The answer is A: Studies have not identified any consistent psychiatric diagnoses among abusers, but abusive men share some common characteristics such as rigid sex role stereotypes, low self-esteem, depression, a high need for power and control, a tendency to minimize and deny their problems or the extent of their violence, a tendency to blame others for their behavior, violence in the family of origin (particularly witnessing parental violence), and drug and alcohol abuse (which are not causative but are often associated). Men who have alcoholism combined with a major depressive disorder or antisocial personality disorder are more likely to commit domestic violence than are men with either of these conditions alone.

Most researchers believe that abusive behavior is the result of multiple factors, including individual characteristics, a family history of violence, and the culturally rooted belief that violence is an acceptable means of solving problems and that violence toward women is acceptable or tolerated. Factors that specifically relate to partner abuse include the following:

- A power differential in the relationship in which one partner is financially or emotionally dependent on the other
- A temporary or permanent disability (including pregnancy)
- A force orientation—a belief on the part of the perpetrator that violence is an acceptable solution to conflicts and problems
- A personal or family history of abuse

Signs that often indicate a need to further assess the risk of abuse include excessive work loss, sleep disturbances, substance abuse, anxiety, sexual dysfunction, depression, frequent injuries, or being "accident prone." It is imperative to discuss events noted in these records with the patient and to assess any discrepancy between an injury and its reported causative mechanism because injuries that are related to battering are often attributed to falling on the stairs or some other household accidents. In such cases, the patient should be asked to describe the accident in more detail, or the physician should ask about precipitating factors (eg, "Were you pushed?").

Ancillary tests should be obtained as indicated for the specific injury or infection. The physician should be especially alert for pregnancy complications and sexually transmitted infections, including human immunodeficiency virus infection.

Additional Reading: Intimate partner violence. *Am Fam Physician*. 2016;94(8):646-651.

4. Kava is marked as an herbal remedy and it has been found to be useful to the treatment of which one of the following conditions?

A) Anxiety
B) Attention-deficit disorder
C) Depression
D) Impotence
E) Memory loss

The answer is A: Kava or kava-kava is a supplement derived from the roots of the *Piper methysticum* plant, which is found in the western Pacific islands. Kava active ingredients are called kavalactones, which have anesthetic and sedating effects.

The drug appears beneficial in the management of anxiety and tension of nonpsychotic origin and does not adversely affect cognitive function, mental acuity, or coordination. A Cochrane systematic review concluded it was likely to be more effective than placebo for treating short-term anxiety. The long-term use of high doses has been associated with scaling of the skin on the extremities. Kava may potentiate the action of other centrally mediated agents and interact with alcohol. Kava has been associated with liver toxicity as well.

Additional Reading: Complementary/integrative therapies that work: a review of the evidence. *Am Fam Physician*. 2016;94(5):369-374.

5. Individuals with intellectual and developmental disabilities are at risk for various medical conditions due to underlying disabilities and the long-term use of medications. Which one of the following conditions is commonly seen in patients with intellectual and developmental disabilities, regardless of the underlying disorder?

A) Diabetes mellitus
B) Hyperthyroidism
C) Hyperparathyroidism
D) Osteoporosis
E) Pernicious anemia

The answer is D: Osteoporosis is a common condition seen in patients with intellectual and developmental disabilities, particularly among non–weight-bearing patients. It has been estimated that as many as 50% of such adults have osteoporosis or osteopenia. Conditions associated with an increased risk of osteoporosis include cerebral palsy, Down syndrome, use of antiepileptics, special diets (eg, ketogenic diet for seizure control), and hypogonadism.

Aggressive evaluation of traumatic injuries with radiographic studies may be justified even when there are few physical findings. Furthermore, osteoporosis and use of antiepileptics may predispose patients to degenerative disk disease with spinal cord compromise, leading to functional decline.

Additional Reading: Primary care of the adult with intellectual and developmental disabilities. In: *UpToDate*. 2022.

➜ **Osteoporosis is a common condition seen in patients with intellectual and developmental disabilities, particularly among non–weight-bearing patients.**

6. Valerian is derived from the perennial herb *Valeriana officinalis* and has been suggested for use in various mental health and behavioral disorders. In which one of the following conditions has valerian been found to be helpful?

A) Bulimia
B) Depression
C) Insomnia
D) Mania
E) Menstrual disorders

The answer is C: Valerian has been used to ease insomnia, anxiety, and nervous restlessness for centuries. Some research suggests that valerian may help people with insomnia. Germany's Commission E approved valerian as an effective mild sedative and the US Food and Drug Administration listed valerian as "Generally Recognized as Safe."

It is believed that valerian acts by increasing the amount of γ-aminobutyric acid (GABA) in the brain. GABA helps regulate nerve cells and has a calming effect on anxiety. Valerian may potentiate the effects of other central nervous system depressants.

Additional Reading: Complementary/integrative therapies that work: a review of the evidence. *Am Fam Physician*. 2016;94(5):369-374.

7. An extract of the *Ginkgo biloba* leaf from the maidenhair tree is marketed as a dietary supplement for several health concerns, but it has been associated with some adverse effects. Patients with which of the following conditions should use *G biloba* with caution?

A) Cardiac conduction defects
B) Epilepsy
C) Peripheral neuropathy
D) Prior deep venous thrombosis
E) Renal insufficiency

The answer is B: An extract of the dried *G biloba* leaves is used to alleviate symptoms that are associated with a range of cognitive problems and has been approved in Germany for the treatment of dementia. Ginkgo is thought to have antioxidant properties; however, its exact mechanism of action is unclear.

Numerous clinical trials have been performed using *G biloba* for various central nervous system and vascular conditions. It is thought that there are two main groups of active constituents responsible for its medicinal effects: terpene lactones and ginkgo flavone glycosides, which are present in varying concentrations in the leaf of the ginkgo tree.

Safety in pregnancy and in lactation has not been determined. The most common adverse effect is headache. Isolated reports of seizure associated with ginkgo use have been published but whether ginkgo lowers seizure threshold is uncertain. The use of ginkgo in patients with seizure disorders should therefore be done with caution. Caution should also be exercised when using ginkgo combined with anticoagulant treatment, including aspirin, when there is risk of bleeding, as in peptic ulcer disease and subdural hematoma.

Additional Reading: Complementary/integrative therapies that work: a review of the evidence. *Am Fam Physician*. 2016;94(5):369-374.

8. Yohimbine is obtained from the bark of the West African yohimbe tree and is marketed for the treatment of impotence. This natural supplement has been associated with which one of the following side effects?

A) Cataract formation
B) Colon polyps
C) Priapism
D) Hypertensive complications
E) Skin pigmentation

The answer is D: Yohimbine is an indole alkaloid that is obtained from the bark of a West African tree (*Pausinystalia yohimbe*). The product is an α-adrenergic receptor antagonist that is marketed for the treatment of impotence, and studies have shown that it can enhance erectile functioning.

Yohimbine increases sympathetically mediated plasma norepinephrine, which in turn produces a pressor response. Therefore, yohimbine should be administered with caution to patients with hypertension or those who are undergoing concomitant treatment with tricyclic antidepressants or other drugs that interfere with neuronal uptake or metabolism of norepinephrine. The drug may induce panic attacks in patients with anxiety disorders.

Additional Reading: Management of erectile dysfunction. *Am Fam Physician*. 2010;81(3):305-312.

9. Adenosylmethionine (S-adenosylmethionine [SAMe]) is an alternative medication that is used for the treatment of depression. The mechanism of action is thought to affect levels of which one of the following neurotransmitters?

A) Acetylcholine
B) γ-aminobutyric acid
C) Norepinephrine
D) Serotonin

The answer is D: SAMe is a metabolite of folate that facilitates the synthesis of neurotransmitters (including dopamine, norepinephrine, and serotonin) and may be effective and well tolerated for treatment-resistant depression. Oral and intravenous SAMe supplementation has been shown to increase SAMe levels significantly in cerebrospinal fluid, indicating SAMe's crossover through the blood-brain barrier. This has been associated with increased levels of serotonin metabolites in cerebrospinal fluid.

Depressed patients may have low serotonin levels associated with low levels of SAMe. A few randomized trials have compared adjunctive SAMe with placebo among patients with unipolar major depression and found it effective with lower rates of discontinuation due to side effects. However, because no studies have yet validated the long-term safety or efficacy of SAMe, further large long-term studies should be conducted before it receives widespread recommendation.

Additional Reading: S-adenosyl methionine (SAMe) for depression in adults. *Cochrane Database Syst Rev*. 2016.

10. St. John's wort is a plant that has been used for centuries for health purposes. The most common side effect of high-dose St. John's wort is which one of the following conditions?

A) Hoarseness
B) Hypertension
C) Myalgias
D) Photosensitivity
E) Tremor

The answer is D: St. John's wort appears to be useful for mild depression, similar to treatment with standard prescription antidepressants, but the evidence is limited. Transient photosensitivity is generally the most common side effect of St. John's wort and occurs more commonly at higher dosages. Other side effects include gastrointestinal upset, increased anxiety, minor palpitations, fatigue, restlessness, dry mouth, headache, and increased depression.

Additional Reading: Complementary/integrative therapies that work: a review of the evidence. *Am Fam Physician*. 2016;94(5):369-374.

11. Although an herb, St. John's wort can still cause side effects and drug-drug interactions. Which one of the following medications is affected by the concurrent use of this herb?

A) Amoxicillin
B) Gabapentin
C) Glipizide
D) Hydrochlorothiazide
E) Oral contraceptives

The answer is E: Because of the induction of CYP 3A4, concurrent use of St. John's wort may reduce the effectiveness of oral contraceptives. There are case reports of breakthrough bleeding and undesired pregnancy in women taking oral contraceptive pills, presumably due to lowering of ethinyl estradiol concentrations. Women using oral contraceptives should be counseled regarding possible breakthrough bleeding and might consider a barrier method of contraception when taking St. John's wort. Additionally, St. John's wort should not be combined with other antidepressants to avoid the possibility of serotonin syndrome.

Additional Reading: Complementary/integrative therapies that work: a review of the evidence. *Am Fam Physician*. 2016;94(5):369-374.

12. Men die by suicide four times as often as women. Which one of the following methods is the most common means for suicide completion among men?

A) Carbon monoxide poisoning
B) Firearms
C) Hanging
D) Illicit drug overdose
E) Prescription medication overdose

The answer is B: Access to a means to attempt suicide is an important precipitating cause in suicide. This is true even after controlling for other risk factors such as depression or substance use. Firearms are the most common means for suicide completion among men. Other means include medications, illicit drugs, toxic chemicals, carbon monoxide, hanging, and cutting.

Men die by suicide four times as often as women, whereas women attempt suicide two to three times as often as men. Poisoning is the most common means among women. Almost anything can be used as a means to attempt suicide, but access to the most lethal means often results in death.

Additional Reading: Screening for suicide risk in adolescents, adults, and older adults in primary care: recommendation statement. *Am Fam Physician*. 2015;91(3):190F–190I.

The USPSTF concluded that the evidence on screening for suicide risk in primary care is insufficient and that the balance of benefits and harms cannot be determined.

13. The term "intimate partner violence" (IPV) refers to physical, sexual, or psychologic harm inflicted by a current or former partner or spouse. Which one of the following statements is true regarding IPV?

A) IPV is higher among Caucasian women compared with other ethnic classes.
B) IPV affects men and women equally.
C) IPV is rarely seen in the elderly.
D) IPV increases during pregnancy.

The answer is D: Studies show that women are much more likely than men to be the victims of IPV. The Centers for Disease Control and Prevention's report on the National Intimate Partner and Sexual Violence Survey of 2010 estimates that more than one in three women (35.6%) have experienced IPV in their lifetime. Screening for IPV during pregnancy is important because pregnancy may be one of the only times women, especially of lower socioeconomic status, are connected with health care.

The U.S. Preventive Services Task Force (USPSTF) recommends that clinicians screen women of childbearing age for IPV (group A recommendation) and provide or refer women who screen positive to intervention services (group C recommendation). This recommendation applies to women who do not have signs or symptoms of abuse. However, the USPSTF concluded that the current evidence is insufficient to assess the balance of benefits and harms of screening all elderly or vulnerable adults (physically or mentally dysfunctional) for abuse and neglect.

IPV among gay and lesbian relationships appears to be as common as in heterosexual relationships and is also a significant problem among the elderly. Elder abuse is associated with an increase in reports of chronic pain, depression, number of health conditions, and an increased mortality.

The abuser is most commonly a relative (usually the spouse). Domestic violence often begins or, if already present, increases during pregnancy and the postpartum period. IPV is much more common among black, Hispanic, and Native American women compared with Caucasian women.

Additional Reading: Intimate partner violence. *Am Fam Physician*. 2016;94(8):646-651.

14. In assessing the risk for suicide in a depressed patient, understanding risk factors can be helpful in deciding the best course of treatment. All of the following are considered risk factors for suicide; identify which one is associated with the greatest risk for suicide?

A) A low-income status
B) Being single (never married)
C) Current unemployment
D) Previous psychiatric admission
E) Residing in an urban area

The answer is D: Each year, about 30,000 people in the United States die by suicide, and the strongest single factor predictive of suicide is a history of attempted suicide in the past.

Suicide rates are higher in residents of urban areas and increased with unemployment, single status (never married), low income, and receipt of pension or social security benefit. However, the strongest risk factor is having a psychiatric illness, and the severity of psychiatric illness is associated with the risk of suicide. More specifically, admission to a psychiatric hospital is a significant risk factor for suicide, with one study revealing that one-half of the persons who committed suicide had a history of admission to a psychiatric facility.

One meta-analysis found that the lifetime risk of suicide is 8.6% in patients who have had a psychiatric inpatient admission involving suicidal ideation, 4% in patients who have had a psychiatric admission for an affective disorder without suicidality, 2.2% in psychiatric outpatients, and less than 0.5% in the general population. Regardless of diagnosis, the greatest risk was during hospital admission and in the first week following discharge.

Additional Reading: Screening for suicide risk in adolescents, adults, and older adults in primary care: recommendation statement. *Am Fam Physician*. 2015;91(3):190F–190I.

➔ The strongest single factor predictive of suicide is a history of attempted suicide in the past.

15. A middle-aged man who drives a truck for a living presents for a Department of Transportation (DOT) physical examination certification. Which one of the following conditions would disqualify this patient from obtaining the DOT certification?

A) Having Type 1 diabetes
B) Having a blood pressure (BP) reading of 158/94 mm Hg
C) Requiring the use of a hearing aid
D) A vision screen with 20/40 in both eyes
E) A field of vision measured at 70° in each eye

The answer is A: Many physicians perform DOT certification physical examinations. A patient taking insulin cannot be certified for interstate driving; it is considered a disqualifying condition. However, a driver who has diabetes controlled by oral medications and diet may be qualified if the disease is well controlled and the driver is under medical supervision. If diabetes is untreated or uncontrolled, certification should not be given.

From a cardiac standpoint, any condition known to be accompanied by sudden and unexpected syncope, collapse, or congestive heart failure is disqualifying. Conditions such as myocardial infarction, angina, and cardiac dysrhythmias should, in most cases, be evaluated by a cardiologist before certification is issued. Holter monitors and exercise stress tests may be needed when a driver has multiple risk factors. Tachycardia or bradycardia should be investigated to rule out underlying cardiac disease. Asymptomatic dysrhythmia with no underlying disease process should not be disqualifying.

With regard to BP, if the BP is 159/99 mm Hg or lower, a full 1-year certification is appropriate. If the BP is >160-179/100-109 mm Hg, temporary certification may be granted for 3 months to allow time for the driver to be evaluated and treated. If the initial BP is 180/110 mm Hg or higher, the driver should not be certified. Once the driver's BP is under control, certification can be issued for no more than 1 year at a time. Several readings should be taken over several days to rule out "white coat" hypertension. Significant target organ damage and additional risk factors increase the risk of sudden collapse (syncope) and should be disqualifying.

Vision must be at least 20/40 in each eye with or without correction. Certification can be given once vision has been corrected, but not until. The driver should be advised to have his or her eyes evaluated, obtain corrective lenses, and then return for certification. Field of vision must be at least 70° in each eye. Color vision must allow recognition of standard traffic signals (ie, red, green, and amber).

The driver should pass a whispered voice test at 5 ft in at least one ear. A hearing aid may be worn for the test. If the test result is questionable, an audiogram is recommended. The better ear must not have an average hearing loss of more than 40 dB at 500, 1000, and 2000 Hz (to obtain an average, add the 3 decibel losses together and divide by 3).

Additional Reading: Commercial driver's license examination. In: *UpToDate*. 2022.

16. Understanding basic statistical analysis is useful in caring for patients with an evidence-based approach. Which term below is used to refer to the proportion of patients with a disease in whom a test result is positive?

A) Reliability
B) Sensitivity
C) Specificity
D) The *P* value
E) Variability

The answer is B: Sensitivity (the true positive rate) is defined as the proportion of people who are affected by a given disease and who test positive for that disease. For example, the proportion of patients who actually have coronary artery disease and also test positive with a treadmill exercise test would be defined as the sensitivity. Typically, the sensitivity for treadmill exercise testing is 72% to 96%.

Specificity (the true negative rate) is defined as the proportion of people who do not have a given disease and who test negative for that disease.

The *P*-value is the probability that, using a given statistical model, the null hypothesis is true. That is the finding is not due to chance. In clinical medicine, a *P*-value <0.05 is considered significant, and the smaller the *P*-value, the more statistically significance the finding. However, statistical significance only relates to the quality of the testing; it does not equate to clinical significance.

Additional Reading: Terms used in evidence-based medicine. *Am Fam Physician*. www.aafp.org/journals/afp/authors/ebm-toolkit/glossary.html

17. Which one of the following patients is eligible for the Medicare hospice benefit?

A) A patient with end-stage chronic obstructive pulmonary disease with a life expectancy of 6 months
B) A patient with amyotrophic lateral sclerosis with a life expectancy of 9 months
C) A patient on hemodialysis with a life expectancy of 12 months
D) A patient with stage IV breast cancer with a life expectancy of 18 months

The answer is A: Patients with a life expectancy of 6 months or less are eligible for the Medicare hospice benefit. This benefit allows patients to receive hospice care in either the home or hospital setting. In addition to patients with terminal cancer, patients with end-stage cardiac, pulmonary, and chronic debilitating diseases are eligible. Approximately two-thirds of patients enrolled in hospice die from non–cancer-related diagnoses, and approximately 60% of Medicare patients are not enrolled in hospice at the time of their death.

Additional Reading: The use of hospice care for patients without cancer. *Am Fam Physician*. 2010;82(10):1196.

18. In a placebo-controlled trial involving 100 patients, 30 patients died during the study period. Of the 30 patients, 10 had received the active drug and 20 had received a placebo; thus, the mortality rate was 40% for those treated with the placebo, but one-half of that, 20%, for those who received the active drug. The number needed to treat (NNT) can be calculated, and for this drug the NNT is which one of the following?

A) 5
B) 10
C) 25
D) 50
E) 100

The answer is A: The benefit of an intervention can be expressed by NNT. NNT is the reciprocal of the absolute risk reduction (ARR) (the absolute adverse event rate for placebo minus the absolute adverse event rate for treated patients). In this case, the risk of death without treatment was 40% (the placebo group), and the risk of death was reduced to 20% when treated. Thus, the ARR was 20% (40% − 20% = 20%). The relative risk reduction was 50%, a drop from 40% to 20%. Relative risk reduction often exaggerates the benefit.

Once you have calculated the ARR—in this case 0.20 (20%), you can calculate the NNT, which is the reciprocal 1/0.2 = 5. Thus, one can interpret the findings as "This study suggests that you have to treat five patients with this drug to prevent one death."

NNT varies for medical treatments—an NNT of 5 represents an effective medication.

Additional Reading: EBM glossary. *Am Fam Physician*. www.aafp.org/journals/afp/authors/ebm-toolkit/glossary.html

19. Personalized medicine refers to using a patient's genetic information (such as having a *BRCA* gene mutation) to predict their risk of disease and to customize treatments. The *BRCA* genetic locus has been linked with all of the listed cancers except which one?

A) Breast cancer
B) Colon cancer
C) Gastric cancer
D) Ovarian cancer
E) Prostate cancer

The answer is C: Discovered in the 1980s, *BRCA1* is a gene on chromosome 17 that is known to be involved in tumor suppression. A woman with certain known mutations in *BRCA1* has an increased risk for breast cancer and ovarian cancer. There is a higher risk in Ashkenazi Jewish women (most Jewish people in the United States are of this Eastern European origin). *BRCA2* is another susceptibility gene for breast cancer and is found on chromosome 13. Mutations in *BRCA2* confer an elevated breast cancer risk similar to that occurring with *BRCA1* mutations.

In a family with a history of breast and/or ovarian cancer, the family member who has breast or ovarian cancer should be tested first; if found to have a harmful *BRCA1* or *BRCA2* mutation, then other family members can be tested to see if they also have the mutation.

As many as one-third of women below age 29 years with breast cancer carry a *BRCA1* or *BRCA2* mutation, but only 2% of women aged 70 to 79 years with breast cancer carry such a mutation. Genetic studies in high-risk families suggest that *BRCA1* and *BRCA2* mutations may account for 50% of inherited breast and ovarian cancers and are also associated with an increase in prostate and colon cancers.

Known carriers should begin performing monthly breast self-examinations at age 18 years and should begin having annual clinical examinations at age 25 years. Annual mammography is also recommended beginning at age 25 years. Insufficient evidence exists to recommend for or against prophylactic mastectomy. Even this invasive procedure does not appear to provide definitive treatment because cases have been reported of breast cancer occurring after bilateral mastectomies.

Currently, the U.S. Preventive Services Task Force (USPSTF) recommends against routine referral for genetic counseling or routine breast cancer susceptibility gene (*BRCA*) testing for women whose family history is *not* associated with an increased risk for deleterious mutations in breast cancer susceptibility gene 1 (*BRCA1*) or breast cancer susceptibility gene 2 (*BRCA2*). Additionally, the USPSTF recommends that women whose family history is associated with an increased risk for deleterious mutations in *BRCA1* or *BRCA2* genes be referred for genetic counseling and evaluation for *BRCA* testing.

Additional Reading: Breast cancer screening update. *Am Fam Physician*. 2013;87(4):275-278.

20. The Health Insurance Portability and Accountability Act (HIPAA) of 1996 was updated in 2013 via the Final Omnibus Rule and enacted which one of the following measures?

A) Mandatory health insurance for all people earning less than $12,000 per year
B) A stringent code for the uniform transfer of medically related data
C) To allow health maintenance organizations more diagnostic testing of patients and less scrutiny of physicians
D) To allow all Americans to invest in a medical savings account
E) Improved access of third parties to patients' medical records

The answer is B: The HIPAA 1996 includes the "portability" aspect of the law (which protects the ability of people with current or preexisting medical conditions to get health insurance) and the "accountability" aspects of the law (which include enforcement). Its multiple provisions include strict codes for the uniform transfer of electronic data, including billing and other routine exchanges, and new patient rights regarding personal health information, including the right to access this information and to limit its disclosure. Also outlined are specific physical, procedural, and technological security protections that all health care organizations must take to ensure the confidentiality of patients' medical information. Every medical practice in the United States must comply with HIPAA regulations, including transaction standards (ie, the rules standardizing electronic data exchange of health-related information).

Additional Reading: HIPAA again: confronting the updated privacy and security rules. *Fam Pract Manag.* 2013;20(3):18-22.

21. The residents in your family practice are working on a quality improvement project and want to start exploring how an intervention could improve A1C levels in patients with type 2 diabetes. You ask them to run some reports for the practice using the electronic health record (EHR) to get a baseline first. What is the key purpose of using a registry?

A) To identify and eliminate care gaps, especially for high-risk patients.
B) To access shared patient data from hospitals and other providers.
C) To ease electronic health record documentation
D) To improve billing.

The answer is A: A registry is a population health tool that organizes data for a group of patients and provides timely, actionable reports that can be used to close care gaps or identify high-risk patients who may need more intense care.

A registry may be a simple spreadsheet populated from paper or electronic records, or it may be a more robust application available through an EHR or a third-party vendor.

Data validation ensures accuracy of the information so that practices can be confident using the registry to report quality measures.

Additional Reading: Put Your Clinical Data to Work with a Registry. *Fam Pract Manag.* 2021;28(6):21-24.

22. Approximately what percentage of antibiotic prescriptions in the ambulatory visit setting are considered unnecessary?

A) 5%
B) 10%
C) 30%
D) 55%

The answer is C: 30%.

Additional Reading: Antibiotic stewardship throughout the primary care visit: opportunities for office staff. *Fam Pract Manag.* 2021;28(6):10-14.

Section IV. Mental Health

Each of the following questions or incomplete statements is followed by suggested answers or completions. Select the ONE BEST ANSWER in each case.

1. The following are components of cognitive behavioral therapy (CBT) expect:

A) Weekly homework assignments
B) Treatment is goal oriented and collaborative; patient is expected to be an active participant.
C) One 60- to 90-minute in-person or virtual session per week, typically for 8 to 12 weeks.
D) Sessions that primarily focus on identifying the unconscious origin of the thoughts that affect the patient's actions.

The answer is D: Cognitive therapy is a psychological treatment method that helps patients correct false self-beliefs that contribute to certain moods and behaviors. The basic principle behind cognitive therapy is that a thought precedes a mood and that both are interrelated with a person's environment, physical reaction, and subsequent behavior. Therefore, changing a thought that arises in a given situation changes mood, behavior, and physical reaction. Although it is unclear who benefits most from cognitive therapy, motivated patients who have an internal center of control and the capacity for introspection likely would benefit most.

Understanding the subconscious or unconscious origins of the thoughts that affect the patient's actions is the focus of psychoanalytic therapy. This type of therapy may be the best fit for those who have undergone therapy for a long time and want to go deeper to understanding the unconscious mind.

Additional Reading: Common questions about cognitive behavior therapy for psychiatric disorders. *Am Fam Physician.* 2015;92(9):807-812.

2. Specific signs and symptoms can assist physicians in distinguishing between delirium and a preexisting psychiatric disorder in patients who are exhibiting unusual behaviors. Which one of the following is associated with delirium?

A) Auditory hallucinations
B) Feelings of hopelessness
C) Memory impairment
D) Slow onset with a variable course
E) Slowing on electroencephalography (EEG) recordings

The answer is E: EEG recordings can be useful in differentiating delirium from other conditions. In patients with delirium, the EEG displays a diffuse slowing of the background rhythm. An exception is patients with delirium tremens, where the EEG shows fast activity. EEGs are also useful in detecting ictal and postictal seizure activity, as well as nonconvulsive status epilepticus, all of which can present as delirium. Abnormal EEG readings would not be expected in patients with psychotic disorders or depression. However, slowing may occur in patients with dementia.

Visual hallucinations are an indicator of an underlying metabolic disturbance or adverse effect of medication or substance abuse. Although visual hallucinations can occur in patients with primary psychiatric illnesses such as schizophrenia, they are much less common than auditory hallucinations. Visual hallucinations that occur in patients with delirium can be formed (eg, people and animals) or unformed (eg, spots and flashes of light).

Additionally, the acute onset and fluctuating nature of delirium are hallmark features in distinguishing it from primary psychiatric disorders. Patients are often unable to provide an adequate history. It is important to interview family members and caregivers to determine the time of onset of symptoms and other pertinent medical and psychiatric information, including a review of medications and a history of substance abuse. It is also important to know how patients are currently different from their normal cognitive state. Psychiatric symptoms that arise in persons 50 years and older without a prior psychiatric history or the development of new symptoms in patients with pre-existing psychiatric illness should undergo a thorough medical workup.

Additional Reading: Delirium in older persons: evaluation and management. *Am Fam Physician*. 2014;90(3):150-158.

3. Obsessive-compulsive disorder (OCD) is characterized by recurrent obsessions and compulsive behaviors such as repeated hand washing and checking routines. Which of the following statements regarding the disorder is true?

A) CBT is rarely helpful in treatment.
B) Patients diagnosed with OCD rarely know they are affected.
C) Selective serotonin reuptake inhibitors (SSRIs) are often first-line therapy.
D) Structural changes are not found in the brain.
E) Successful treatment leads to symptom resolution.

The answer is C: OCD typically appears during the young adult years and has a chronic variable course. Although treatment can lessen the severity of the disorder, patients typically have some residual symptoms. It is often many years before affected patients are properly diagnosed and treated. OCD appears to have a genetic basis. Although some neurologic findings have been associated with OCD, such as increased gray matter and decreased white matter on brain imaging, the diagnosis remains a clinical one.

Patients with OCD are plagued by recurrent obsessions and often perform compulsive washing and checking rituals in an attempt to deal with the anxiety provoked by their obsessions. Those affected by OCD usually are aware that their behavior is irrational and may spend a lot of effort to hide their symptoms from others.

CBT is helpful in the treatment of OCD. In most patients, combining medication with behavioral therapy produces the best results. SSRIs should be utilized first, with other psychotropic agents added if initial therapy fails. The optimal SSRI dose for OCD tends to be higher than the dose used to treat depression, and an adequate trial of medication may take up to 12 weeks.

Additional Reading: Obsessive-compulsive disorder: diagnosis and management. *Am Fam Physician*. 2015;92(10):896-903.

4. The American Psychiatric Association's *DSM* outlines the criteria for diagnosing behavioral and mental health disorders. Which of the following is the *DSM* definition for an adjustment disorder with depressed mood?

A) A lifetime obsession with morbid thoughts
B) Tearfulness related to the death of a loved one over 1 year ago
C) Thoughts of death and morbid preoccupation with worthlessness with no obvious triggering event
D) Transient, normal depressive responses or mood changes to stress
E) The development of low mood, tearfulness or hopelessness, or behavioral symptoms in response to an identifiable stressor that occurs within 3 months of the onset of the stressor

The answer is E: Adjustment disorder with depressed mood is defined as development of emotional or behavioral symptoms in response to an identifiable stressor that occurs within 3 months of the stressor. Symptoms include depressed mood, tearfulness, and hopelessness and occur out of proportion to the severity or intensity of what would usually be expected from exposure to the stressor and cause significant impairment in social and occupational/academic functioning. Once the stressor (or its consequences) has terminated, the symptoms resolve within 6 months.

Additional Reading: American Psychiatric Association. *Diagnostic and Statistical Manual of Mental Disorders*. 5th ed. American Psychiatric Publishing; 2013.

5. Medications have various side effects, some of which can be life threatening. Which one of the following medications is limited by potentially life-threatening rashes?

A) Lamotrigine (Lamictal)
B) Fluoxetine (Prozac)
C) Gabapentin (Neurontin)
D) Phenytoin (Dilantin)
E) Tramadol (Ultram)

The answer is A: Lamotrigine is an anticonvulsant drug used in the treatment of epilepsy and bipolar depression. Many rapid cycling bipolar patients with major depression do not respond to a first-line treatment with quetiapine, and for these patients, treatment with lamotrigine is indicated.

Lamotrigine has also been proved to be modestly effective in patients with trigeminal neuralgia, neuropathy associated with human immunodeficiency virus infection, and poststroke pain. The drug is ineffective in patients with unspecified refractory neuropathic pain.

However, the use of lamotrigine is limited by potentially life-threatening rashes, which may develop in up to 10% of patients during the initial 1 to 2 months of therapy and necessitates discontinuation of the drug. The risk of developing a life-threatening rash such as Stevens-Johnson syndrome, toxic epidermal necrolysis, or angioedema is approximately 1 in 1000 adults.

Gabapentin is associated with the central nervous system and respiratory depression. Fluoxetine is associated with QT prolongation and increased suicidal ideation. Phenytoin is associated with severe hypotension and cardiac arrhythmias when administered via rapid infusion.

Additional Reading: Bipolar disorder in adults: pharmacotherapy for acute depression. In: *UpToDate*. 2022.

6. Postpartum psychosis (puerperal psychosis) is a psychiatric condition, which occurs after birth in a small percentage of women. This condition typically develops how soon after delivery?

A) During the first 1 to 3 months after delivery
B) 4 to 6 months after delivery
C) 6 to 12 months after delivery
D) After the child has reached the age of 1 year

The answer is A: The onset of puerperal psychosis occurs in the first 1 to 4 weeks after childbirth. The data suggest that this may be a presentation of bipolar disorder that is triggered by the hormonal shifts that occur after delivery. The patient develops frank psychosis, cognitive impairment, and grossly disorganized behavior that represent a complete change from previous functioning. When trying to determine if the presence of a symptom is a sign of depression or a normal postpartum reaction, the physician should consider the circumstances. Loss of energy and diminished concentration are frequently the result of sleep deprivation. A postpartum woman who has no energy or difficulty in concentrating or in making decisions is cause for concern. Determining how much time has elapsed since delivery helps the physician to distinguish the condition from subclinical mood fluctuations, which occur with such frequency during the first 2 weeks after delivery that they are considered part of the normal postpartum experience.

Postpartum "blues" is a transient condition characterized by mild, although often rapid, mood swings from elation to sadness, irritability, anxiety, decreased concentration, insomnia, tearfulness, and crying spells. 40% to 80% of postpartum women develop these mood changes, generally within 2 to 3 days of delivery, with symptoms peaking on the fifth postpartum day and resolution of symptoms within 2 weeks. Women who experience them have an increased risk for depression later in the postpartum period, especially if the symptoms were severe.

Subclinical mood swings in either direction (high vs low) after delivery are an indication for more intensive follow-up later in the postpartum period, and clinicians are encouraged to screen for depression and related symptoms at the first postpartum follow-up visit or at least by 6 weeks' postpartum. Finally, depression must be distinguished from puerperal psychosis. Most puerperal psychoses have their onset within the first month of delivery and are related to mania. An inability to sleep for several nights, agitation, expansive or irritable mood, and avoidance of the infant are early warning signs that herald the onset of puerperal psychosis.

Because the woman is at risk of harming herself or her baby (or both), postpartum psychosis is a medical emergency. Most patients with puerperal psychosis require inpatient treatment in a hospital with neuroleptic agents and mood stabilizers. Before a definitive diagnosis is made, depression caused by a medical condition such as thyroid dysfunction or anemia must be ruled out.

Additional Reading: Identification and management of peripartum depression. *Am Fam Physician*. 2016;93(10):852-858.

> **Postpartum "blues" is a transient condition characterized by mild, although often rapid mood, swings from elation to sadness, irritability, anxiety, decreased concentration, insomnia, tearfulness, and crying spells. 40% to 80% of postpartum women develop such mood changes, generally within 2 to 3 days of delivery, with symptoms peaking on the fifth postpartum day and resolution within 2 weeks.**

7. Haloperidol is a typical antipsychotic medication used in the treatment of schizophrenia, mania in bipolar disorder, and acute psychosis. Which one of the following statements is true regarding the use of haloperidol?

A) Haloperidol is US Food and Drug Administration (FDA)–approved for intravenous (IV) use.
B) Haloperidol is considered safe in those with a known seizure disorder.
C) Haloperidol can cause prolongation of the QT interval.
D) Electrocardiogram monitoring is not necessary when the drug is given orally.
E) None of the above.

The answer is C: Although haloperidol has not been FDA approved for IV use, it is commonly used intravenously and is generally thought to be safe. Haloperidol may alter cardiac conduction and prolong the QT interval leading to life-threatening arrhythmias. It should be used with caution or avoided in patients with electrolyte abnormalities. Electrocardiographic monitoring is always necessary. Haloperidol should be avoided if possible in patients with a known seizure disorder as it may lower the seizure threshold.

Additional Reading: Haloperidol: drug information. In: *UpToDate*. 2022.

8. Sexual dysfunction is a common side effect of psychotropic medications, including those listed below. Which one of the following medications is least likely to cause problems with libido?

A) Bupropion
B) Cimetidine
C) Citalopram
D) Fluoxetine
E) Risperidone

The answer is A: Consistent evidence shows that, with the exception of bupropion, mirtazapine, and trazodone, most antidepressant medications may cause a decline in libido or sexual functioning despite improvement of depression. Up to one-half of patients surveyed before and after starting therapy with the selective serotonin reuptake inhibitors such as fluoxetine, paroxetine, fluvoxamine, citalopram, and sertraline reported a decline in libido with medication use.

Even when patients report improvements in depression with treatment, some continue to experience a lowered libido. Sexual dysfunction, including low sexual desire, in men and women may be the consequence of psychologic or emotional factors, hormonal abnormalities, autonomic neuropathy, vascular insufficiency, or drug side effects.

Several antipsychotic agents, including haloperidol, thioridazine, and risperidone, can decrease libido. Cimetidine, in contrast to ranitidine, has been found to lower libido and cause erectile dysfunction.

Psychologic and interpersonal factors commonly affect sexual desire. These factors include stressful life events (loss of job or family trauma), life milestones (children leaving home), fatigue, lack of privacy, and ongoing relationship problems. Alcohol and narcotics are also known to decrease libido, arousal, and orgasm.

Additional Reading: Sexual dysfunction caused by SSRIs: management. In: *UpToDate*. 2022.

9. When considering light therapy for seasonal affective disorder (SAD), which one of the following conditions is not a factor in predicting a positive result?

A) A history of reactivity to ambient light
B) A positive family history of SAD
C) An increased intake of sweet foods later in the day
D) Having a high number of vegetative symptoms
E) The presence of hypersomnia

The answer is B: SAD is a mood disturbance with a seasonal pattern, typically occurring in the autumn and winter with remission in the spring or summer. Light therapy is a generally well-tolerated treatment, with most patients experiencing clinical improvement within 1 to 2 weeks after the start of therapy.

Light therapy involves exposure to minimum 2500 lux of visible light. 10,000 lux for 30 min/d has been shown to be effective. Factors that have predicted a positive response to light therapy include hypersomnia, high rate of vegetative symptoms, an increased intake of sweet foods in the afternoon, and a history of reactivity to ambient light. A positive family history does not necessarily increase a positive response to light therapy.

Additional Reading: Seasonal affective disorder. *Am Fam Physician*. 2012;86(11):1037-1041.

10. Assessing behaviors is useful to categorize various patient actions. Urges or impulses to repeat behaviors in a stereotyped manner in an attempt to relieve anxiety are consistent with which one of the following terms?

A) Adaptation
B) Congruence
C) Compulsion
D) Obsession
E) Transference

The answer is C: Compulsions are (1) repetitive behaviors or mental acts (eg, hand washing, ordering, and checking) that the individual feels driven to perform in response to an obsession or according to rules that must be rigidly applied and (2) the behaviors or mental acts that are aimed at preventing or reducing anxiety or distress or preventing some dreaded situation (even though they are not connected in any realistic way with what they are designed to neutralize or prevent, or are clearly excessive).

An obsession is a persistent thought, urge, or image that is experienced as intrusive and unwanted and that in most people is associated with marked anxiety or distress. The person tries to suppress such thoughts, urges, or images with some other thoughts or actions (eg, compulsion). In many cases, these obsessions have a theme that an insignificant oversight will result in tremendous catastrophe. Other common themes are contamination, a need for ordering things, aggressive impulses, and sexual imagery.

Additional Reading: American Psychiatric Association. *Diagnostic and Statistical Manual of Mental Disorders*. 5th ed. American Psychiatric Publishing; 2013.

11. Which of the following medications is used in the classic treatment of bipolar I disorder and mania?

A) Alprazolam
B) Amitriptyline
C) Lithium
D) Phenytoin
E) Sertraline

The answer is C: Lithium is considered a first-line medication for bipolar I disorder and has been more widely studied than any other maintenance treatment for bipolar I disorder and is consistently supported across multiple randomized trials. Bipolar I disorder is most commonly diagnosed in persons between 18 and 24 years of age, with the mean age of onset for a first manic, hypomanic, or depressive episode at 18 years of age.

The clinical presentations of this disorder are diverse and include mania, hypomania, and psychosis. Frequently associated conditions include substance abuse, attention-deficit/hyperactivity disorder, anxiety disorders, and other mood disorders. Patients with acute mania must be evaluated urgently. Treatment involves the use of mood stabilizers such as lithium, valproic acid, and carbamazepine.

Additional Reading: Bipolar disorders: a review. *Am Fam Physician*. 2012;85(5):483-493.

12. Which one of the following statements best describes cognitive behavioral therapy (CBT)?

A) A treatment process that helps patients reverse unhelpful beliefs that lead to distressing moods and behaviors
B) A confrontation with the patient that exposes certain inadequacies in social interaction
C) A process of introspective review of past behaviors that highlights poor judgment
D) Therapy that involves a repeated exposure to one's fears to overcome associated anxiety
E) Therapy that involves an exhaustive review of past events to outline previous failures

The answer is A: Cognitive therapy is defined as a treatment process that helps patients identify and change unhelpful beliefs that lead to problematic moods and behaviors. The basic principle behind cognitive therapy is that a thought comes before an emotion and that both are associated with a person's environment, physical reaction, and subsequent behavior. As a result, changing a thought that arises in a given situation can alter one's emotions, behavior, and physical reactions. Motivated patients who have an internal locus of control and the capacity for introspection tend to benefit most.

During cognitive therapy, the therapist assists the patient with several steps. First, the patient accepts that some of his or her perceptions and interpretations of reality may not be entirely true (because of past experience or hereditary or biologic reasons) and that these interpretations lead to negative thoughts. Next, the patient learns to recognize the negative (surface or "automatic") thoughts and discovers alternative thoughts that reflect reality more closely. The patient then decides internally whether the evidence supports the negative thought or the alternative thought.

Ideally, the patient will recognize distorted thinking and "reframe" the situation. As cognitive therapy progresses, it focuses more on reframing deeply held or "core" beliefs about self and the world.

In CBT for depression, behavioral principles are used to overcome a patient's reluctance at the beginning of therapy and to reinforce positive activities. An important part of CBT for depression is having the patient participate in pleasurable activities, especially with others, which usually give positive reinforcement.

Additional Reading: Common questions about cognitive behavior therapy for psychiatric disorders. *Am Fam Physician*. 2015;92(9):807-813.

13. You are seeing a middle-aged woman who is dying from ovarian cancer. She appears sad today and reports feeling tired. She questions whether she is developing depression. Which one of the following is used to detect depression in a dying patient?

A) Concern over being a burden
B) Crying spells
C) Dependency feelings
D) Pervasive hopelessness
E) Weight loss

The answer is D: Serious and progressive illness evokes distress in patients, families, and clinicians, often engendering fear, anxiety, anger, dread, sadness, helplessness, and uncertainty. Hope permits patients, their families, and loved ones to cope with these difficult emotions and helps them endure the stresses of treatment. A person who is grieving maintains a sense of hope. Hope may change from the hope for a cure to the hope for prolonging life to the hope to live comfortably and without pain for the duration of life, but it is not lost in persons who are dying.

Grief is an adaptive, universal, and highly personalized response to the multiple losses that occur at the end of life. The symptoms of grief may overlap with those of major depression or a terminal illness or its treatment; however, grief is a distinct entity, separate from depression.

Feelings of pervasive hopelessness, helplessness, worthlessness, guilt, lack of pleasure, and suicidal ideation are present in patients with depression, but not in those experiencing grief. Pervasive hopelessness is a hallmark of depression.

Additional Reading: Managing grief and depression at the end of life. *Am Fam Physician*. 2012;86(3):259-264.

14. A young woman presents with a history of binge eating, after which she vomits. You obtain a metabolic panel and expect to see which one of the following electrolyte abnormalities in a bulimic patient such as this individual?

A) Metabolic acidosis
B) Respiratory acidosis
C) Metabolic alkalosis
D) Respiratory alkalosis
E) Normal electrolytes

The answer is C: Bulimia nervosa involves the uncontrolled eating of an abnormally large amount of food in a short period, followed by compensatory behaviors, such as self-induced vomiting, laxative abuse, or excessive exercise. Symptoms and signs of bulimia include reflux esophagitis, abdominal cramping, diarrhea, and rectal bleeding. Electrolyte abnormalities and metabolic alkalosis signal extreme purging habits in a bulimic patient. Patients with anorexia generally have laboratory test results within normal limits until the late stage of the condition.

Additional Reading: Initial evaluation, diagnosis, and treatment of anorexia nervosa and bulimia nervosa. *Am Fam Physician*. 2015;91(1):46-52.

15. A 39-year-old woman is asking if you can refill her antidepressant. It was prescribed by a psychiatrist to treat severe depression, but he has retired. The patient cannot recall the medication that she is taking, but she remembers that the psychiatrist told her to avoid red wine and cheese. Which one of the following classes of psychotropic medication is this patient most likely taking?

A) An anxiolytic
B) A neuroleptic
C) A monoamine oxidase inhibitor (MAOI)
D) A selective serotonin reuptake inhibitor (SSRI)
E) A TCA

The answer is C: Antidepressant medications have various actions, and drug selection should depend on the symptoms and the side effect profile of the medication:

- MAOIs: These include phenelzine and tranylcypromine. MAOIs are not used frequently for the treatment of depression because of the potential for severe side effects. Interactions with sympathomimetic medications or tyramine-containing foods (eg, cheeses, wines, beers, aged meats and fruits, beans, liver, and yeast extracts) can lead to a hypertensive crisis. Orthostatic hypotension, nausea, insomnia, and sexual dysfunction are also common
- Tricyclic antidepressants (TCAs): These include amitriptyline, imipramine, nortriptyline, and desipramine. TCAs have been commonly used in the treatment of depression since the mid-1980s. These medications may require 2 to 6 weeks before full therapeutic effect is noted. Many have anticholinergic side effects. Amitriptyline has the most anticholinergic properties, including dry mouth, blurred vision, constipation, ileus, urinary retention, and even delirium. In most cases, these side effects improve with time.
- SSRIs: These include fluoxetine, paroxetine, citalopram, escitalopram, and sertraline. SSRIs are effective in the treatment of depression and have a lower incidence of side effects compared with TCAs. The risk of death from overdose is also low with these medications. They are activating and should be given during the day.
- Serotonin-norepinephrine reuptake inhibitors: This group includes venlafaxine and duloxetine. They have dual serotonin and norepinephrine mechanism of action.
- Norepinephrine-dopamine reuptake inhibitors: The only antidepressant in this class is bupropion.
- Serotonin modulators: These medications primarily block the serotonin-2 receptor and inhibit reuptake of serotonin and norepinephrine. The group includes nefazodone, trazodone, and mirtazapine.

Additional Reading: Drugs for depression. *Med Lett Drugs Ther*. 2020 (1592).

16. A 27-year-old woman presents with complaints of fatigue, a decreased appetite, and insomnia. She also reports trouble concentrating at work, and although she is an avid hiker, she has not been interested in any recent excursions arranged by her friends. The most likely diagnosis to explain her presentation is which one of the following conditions?

A) Anorexia nervosa
B) Bulimia
C) Cyclothymia
D) Depression
E) Somatoform disorder

The answer is D: Common symptoms that are associated with clinical depression include depressed mood, diminished interest or pleasure, significant appetite or weight change, sleep disturbances, agitation, fatigue, feelings of worthlessness or guilt, difficulty with concentration, or suicidal thoughts. Symptoms must be present for at least 2 weeks before the diagnosis is made. In addition, symptoms must be present almost daily and must represent a change from the patient's previous level of functioning. Other contributing causes must be ruled out. Either a depressed mood or anhedonia (a loss of pleasure in previously enjoyable activities) must also be present for the diagnosis.

Cyclothymia (cyclothymic disorder) is associated with emotional ups and downs, but they are not as extreme as those in bipolar I or II disorder.

Somatoform disorder presents with various bodily symptoms, such as pain, gastrointestinal complaints, and sexual issues. The symptoms may or may not be traceable to a physical cause, but they are associated with disproportionate levels of distress. Many individuals also suffer with anxiety.

Additional Reading: American Psychiatric Association. *Diagnostic and Statistical Manual of Mental Disorders*, 5th ed. American Psychiatric Publishing; 2013.

17. You have been caring for a young woman with an eating disorder, who is slowly recovering. She stopped menstruating a year ago and now she is regaining weight. She is asking at what point she can expect her menstrual periods to resume. You tell her that she should expect her periods to return when she is regained enough weight to be at what percent of her ideal body weight?

A) 75% of ideal body weight
B) 80% of ideal body weight
C) 90% of ideal body weight
D) 100% of body weight
E) As it has been more than a year, she is unlikely to resume menstruating

The answer is C: Menstruation usually resumes in women affected with anorexia when the patient approaches 90% of ideal body weight.

Additional Reading: Initial evaluation, diagnosis, and treatment of anorexia nervosa and bulimia nervosa. *Am Fam Physician*. 2015;91(1):46-52.

18. Various behaviors are seen in a patient with bulimia. Which of the following are associated with bulimia?

A) Anxiety
B) Mood disorders
C) Poor impulse control
D) Substance abuse
E) All of the above

The answer is E: Young women with bulimia characteristically have psychiatric comorbidities, across a wide range of mental disorders. There is an increased frequency of depressive symptoms, low self-esteem, and bipolar and depressive disorders. There is also an increased frequency of anxiety disorders as well as substance use disorders, especially alcohol and stimulant use. Poor impulse control is associated with bulimia nervosa, which might result in patients engaging in risky behaviors such as unprotected sexual activity, self-mutilation, and suicide attempts.

Additional Reading: American Psychiatric Association. *Diagnostic and Statistical Manual of Mental Disorders*. 5th ed. American Psychiatric Publishing; 2013.

19. Obsessive-compulsive disorder (OCD) can be difficult for physicians to address and causes significant distress for patients and families. Which one of the following statements regarding this condition is true?

A) Anxiety is a central feature.
B) Compulsions are thoughts or ideas that recur.
C) Most affected patients have obsessions as well as compulsions.
D) Obsessions are repetitive behaviors.
E) Patients are usually unaware of their actions and thoughts and are resistant to them.

The answer is A: OCD is characterized by the presence of obsessions and/or compulsions (ie, recurrent actions or ideas that interfere with normal daily activities). Anxiety is a central feature of this disorder, but it is generated by internal thoughts as opposed to external circumstances. The patient is usually aware of the actions and thoughts and feels a strong inner resistance toward them.

Obsessions are defined as thoughts or ideas that recur, and the patient tries to repress them. Common obsessions include fear of dirt, germs, or contamination; disgust with bodily waste or secretions; fear of harming a family member or friend; concern with order, symmetry (balance), and exactness; worry that a task has been done poorly, even when the person knows this is not true; fear of thinking evil or sinful thoughts; constantly thinking about certain sounds, images, words, or numbers; or a constant need for reassurance.

Compulsions are repetitive behaviors that are performed in response to the obsessions. Common compulsions include cleaning and grooming rituals, such as excessive hand washing, showering, and toothbrushing; checking rituals involving drawers, door locks, and appliances to ensure they are shut, locked, or turned off; repeating rituals, such as going in and out of a door, sitting down and getting up from a chair, and touching certain objects several times; putting items in a certain order or arrangement; counting over and over to a certain number; saving newspapers, mail, or containers when they are no longer needed; or seeking reassurance and approval.

Obsessions and compulsions can have an aggressive or sexual attachment. Fewer than 10% of patients have both obsessions and compulsions; however, individuals may exhibit multiple obsessions or multiple compulsions.

The neurosis affects men and women equally and is often found in those of a higher socioeconomic class with above-average intelligence. The condition usually becomes apparent in childhood. Clomipramine (Anafranil) helps many people with OCD and usually decreases symptoms to mild levels. Side effects from this drug, such as dry mouth, constipation and drowsiness, and sometimes an inability to achieve orgasm, are common. Fluoxetine, sertraline, paroxetine, and fluvoxamine (Luvox) can also help some patients with OCD.

Additional Reading: American Psychiatric Association. *Diagnostic and Statistical Manual of Mental Disorders*. 5th ed. American Psychiatric Publishing; 2013.

Obsessions are thoughts or ideas that recur, and the patient tries to repress them. Compulsions are repetitive behaviors that are performed in response to the obsessions.

20. A manic patient has been admitted and treated with intramuscular doses of haloperidol. You are called by the nursing staff because he has now developed a high fever, tachycardia, tachypnea, diaphoresis, and hypertension. You suspect that he has developed which one of the following syndromes?

A) Malignant hyperthermia
B) Neuroleptic malignant syndrome
C) Rhabdomyolysis
D) Sepsis
E) Serotonin syndrome

The answer is B: Neuroleptic malignant syndrome is an uncommon idiosyncratic condition that is associated with the use of dopamine antagonist (ie, antipsychotic medications). It is usually associated with the more potent typical antipsychotics, such as haloperidol and the piperazine phenothiazines (perphenazine, fluphenazine, trifluoperazine).

The symptoms include high fever (102-104 °F), tachycardia, tachypnea, diaphoresis, autonomic dysfunction, mental status changes, hypertension or hypotension, tremors, and leukocytosis. Seizures can be precipitated as well. Significant elevations of serum creatine kinase may signal rhabdomyolysis as a complication of muscle rigidity. Other complications include respiratory failure, myocardial infarction, and renal and hepatic failure. Disseminated intravascular coagulopathy may also occur.

Treatment involves stopping the antipsychotic, supportive care, and the use of intravenous dantrolene. Bromocriptine, amantadine, and benzodiazepines can also be used. Mortality approaches 30%.

Additional Reading: Adverse effects of antipsychotic medications. *Am Fam Physician*. 2010;81(5):617-622.

21. As much as a third of the population may have a panic attack during any year, but far fewer are affected with panic disorder. Panic disorder is defined as recurrent, unexpected attacks that may involve which one of the following symptoms?

A) Flight of ideas
B) Hallucinations
C) Feelings of choking
D) Feelings of envy
E) Feelings of loss

The answer is C: According to the *DSM 5*, the definition of panic attack is a sudden surge of intense fear or intense discomfort that reaches a peak within minutes and is accompanied by at least four of the following symptoms:

- Palpitation, pounding heart, or accelerated heat rate
- Sweating
- Trembling or shaking
- Sensations of shortness of breath or smothering
- Feelings of choking
- Chest pain or discomfort
- Nausea or abdominal distress
- Feeling dizzy, lightheaded, unsteady, or faint
- Chills or heat sensations
- Paresthesias
- Derealization
- Fear of losing control or going crazy
- Fear of dying

Panic disorder is diagnosed when there are recurrent unexpected panic attacks, and at least one of the attacks has occurred after at least a month of one or both the following:

- Persistent concern or worry about additional attacks or its consequences
- Significant maladaptive change in behavior related to the attacks

Treatment for panic disorders involves counseling, antidepressants (eg, paroxetine and buspirone), and benzodiazepines (eg, alprazolam).

Additional Reading: American Psychiatric Association. *Diagnostic and Statistical Manual of Mental Disorders*. 5th ed. American Psychiatric Publishing; 2013.

22. You are seeing an older man who has been suffering from Parkinson disease (PD). Recently, his wife has been concerned because he has been experiencing some hallucinations and voicing paranoid thoughts. Which one of the following medications is best indicated in a patient with PD who experiences psychosis?

A) Haloperidol (Haldol)
B) Olanzapine (Zyprexa)
C) Quetiapine (Seroquel)
D) Risperidone (Risperdal)
E) Thioridazine (Mellaril)

The answer is C: Psychosis is a frequent complication of PD, and hallucinations are the most common manifestation, affecting up to 40% of patients with PD, particularly those at an advanced stage of illness. The most important triggers are antiparkinson medications; other triggers include infection, delirium, or dementia.

Quetiapine (Seroquel) has shown promise in the treatment of psychosis in elderly patients with Alzheimer disease and PD. It improves psychosis in patients with PD without exacerbating movement disorders. This feature has led some experts to recommend it as the first-line agent for treatment of psychosis in patients with PD.

Haloperidol and thioridazine can cause drug-induced parkinsonism, akathisia, acute dystonia, and tardive dyskinesia. Risperidone exacerbates movement disorders in patients with PD. In patients with PD, olanzapine was found to increase motor symptoms.

Additional Reading: Parkinson disease. *Am Fam Physician*. 2020;102(11):679-691.

23. Quetiapine (Seroquel) is a second-generation or "atypical" antipsychotic and like other agents in this class has side effects. Which one of the following is a potential side effect of quetiapine?

A) Agranulocytosis
B) Cataract formation
C) Hepatotoxicity
D) Thrombocytopenia
E) Weight gain

The answer is B: Common side effects for quetiapine (Seroquel) include sedation, headache, and orthostatic hypotension. Cataract formation was noticed in premarketing studies, but a causal relationship has not been found. However, screening for cataract formation is recommended at the initiation of therapy and at 6-month intervals thereafter.

Additional Reading: *Quetiapine: drug information*. In: *UpToDate*. 2022.

24. Fluoxetine (Prozac) is a selective serotonin reuptake inhibitor (SSRI) antidepressant. Which one of the following statements about this medication is true?

A) Side effects often include dry mouth, urinary retention, and blurred vision.
B) The treatment of panic disorder typically requires higher doses than the recommended starting dose for depression.
C) The mechanism of action includes the reuptake of dopamine at the postsynaptic junction.
D) The drug has significant anticholinergic activity.
E) Treatment of bulimia typically requires higher doses than the recommended starting dose for depression.

The answer is E: Fluoxetine is US Food and Drug Administration approved for the treatment of depression, obsessive-compulsive disorder (OCD), premenstrual dysphoric disorder, panic disorder, and bulimia nervosa. Other uses include the treatment of dysthymic disorder, posttraumatic stress disorder, social phobia, and bipolar disorder depression in combination with other medication, fibromyalgia, and Raynaud phenomenon.

The medication is an SSRI, which has little anticholinergic activity (which can cause blurred vision, urinary retention, and dry mouth). The starting dose of fluoxetine is usually 10 to 20 mg/d, which can then be titrated up to achieve a clinical response; 80 mg/d is the maximum dosage. The full therapeutic response may take up to 4 weeks. Higher dosages (60 mg/d or more) are recommended for the treatment of bulimia and OCD. The treatment of panic disorder often requires smaller initial doses. Initial doses of 20 mg may precipitate panic attacks and lead to a high discontinuation rate; therefore, starting at 10 mg/d for patients with panic disorder can be helpful.

Side effects include headaches, anxiety, nervousness, excessive sweating, insomnia, anorexia, weight loss, nausea, diarrhea, and rash. Depressed patients should be monitored closely for suicidal thoughts or gestures, especially once their depression starts to improve. In most cases, medication for depression is complemented with counseling and is more effective than medication alone.

Additional Reading: Fluoxetine: drug information. In: *UpToDate*. 2022.

25. Seasonal affective disorder (SAD) is a depressive disorder that has seasonal variations. The treatment of choice for this disorder is which one of the following therapies?

A) Electroconvulsive shock treatment
B) Intense white light therapy
C) Psychotherapy
D) Monoamine oxidase inhibitors
E) Tricyclic antidepressants

The answer is B: SAD is a pattern of major depressive episodes that occur and remit with changes in seasons. Two patterns have been identified. The most often recognized is the fall-onset type, also known as winter depression, in which major depressive episodes begin in the late fall to early winter months and remit during the summer months. Atypical signs and symptoms of depression predominate in cases of winter depression and include the following:

- Increased rather than decreased sleep
- Increased rather than decreased appetite and food intake with carbohydrate craving
- Marked increase in weight
- Irritability
- Interpersonal difficulties (especially rejection sensitivity)
- Leaden paralysis (a heavy, leaden feeling in the arms or legs)

A spring-onset pattern (summer depression) also has been described in which the severe depressive episode begins in late spring to early summer and is characterized by typical vegetative symptoms of depression, such as decreased sleep, weight loss, and poor appetite.

Patients with winter depression usually reside in the more northern regions, and symptoms tend to develop when the days become shorter and nighttime is more prolonged. Treatment with intense white light has proved to be successful in controlling symptoms. Light therapy is initiated with a 10,000-lux light box directed toward the patient at a downward slant. The patient's eyes should remain open throughout the treatment session; however, staring directly into the light source is unnecessary and is not advised. The patient should start with a single 10- to 15-minute session per day, gradually increasing the session's duration to 30 to 45 minutes. Sessions should be increased to twice a day if symptoms worsen. Ninety minutes a day is the conventional daily maximum duration of therapy, although there is no reason to limit the duration of sessions if side effects are not severe.

Additional Reading: Seasonal affective disorder. *Am Fam Physician*. 2012;86(11):1037-1041.

26. Personality disorders can be difficult to treat. Which one of the following is a characteristic of antisocial personality disorder?

A) Adolescents under the age of 18 are commonly affected.
B) Many have a record of stealing, fighting, rape, or arson.
C) Symptoms include severe agoraphobia.
D) Schizophrenia may coexist.
E) Those who are affected suppress their conflicts.

The answer is B: Patients with antisocial personality disorder are often impulsive, reckless, and immoral. They often had previous problems concerning truancy, cruelty to animals and other individuals, and initiation of fights and use of weapons with fighting. They usually have a record of stealing, possibly rape, arson, and falsifying the truth since childhood.

Although *DSM* diagnostic criteria state that someone must be above 18 years of age, the definition also requires that a pattern of irresponsible behavior must be present since the age of 15, with school suspension, employment problems, poor parenting, lack of monogamy (no monogamous relationship lasting more than 1 year), and failed financial obligations in the absence of schizophrenia or manic episodes.

People with antisocial personality disorder act out their conflicts or go against the rules of social normalcy and, in many cases, those affected lack regard for other people's rights.

Additional Reading: American Psychiatric Association. *Diagnostic and Statistical Manual of Mental Disorders*. 5th ed. American Psychiatric Association; 2013.

27. All of the following medications are classified as selective serotonin reuptake inhibitors (SSRIs), except which one?

A) Escitalopram (Lexapro)
B) Fluoxetine (Prozac)
C) Mirtazapine (Remeron)
D) Paroxetine (Paxil)
E) Sertraline (Zoloft)

The answer is C: Mirtazapine (Remeron) is a tetracyclic antidepressant unrelated to tricyclic antidepressants and SSRIs. It is unique in its action among the currently available antidepressants. It is referred to as a serotonin modulator. Mirtazapine is a presynaptic α_2-adrenergic receptor antagonist plus a potent antagonist of postsynaptic serotonin-2 and serotonin-3 receptors. The net outcome of these effects is stimulation of the release of norepinephrine and serotonin. The drug has antidepressant and anxiolytic effects. It can cause sedation and weight gain but does not cause sexual dysfunction.

Additional Reading: Atypical antidepressants: pharmacology, administration, and side effects. In: *UpToDate*. Waltham, MA: 2022.

28. Many medications cause withdrawal symptoms, including selective serotonin reuptake inhibitors (SSRIs). Which one of the following SSRIs is most likely to cause withdrawal symptoms with abrupt discontinuation?

A) Citalopram (Celexa)
B) Fluoxetine (Prozac)
C) Paroxetine (Paxil)
D) Sertraline (Zoloft)

The answer is C: Studies have shown that when comparing fluoxetine, sertraline, paroxetine, and citalopram, withdrawal from paroxetine was shown to cause more severe symptoms that may occur more quickly, even after the second missed dose. Withdrawal symptoms can include dysphoric mood, irritability, agitation, dizziness, sensory disturbances (eg, electric shocklike sensations), anxiety, confusion, headache, lethargy, emotional lability, insomnia, hypomania, tinnitus, and seizures.

Fluoxetine may have the least severe withdrawal symptoms because of its long half-life. Methods to prevent antidepressant discontinuation syndrome include tapering the drug and educating the patient to avoid sudden cessation of the medication. Reintroduction of the medication will usually reverse severe symptoms within 24 hours.

Additional Reading: Drugs for depression. *Med Lett Drugs Ther*. 2020 (1592).

29. Which of the following factors is associated with persistent depressive disorder?

A) Flight of ideas
B) Mania
C) Myasthenia gravis
D) Sleep disturbances
E) Substance abuse

The answer is D: Persistent depressive disorder, also referred to as dysthymia, is known as a condition characterized by depressed mood for at least 2 years with concomitant impairment in some areas of functioning. The *DSM 5* consolidated major depressive disorder and dysthymia into a diagnosis called persistent depressive disorder. Persistent depressive disorder is characterized by depressed mood for most of the day, more days than not, for at least 2 years. Although depressed, two or more of the following must also be present:

- Appetite changes
- Sleep disturbances
- Low energy or fatigue
- Low self-esteem
- Poor concentration/difficulty making decisions
- Feelings of hopelessness

In this new diagnosis, criteria for major depressive disorder can be present continuously but the symptoms must not have another medical cause or be explained by the use of substances. The patient cannot have a history of mania, hypomania, or cyclothymia.

Additional Reading: American Psychiatric Association. *Diagnostic and Statistical Manual of Mental Disorders*. 5th ed. American Psychiatric Association; 2013.

30. A 24-year-old nonbinary graduate student presents to your clinic with concerns about having attention-deficit/hyperactivity disorder (ADHD) after watching a video on social media. They report inattentiveness and a lack of concentration for the last few years resulting in poorer academic performance than when they were an undergraduate. They say their husband also complains of their lack of focus and attentiveness when attending to household chores. They do not recall having similar problems when they were younger.

In order to diagnose adult ADHD you need:

A) Evidence of symptoms of ADHD present before age 12
B) Evidence of symptoms of ADHD present before age 6
C) A therapeutic trial of short-acting stimulant like Adderall.
D) A therapeutic trial of a medication like Atomoxetine.

The answer is A: ADHD affects 4% to 5% of US adults and can cause significant personal distress and negative impact on work performance and relationships. When evaluating an adult for a new diagnosis of ADHD, it is important to consider a differential diagnosis with other considerations that have similar symptoms like hearing impairment, a history of head trauma, drug side effects, thyroid disease, sleep apnea, hepatic disease, and lead toxicity. Diagnosing an adult with ADHD is challenging and often involves obtaining a longitudinal history starting with primary school years and obtaining collateral information.

Additional Reading: Diagnosis and management of attention-deficit/hyperactivity disorder in adults. *Am Fam Physician*. 2012;85(9):890-896.

31. You are seeing a patient with a major depressive disorder. His psychiatrist has suggested a trial of a monoamine oxidase inhibitor (MAOI), in place of his current fluoxetine, which has not been effective. How long should a patient be off fluoxetine, before taking an MAOI?

A) 1 day
B) 3 days
C) 1 week
D) 1 month
E) No delay is necessary

The answer is D: Because of fluoxetine's long half-life, patients should allow at least a 4-week elapse between the discontinuation of fluoxetine and commencement of MAOI therapy. Because the combination of MAOIs and other antidepressants can result in severe toxicity (eg, hypertensive crisis and serotonin syndrome), it is recommended that 2 weeks elapse between discontinuing an MAOI and starting a different antidepressant. Two weeks should also elapse between discontinuing a tricyclic antidepressant, selective serotonin reuptake inhibitor (other than fluoxetine), venlafaxine, duloxetine, or mirtazapine and starting an MAOI. When switching between MAOIs, we recommend that 2 weeks elapse between discontinuing the first MAOI and starting the second as well.

Additional Reading: Antidepressant medication in adults: switching and discontinuing medication. In: *UpToDate*. 2022.

32. Which one of the following statements is associated with an adjustment disorder?

A) Depression and anxiety are commonly associated.
B) Medication is usually indicated for treatment.
C) Support groups are rarely of any benefit.
D) The patient has an expected reaction to a known stressor.
E) The condition is usually long term, lasting for several years or more.

The answer is A: An adjustment disorder is defined as an excessive maladaptive reaction to an identifiable psychosocial stressor (eg, death of a loved one, loss of a job, marital discord, or divorce) that has occurred within the previous 3 months. The reaction may affect social relationships or the ability to function effectively at work or school. The disturbance cannot last for more than 6 months, and other mental disorders must be ruled out. In most cases, depression and anxiety are major manifestations. The best treatment is psychosocial support to help enhance the patient's ability to cope and adapt to stressful conditions. In most cases, medication is not necessary; rather, psychotherapy (individual, family, behavioral, and self-help groups) is used in treatment.

Additional Reading: *American Psychiatric Association. Diagnostic and Statistical Manual of Mental Disorders*. 5th ed. American Psychiatric Publishing; 2013.

An adjustment disorder is an excessive maladaptive reaction to an identifiable psychosocial stressor (eg, death of a loved one, loss of a job, marital discord, and divorce) that has occurred within the previous 3 months.

33. Which one of the following is true about somatization disorder, now called somatic symptom disorder in *DSM 5*?

A) Men are more commonly affected than women.
B) Patients exhibit multiple physical complaints that usually have an identifiable physiologic basis.
C) Symptoms rarely affect the patient's interpersonal relationships.
D) The condition usually develops after the age of 50 years.
E) Treatment involves frequent office visits and reassurance to the patient.

The answer is E: Somatic symptom disorder (previously called somatization disorder) is a condition characterized by one or more somatic complaints that are distressing and result in disruption of daily life. Excessive thoughts, feelings, or behaviors related to the somatic symptoms are manifested as one or more of the following: disproportionate and persistent thoughts about the seriousness of one's symptoms; persistent high levels of anxiety about health or symptoms; and excessive time and energy devoted to these symptoms or health concerns.

The condition generally develops in the teen years and almost always before 30 years of age. Women are more commonly affected than men, and there is usually a positive family history. The symptoms generally interrupt one's job and interpersonal relationships. Because there is an increased association with depressive disorders, there is also a corresponding increased suicide risk.

Diagnosis should specify if pain is a predominant symptom, if the symptoms are persistent or episodic, and level of severity (mild, moderate, or severe). With regard to treatment, reassurance with frequent office visits and sensitivity to the patient's needs is usually beneficial. Costly tests and repeated subspecialty consultations are discouraged unless there are questions with the diagnosis.

Additional Reading: American Psychiatric Association. *Diagnostic and Statistical Manual of Mental Disorders*. 5th ed. American Psychiatric Association; 2013.

34. Buspirone (Buspar) is an antianxiety medication that is structurally different than the benzodiazepines. Which one of the following statements about the use of buspirone is true?

A) The drug is used in the treatment of acute anxiety.
B) The drug may cause displacement of tightly bound drugs, such as phenytoin and warfarin, leading to toxicity.
C) Side effects include dizziness, fatigue, nervousness, and headache.
D) The medication is commonly associated with abuse.
E) The drug can be used in combination with monoamine oxidase inhibitors (MAOIs) to treat resistant depression.

The answer is C: Buspirone (Buspar) is an antianxiety medication that is used to treat chronic anxiety. It is not associated with abuse, drowsiness, or functional limitations. Buspirone is not useful in the treatment of acute anxiety because it often takes several days to weeks to produce its therapeutic effect.

The drug's mechanism of action is unknown but primarily involves serotonin and dopamine receptors, and it indirectly affects γ-aminobutyric acid receptors. The medication does not affect other tightly bound drugs, such as warfarin, propranolol, or phenytoin, but may affect less tightly bound drugs, such as digoxin.

Patients receiving MAOIs should not use buspirone because of the risk of elevated blood pressure and hypertensive crisis. Side effects reported with the use of buspirone include dizziness, fatigue, nervousness, headache, decreased concentration, palpitations, nausea, and abdominal complaints.

Additional Reading: Diagnosis and management of generalized anxiety disorder and panic disorder in adults. *Am Fam Physician*. 2015;91(9):617-624.

35. A 42-year-old woman presents to your office. Her life appears chaotic, and she transfers many of her dysfunctional feelings and conflicts to you, her physician. She is, at times, paranoid, depressed, and angry. She has a history of multiple unstable interpersonal relationships. The most likely diagnosis for her presentation is which one of the following conditions?

A) Antisocial behavior
B) Borderline personality disorder
C) Histrionic disorder
D) Narcissistic disorder
E) None of the above

The answer is B: Borderline personality disorder is a pattern of instability in interpersonal relationships, self-image, and affects, with marked impulsivity beginning in early adulthood and present in various contexts. Treating borderline personality disorder can be difficult and challenging; patients can present with a wide range of symptoms, including depression, anger, paranoia, extreme dependency, self-mutilation, and alternating idealization and devaluation of the physician. Their lives tend to be chaotic. They transfer many of their dysfunctional feelings and conflicts to the treating physician and the medical encounter.

There are a number of common co-occurring disorders with borderline personality disorder, including mood disorders, substance use disorders, bulimia nervosa, posttraumatic stress disorder, and attention-deficit/hyperactivity disorder. A detached professional stance and clear limit setting in terms of availability, appointment frequency, appropriate behavior, and medication use are necessary to manage these patients successfully. It is important to monitor one's own feelings and to refrain from responding inappropriately to verbal attacks and manipulation.

Dialectical behavior therapy is a combination of cognitive behavioral therapy and mindfulness to alter maladaptive thoughts leading to moods and behaviors while staying present in the moment. The development of a formal behavioral treatment plan and insistence on participation in behavioral health/psychiatric care may be helpful to establish an effective working relationship.

Additional Reading: Treating patients with borderline personality disorder in the medical office. *Am Fam Physician*. 2013;88(2):140-141.

36. Which one of the following therapies is the primary treatment for patients with schizophrenia?

A) Behavioral therapy
B) Cognitive therapy
C) Interpersonal therapy
D) Pharmacotherapy
E) Psychodynamic psychotherapy

The answer is D: Schizophrenia is a psychiatric disorder involving chronic or recurrent psychosis. It is commonly associated with impairments in social and occupational functioning and is the most disabling and economically catastrophic medical disorder, ranked by the World Health Organization as one of the top 10 illnesses contributing to the global burden of disease.

Pharmacotherapy is the primary treatment for schizophrenia and other psychotic disorders, specifically antipsychotic medications. They have been shown in clinical trials to be effective in treating symptoms and behaviors associated with the disorder.

Antipsychotic medications have significant side effects; assessment and management of these adverse effects are an important part of treatment. Evidence-based psychosocial interventions in conjunction with pharmacotherapy can also help patients achieve recovery.

Additional Reading: Schizophrenia. *Am Fam Physician*. 2014;90(11):775-782.

37. A 31-year-old woman whom you are treating is emotional and seductive in her behavior toward you. She is focused on her appearance to others and wants to be the center of attention. You note that she has a difficult time making decisions. The most likely diagnosis is to account for these behaviors is which one of the following disorders?

A) Antisocial behavior
B) Borderline personality disorder
C) Histrionic disorder
D) Narcissistic disorder
E) None of the above

The answer is C: The essential feature of histrionic personality disorder is pervasive and excessive emotionality and attention-seeking behavior in various contexts. Histrionic patients are often not satisfied if they are not the center of attention. They tend to be emotional and seductive, suggestible, and use their appearance to attract the attention of others. As a result, the implications of illness and aging may have a profound impact on their psychological functioning.

When faced with these patients, the physician should maintain an awareness of the patients' interpersonal style and be empathetic to their issues, while avoiding inappropriate emotional or seductive behaviors. Additionally, these patients have difficulties in dealing with facts, details, and decision-making. As a result, they may require extra assistance in processing medical information.

Additional Reading: Personality disorders: review and clinical application in daily practice. *Am Fam Physician*. 2011;84(11):1253-1260.

38. Before the diagnosis of posttraumatic stress disorder (PTSD) can be made, the patient should report symptoms that have been present for at least what amount of time?

A) 1 week
B) 1 month
C) 3 months
D) 6 months
E) 1 year

The answer is B: PTSD can occur after any major traumatic event (exposure to actual or threatened death, serious injury, or sexual violence). Exposure can be from direct experience, witnessing the event, learning that the traumatic event occurred, or experiencing extreme repeated or extreme exposure to aversive details of the traumatic event.

Symptoms include intrusive symptoms such as disturbing thoughts and nightmares about the traumatic event, dissociative reactions (flashbacks), and reactions to cues/triggers that symbolize the event; avoidance symptoms such as avoiding memories or external reminders; negative alterations in cognitions and mood; and marked arousal and reactivity.

The symptoms must be present for at least 1 month; and the symptoms must cause clinically important distress or reduced day-to-day functioning. Acute stress disorder occurs immediately after a trauma and lasts at least 3 days but up to 1 month after a major traumatic event. Different types of trauma lead to a similar clinical presentation of PTSD, and there is a lot of evidence that PTSD is associated with numerous health conditions and poor health outcomes.

Treatments for PTSD can include selective serotonin reuptake inhibitor medication, cognitive processing therapy, prolonged exposure therapy, and other medications to manage symptoms. However, benzodiazepines should be avoided in patients with PTSD.

Additional Reading: Identifying and managing posttraumatic stress disorder. *Am Fam Physician*. 2013;88(12):827-834.

39. All of the following statements about bipolar disorder are true, except which one?

A) Bipolar disorder is characterized by one or more episodes of mania.
B) Depression is required for a diagnosis of bipolar I disorder.
C) The mean age of onset for the first symptoms of bipolar I disorder is 18 years.
D) Bipolar II is typically brought to medical attention when the patient is depressed.
E) Lithium is a first-line treatment for bipolar disorder.

The answer is B: Bipolar disorder is characterized by one or more episodes of mania (ie, a distinct period during which there is an abnormal, persistently elevated, expansive, or irritable mood and persistently increased activity or energy that is present for most of the day, nearly every day, for a period of at least 1 week). Manic episodes may involve flight of ideas, excessive spending, aggressive and grandiose behavior, little sleep, and activities that are later regretted.

In bipolar I, there are typically episodes of major depression as well (eg, anhedonia, inability to concentrate, withdrawal from activities, chronic fatigue, loss of sexual drive, insomnia, and anorexia with weight loss); however, this is not required for diagnosis. The mean age of onset for the first manic, hypomanic, or depressive episode among patients with bipolar I disorder is 18 years.

Bipolar II disorder is characterized by meeting criteria for a current or past hypomanic episode and a current or past episode of major depression. Bipolar II is typically brought to medical attention when the patient is depressed. A careful history usually illuminates the diagnosis revealing episodes of hypomania. Some depressed patients will develop hypomania when given antidepressants.

Lithium is a first-line treatment for bipolar disorder. It is important to remember that lithium levels need to be followed, and abnormalities associated with the kidneys and thyroid can be induced with medication. Valproic acid (Depakene) can also be used to treat the manic symptoms. If the patient is psychotic, a neuroleptic medication may also be given. Long-acting benzodiazepines can be used for treating agitation. However, in patients with a substance abuse history, benzodiazepines should be used with caution because of the addictive potential of these agents. When the patient with bipolar disorder becomes depressed, a selective serotonin reuptake inhibitor or bupropion is recommended. The use of tricyclic antidepressants should be avoided because of the possibility of inducing rapid cycling of symptoms.

Additional Reading: Bipolar disorders: a review. *Am Fam Physician*. 2012;85(5):483-493.

The lifetime risk of suicide among patients with bipolar disorder is estimated to be at least 15 times greater than the general population. Co-occurring mental disorders are common.

40. Tardive dyskinesia (TD) is a condition characterized by repetitive, involuntary movements. It is associated with which one of the following?

A) Antiparkinsonian medications
B) Chronic blockade of dopaminergic receptors
C) Long-term (>2 years) use of lithium
D) Long-term (>2 years) use of serotonin reuptake inhibitors
E) Short-term (<3 months) use of phenothiazine neuroleptics

The answer is B: TD is a condition characterized by repetitive, involuntary, and purposeless choreiform movements of the extremities and buccal, oral, and lingual structures. Although often considered an extrapyramidal symptom, TD is a separate, mechanistically distinct phenomenon. The condition is thought to be secondary to chronic blockage of dopamine receptors in the brain. It is usually associated with side effects of long-term use of phenothiazine neuroleptics and anticholinergic medication.

Older patients and those with previous brain injury have a higher incidence of TD. In most cases, the symptoms do not resolve when the medication is discontinued.

Prevention of TD and the early detection and treatment of potentially reversible cases of TD are therefore of paramount importance. The only certain method of TD prevention is to avoid treatment with antipsychotic drugs. However, sometimes the benefits outweigh the risks. Patients on antipsychotic drugs, particularly for longer than 3 months, require careful and continuous evaluation.

Additional Reading: Adverse effects of antipsychotic medications. *Am Fam Physician*. 2010;81(5):617-622.

41. Anorexia nervosa is a psychiatric problem that includes severe dieting, which leads to a significantly low body weight. When evaluating a patient with anorexia, all of the listed abnormalities can be seen except which one?

A) Hypokalemia
B) Leukopenia
C) Prolonged QT interval on electrocardiogram (ECG)
D) Metabolic alkalosis
E) Elevated sedimentation rate

The answer is E: Anorexia nervosa is a psychiatric problem that centers on restriction of energy intake that leads to a significantly low body weight, intense fear of gaining weight or becoming fat, and persistent behavior that interferes with weight gain, as well as disturbance in the way one's body weight and shape are experienced. This results in the undue influence of body weight or shape on self-evaluation, and a persistent lack of recognition of the seriousness of the low body weight. Among women, the lifetime prevalence of anorexia nervosa is 0.5% to 3.7%.

Symptoms can include binge eating and self-induced vomiting or extreme restriction through dieting, exercise, and fasting. Women account for 95% of those affected. Onset is usually during adolescence but can occur earlier. Severe cases can be fatal. Most patients are described as being compulsive, intelligent, and meticulous; they are usually high achievers.

Physical findings include cachexia (>15% less than ideal weight), amenorrhea, loss of sexual desire, low body temperature, cold intolerance, bradycardia, dental erosions, hypotension, hypothermia, edema, and hirsutism. Depression may also be present.

Laboratory findings include electrolyte disorders (eg, hypokalemia), metabolic alkalosis, increased blood urea nitrogen secondary to dehydration, thrombocytopenia, leukopenia, low or normal erythrocyte sedimentation rate, and prolonged QT interval on ECG.

Short-term treatment involves active intervention to restore weight (which may require hospitalization), correction of electrolytes, and preservation of vital functions; long-term treatment involves psychiatric and psychological treatment including family therapy to restore a healthy body image and to treat possible underlying depression.

The goals of treatment for anorexia nervosa are to restore patients to a healthy weight, treat the physical complications, enhance the patient's motivation to cooperate with treatment, and provide education about healthy nutrition and eating habits. Other goals of treatment include correcting maladaptive thoughts, attitudes, and feelings related to the eating disorder; treating associated psychiatric conditions; enlisting family support; and attempting to prevent relapse. Medication should be considered in the treatment of anorexia but should not be the sole or primary treatment.

Additional Reading: Initial evaluation, diagnosis, and treatment of anorexia nervosa and bulimia nervosa. *Am Fam Physician*. 2015;91(1):46-52.

42. An 82-year-old woman is hospitalized with urosepsis. On the second day of her hospitalization, the nurse calls and tells you that she has become confused, is yelling, and has made multiple attempts to leave her room. You suspect delirium. She has no history of drug or alcohol abuse. Appropriate medication to administer at this time would be which one of the following?

A) Diazepam
B) Lorazepam (Ativan)
C) Fluoxetine
D) Haloperidol
E) Mirtazapine

The answer is D: The management of delirium involves identifying and correcting the underlying medical problem and symptomatically managing any behavioral or psychiatric symptoms. Low doses of antipsychotic drugs (eg, haloperidol) can help to control agitation. The use of benzodiazepines should be avoided except in cases of alcohol or sedative-hypnotic withdrawal because these can exacerbate symptoms. Environmental interventions, including frequent reorientation of patients by nursing staff and education of patients and families, should be instituted in all cases.

Additional Reading: Delirium in older persons: evaluation and management. *Am Fam Physician*. 2014;90(3):150-158.

43. A middle-aged white woman, whom you have been treating for a mental illness, presents with concern that she is having a milky white nipple discharge and you diagnose her with galactorrhea. Which one of the following classes of medication is associated with this occurrence?

A) Antipsychotic medication
B) Benzodiazepines
C) Dopamine agonist
D) Monoamine oxidase inhibitors
E) Tricyclic antidepressants

The answer is A: Antipsychotic (neuroleptic) medications are dopamine receptor antagonist(s) and include the following:

- Phenothiazines—chlorpromazine, thioridazine, mesoridazine (Serentil), perphenazine (Trilafon), trifluoperazine (Stelazine), and fluphenazine (Prolixin)
- Thioxanthenes—thiothixene (Navane)
- Butyrophenones—haloperidol
- Dihydroindolones—molindone (Moban)
- Dibenzoxazepine—loxapine (Loxitane)

Side effects of these medications are extensive and include anticholinergic effects such as dry mouth, blurred vision, urinary retention, delayed gastric emptying, acute glaucoma in patients with narrow anterior chamber angles, orthostatic hypotension, sexual dysfunction, cardiac arrhythmias, and endocrine abnormalities (hyperglycemia and hyperprolactinemia with galactorrhea).

Extrapyramidal symptoms include akathisias (the desire to be in constant motion), acute dystonias (bizarre muscle spasms of the head, neck, and tongue), drug-induced parkinsonism (pill-rolling tremor, rigidity, and bradykinesia), and tardive dyskinesia (TD) (abnormal repetitive movements of the face, tongue, trunk, or limbs). The medications are indicated in the treatment of schizophrenia, psychoses, and mania. The risk for TD increases with age and the length of administration of the medication. Neuroleptic malignant syndrome is a severe life-threatening side effect of antipsychotics that requires prompt recognition and treatment. Newer atypical antipsychotics have fewer side effects, but patients still need to be monitored for adverse events.

Additional Reading: Evaluation and management of galactorrhea. *Am Fam Physician*. 2012;85(11):1073-1080.

44. Depression is one of the most common problems seen by family physicians and can present with various symptoms. Which one of the following is a recognized symptom of depression?

A) A sense of entitlement
B) Changes in appetite or eating habits
C) Depersonalization
D) Flight of ideas
E) Hallucinations

The answer is B: Women are more often affected by depression than men, and the most common age range is 20 to 50 years. *DSM 5* requires that the patient must show either anhedonia or depressed mood, along with at least five of the following symptoms for 2 weeks or more to make the diagnosis.

- Depressed or irritable mood, or both (most of the day)
- Anhedonia (diminished interest or pleasure, or both, in most activity)
- Significant change in weight or appetite, or both, with no effort
- Insomnia; hypersomnia
- Psychomotor retardation or agitation
- Fatigue; decreased activity
- Feelings of worthlessness or inappropriate guilt
- Poor concentration; indecisiveness
- Recurrent thoughts of death or suicide, or both

The patient must have no evidence of previous psychiatric diagnosis, no organic contributing cause, and no recent emotional loss.

Many patients have a family history of depression and substance abuse. Evaluation should be performed to rule out causative factors such as anemia, infections, hypothyroidism, medication-related side effects, and alcohol or illegal drug abuse.

Psychotherapy and antidepressant medication are the mainstays of treatment. Electroconvulsive therapy is reserved for severe cases refractory to other treatments. Hospitalization is indicated if a patient is suicidal.

Additional Reading: American Psychiatric Association. *Diagnostic and Statistical Manual of Mental Disorders*. 5th ed. American Psychiatric Association; 2013.

45. An older patient whose spouse recently died is seen for follow-up of her hypertension. She is complaining of anxiety, insomnia, depressed mood, and anorexia. She reports that she continues to work and remains active playing cards with her friends. The most appropriate treatment at this time would be which one of the following?

A) Admit for inpatient psychiatric treatment.
B) Encourage frequent office visits for biofeedback.
C) Offer normalization of symptoms, reassurance, and emotional support.
D) Prescribe an antidepressant.
E) Prescribe a tranquilizer.

The answer is C: Grief or bereavement reaction occurs in response to significant loss or separation. Situations such as the death of a loved one, marital separation, loss of a girlfriend or boyfriend, or a move to a different and unfamiliar location can give rise to the condition. The reaction is a normal process that usually improves with time. Symptoms include anxiety, insomnia, depressed mood, anorexia, and mood swings.

Treatment involves frequent, short office visits to allow patients to express their grief or referral to a behavioral health provider. Patients should be encouraged to maintain regular patterns of activity, sleep, exercise, and nutrition as much as possible because these activities appear to enhance adaptation during bereavement.

The use of major tranquilizers and antidepressants is unnecessary and may interfere with the normal grieving process. Sleep disruption is a common symptom of grief, and the short-term prescription of a hypnotic may be effective in promoting sleep. For individuals who experience high levels of anxiety, a time-limited prescription of an anxiolytic can be useful as a crisis measure. However, these medications generally should not be prescribed at high doses or for long periods because their use has the potential to retard and inhibit the grieving process.

Patient reassurance is usually all that is needed. It is common for grief to intensify during the holidays or special events. In severe cases, in which there is significant functional impairment over a longer period of time or psychomotor retardation, antidepressants may become necessary.

Additional Reading: Grief and major depression—controversy over changes in DSM-5 diagnostic criteria. *Am Fam Physician*. 2014;90(10):690-694.

46. A 29-year-old man is having job-related problems because of a pattern of grandiosity with a lack of empathy; furthermore, his coworkers report that he frequently takes advantage of others for his own self-promotion, yet he is extreme sensitive to any perceived criticism. The most likely diagnosis to account for these behaviors is which one of the following disorders?

A) Antisocial personality disorder
B) Borderline personality disorder
C) Bipolar disorder
D) Narcissistic personality disorder
E) Paranoid personality disorder

The answer is D: Patients who are affected with narcissistic personality disorder exhibit impairment in social or job situations with a pervasive pattern of grandiosity, need for admiration, lack of empathy, and extreme sensitivity to the evaluation and judgment of others. They must exhibit at least five of the following *DSM 5* criteria:

- Shows arrogant, haughty behaviors or attitudes
- Interpersonally explosive (takes advantage of others for self-promotion)
- Requires constant attention and admiration of others
- Lacks empathy toward others
- Obsessed with feelings of envy
- Possesses a sense of entitlement
- Possesses a grandiose sense of self-importance
- Remains preoccupied with fantasies of unlimited success
- Believes he or she is unique and can only be understood by other special people

Many highly successful people exhibit traits that are considered narcissistic; however, only when these traits are inflexible, maladaptive, and persistent, despite impairment and distress, they are clinically significant. Patients with narcissistic personality disorder often experience depression and severe bouts of envy toward others. Occasionally, those who are affected become delusional in their thoughts. Criticism may leave patients with narcissistic personality disorder feeling degraded and humiliated, and they may react with disdain, rage, or defiance. The course of this disease is long term; however, narcissistic symptoms tend to diminish after the age of 40 years, when pessimism usually develops.

Additional Reading: Narcissistic personality disorder. In: Domino F, ed. *The 5-Minute Clinical Consult*. Wolters Kluwer; 2022.

47. The Mini-Mental State Examination (MMSE) is a widely used measure to assess cognition in clinical practice when there is a concern for dementia. Traditionally, what MMSE cutoff score is indicative of a significant cognitive impairment?

A) 15
B) 18
C) 24
D) 27
E) 30

The answer is C: Although primary care physicians often do not recognize cognitive impairment in a brief office visit, the MMSE can serve as a useful screening tool. This scale can be easily administered in the office in about 10 minutes to assess orientation, memory, attention and calculation, language, and visual construction. Patients score between 0 and 30 points, and cutoffs of 23/24 have typically been used to show significant cognitive impairment. Using a cutoff of 24 points, the MMSE had a sensitivity of 87% and a specificity of 82% in a large population-based sample.

However, the test is not sensitive for mild dementia, and scores may be influenced by age and education, as well as language, motor, and visual impairments. The MMSE can also show a ceiling effect allowing those with a higher level of education, even those with cognitive impairment, to have a perfect score of 30/30. This ceiling effect may limit the sensitivity of the MMSE, especially for individuals with mild cognitive impairment or mild dementia.

Other screening tools for dementia in primary care are available, such as having the patient draw a clock. This single task covers multiple cognitive domains and screens for cognitive problems. Clock drawings are helpful in 1- to 3-minute forms but must be scored appropriately, and sensitivity to mild forms of impairment can be low.

The Montreal Cognitive Assessment is another tool that was originally developed to help screen for mild cognitive impairment. It can be used in about 10 minutes by any clinician. It assesses attention/concentration, executive functions, conceptual thinking, memory, language, calculation, and orientation. A score of 25 or lower (from maximum of 30) is considered significant cognitive impairment. It performs as well as the MMSE, including screening for dementia. It has been widely translated as it also is utilized to assess executive function. It is particularly useful to evaluate patients with vascular impairment and vascular dementia. As it assesses executive function, it is particularly useful for patients with vascular impairment, including vascular dementia.

Additional Reading: Evaluation of suspected dementia. *Am Fam Physician*. 2011;84(8):895-902.

48. Conversion disorder can be difficult to diagnose. Which one of the following statements about this disorder is true?

A) Men are more commonly affected than women.
B) Neurological or other medical conditions rarely coexist with conversion disorder.
C) Symptoms have a definitive pathophysiologic explanation.
D) Those who are affected often subject themselves to unnecessary medical testing.
E) Treatment usually involves pharmacotherapy.

The answer is D: Patients with conversion disorder, also known as functional neurological symptom disorder, present with symptoms of altered voluntary motor or sensory function in which the symptoms/clinical findings are incompatible with a recognized neurological or medical condition. Motor symptoms can include weakness or paralysis, abnormal movements (tremors, dystonic movements), gait abnormalities, and abnormal limb posturing. Sensory symptoms include altered, reduced, or absent skin sensation, vision, or hearing. Episodes of psychogenic or nonepileptic seizures are also common.

Although the diagnosis requires that the symptom is not explained by neurological disease, it should not be made simply because results from investigations are normal or because the symptom is "bizarre." The diagnosis of conversion disorder should be based on the overall clinical picture and not on a single finding. The phenomenon of *la belle indifference* (ie, lack of concern about the nature or implications of the symptom) has been associated with conversion disorder but it is not specific for conversion disorder and should not be used to make the diagnosis.

Conversion disorder is two to three times more prevalent in women, and onset has been reported throughout the lifespan. Onset may be associated with stress or trauma (psychologic or physical) but is not exclusive to the occurrence. The diagnosis may be difficult initially because the patient believes that the symptoms stem from a physical disorder and that other neurological or medical conditions commonly do coexist with conversion disorder.

As physicians are taught almost exclusively to consider (and exclude) physical disorders as the cause of physical symptoms, the diagnosis is often considered only after extensive physical examinations and laboratory tests fail to reveal a disorder that can fully account for the symptom and its effects. Although ruling out a possible underlying physical disorder is crucial, early consideration of conversion may avoid tests that increase the costs and risks to the patient and that may unduly delay diagnosis.

The best clue is that conversion symptoms rarely conform fully to known anatomic and physiologic mechanisms. Many patients, because of their complaints, subject themselves to unnecessary medical tests. Treatment usually involves psychotherapy. Medication is generally not warranted.

Additional Reading: Somatization and conversion disorder. *Can J Psychiatry*. 2004;49(3):172-178.

49. You prescribed a selective serotonin reuptake inhibitor to a young woman for depression yesterday and her partner calls today to report that she is not feeling well. She has a fever, with sweating, and is tremulous. You suspect serotonin syndrome. Which one of the following should be used initially in conjunction with benzodiazepines in the treatment of this condition?

A) Cyproheptadine
B) Dantrolene
C) Diphenhydramine
D) Nitroprusside
E) Prednisone

The answer is A: The onset of serotonin syndrome is usually within 24 hours with 60% of cases occurring within 6 hours of exposure to, or change in, dosing of a serotonergic agent. Rarely, cases have been reported weeks after discontinuation of serotonergic agents.

The initial pharmacologic treatment of serotonin syndrome is with benzodiazepines and cyproheptadine (an antihistamine with serotonin antagonist properties). Other medications may include dantrolene and methysergide. If muscular rigidity and hyperthermia do not respond to these interventions, neuromuscular paralysis with endotracheal intubation is appropriate.

In addition to tachycardia, hypertension, and hyperthermia (severe cases), the clinical findings associated with this syndrome include the following:

- Neuromuscular findings (seen in above half of patients with serotonin syndrome)
- Hyperreflexia (greater in lower extremities)
- Clonus (involuntary muscle contractions, most commonly tested by flexing foot upward rapidly; includes ocular)
- Myoclonus (greater in lower extremities)
- Tremor (greater in lower extremities)
- Hypertonia
- Bilateral Babinski sign
- Akathisia
- Tonic-clonic seizures (severe cases)
- Autonomic signs
- Diaphoresis
- Mydriasis
- Flushing
- Dry mucous membranes
- Vomiting, diarrhea, increased bowel sounds
- Mental status changes: anxiety, disorientation, delirium
- Severe cases have led to altered level of consciousness, rhabdomyolysis, metabolic acidosis, and disseminated intravascular coagulation

Additional Reading: Serotonin syndrome. In: Domino F, ed. *The 5-Minute Clinical Consult*. Wolters Kluwer; 2022.

Serotonin syndrome usually presents within 24 hours of exposure to or change in dosing of a serotonergic agent.

50. Lithium is a useful medication in the treatment of bipolar disorder yet is associated with various worrisome side effects. Which one of the following statements is true regarding lithium administration?

A) Long-term lithium use may affect thyroid function.
B) Drug levels remain constant and do not need routine monitoring.
C) Hepatotoxicity can develop after 4 weeks of therapy.
D) Peripheral neuropathy is a common side effect.
E) Renal function is not affected by the use of lithium.

The answer is A: Side effects of lithium use include tremor, polydipsia, polyuria, gastrointestinal irritation, and diarrhea. Hypothyroidism and renal toxicity are other complications of lithium administration. Toxicity is characterized by lethargy, seizures, nephropathy, and coma. Therefore, lithium blood levels should be monitored carefully and adjusted as necessary. In addition, serum creatinine and thyroid function tests should be evaluated periodically. Drugs that decrease renal clearance, such as nonsteroidal anti-inflammatory agents, should be used cautiously in patients receiving lithium.

Additional Reading: Bipolar disorders: a review. *Am Fam Physician*. 2012;85(5):483-493.

51. A 32-year-old woman, who has had problems with drinking in the past, presents once again with vague somatic complaints that are out of proportion to any medical findings. In addition, she has had frequent mood swings and reports difficult interpersonal relationships. She is always interested in your personal life and thinks you are a "wonderful doctor" as she asked for your help again today. The most likely diagnosis to explain this presentation is that she has which one of the following disorders?

A) Bipolar disorder
B) Borderline personality disorder
C) Dysthymic disorder
D) Narcissistic personality disorder
E) Schizophreniform disorder

The answer is B: Patients with borderline personality disorder are often encountered in the family physician's office. Characteristics of this disorder include impulsiveness, unstable and intense interpersonal relationships, substance abuse, and self-destructive behavior with accident proneness. Those who are affected lack self-control, lack self-fulfillment, and have identity problems. Their behaviors include aggressive and suicidal actions with frequent mood swings.

In many cases, they present with vague, unexplainable somatic complaints; do not follow therapeutic recommendations; and can be frustrating to their physicians. Most affected persons present during adolescence.

Treatment involves adequate communication, supportive limit setting, frequent office visits, and occasionally medication. Acute crisis may require hospitalization. Patients with this disorder have high comorbidity with other psychiatric disorders and high rates of suicidal ideation, and they cause particular treatment difficulties, including hostility toward caregivers and low rates of treatment compliance.

The central feature of patients with borderline personality disorder is a morbid fear of abandonment, with consequential pathologic responses to perceived rejection. Such patients may demand inappropriate amounts of time or support from a primary care physician, and they may become hostile and demanding or suicidal if these needs are not met.

The family practitioner should be alert to the following "red flags": a history of doctor shopping; a history of legal suits against physicians or other professionals; a history of suicide attempts; a history of several brief marriages or intimate relationships; an immediate idealization of you as a "wonderful doctor," especially if the patient compares you with disappointing caregivers of the past; and excessive interest in your personal life, eventually leading to invitations to socialize with you. Behavior of this type implies boundary violations, and its purpose is to cement a relationship with the physician, allaying the patient's ever-present fear of abandonment.

Additional Reading: Borderline personality disorder. In: Domino F, ed. *The 5-Minute Clinical Consult*. Wolters Kluwer; 2022.

52. A young woman reports that she has premenstrual syndrome (PMS) and feels lousy every month, to the extent that she feels so depressed that she struggles to get out of bed, yet she is fine a couple of days after her menses begins. She is asking if there is a medication that she could take to help with her symptoms. You believe that she is suffering from premenstrual dysphoric disorder. Which one of the following medications has been shown to be beneficial in the treatment of this disorder?

A) Fluoxetine
B) Furosemide
C) Haloperidol
D) Lithium
E) Progesterone

The answer is A: PMS is a complex of physical and emotional symptoms sufficiently severe to interfere with everyday life, which occurs cyclically during the luteal phase of menses. PMDD is a severe form of PMS characterized by severe recurrent depressive and anxiety symptoms, with premenstrual (luteal phase) onset, which remits a few days after the start of menses.

PMDD's mood-related symptoms leading to functional impairment are what distinguish it from PMS. The core feature of PMDD is the recurrent expression of symptoms during the end of the luteal phase of the menstrual cycle with a symptom-free period shortly after the onset of menses. According to *DSM 5*, patients with PMDD must have a symptom-free postmenstrual week, and they typically experience the symptom of being overwhelmed or out of control during the most affected time. At least one of the following must be present to make the diagnosis: mood swings; marked irritability or anger; marked depressed mood or hopelessness; and marked anxiety or tension. The time of greatest well-being is just before ovulation.

The average age of presentation is 36 years. Many report that their symptoms began when they were in their 20s and worsened over time. Those who are affected are at higher risk for development of a major depressive disorder. Fluoxetine (Prozac) has been found to be beneficial in treating symptoms, as has sertraline.

Additional Reading: Premenstrual syndrome (PMS) and premenstrual dysphoric disorder (PMDD). In: Domino F, ed. *The 5-Minute Clinical Consult*. Wolters Kluwer; 2022.

53. You have treated a middle-aged man with a tricyclic antidepressant (TCA), who took the entire bottle of his medication in an unsuccessful suicide attempt. In assessing his cardiac status, which of the following electrocardiogram findings is most commonly associated with TCA toxicity?

A) Prolongation of the PR interval
B) Prolongation of the QT interval
C) Third-degree atrioventricular block
D) T-wave elevations across the precordial leads
E) Widened QRS interval

The answer is B: The TCAs have been used less frequently as first-line agents for depression with the development of the selective serotonin reuptake inhibitors (SSRIs). This is mainly due to the side effect profile of the TCAs. These drugs interact with a wide variety of brain receptor types that result in their antidepressant efficacy and side effect profiles. Most serious is the toxicity of the cyclic antidepressants in overdose. In comparison with the SSRIs, the cyclic antidepressants can be fatal in doses as little as five times the therapeutic dose. The toxicity is usually due to prolongation of the QT interval, leading to arrhythmias.

Additional Reading: Common questions about the pharmacologic management of depression in adults. *Am Fam Physician*. 2015;92(2):94-100.

54. A 42-year-old teacher presents with feelings of getting "choked up." The symptoms are constant and are not made worse with swallowing; indeed, he has not felt that food is stuck in his throat. Eating and drinking actually seem to help relieve his symptoms. He has had no recent weight changes. The most likely diagnosis to account for his presentation is which one of the following?

A) Barrett esophagus
B) Globus hystericus
C) Panic attacks
D) Reflux esophagitis
E) Zenker diverticulum

The answer is B: Globus hystericus (globus sensation) is defined as the subjective sensation of a lump or mass in the throat. No specific cause or mechanism has been determined; however, there is some evidence to suggest that increased cricopharyngeal (upper esophageal sphincter) pressures or abnormal hypopharyngeal motility may be present during the time of symptoms. The sensation may result from gastroesophageal reflux or from frequent swallowing and drying of the throat associated with anxiety or other emotional states.

Although not related to a specific psychiatric disorder, globus may be a symptom of certain mood states. Suppression of sadness is most often implicated. Symptoms resemble the normal sensation of being "choked up." With globus, symptoms do not become worse during swallowing, food does not stick in the throat, and eating or drinking often provides relief. No pain or weight loss occurs. Chronic symptoms may be experienced during grief reactions and may be relieved by crying.

The diagnosis is based on the history and physical examination and is a diagnosis of exclusion. The treatment involves treating the underlying psychologic condition.

Additional Reading: Globus sensation. In: *UpToDate*. 2022.

55. A young man is asking if a medication will help treat his premature ejaculation because he is frustrated and feels that this has interfered with his ability to develop a relationship. Which one of the following medications can be prescribed to help with this situation?

A) Finasteride (Proscar)
B) Progesterone (Provera)
C) Sildenafil (Viagra)
D) Sertraline (Zoloft)
E) Tamsulosin (Flomax)

The answer is D: Premature ejaculation is best defined as persistent or recurrent ejaculation with minimal stimulation before, on, or shortly after penetration and before the sexual partner wishes it. Premature ejaculation is thought to be the most common form of male sexual dysfunction, with an estimated prevalence of up to 40%.

Treatment of ejaculatory dysfunction centers on relationship counseling, behavioral therapy, and pharmacologic interventions.

Behavioral therapy has been considered the gold standard of treatment. Techniques include the Semen Pause Maneuver, the Masters and Johnson Pause-Squeeze Technique, and the Kaplan Stop-Start Method. These techniques are directed at the induction of male sexual arousal to the point of ejaculation followed by relaxation before orgasm is allowed to occur. The methods can be self-applied, however, with suboptimal outcomes; hence, involvement of the sexual partner is essential.

Because of the limitations of behavioral therapy, pharmacologic interventions are often used to treat premature ejaculation. Anorgasmia and delayed ejaculatory response are well-known side effects of TCAs (clomipramine) and selective serotonin reuptake inhibitors. Recent studies have shown that these drugs modify the ejaculatory response in men with premature ejaculation. Results appear better with clomipramine, but sertraline was better tolerated and had a better safety profile.

Additional Reading: Ejaculatory disorders. In: Domino F, ed. *The 5-Minute Clinical Consult*. Wolters Kluwer; 2022.

56. Although useful, like all medications, antidepressants can cause several drug-drug interactions. Which one of the following antidepressant medications has the lowest risk for such complications?

A) Amitriptyline
B) Citalopram
C) Fluoxetine
D) Paroxetine
E) Sertraline

The answer is B: Most selective serotonin reuptake inhibitors (SSRIs) are associated with significant drug interactions. The SSRIs may inhibit hepatic cytochrome P450 enzymes that metabolize other medications, thereby causing drug-drug interactions. Fluoxetine, paroxetine, and, to a lesser extent, sertraline can inhibit the metabolism of warfarin (Coumadin), cisapride (Propulsid), benzodiazepines, quinidine, TCAs, theophylline, and some statins. In patients who are at risk for these interactions, citalopram may offer an advantage.

Studies have shown that compared with other SSRIs, citalopram and escitalopram have less of an inhibitory effect on the cytochrome P450 system. They are as effective as fluoxetine and sertraline in the treatment of depression and thus good choices for situations in which drug-drug interactions are a concern.

Additional Reading: Drugs for depression. *Med Lett Drugs Ther*. 2020 (1592).

57. A 49-year-old accountant complains of a depressed mood with low energy and poor self-esteem for the past few years. Although he feels out of sorts, he has continued to work and attend to his family life. His presentation is consistent with which one of the following disorders?

A) Attention-deficit disorder
B) Dissociation disorder
C) Introvert personality disorder
D) Major depressive disorder
E) Persistent depressive disorder

The answer is E: Persistent depressive disorder (previously called dysthymia in *DSM-IV-TR*) is a chronic, low-intensity mood disorder. By definition, symptoms must be present consecutively for more than 2 years. It is characterized by anhedonia, low self-esteem, and low energy. It may have a more psychologic than biologic explanation and tends to respond to medication and psychotherapy equally. Long-term psychotherapy is frequently able to establish a permanent change in dysthymic individuals.

Additional Reading: Depression. In: Domino F, ed. *The 5-Minute Clinical Consult*. Wolters Kluwer; 2022.

58. Bupropion is a norepinephrine-dopamine reuptake inhibitor (NDRI) that is primarily used as an antidepressant and for smoking cessation. This drug is structurally related to which one of the following medication classes?

A) Anxiolytics
B) Alcohols
C) Antibiotics
D) Barbiturates
E) Stimulants

The answer is E: Bupropion is a monocyclic aminoketone that is structurally related to amphetamine. Some authorities classify the drug as an NDRI because it inhibits presynaptic reuptake of dopamine and norepinephrine (with a greater effect on dopamine). The drug has little effect on other neurotransmitters and little to no affinity for postsynaptic receptors.

Bupropion is used to treat major depression, seasonal affective disorder, attention-deficit/hyperactivity disorder, tobacco dependence, hypoactive sexual disorder, and obesity. Contraindications include bulimia nervosa, anorexia nervosa, use of monoamine oxidase inhibitors in the past 2 weeks, seizure disorders, and abrupt withdrawal from alcohol, benzodiazepines, or other sedatives.

The most common adverse reactions include tremor, headaches, rash, and urticaria. Other adverse effects include insomnia and dry mouth. Bedtime administration should be avoided.

Additional Reading: Drugs for depression. *Med Lett Drugs Ther*. 2020 (1592).

59. The following nonpharmacological approaches to depression have been shown to have some level of evidence in reducing symptoms of depression except:

A) Exercise
B) Yoga
C) Tai Chi
D) Qi Gong
E) Acupuncture

The answer is E: Many people with depression or anxiety turn to nonpharmacologic and nonconventional interventions, including exercise, yoga, meditation, tai chi, or qi gong. Meta-analyses and systematic reviews have shown that these interventions can improve symptoms of depression and anxiety disorders.

Additional Reading: Depression and anxiety disorders: benefits of exercise, yoga, and meditation. *Am Fam Physician*. 2019;99(10):620-627.

Emergent and Surgical Care

CHAPTER 5

The questions in this chapter are separated into two sections: Emergent Care and Surgical Care. Many of the emergent care topics are urgent in nature and some of the surgical care questions are emergent by their nature but are grouped this way to help focus your studying as you prepare for the American Board of Family Medicine examination. Additionally, each question is annotated to note which organ system it also relates to; if you are concerned about a particular area, paying attention to which organ system is represented can help you to identify areas of weakness as well.

Section I. Emergent Care

Each of the following questions or incomplete statements is followed by suggested answers or completions. Select the ONE BEST ANSWER in each case.

1. A 53-year-old carpenter presents with complaints of pain in his right wrist and weakness in his grip, making it harder for him to work. On examination, he has pain over the radial aspect of the wrist that is aggravated by flexing the thumb and applying ulnar flexion. The most likely diagnosis to account for such a presentation is which one of the following conditions?

A) Boxer's fracture
B) Hamate fracture
C) Scaphoid fracture
D) Carpal tunnel syndrome
E) de Quervain tenosynovitis

The answer is E: The combination of wrist pain and grip weakness is a characteristic of de Quervain tenosynovitis. Local tenderness is present over the distal portion of the radial styloid adjacent to abductor pollicis longus tendon. The pain is generally reproduced with direct palpation of the involved tendons. Pain is aggravated by passively stretching the thumb tendons over the radial styloid in thumb flexion (the Finkelstein maneuver).

Carpal tunnel syndrome will present with paresthesia and/or weakness primarily in the distribution of the median nerve, which would include the thumb and index finger. Phalen maneuver is a diagnostic test for carpal tunnel syndrome.

A scaphoid fracture presents with mild, dull pain, deep in the radial wrist that is worsened when making a grip. On examination, there is tenderness to palpation in the anatomical "snuff box"—this is a sensitive but not specific test. A boxer's fracture refers to a fracture of the midshaft of the fifth metacarpal (typically following a blow with a closed fist). A hamate fracture presents with pain along the ulnar side of the hand and is frequently seen in sports that require swinging of bats or racquets.

Additional Reading: de Quervain's Tenosynovitis. In: *UpToDate*. 2022.
Category: Musculoskeletal system

Finkelstein test is used to diagnose de Quervain tenosynovitis. Grasp the patient's thumb and deviate the hand sharply toward the ulna (ulnar deviation). If sharp pain occurs along the distal radius, the test is considered positive and de Quervain tenosynovitis is likely.

2. A 25-year-old gardener presents with a red eye; he reports having gotten a scratch when pruning some bushes earlier in the day. On examination, you detect a corneal abrasion. Which one of the following statements is true regarding corneal injuries?

A) Foreign bodies should not be removed to avoid the potential for further corneal injury.
B) Patients should have the affected eye patched for 24 hours.
C) Topical antibiotics are recommended to prevent superinfection.
D) Topical anesthetics should be given to treat the discomfort.
E) None of the above.

The answer is C: Patients should be treated with topical antibiotics to prevent superinfection. Antibiotics ointment is better than drops. However, controlled studies have not found patching to improve the rate of healing or comfort in patients with traumatic or foreign body abrasions and should be avoided. If a corneal foreign body is detected, an attempt can be made to remove it by irrigation. The administration of topical anesthetics is controversial. Animal studies showed that it can delay corneal epithelial healing. In humans, some studies showed that dilute solutions of proparacaine 0.05% provide analgesia without impairing healing after several days of treatment.

Additional Reading: Evaluation and management of corneal abrasions. *Am Fam Physician*. 2013;87(2):114-120.
Category: Special sensory systems

3. You are assessing a high school football player who is complaining of finger pain and swelling after a tackle. He has grabbed his opponent by the jersey and felt the pain immediately after falling to the ground. You suspect "jersey finger." Which finger is most likely to be involved with this type of injury?

A) Thumb
B) Index finger
C) Middle finger
D) Ring finger
E) Fifth finger ("pinky")

The answer is D: Disruption of the flexor digitorum profundus tendon, also known as "jersey finger," commonly occurs when an athlete's finger catches on another player's clothing, usually while playing a tackling sport such as football or rugby. The injury causes forced extension of the distal interphalangeal (DIP) joint during active flexion. The ring finger is the weakest finger and accounts for 75% of jersey finger cases. Acute pain and swelling over the volar aspect of the DIP joint and distal phalanx are characteristics. The characteristic finding of jersey finger is the inability to actively flex the DIP joint.

Additional Reading: Common finger fractures and dislocations. *Am Fam Physician*. 2022;105(6):631-639.
Category: Musculoskeletal system

➔ **The "jersey finger" is a common sports injury. It can happen when one player grabs another player's jersey and a finger (usually the ring finger) gets caught and pulled. The flexor digitorum profundus tendon is pulled off the bone, with an inability to flex the finger at the DIP joint.**

4. A 19-year-old basketball player presents with complaints of pain and difficulty in fully extending his middle finger after a "jam" injury when trying to catch the ball. On examination, you detect an injury to the extensor tendon at the distal interphalangeal (DIP) joint of his middle finger; this type of injury is also known as which one of the following?

A) A boutonnière deformity
B) A jersey finger
C) A mallet finger
D) Swan necking

The answer is C: Injury to the extensor tendon at the DIP joint is also known as a mallet finger. The condition is the most common closed tendon injury of the finger. Mallet finger is usually caused by an object (eg, a ball) striking the finger, creating a forced flexion of an extended DIP. The extensor tendon may be strained, partially torn, or completely ruptured or separated by a distal phalanx avulsion fracture. Those affected with mallet finger complain of pain at the dorsal DIP joint, inability to actively extend the joint, and, often, with a characteristic flexion deformity. It is necessary to isolate the DIP joint during the evaluation to ensure extension is from the extensor tendon and not the central slip. The absence of full passive extension may indicate bony or soft tissue entrapment requiring surgical intervention. Mallet finger most often involves the middle finger and the next.

A boutonnière deformity refers to flexion of the proximal interphalangeal joint and hyperextension of the DIP joint. A swan neck deformity refers to hyperextension of the proximal interphalangeal joint and flexion of the DIP joint. These types of deformity are commonly caused by inflammatory joint destruction as seen with rheumatoid arthritis but may also occur with trauma.

Additional Reading: Common finger fractures and dislocations. *Am Fam Physician*. 2022;105(6):631-639.
Category: Musculoskeletal system

5. Where are most Morton neuromas found?

A) In the tarsal tunnel of the third toe
B) At the first metatarsal phalangeal joint
C) Between the third and fourth toes
D) At the attachment of the plantar fascia
E) At the head of the fifth metatarsal

The answer is C: Morton neuromas are typically found between the metatarsal of the third and fourth toes or at the bifurcation of the fourth plantar digital nerve. The second and third common digital branches of the medial plantar nerve are the most frequent sites for development of interdigital neuromas. Morton neuromas develop as a result of chronic trauma and repetitive stress, because it occurs in persons wearing tight-fitting or high-heeled shoes. Pain and paresthesias are usually mild at onset and are located in the interdigital space of the affected nerve. In some cases, the interdigital space between the affected toes may be widened because of an associated ganglion or synovial cyst. Pain is noted in the affected interdigital space when the metatarsal heads of the foot are squeezed together. Injection with 1% lidocaine can assist in confirming the diagnosis.

Additional Reading: Pinpoint foot pain at the base of the phalanx. *Am Fam Physician*. 2022;105(6):673-674.
Category: Musculoskeletal system

6. A patient with a history of kidney stones presents with complaints of left-sided flank pain and is concerned that he has another stone. Which one of the following tests is the most sensitive and specific for the detection of renal stones?

A) A kidney, ureter, and bladder (KUB) plain abdominal x-ray
B) A noncontrast helical computed tomography (CT)
C) An abdominal ultrasonography
D) Intravenous (IV) pyelography

The answer is B: A noncontrast helical CT can detect both stones and urinary tract obstruction and has become the gold standard for the diagnosis of urinary stones. The specificity of helical CT is nearly 100%. Ultrasonography is the procedure of choice for patients who should avoid radiation, including pregnant women and possibly women of childbearing age. It is sensitive for the diagnosis of urinary tract obstruction and can detect radiolucent stones missed on KUB plain abdominal x-ray. IV pyelogram has a higher sensitivity and specificity than an abdominal plain film for the detection of stones and provides data about the degree of obstruction.

Additional Reading: Kidney stones: treatment and prevention. *Am Fam Physician*. 2019;99(8):490-496.
Category: Nephrologic system

7. A 31-year-old man is seen in the emergency department for lateral foot pain that occurred when he fell down while playing basketball. X-ray images of the foot confirm a displaced fracture of the proximal fifth metatarsal. Appropriate management consists of which one of the following?

A) Nonsteroidal anti-inflammatory drugs and limited weight-bearing with a gradual return to usual activities in 2 to 4 weeks
B) Crutches with no weight-bearing for 4 to 6 weeks
C) Short leg walking cast for 6 to 8 weeks
D) External reduction followed by casting for 6 to 8 weeks with limited weight-bearing
E) Orthopedic referral

The answer is E: Fractures of the proximal portion of the fifth metatarsal may be classified as avulsions of the tuberosity or fractures of the shaft within 1.5 cm of the tuberosity. The tuberosity, or styloid, is the most proximal portion of the fifth metatarsal. It protrudes in the lateral and plantar planes.

Fractures of the tuberosity are the most common among lower extremity fractures. Tuberosity avulsion fractures cause pain and tenderness at the base of the fifth metatarsal. Bruising, swelling, and other injuries may be present. Nondisplaced tuberosity fractures are usually treated conservatively and heal without difficulty; however, orthopedic referral is indicated for (1) fractures that are comminuted or displaced, (2) fractures that involve more than 30% of the cubometatarsal articulation surface, and (3) fractures with delayed union.

Management and prognosis of acute (Jones fracture) and stress fracture of the fifth metatarsal within 1.5 cm of the tuberosity depend on the type of fracture, on the basis of classification. Simple fractures are generally treated conservatively with a non–weight-bearing short leg cast for 6 to 8 weeks. Fractures with delayed union may also be treated conservatively or may be managed surgically, depending on patients' preference and other factors.

All displaced fractures and nonunion fractures should be managed surgically. Although most fractures of the proximal portion of the fifth metatarsal respond well to appropriate management, delayed union, muscle atrophy, and chronic pain may be long-term complications.

Additional Reading: Diagnosis and management of common foot fractures. *Am Fam Physician*. 2016;93(3):183-191.
Category: Musculoskeletal system

8. A 2-year-old child is seen in the emergency department and diagnosed with a spiral-type fracture of the left radius secondary to falling down the stairs at home. You also observe multiple contusions in various stages of healing. The most appropriate initial treatment for this child is which one of the following?

A) Splinting of the fracture with orthopedic referral
B) Hospitalization
C) Social service consultation
D) Immediate reduction of the fracture and safety counseling for the child's parents
E) Open reduction and internal fixation and follow-up in 3 days

The answer is B: Child abuse is a difficult problem that must be identified as quickly as possible. Children younger than 3 years are the most commonly abused, and most children who die of child abuse are younger than 5 years. Most child abuse takes place in the home and is instituted by persons known to and trusted by the child. Although widely publicized, abuse in day care and foster care settings accounts for only a minority of confirmed cases of child abuse. Child abuse is 15 times more likely to occur in families in which spousal abuse occurs. Children are three times more likely to be abused by their fathers than by their mothers.

Once a health care worker has any suspicion of child abuse, he or she is legally required to report the case for investigation. Protection of the child is the most important goal. The child should be hospitalized in a safe environment, while further investigation by social workers is performed.

Clinical findings include multiple fractures (especially spiral-type fractures), multiple bruises in different stages of healing, intestinal trauma injuries, burns, poor nutrition, poor development, and bizarre accidents reported by parents. More than 50% of fractures in children younger than 1 year are secondary to abuse.

Before discharge from the hospital, the child's home environment must be determined to be safe by the appropriate protection agency. Further counseling for the child and family should be initiated after discharge. Unfortunately, therapy for child-abusing adults fails in approximately 33% of cases. As adults, children who were abused have a higher incidence of depression and drug abuse.

Additional Reading: Diagnosis and management of physical abuse in children. *Am Fam Physician*. 2013;88(10):669-675.
Category: Patient/population-based care

9. You are on call for the nursery and are paged about a newborn who is vomiting bile-stained emesis. The delivery was uneventful, and the mother is breastfeeding her newborn. The most appropriate management in response to this page is to order which one of the following?

A) Administer a promethazine rectal suppository.
B) Decrease the feeding frequency.
C) Obtain an upper gastrointestinal (GI) barium study.
D) Obtain a barium enema.
E) Place a nasogastric tube.

The answer is C: The diagnosis of intestinal malrotation should be suspected in any infant who presents with bilious emesis, acute duodenal obstruction, or abdominal tenderness associated with hemodynamic deterioration. Intestinal malrotation is a condition that occurs during development of the fetus. As the bowel develops outside the abdomen, it returns to the body cavity with a counterclockwise rotation. When malrotation occurs, no rotation occurs as the bowel returns to the abdomen. When this happens, the root of the mesentery is no longer broad and splayed across the retroperitoneum. Instead, there is a narrow stalk on which the bowel can easily twist. This can lead to a life-threatening volvulus. Presenting symptoms include vomiting of bile-stained material, abdominal distension, and dehydration soon after birth.

Barium enema may be misleading in the diagnosis of malrotation and is used only as an adjunct to the upper GI series. Barium enema can be helpful in the diagnosis of volvulus if it shows complete obstruction of the transverse colon, particularly if the head of the barium column has a beaked appearance.

Additional Reading: Intestinal malrotation in children. In: *UpToDate*. 2022.
Category: Gastroenterology system

10. A 37-year-old carpenter is being evaluated for low back pain, and he is concerned that he has a "slipped" disk because the pain started after he lifted a heavy wooden beam. Which one of the following statements about lumbar disk disease is true?

A) Forward flexion of the trunk often helps relieve symptoms.
B) Symptoms are typically due to anterior herniation of the nucleus pulposus.
C) The L5-S1 interspace is usually involved.
D) Treatment usually requires surgical intervention.
E) Treatment involves strict bed rest for 1 to 2 weeks.

The answer is C: Lumbar disk disease usually results from posterior herniation of the nucleus pulposus that impinges on the spinal cord. The most common site is the L5-S1 interspace, which affects the first sacral nerve root. Patients typically recall a precipitating event such as lifting a heavy object. Symptoms include severe back pain that radiates to the legs and that is aggravated by coughing, sneezing, or forward flexion of the trunk. The condition is the most common cause of sciatica. Examination may show decreased sensation in a dermatome pattern, weakness, decreased reflexes, and a positive straight leg raising test. In severe cases, patients may experience bowel or bladder incontinence.

Radiographs and laboratory tests are generally unnecessary, except in the few patients in whom a serious cause is suspected on the basis of a comprehensive history and physical examination. Surgical evaluation is indicated in patients with worsening neurologic deficits or intractable pain that is resistant to conservative treatment.

Bed rest should not be recommended for patients with nonspecific acute low back pain. Moderate-quality evidence suggests that bed rest is less effective in reducing pain and improving function at 3 to 12 weeks than staying active. Prolonged bed rest can also cause adverse effects such as joint stiffness, muscle wasting, loss of bone mineral density, pressure ulcers, and venous thromboembolism.

The treatment plan should be reassessed in patients who do not return to normal activity within 4 to 6 weeks. Most mild cases can be treated with the limitation of aggravating activity, anti-inflammatory agents, and muscle relaxants.

Additional Reading: Diagnosis and treatment of acute low back pain. *Am Fam Physician*. 2012;85(4):343-350.
Category: Musculoskeletal system

Red flags that suggest the need for imaging include pain that lasts more than 6 weeks, pain in persons younger than 18 years or older than 50 years, a history of trauma, constitutional symptoms, atypical pain (eg, pain that occurs at night or that is unrelenting), the presence of a severe or rapidly progressive neurologic deficit, urinary and/or fecal incontinence, poor rectal tone, and a history of malignancy.

11. A 5-year-old boy is brought to the emergency department by his frantic mother. He is having trouble breathing and has a high fever. On examination, you hear inspiratory and expiratory stridor and he is drooling. Initial treatment for this child would be which one of the following?

A) Administer epinephrine.
B) Administer inhaled bronchodilators.
C) Administer oxygen therapy.
D) Provide airway management by trained personnel.
E) Position the child in the supine position.

The answer is D: Epiglottitis is a severe, life-threatening condition usually seen in children between 3 and 10 years of age. The condition was usually the result of a *Haemophilus influenzae* type B (Hib) infection. In recent years, the occurrence of epiglottitis has been reduced dramatically by the widespread use of the Hib vaccine. Other causes include bacterial infections by *Streptococcus* and *Staphylococcus* species.

Manifestations include stridor with inspiration and expiration, high fever, dysphagia, drooling, and toxic appearance. Children may lean forward with their neck outstretched to minimize airway obstruction.

Laboratory findings include an elevated white blood cell count and positive blood cultures. Arterial blood gases may show hypoxia. Lateral neck radiographs show a swollen epiglottis with obstruction of the airway (positive thumb sign).

Treatment involves securing the child's airway, but this should be accomplished only by trained personnel. Before intubation, the child should not be moved, nor should the child be placed in a supine position. Oxygen should also be avoided because of the risk of aggravating the child and possible complete obstruction of the airway. Intravenous antibiotics should be started immediately, and the child should be monitored in an intensive care setting.

Additional Reading: Epiglottitis, pediatric. In: *The 5-Minute Clinical Consult*. Wolters Kluwer; 2022.
Category: Respiratory system

12. You are preparing to repair a laceration on the knee of a young child and want to use a local anesthetic with a long duration of action. Which one of the following agents has the longest duration of action?

A) Bupivacaine
B) Lidocaine
C) Mepivacaine
D) Procaine
E) Tetracaine

The answer is A: Of the listed agents, bupivacaine has the longest duration of action. Bupivacaine has a longer onset of action (5 minutes) compared to lidocaine (2 minutes). Mixing 50/50 bupivacaine and lidocaine is a practice that allows for fast onset and long duration of local anesthetic.

- Lidocaine and mepivacaine 1 to 3 hours depending on whether it is mixed with epinephrine.
- Bupivacaine duration 4 to 8 hours.

Additional Reading: *Infiltration of local anesthetics*. In: *UpToDate*. 2022.
Category: Integumentary system

13. A 29-year-old mother of three children presents to your office with complaints of a painful "red eye." She denies any recent trauma or injury. On examination, you note left eye redness with pain. Which one of the following should be performed initially?

A) Application of a local anesthetic
B) Fluorescein staining
C) Funduscopic examination
D) Irrigation
E) Visual acuity testing

The answer is E: Almost all patients with ocular problems should have visual acuity testing before anything else is done. If this is difficult, a local anesthetic may be applied. The main exception to this rule is a chemical burn of the eye, which should be irrigated for 30 minutes before further evaluation or treatment is undertaken.

Additional Reading: Ocular emergencies. *Am Fam Physician*. 2007;76(6):829-836.
Category: Special sensory systems

14. A 37-year-old woman presents to the emergency department with complaints of abdominal pain. She has a history of unexplained physical symptoms that began in her late teenage years. She is somewhat vague concerning past medical evaluations, but a review of her extensive medical record reveals numerous normal laboratory and imaging tests and several surgical procedures that have failed to alleviate her symptoms, along with frequent requests for refills of narcotics. This history is most compatible with which one of the following?

A) Generalized anxiety disorder
B) Hypochondriasis
C) Malingering
D) Panic disorder
E) Somatization disorder

The answer is E: Somatization disorder usually begins in the teens or twenties and is characterized by multiple unexplained physical symptoms, insistence on surgical procedures, and an imprecise or inaccurate medical history. Abuse of alcohol, narcotics, or other drugs is also commonly seen.

Hypochondriacs are overly concerned with bodily functions and often provide extensive, detailed medical histories. Malingering is an intentional pretense of illness to obtain personal gain. Patients with panic disorder have episodes of intense, short-lived attacks of cardiovascular, neurologic, or gastrointestinal symptoms. Generalized anxiety disorder is characterized by unrealistic worry about life circumstances accompanied by symptoms of motor tension, autonomic hyperactivity, or vigilance and scanning.

Additional Reading: Somatic symptom disorder. *Am Fam Physician*. 2016;93(1):49-54A.
Category: Psychogenic disorders

15. An ambulance brings a 34-year-old man to the emergency department, following a motor vehicle crash. On examination, you notice that he has paradoxical respirations, as his chest expands with expiration and contracts with inspiration. The most likely diagnosis to explain this presentation is which one of the following?

A) Cardiac contusion
B) Flail chest
C) Pneumothorax
D) Ruptured thoracic aorta
E) Ruptured esophagus

The answer is B: In cases of severe blunt trauma to the chest, multiple rib fractures may lead to flail chest. By definition, a flail chest occurs in the presence of two or more fractures in three or more consecutive ribs, causing instability of the chest wall; however, the condition can also occur after costochondral separation.

The diagnosis is made by noting paradoxical chest wall motion in which the chest wall depresses with inspiration and expands with expiration. There may be coexisting intrathoracic or intra-abdominal injuries, and the mortality rate for patients with flail chest exceeds 50% in some series.

Initial management of flail chest consists of oxygen and close monitoring of early signs of respiratory compromise, ideally using both pulse oximetry and capnography. Importantly, multimodal analgesia is vitally important for complex chest injuries, especially in the elderly. This includes standing Tylenol, nonsteroidal anti-inflammatory drugs, opioids, Gabapentin, lidocaine patches, and frequently regional blocks by anesthesia. When the mechanics of respiration are altered, such as with this patient, and patients are not breathing deeply due to pain (ie, splinting), atelectasis sets in which can lead to pneumonia, acute respiratory distress syndrome, and death. There is a stepwise increase in the risk for mortality as the number of ribs broken increases.

Noninvasive positive airway pressure by mask may obviate the need for endotracheal intubation in alert patients. Patients with severe injuries, respiratory distress, or progressively worsening respiratory function require endotracheal intubation in alert patients. Patients with flail chest that fail conservative management may progress to needing rib plating by a thoracic surgeon.

Additional Reading: Flail chest, emergency medicine. In: *The 5-Minute Clinical Consult*. Wolters Kluwer; 2022.

16. An 18-month-old child is brought into the emergency department after being involved in a motor vehicle crash. He is lethargic, with a low blood pressure (BP) and tachycardia. His capillary refill is delayed, and his mucous membranes are dry. Appropriate management at this time would be which one of the following interventions?

A) Administer intravenous (IV) lactated Ringer's solution as a 20 mL/kg bolus.
B) Administer IV D5W (20 mL/kg) for 30 to 60 minutes.
C) Administer IV 0.45 normal saline (20 mL/kg) for 30 to 60 minutes.
D) Administer IV D5W with normal saline (20 mL/kg) for 30 to 60 minutes.
E) Provide an oral rehydration solution.

The answer is A: Emergent resuscitation of infants and children typically involves fluid replacement. Fluid deficits can result from a host of conditions including infection, trauma, or dehydration. A short-term weight loss >1% body weight per day is presumed to represent a fluid deficit. The rate at which the deficit is replaced depends on the severity of dehydration and the rate of fluid loss.

In general, when signs of circulatory compromise exist, 20 mL/kg of lactated Ringer's solution or 0.9% sodium chloride solution is rapidly infused intravenously to restore adequate perfusion. Children in severe hypovolemic shock may require and tolerate fluid boluses totaling 60 to 80 mL/kg within the first 1 to 2 hours of presentation. The need for additional fluid should alert the physician to anticipate complications of acute shock. The remainder of the deficit can be replaced over 8 to 48 hours, depending on the clinical need.

There are some unique attributes of trauma patients that should be appreciated when resuscitating a trauma patient in extremis, such as this. Family medicine physicians often manage trauma outside of mature trauma systems where blood would otherwise be immediately available in a trauma bay. For any trauma patients in extremis, whole blood or balanced blood product resuscitation is preferred over any crystalloid. It is important to appreciate two things about crystalloid in trauma: (1) acidosis contributes to coagulopathy and normal saline is 100 times more acidic than lactated Ringer's, which is why surgeons prefer lactated Ringer's over normal saline, and (2) crystalloids lack oxygen-carrying capacity and coagulation factors, which are what bleeding patients need. In the community hospital, bolusing lactated Ringer's while blood is being prepared may be required to stabilize a patient.

Additional Reading: Deficit Therapy. In: *UpToDate*. 2022.
Category: Nonspecific system

17. When determining the diagnosis in a patient with an acute abdomen, which one of the following imaging studies has the highest accuracy rate to diagnose appendicitis?

A) Abdominal ultrasonography
B) Barium enema
C) Computed tomography (CT) of the abdomen
D) Hepatobiliary iminodiacetic acid scan
E) Plain films of the abdomen

The answer is C: Acute appendicitis is the most common reason leading to emergent abdominal surgery. The overall diagnostic accuracy achieved by traditional history, physical examination, and laboratory tests has been approximately 80%. The accuracy of diagnosis varies and is more difficult in women of childbearing age, children, and elderly persons. If the diagnosis of acute appendicitis is clear from the history and physical examination, prompt surgical referral is warranted.

In atypical presentations, ultrasonography and CT may help lower the rate of false-negative appendicitis diagnoses, reduce morbidity from perforation, and lower medical expenses. Ultrasonography is safe and readily available, with a sensitivity of 86% and a specificity of 81%; however, CT scan has a better specificity (91%-98%) and sensitivity (95%-100%). Disadvantages of CT include radiation exposure, cost, and possible complications from contrast media.

Additional Reading: Appendicitis, acute. In: Domino F, ed. *The 5-Minute Clinical Consult*. Wolters Kluwer; 2022.
Category: Gastroenterology system

18. A patient presents following an injury and has pain with palpation over the anatomic "snuff box" (the area between the extensor pollicis brevis and the extensor pollicis longus tendons). This finding typically is indicative of which one of the following fractures?

A) Boxer's fracture
B) Colles fracture
C) Cuboid fracture
D) Hook of the hamate fracture
E) Scaphoid fracture

The answer is E: Scaphoid fractures account for approximately 60% of carpal bone fractures and are often missed on the initial radiograph. They frequently occur following a fall onto an outstretched hand. Symptoms include pain over the area with radial deviation of the wrist. Reduction is seldom necessary; however, the arm, wrist, and thumb should be immobilized with a thumb spica cast for at least 6 weeks. If pain persists for longer than 4 months, there is an increased risk of nonunion or avascular necrosis with development of arthritis. Surgery may be indicated for this condition.

If clinically suspected, radiographs (including scaphoid views) should be performed initially. Plain wrist films usually do not detect these fractures. In some cases, a bone scan or tomograms may be necessary to confirm the diagnosis. Bony electrical stimulation has also been shown to be effective in the healing of scaphoid fractures. Displaced fractures require open reduction with screw fixation.

Additional Reading: Evaluation and diagnosis of wrist pain: a case-based approach. *Am Fam Physician*. 2013;87(8):568-573.
Category: Musculoskeletal system

19. A felon is a clinical term that refers to which one of the following conditions?

A) Asymmetric nevus
B) Herpetic infection associated with a phalanx
C) Infection of the distal pulp space of a phalanx
D) Neuroma associated with the flexor tendon
E) Prominence of the distal fifth toe

The answer is C: A felon is an infection of the pulp space of a phalanx. A felon is usually caused by inoculation of bacteria into the fingertip through a penetrating trauma. The most commonly affected digits are the thumb and index finger. Predisposing causes include splinters, bits of glass, abrasions, and minor trauma. A felon may also arise when an untreated paronychia spreads into the pad of the fingertip. The most common site is the distal pulp, which may be involved centrally, laterally, and apically. The septa between pulp spaces ordinarily limit the spread of infection, resulting in an abscess, which creates pressure and necrosis of adjacent tissues. The underlying bone, joint, or flexor tendons may become infected, and intense throbbing pain and a swollen pulp are present.

If diagnosed in the early stages of cellulitis, a felon may be treated with elevation, oral antibiotics, and warm water or saline soaks. Radiographs should be obtained to evaluate for osteomyelitis or a foreign body. Tetanus prophylaxis should be administered when necessary. If fluctuance is present, incision and drainage are appropriate along with the administration of appropriate antibiotics (usually a cephalosporin or antistaphylococcal penicillin).

Additional Reading: Common acute hand infections. *Am Fam Physician*. 2003;68:2167-2176.
Category: Integumentary system

20. A patient is found to have a whitish lesion on his buccal mucosa during a general medical examination. It is not painful and does not change when wiped with a gauze pad. The most likely diagnosis for such a finding is which one of the following?

A) Gingivitis
B) Leukoplakia
C) Periodontitis
D) Squamous cell carcinoma
E) Thrush

The answer is B: Leukoplakia is a precancerous lesion that appears as a white, elevated, plaquelike growth that usually has asymmetric borders and usually affects the oral mucosa. It cannot be wiped off. The lesions tend to occur on the lip, mouth, buccal mucosa, or vaginal mucosa. Those at risk are cigarette smokers, pipe smokers, smokeless tobacco users, and heavy alcohol users. Others at risk include those with chronic oral infections, chronic malocclusion, or long-term ultraviolet light exposure. Approximately 10% may show malignant transformation. If suspected, these lesions should be biopsied to rule out malignancy.

Thrush, which is the result of *Candida* infections, can resemble leukoplakia, but *Candida* can be removed using a gauze pad.

Periodontitis is a chronic inflammatory disease that destroys bone and gum tissues that support the teeth. If only the superficial gums are involved in this breakdown, the disease is referred to as gingivitis. If it is more advanced and involves the connecting tissues and bone, then it is called periodontitis.

Additional Reading: Common oral lesions: part II. Masses and neoplasia. *Am Fam Physician*. 2007;75(4):509-512.
Category: Integumentary system

21. A 2-year-old child is brought into your office by his mother, who reports that he fell off his bed and has been limping for the past couple of days. She stated that he had hit his head but had no loss of consciousness and has been acting normally since his fall. You note retinal hemorrhages and several areas of bruising on the head, legs, thighs, and arms in varying stages of healing. The most likely explanation for his presentation is which one of the following?

A) Autism
B) Abuse
C) Hemophilia
D) Leukemia
E) Poor coordination

The answer is B: Head injuries in children are often accidental; however, such injuries can be the result of physical abuse. Children with head injuries related to abuse tend to be younger than those with accidental injuries. Boys are more frequently affected. Subdural hematoma, subarachnoid hemorrhage, and retinal hemorrhage are more common in abused children. Child abuse should be strongly suspected when such injuries are present in a child without a history of a fall or with a history of a fall from a relatively low height. Multiple injuries in various stages of healing should also alert the clinician to the possibility of abuse. A skeletal survey for children younger than 3 years should be performed when inflicted head injuries are suspected.

Additional Reading: Child abuse: approach and management. *Am Fam Physician*. 2007;75(2):221-228.
Category: Nonspecific system

22. A 67-year-old man presents to your office because he has not been feeling well and complaining of abdominal pain. His past medical history is relatively unremarkable, although he is a smoker. On examination, his vital signs are stable, and his abdominal examination is benign, but you detect a pulsatile mass in his midabdomen. The most appropriate test at this time would be to do which one of the following?

A) Order a magnetic resonance imaging of the abdomen.
B) Order an ultrasonography of the abdomen.
C) Order an upper gastrointestinal x-ray series.
D) Order a barium enema.
E) Obtain a complete blood count, electrolytes, and erythrocyte sedimentation rate.

The answer is B: An abdominal aortic aneurysm (AAA) is defined as a dilated aorta with a diameter of at least 1.5 times the diameter measured at the level of renal arteries. AAAs result from a weakening in the wall of the aorta. Most cases occur inferior to the renal arteries and are asymptomatic; however, back pain or abdominal pain may precede rupture. Most aneurysms are the result of atherosclerotic disease that results in weakening of the vessel. Strong evidence suggests a genetic susceptibility to AAAs. Patients with these aneurysms have a 20% chance of having a first-degree relative with the same condition. Male siblings are at particular risk. Approximately 75% of AAAs are asymptomatic and are detected during routine physical examination or during an unrelated radiologic or surgical procedure.

Symptoms of an AAA may result from expansion or rupture of the aneurysm, pressure on adjacent structures, embolization, or thrombosis. The most commonly reported symptom is any type of abdominal, flank, or back pain. Pressure on adjacent viscera may result in compression of the bowel. Patients may present with early satiety and, occasionally, nausea and vomiting. Rarely, ureteral compression may result in a partial ureteral obstruction. Thrombus and atheromatous material, which line nearly all AAAs, may occasionally result in distal arterial embolization and, rarely, aneurysm thrombosis. The abrupt onset of severe, constant pain in the abdomen, flank, or back, unrelieved by positional changes, is a characteristic of expansion or rupture of the aneurysm.

Physical examination often reveals a pulsating abdominal mass. Obesity, uncooperativeness, ascites, tortuosity of the aorta, and excessive lumbar lordosis are conditions that may make diagnosis by palpation difficult. Examination of the abdominal aorta is facilitated by having the patient lie on the examination table with the knees slightly flexed. The aorta is palpated during exhalation. A pulsatile abdominal mass left of midline—between the xiphoid process and the umbilicus—is highly suggestive of an AAA.

Diagnosis is made with ultrasonography or CT examination. B-mode ultrasonography is the screening method of choice for asymptomatic AAAs. It is inexpensive and does not require ionizing radiation yet reveals details of the vessel wall and whether it is associated with an atherosclerotic plaque, along with an accurate measurement of the longitudinal and transverse dimensions of the aneurysm.

Typically, aneurysms >5.5 to 6 cm are treated surgically, whereas smaller aneurysms are observed for any changes. If they grow 1 cm/y, larger surgery is recommended. Endovascular repair is safer, results in shorter hospital stays and quicker recovery, and translates into significant cost savings when compared with conventional surgery. The operative mortality rate is usually <5%. The mortality rate of patients with aneurysms >6 cm is approximately 50% in 1 year without repair; patients with aneurysms between 4 and 6 cm have a mortality rate of 25% in 1 year.

Additional Reading: *Recommendation:* Abdominal Aortic Aneurysm – Screening | United States Preventive Services Taskforce (uspreventiveservicestaskforce.org)
Category: Cardiovascular system

The U.S. Preventive Services Task Force recommends one-time screening for AAA with ultrasonography in men aged 65 to 75 years who have ever smoked (grade B recommendation).

23. A 53-year-old woman presents to the office complaining of right-upper-quadrant, colicky abdominal pain for the past few days and now she is feeling nauseous and has vomited. On examination, there is significant pain elicited when palpating the right upper quadrant. Laboratory findings include an elevated white blood cell (WBC) count, alkaline phosphatase, and bilirubin level. The most likely diagnosis to account for her presentation is which one of the following?

A) A dissecting abdominal aneurysm
B) A perforated duodenal ulcer
C) Acute viral gastroenteritis
D) Acute pancreatitis
E) Acute cholecystitis

The answer is E: Cholecystitis is an acute inflammation of the gallbladder wall. The condition usually results from an obstruction of the bile ducts as a result of biliary stones (most commonly cholesterol). Risk factors for cholesterol gallstone formation include age, obesity, rapid weight loss, pregnancy, female sex, use of exogenous estrogens, diabetes, certain gastrointestinal conditions, and certain medications. Symptoms include colicky right-upper-quadrant abdominal pain that starts out mild and crescendoes into more severe pain that may last several hours before resolving spontaneously. Patients may also report nausea and vomiting, and low-grade fevers.

Physical examination usually shows marked right-upper-quadrant tenderness with a positive Murphy sign (marked abdominal pain and inspiratory arrest with palpation of the right upper quadrant). A palpable gallbladder is present in as many as 30% to 40% of patients. Laboratory findings include an elevated WBC count and increased serum transaminase, alkaline phosphatase, bilirubin levels, and, in some cases, amylase levels. Jaundice or substantially elevated bilirubin suggest obstruction of the common bile duct and warrants further workup with endoscopic retrograde cholangiopancreatography (ERCP) or magnetic resonance cholangiopancreatography, as endoscopic intervention would generally trump surgical intervention. The diagnosis is usually made with ultrasonography, which has 84% sensitivity and 99% specificity; however, cholescintigraphy (hepatobiliary iminodiacetic acid scan) is the most sensitive test to document obstruction in the cystic duct, with 97% sensitivity and 90% specificity, and is used when there is diagnostic uncertainty given its higher cost than ultrasound. In the gallbladder, stones <2 mm in diameter may be missed or misdiagnosed as sludge. ERCP is the test of choice to detect stones in the common bile duct.

Additional Reading: Appropriate and safe use of diagnostic imaging *Am Fam Physician*. 2013;87(7):494-501.
Category: Gastroenterology system

24. A patient comes in concerned over a mole on his back, which he thinks has been changing over the past couple of months. He is worried about a melanoma because his aunt had died of melanoma a couple of years ago. The most common form of malignant melanoma is which one of the following?

A) Acral lentiginous melanoma
B) Lentigo maligna melanoma
C) Nodular melanoma
D) Superficial spreading melanoma

The answer is D: Cutaneous malignant melanoma accounts for 3% to 5% of all skin cancers and is responsible for approximately 75% of all deaths from skin cancer. It is a serious and life-threatening condition because of the potential for distant metastasis. Studies have shown that the prevalence of melanoma increases with proximity to the equator. Persons with skin types that are sensitive to the effects of ultraviolet radiation—red or blond hair, freckles, and fair skin that burns easily and tans with difficulty—are at higher risk. Although cumulative sun exposure is linked to nonmelanoma skin cancer, intermittent intense sun exposure seems to be more related to melanoma risk. Persons with an increased number of moles, dysplastic nevi, or a family history of the disease and immunosuppression are at increased risk compared with the general population. Melanomas are classified into the following:

Lentigo maligna melanoma: This usually affects older patients in their 60s and 70s. These lesions usually show variegation of color including black, brown, and reddish lesions and are large (measuring 2-6 cm).

Superficial spreading melanoma: This is the most common type. These lesions are usually smaller (2-3 cm in diameter) and tend to affect patients in their 50s and 60s.

Nodular melanoma: These patients are usually younger (average age, 30-50 years). These lesions are usually smaller than the other two types and are slightly raised and uniform in color. Unfortunately, these lesions tend to spread deeply into the underlying tissue and have the worst prognosis.

Acral lentiginous melanoma: This condition is rare and is associated with lesions affecting the palmar and plantar surface of the extremities as well as the subungual skin. It is similar to lentigo maligna melanoma.

The ABCDE mnemonic stands for the following:

Asymmetry
Border irregularities
Color variation
Diameter
Evolution/**E**levation

Any suspicious pigmented lesion should be biopsied. Malignant melanoma may tend to bleed or ulcerate. Early metastasis occurs through the lymph nodes, whereas late metastasis occurs through a hematogenous route and may affect the skin, liver, or lungs.

A properly performed biopsy is essential for the diagnosis. If melanoma is diagnosed, the histologic interpretation of the biopsy determines the prognosis and treatment plan. General recommendations include performing an excisional biopsy whenever possible. Accepted techniques for biopsy include punch, saucerization, and elliptic excision. Shave biopsy will not miss a diagnosis of melanoma but may interfere with the staging process of determining the depth of invasion, the Breslow depth. The Breslow depth is the most important prognostic parameter in evaluating the primary tumor. Because early detection and treatment can lead to identification of thinner lesions, which may increase survival, it is critical that physicians be comfortable with evaluating suspicious pigmented lesions and providing treatment or referral as necessary.

Additional Reading: Cutaneous malignant melanoma: a primary care perspective. *Am Fam Physician*. 2012;85(2):161-168.
Category: Integumentary system

25. A 27-year-old man is brought to the emergency department after being involved in a high-speed motor vehicle crash. He is conscious but complains of abdominal pain. On examination, he is found to have abdominal tenderness. He is hypotensive with low-grade tachycardia. After calling for 2 units of emergency release blood to be transfused, the most appropriate management at this time would be which one of the following?

A) Perform a peritoneal lavage.
B) Obtain an emergent abdominal computed tomographic (CT) scan.
C) Obtain a flat and upright abdominal x-ray series.
D) Perform a bedside ultrasound focused assessment with sonography in trauma (FAST) examination.
E) Perform an exploratory laparotomy.

The answer is D: Patients who have experienced significant abdominal trauma and who have abdominal pain with vital signs derangements should receive a bedside "eFAST," which stands for extended FAST. This study involves six views: a cardiac/subxiphoid view looking for pericardial tamponade; right-upper-quadrant and left-upper-quadrant views looking for free fluid in the hepatorenal and splenorenal spaces, respectively; a pelvic view looking or free fluid in the pelvis; and bilateral lung views to assess for the absence of lung sliding, which is diagnostic of pneumothorax. Free fluid on eFAST examination with hypotension refractory to transfusion would be a hard indication for the patient to go to the operating room with a surgeon. Historically, diagnostic peritoneal lavage was advocated in this setting, but this has been replaced by ultrasound, which is ubiquitous and can be performed rapidly with excellent sensitivity (~75%) and specificity (~95%). While surgically opening the abdomen may seem reasonable, in reality, gaining safe access to the abdominal cavity is fraught with unnecessary risk for the patient, particularly in the setting of prior abdominal surgery or obesity.

Patients who are clinically stable may undergo CT scan to further evaluate the abdomen when blunt trauma has occurred.

Additional Reading: Initial evaluation and management of blunt abdominal trauma in adults. In *UpToDate*. 2022.
Category: Nonspecific system

26. A 34-year-old homeless man presents to the emergency department with a cut on his right hand. The injury occurred while collecting cans from a garbage bin. He does not know if he had a tetanus vaccine before. The most appropriate immunization to administer in this situation is which one of the following?

A) Adult diphtheria tetanus toxoid.
B) Diphtheria-tetanus-acellular pertussis vaccine.
C) Diphtheria tetanus toxoid and tetanus immunoglobulin.
D) No immunization is necessary at this time.

The answer is C: Tetanus immunization should be administered to those who have completed only the primary series of immunization or who received a booster immunization more than 5 years previously. Tetanus toxoid (0.5 mL intramuscularly) and tetanus immune globulin (250 units intramuscularly) should be given to patients with a dirty wound who have received fewer than three doses of tetanus toxoid or whose prior immunization status is uncertain.

Additional Reading: Tetanus. In: Domino F, ed. *The 5-Minute Clinical Consult*. Wolters Kluwer; 2022.
Category: Nonspecific system

27. A 60-year-old woman is being assessed after a fall on the ice and is diagnosed with a hip fracture. Which one of the following statements is true regarding hip fractures?

A) Avascular necrosis of the femoral head is a serious complication.
B) Location of the fracture has no bearing on the outcome.
C) Most hip fractures do not require surgery for repair.
D) Nonunion or malunion does not occur with hip fractures.
E) None of the above statements are true.

The answer is A: The distinction between intracapsular and extracapsular hip fracture has prognostic value for the patient's outcome. Early detection of intracapsular fractures is especially important because these fractures are prone to complications for two primary reasons. First, interruption of the blood supply to the femoral head frequently occurs and can lead to avascular necrosis. Second, the head fragment of the fracture is often a shell containing fragile cancellous bone that provides poor attachment for a fixation device, a situation that often increases the possibility of nonunion or malunion.

Asymptomatic lesions of the femoral head, which involve less than 15% of the femoral head, may resolve without surgical intervention and may, therefore, be treated nonoperatively. However, asymptomatic avascular necrosis that involves more than 30% of the femoral head is likely to collapse despite surgical interventions; thus, these patients may also be nonoperatively managed at the outset with anticipation of eventual total hip arthroplasty.

Additional Reading: Hip fracture: diagnosis, treatment, and secondary prevention. *Am Fam Physician*. 2014;89(12):945-951.
Category: Musculoskeletal system

28. A 51-year-old man complains of rectal discomfort and bleeding aggravated by bowel movements. He reports a long history of constipation. On examination, there is a small fissure at the lateral 9 o'clock position. Which of the following statements is true about his condition?

A) A cause other than passage of hard stool should be considered.
B) Bowel movements help relieve symptoms.
C) Corticosteroid creams should be avoided because of the risk of bacterial overgrowth.
D) Exercise often leads to development of fissures.
E) Rectal spasms increase blood flow and accelerate healing.

The answer is A: Anal fissures are small tears in the mucosa of the anal canal. Symptoms include rectal pain and bleeding, which is aggravated by bowel movements. They often produce pain disproportionate to the size of the lesion, and the cause is thought to be secondary to traumatic tearing of the mucosa with the passage of large, hard stools. Other causes include proctitis as a result of previous rectal surgery, hemorrhoids, or rectal cancer. Because of its location in the area of the rectal sphincter, spasms may keep the area from healing.

Fissures are most commonly located anterior or posterior to the anus. When fissures are found laterally (as in this case), syphilis, tuberculosis, occult abscesses, leukemic infiltrates, carcinoma, herpes, acquired immunodeficiency syndrome, or inflammatory bowel disease should be considered as causes.

Treatment involves the use of stool softeners and laxatives, a high-fiber diet, hydrocortisone creams, benzocaine ointments, and warm sitz baths, as well as increased oral fluids and adequate exercise. Botulinum toxin injections are also used. Another nonsurgical treatment for anal fissure is nitroglycerin ointment 2% diluted to 0.2% four times a day. Calcium channel blockers, oral or topical, are not better than nitrates but have less side effects. Surgery is indicated for severe cases that are refractive.

Additional Reading: Anal fissure. In: Domino F, ed. *The 5-Minute Clinical Consult*. Wolters Kluwer; 2022.
Category: Gastroenterology system

29. A 39-year-old white woman complains of several episodes of right-upper-quadrant pain during the past year. The episodes typically last 2 to 4 hours and are associated with nausea and vomiting. Her most recent episode occurred 2 weeks ago, and the episodes seem to be happening more often. Which one of the following is most likely to provide an explanation for the patient's symptoms?

A) A bilirubin level
B) An aspartate aminotransferase (AST) level
C) A plain film of the abdomen
D) A hepatobiliary iminodiacetic acid (HIDA) scan
E) Abdominal ultrasonography

The answer is E: Cholecystitis (inflammation of the gallbladder) usually results as a complication of cholelithiasis (gallstones) and irreversible obstruction of the cystic duct by gallstones. This patient, on the other hand, has symptomatic cholelithiasis. The difference is the irreversibility of the cystic duct obstruction and ensuing infection seen in cholecystitis, which does not occur in symptomatic cholelithiasis. The symptoms experienced by this patient are from the intermittent blockage of the cystic duct with stones or from stones passing through the common bile duct. Symptomatic cholelithiasis is managed on an elective surgical basis compared to cholecystitis, which is managed on an urgent/emergent basis. Pain lasting for greater than 6 to 8 hours is reason for these patients to be admitted to the emergency room for evaluation by a surgeon. Intermittent episodes, such as these, can be referred to a surgeon on an outpatient basis with strict return precautions.

In a patient with a typical history for gallstones, an abdominal ultrasonography is likely to show stones and support the diagnosis. Serum bilirubin and AST levels are usually normal except at the time of an attack. Patients with chronic cholecystitis rarely have abnormal laboratory studies. HIDA scans are used in the setting of cholecystitis, as they are only diagnostic when the duct is occluded. Further, even in cholecystitis, HIDA scans are second-line imaging after ultrasound when there remains diagnostic uncertainty. A plain abdominal film will detect only 10% to 15% of cases of cholelithiasis.

Laparoscopic cholecystectomy is the procedure of choice for uncomplicated acute cholecystitis and symptomatic cholelithiasis. Stones can be composed of cholesterol (most common), pigment, and mixed stones. Prophylactic cholecystectomy for asymptomatic cholelithiasis is generally not recommended.

Additional Reading: Cholelithiasis. In: Domino F, ed. *The 5-Minute Clinical Consult*. Wolters Kluwer; 2022.
Category: Gastroenterology system

30. A 31-year-old patient presents after he was bitten on the finger by his neighbor's cat earlier in the day. On examination, he is healthy but has small puncture wounds with minimal inflammation at the site of the bite. He is allergic to penicillin. Appropriate management for this situation includes which one of the following therapies?

A) Administering intravenous ceftriaxone (Rocephin)
B) Applying a topical antibiotic ointment
C) Prescribing oral doxycycline (Vibramycin)
D) Prescribing oral amoxicillin-clavulanate (Augmentin)
E) Observing overnight with reassessment the next day

The answer is C: The oral flora of humans and animals contains a mixture of potential pathogens: *Eikenella corrodens* is frequently isolated from human bites, and *Pasteurella multocida* from many animal bites, particularly those of cats. Antibiotic prophylaxis should be considered for all bites requiring closure and for high-risk bites. All cat bites are considered high risk for infection because they tend to cause deep puncture wounds.

Amoxicillin/clavulanate (Augmentin) is generally considered the first-line prophylactic treatment for animal bites. A 3- to 7-day course of prophylactic antibiotics is likely adequate and was typical in most studies. For patients who are allergic to penicillin, doxycycline is an acceptable alternative, except for children younger than 8 years and pregnant women.

Additional Reading: Dog and cat bites. *Am Fam Physician*. 2014;90(4):239-243.
Category: Nonspecific system

31. A middle-aged man returns with complaints of rectal pain, as it feels like he is "passing glass." Additionally, he notes blood on the toilet paper when he wipes. You had previously diagnosed him with an anal fissure and had prescribed fiber supplements and sitz baths. Which one of the following can interfere with the healing of an anal fissure?

A) External hemorrhoids
B) Internal sphincter spasms
C) Poor blood supply to the dentate line
D) Rectal rugae
E) Sitz baths

The answer is B: Fissures of the anal canal are usually due to traumatic lacerations as a result of chronic constipation with perhaps an underlying infection of the lesion. Other associated conditions include chronic proctitis, rectal carcinoma, hemorrhoids, or previous rectal surgery. The lesion is often associated with the internal sphincter and can cause spasms that can deter healing. Symptoms include a sudden onset, feeling of passing "shards of glass" occurring during bowel movement, with a small amount of bright red blood in stool.

Physical examination usually shows evidence of a linear fissure located in the midline. Treatment involves the use of stool softeners, fiber supplements, sitz baths, and hydrocortisone- or benzocaine-containing cream, which may aid in decreasing any associated pain or inflammation and promote healing. Other options are used to address internal sphincter spasms, which can impair healing; these include topical nitroglycerine 0.2% ointment on a botulinum toxin A (Botox), topical calcium channel blocker, and topical bethanechol. Surgery, targeted at the internal sphincter, is reserved for cases that fail to respond to medical therapy.

Additional Reading: Chronic anal fissures. *Am Fam Physician*. 2016;93(6):498-499.
Category: Gastroenterology system

32. A 17-year-old gymnast fell onto his outstretched hands and immediately had to stop his routine because of pain. On examination, he has pain over his left distal radioulnar joint. Which of the following injuries is most likely?

A) Colles fracture
B) Scaphoid fracture
C) Radius greenstick fracture
D) de Quervain tenosynovitis
E) Triangular fibrocartilage complex (TFCC) injury

The answer is E: Ulnar wrist pain and weakness caused by a fall onto an outstretched hand may result in injury to the TFCC, which is the primary stabilizer of the distal radioulnar joint. The distal radioulnar joint is located just proximally to the wrist joint. It is an articulation between the ulnar notch of the radius and the ulnar head. TFCC injury is common in gymnasts and in racquetball, tennis, and hockey players.

A Colles fracture is one of the most common distal radius fractures in which the broken fragment of the radius tilts upward. A scaphoid fracture frequently occurs following a fall onto an outstretched hand; however, symptoms include pain over the anatomic "snuff box" (area between the extensor pollicis brevis and the extensor pollicis longus tendons) and pain with radial deviation of the wrist. The greenstick fracture is an incomplete fracture that occurs most often during infancy and childhood when bones are soft and that tends to take place in the middle, slower-growing parts of bone.

The combination of wrist pain and grip weakness is characteristic of de Quervain tenosynovitis. Local tenderness is present over the distal portion of the radial styloid, and the pain is generally reproduced with direct palpation of the involved tendons. Pain is aggravated by passively stretching the thumb tendons over the radial styloid in thumb flexion (the Finkelstein maneuver).

Additional Reading: Busconi BD, Stevenson JH. Approach to the patient with TFCC tears. *Sports Medicine Consult: A Problem-Based Approach to Sports Medicine for the Primary Care Physician*. Lippincott Williams & Wilkins; 2009.
Category: Musculoskeletal system

33. You are working in the emergency department, and a gunshot victim, who was bleeding profusely, is brought in. He is being supported with intravenous (IV) fluids, and you call for an immediate blood transfusion. Which one of the following blood types is considered the universal donor?

A) O positive
B) O negative
C) AB positive
D) AB negative
E) B negative

The answer is B: In trauma settings, the use of IV fluid is important to maintain adequate perfusion to vital tissues and organs. The use of blood for fluid replacement requires typing and proper storing, making it impractical to use in emergent settings in which time is extremely valuable. Because of this, a trauma patient should receive two large-bore (16-gauge or larger) IV lines and lactated Ringer's solution until proper blood can be given in a controlled setting. For adults, 1000 mL of crystalloid solution should be given as an initial bolus—children should receive 20 mL/kg. In some emergent situations, O negative blood, the universal donor blood, can be given until the appropriate blood type arrives.

Family medicine physicians often manage trauma outside of mature trauma systems where blood would otherwise be immediately available in a trauma bay. The so-called lethal triad in trauma is hypothermia, coagulopathy, and acidosis, which, when combined, portend a bad outcome. It is important to appreciate that crystalloid is cold, dilutes coagulation factors, lacks oxygen-carrying capacity, and is 100-1000 times more acidotic than blood. Limiting crystalloid administration and transfusing blood early saves lives.

Additional Reading: Initial evaluation and management of shock in adult trauma. In: *UpToDate*. 2022.
Category: Nonspecific system

34. A 3-year-old child is brought into the emergency department by her parents. She has had a high fever and sore throat for 2 days and now is having noisy breathing. On examination, you note that the child is sitting on a stretcher leaning forward with her neck extended. Her breathing is stridorous, and she has a fever. The most likely diagnosis to account for this presentation is which one of the following conditions?

A) Croup
B) Epiglottitis
C) Herpangina
D) Meningitis
E) Strep throat

The answer is B: Epiglottitis is a rapidly progressive and potentially fatal infection that causes swelling of the epiglottis and may lead to compromise of the child's airway. In the past, it was most commonly caused by *H influenzae*. The highest incidence occurs in children between 2 and 5 years of age. In recent years, the occurrence of epiglottitis has been reduced dramatically by the widespread use of the *H influenzae* type B vaccine. Symptoms include a sore throat, high fever, hoarseness, and dysphagia with drooling and stridor. Stridor is an audible, often high-pitched crowing breath sound heard during inspiration; however, it can be heard throughout the respiratory cycle as a patient worsens. Children affected usually lean forward and hyperextend the neck to open the compromised airway.

Because of the rapid course of the infection, the patient should be immediately hospitalized and the airway secured. Inspection of the pharynx can precipitate a complete obstruction of the airway and should not be performed unless there are qualified personnel present who can simultaneously intubate the child during the inspection procedure if necessary. Lateral and anteroposterior soft tissue radiographs should be taken and can confirm the diagnosis. The characteristic "thumb sign" is noted on the lateral radiograph. In addition to securing an airway, parenteral antibiotics should be administered and the child should be monitored closely in an intensive care setting.

Croup is usually due to a parainfluenza virus and is also associated with abnormal breath sounds. Typically, the child will develop coldlike symptoms, and if there is enough inflammation and coughing, they will develop a loud barking cough, a hoarse voice, and a runny nose.

Additional Reading: Antibiotic use in acute upper respiratory tract infections. *Am Fam Physician*. 2012;86(9):817-822.
Category: Respiratory system

35. A 13-year-old patient is brought in with an anaphylactic reaction after having been stung by a bee. Intravenous fluids are being started and you order the immediate administration of which one of the following medications?

A) Diphenhydramine
B) Epinephrine
C) Naproxen
D) Prednisone
E) Propranolol

The answer is B: Anaphylaxis is a life-threatening reaction from an exposure to an allergen that results in respiratory, cardiovascular, cutaneous, gastrointestinal, and neurologic manifestations. Cutaneous and respiratory symptoms are most common, occurring in 90% and 70% of episodes, respectively. With respiratory symptoms, the administration of intramuscular epinephrine (1:1000 dilution dosed at 0.01 mg/kg [maximal dose of 0.3 mg in children and 0.5 mg in adults]), along with appropriate management of airway, breathing, and circulation, is the first and most important therapeutic measure. The allergic response is usually immunoglobulin E–mediated, which leads to mast cell and basophil activation; hence, histamine H1 receptors antagonist (eg, diphenhydramine) and corticosteroids (eg, prednisone) may be useful adjuncts.

The risk of anaphylaxis is doubled in patients with mild asthma and tripled in those with severe disease. The most common triggers are food (egg, fish, food additives, milk, peanuts, sesame, shellfish, tree nuts), latex, insect stings (bee, wasp, fire ant, hymenopteran), medications (allopurinol, angiotensin-converting enzyme inhibitors, β-lactams, aspirin, biologic modifiers, nonsteroidal inflammatory drugs, opioids), radiocontrast media, and animal dander.

The diagnosis of anaphylaxis is typically made when symptoms occur within 1 hour of exposure to a specific antigen. Confirmatory testing using serum histamine and tryptase levels is difficult because blood samples must be drawn with strict time consideration. Allergen skin testing and in vitro assay for serum immunoglobulin E or specific allergens do not reliably predict who will develop anaphylaxis.

Additional Reading: Anaphylaxis: recognition and management. *Am Fam Physician*. 2011;84(10):111-118.
Category: Nonspecific system

36. A middle-aged man is brought to the emergency department with bloody stools, which he had noted over the past couple of hours. He is obviously uncomfortable on examination. The first step in the management of a lower gastrointestinal (GI) hemorrhage is which one of the following measures?

A) Order an emergent computed tomographic scan of the abdomen.
B) Order an emergent bleeding scan.
C) Obtain a surgical consult.
D) Perform a colonoscopy.
E) Resuscitate the unstable patient.

The answer is E: The incidence of massive lower GI bleeding is low (25 episodes per 100,000 persons annually), but the mortality rate is high, with up to 10% of such patients dying. Patients with suspected GI bleeding and hemodynamic instability should have large-bore intravenous access, such as two 18-gauge IV lines or larger, a type and cross for blood products, coagulation labs, Foley catheter, and intra-arterial monitoring, Of note, flow rates are faster through large-bore IV lines than through triple-lumen central venous lines, which is commonly overlooked in the emergency setting. The clinical evaluation of GI bleeding depends on the hemodynamic status of the patient and the suspected source of the bleeding. Patients presenting with upper GI or massive lower GI bleeding, postural hypotension, or hemodynamic instability require inpatient stabilization and evaluation. The immediate response to significant bleeding is to resuscitate the patient if they are unstable. Hospitalization is also required in patients who are hemodynamically unstable or elderly and those who have comorbidities.

GI bleeding suspected from a lower source may be secondary to diverticular disease, angiodysplasia, ulcerative colitis, ischemic colitis, neoplasm, colorectal polyps, proctitis, arteriovenous malformations, anal and rectal neoplasia, and hemorrhoids. However, acute massive rectal bleeding frequently arises from an upper GI source as well.

While colonoscopy identifies bleeding in more than 70% of patients. A technetium-99-tagged red blood cell scan may be helpful in identifying the site of bleeding if the rate of bleeding is greater than 0.1 mL/min. However, positive findings in this type of testing must be verified with an alternative test because of a relatively high number of false-positive results. Angiography may be useful in patients with active bleeding greater than 0.5 mL/min and can identify highly vascular nonbleeding lesions such as angiodysplasia and neoplasms.

Additional Reading: Approach to acute lower gastrointestinal bleeding in adults. In: *UpToDate*. 2022.
Category: Gastroenterology system

37. A 61-year-old man presents to your office with complaints of persistent, severe chest pain, which started this afternoon, following repeated episodes of vomiting earlier in the day. The most appropriate management to address this presentation would be which one of the following?

A) Admit for observation with antiemetics.
B) Administer an intravenous (IV) H_2 antagonist.
C) Administer an IV proton pump inhibitor.
D) Obtain a stat chest x-ray.
E) Perform a treadmill exercise test.

The answer is D: Effort rupture of the esophagus is a spontaneous perforation of the esophagus that most commonly results from a sudden increase in intra-esophageal pressure combined with negative intrathoracic pressure by straining or vomiting. Esophageal rupture, also known as *Boerhaave syndrome*, is a rare, life-threatening condition that can lead to mediastinitis and pleural effusions. Symptoms include midsternal chest pain after a severe episode of vomiting.

A delay in the diagnosis can lead to a poor prognosis, and a stat chest radiograph is warranted. The chest x-ray, or a computed tomographic scan of the chest, will usually show pneumomediastinum. A gastrograffin swallow study showing communication between the esophagus and pleural space can be used to confirm the diagnosis. If the gastrograffin study is nondiagnostic, this can be followed by a thin barium swallow evaluation. Barium evaluation is second line, as it causes significant inflammation when outside of the gastrointestinal tract and thus secondary pleuritis. Treatment involves immediate surgery.

Associated conditions include peptic ulcer disease, alcoholism, and other neurologic disorders. The differential diagnosis includes myocardial infarction, pulmonary embolism, pancreatitis, peptic ulcer disease with rupture, or a dissecting aortic aneurysm.

Additional Reading: Boerhaave's syndrome: effort rupture of the esophagus. In: *UpToDate*. 2022.
Category: Gastroenterology system

38. You have completed suturing a laceration on the cheek of a teenager, and his mother is asking when he should return to have the sutures removed. You inform her that facial sutures should be removed at which one of the following times after placement?

A) 24 hours.
B) 3 to 5 days.
C) 7 to 10 days.
D) 14 days.
E) Only absorbable sutures should be used on the face and do not need removal.

The answer is B: Sutures or staples should typically be removed 7 days after placement, but it is recommended that facial sutures be removed sooner (within 3-5 days) to minimize scarring. Sutures in areas subject to high tension should be left in place for 10 to 14 days.

Sutured or stapled lacerations should be covered with a protective, nonadherent dressing for at least 24 to 48 hours to avoid contamination. Patients should be instructed to observe the wound for the presence of warmth, redness, swelling, or drainage. Postoperative care for lacerations does not include the routine use of prophylactic antibiotics, unless there is evidence of bacterial contamination or a risk factor.

Additional Reading: Essentials of skin laceration repair. *Am Fam Physician*. 2008;78(8):945-951.
Category: Nonspecific system

39. You are examining a patient with complaints of right ear discomfort and observe a cholesteatoma on otoscopic examination. The most appropriate treatment for cholesteatoma is which one of the following measures?

A) Prescribe an oral antibiotic.
B) Prescribe antibiotic ear drops.
C) Prescribe an oral corticosteroid.
D) Refer for surgical removal.
E) Refer for tympanostomy tube placement.

The answer is D: Cholesteatoma is a collection of keratinized, desquamated epithelial cells in the middle ear or mastoid. It can be seen during otoscopic examination as white debris in the middle ear, with destruction of the ear canal bone adjacent to a tympanic membrane perforation. A cholesteatoma can occur as a primary lesion or as the result of chronic otitis media and/or perforation of the tympanic membrane. Prolonged dysfunction of the eustachian tube with the development of chronic negative pressure results in the formation of a squamous epithelial lined sac, which remains chronically infected.

Bone destruction due to an otherwise unsuspected cholesteatoma may be demonstrated on a computed tomographic scan. Cholesteatoma, particularly with perforation, greatly increases the probability of a serious complication (eg, purulent labyrinthitis, facial paralysis, and intracranial suppuration). A cholesteatoma typically erodes the temporal bone and may destroy the small ossicle bones. With time, they can erode into the facial nerve or into the brain. Treatment involves surgical removal.

Additional Reading: Perforated tympanic membrane. In: Domino F, ed. *The 5-Minute Clinical Consult*. Wolters Kluwer; 2022.
Category: Special sensory systems

40. A 27-year-old teacher presents to the emergency department complaining of abdominal pain, anorexia, and vomiting. The pain is periumbilical and achy in nature. Physical findings show a fever (temperature, 101.5 °F), and she has rebound tenderness along with positive psoas and obturator signs. The most likely diagnosis to explain her presentation is which one of the following?

A) A bowel infarction
B) A ruptured ectopic pregnancy
C) Acute appendicitis
D) Acute cholecystitis
E) Acute ovarian torsion

The answer is C: Appendicitis is the most common acute surgical condition of the abdomen. Approximately 7% of the population will have appendicitis in their lifetime, with the peak incidence occurring between the ages of 10 and 30 years. The diagnosis in infants, the elderly, and obese and pregnant patients is often more difficult. The mortality rate in nonperforated appendicitis is less than 1%, but it may be as high as 5% in young and elderly patients in whom diagnosis may often be delayed, thus making perforation more likely.

The diagnosis of appendicitis is based primarily on the patient's history and the physical examination. Although the symptoms are not always consistent, the typical presentation involves dull, periumbilical pain that migrates to the right lower abdomen. Anorexia, nausea, and vomiting usually accompany the onset of the abdominal pain.

Physical findings often include a low-grade fever, right-lower-quadrant pain, rebound tenderness, and spasms of the overlying abdominal muscles with guarding. A positive psoas sign (ie, pain with passive extension of the right hip) and obturator sign (ie, pain with internal and external rotation of the flexed right hip) are strongly supportive of the diagnosis. Rectal examination may reveal localized tenderness.

Laboratory results usually show a moderate leukocytosis (10,000-20,000 white blood cells/mm^3) with a left shift; however, this finding neither confirms nor excludes the diagnosis. Hematuria, proteinuria, and pyuria may be present.

A computed tomographic (CT) scan with contrast (sensitivity ~91%-98%; specificity 95%-99%) is the imaging modality of choice; however, ultrasonography is an alternative in pregnant patients, children, and women with suspected gynecologic pathology. Sensitivity and specificity vary by report, and accuracy depends on the skill of the ultrasonographer. Although ultrasonography can diagnose appendicitis, it does not reliably exclude the diagnosis. Starting with ultrasonography and, if negative, obtaining a CT scan have been proposed as an effective workup strategy.

Additional Reading: Appendicitis, acute. In: Domino F, ed. *The 5-Minute Clinical Consult*. Lippincott Williams & Wilkins; 2022.
Category: Gastroenterology system

41. Tissue adhesives are used to close lacerations and have some advantages and disadvantages when compared with traditional suturing. All of the following statements regarding adhesives are true, except which one?

A) Adhesives are not recommended over high-tension areas.
B) Exposure to water has little effect on adhesives.
C) They are resistant to bacterial growth.
D) They have lower tensile strength when compared with sutures.
E) They are not useful on the hand.

The answer is B: Application of tissue adhesives is useful in repairing lacerations. Adhesives are resistant to bacterial growth; however, they have lower tensile strength when compared with sutures and are not recommended over high-tension areas. Thus, they are not useful on the hand, and exposure to water is contraindicated.

Additional Reading: Common questions about wound care. *Am Fam Physician*. 2015;91(2):86-92.
Category: Nonspecific system

Tissue adhesives can be used as an alternative for closure of simple, noninfected lacerations in which the wound edges are easily approximated in areas of low tension and moisture.

42. A 23-year-old salesman presents with eye pain. He was playing Frisbee with his friends and was hit in the face and now it feels like his eye has been scratched. You suspect a corneal abrasion. This diagnosis can best be accomplished in a family physician's office by performing which one of the following procedures?

A) A slit-lamp examination
B) An ophthalmoscope magnification examination
C) A fluorescein dye examination
D) A peripheral visual field examination
E) Schiotz tonometer measurements

The answer is C: Eye injuries are frequently encountered in the family physician's office, and visual acuity should be tested at the time of presentation. Common injuries include the following:

Corneal abrasions: Corneal abrasions occur when there is localized loss of epithelium from the cornea typically caused by trauma. Symptoms include pain, foreign body sensation, tearing, and injection and history of trauma. A fluorescein dye examination is used to diagnose corneal abrasions. The goals of treatment include pain control, prevention of infection, and healing. Pain relief may be achieved with topical nonsteroidal anti-inflammatory drugs or oral analgesics. Follow-up may not be necessary for a patient with small (4 mm or less), uncomplicated abrasions; normal vision; and resolving symptoms. Contact lens–related abrasions should be treated with topical antipseudomonal antibiotics. Referral is indicated for any patient with symptoms that do not improve or that worsen, a corneal infiltrate or ulcer, significant vision loss, or a penetrating eye injury.

Foreign bodies: Inspection of the entire cornea is necessary to identify foreign bodies. The upper and lower eyelid should also be inspected. Foreign bodies should be removed by flushing with normal saline, a cotton swab, an eye spud, or a 25-gauge needle. Fluorescein dye examination should be performed to rule out an abrasion. Rust rings should be examined for and removed as much as possible by an ophthalmologist; however, complete removal is unnecessary.

Subconjunctival hemorrhage: This condition is present when there is a well-demarcated area of injection from the rupture of small subconjunctival vessels. Causes include trauma, coughing, vomiting, straining, or viral hemorrhagic conjunctivitis. Blood in the anterior chamber indicates a hyphema and requires immediate ophthalmologic referral. Referral is indicated for any patient with symptoms that do not improve or that worsen, a corneal infiltrate or ulcer, significant vision loss, or a penetrating eye injury.

Additional Reading: Evaluation and management of corneal abrasions. *Am Fam Physician*. 2013;87(2):114-120.
Category: Special sensory systems

43. A middle-aged man presents with a recurrent nosebleed. In considering his treatment, which one of the following statements about epistaxis is true?

A) Nasal packs should be left in place for at least 72 hours.
B) In most cases, anterior bleeding originates from Kiesselbach area.
C) The use of silver nitrate or electric cautery is contraindicated in the nose.
D) Antibiotics are only needed when a nasal pack is in place for those with symptoms of sinusitis.
E) Patients with chronic obstructive pulmonary disease are not affected by nasal packing because most patients are mouth breathers.

The answer is B: Epistaxis has been reported to occur in up to 60% of the general population. Nosebleeds can be caused by several different mechanisms including trauma, nose picking, infection, foreign bodies, excessive drying of the nasal mucosa, and bleeding disorders. Most bleeding originates from a plexus of vessels in the anteroinferior septum called *Kiesselbach plexus*. In most cases, pinching the nasal ala together for 10 to 15 minutes stops the bleeding. If nasal bleeding continues, the local and/or systemic source should be identified.

Common local causes of epistaxis include chronic sinusitis, epistaxis digitorum, foreign bodies, intranasal neoplasm or polyps, irritants, medications (topical steroids), rhinitis, septal deviation, septal perforation, trauma, vascular malformation, or telangiectasia. Systemic causes include hemophilia, hypertension, leukemia, liver disease, medications (aspirin, anticoagulants, nonsteroidal anti-inflammatory drugs), platelet dysfunction, and thrombocytopenia.

Once the source is located, nasal packing or cauterization with silver nitrate or electric cautery may be necessary. If the nose is packed, antibiotics such as trimethoprim-sulfamethoxazole should be started while the packing is in place. Packs should not be left in place for more than 48 hours. If bleeding continues, a posterior source is most likely the cause and a posterior pack should be placed. Hospitalization for observation is indicated with serial blood counts in posterior bleeds. For severe nosebleeds, a bleeding time and von Willebrand factor should be checked to rule out bleeding disorders.

Referral to an otolaryngologist is appropriate when bleeding is refractory, complications are present, or specialized treatment (balloon placement, arterial ligation, angiographic arterial embolization) is required.

Additional Reading: Epistaxis. In: Domino F, ed. *The 5-Minute Clinical Consult*. Lippincott Williams & Wilkins; 2022.
Category: Special sensory systems

44. A 62-year-old man presents with complaints of leg pain. He notes that the pain is primarily in his buttocks and thighs. It is worse when he is walking but improved when he sits. On examination, his vital signs are normal, he has no peripheral edema, and his pedal pulses are intact. The most likely diagnosis to explain his symptoms is which one of the following?

A) A dissecting aortic aneurysm
B) An incarcerated inguinal hernia
C) Intermittent claudication
D) Myasthenia gravis
E) Spinal stenosis

The answer is E: Spinal stenosis is a condition characterized by narrowing of the spinal canal and foramen. Pain in the legs, calves, thighs, and buttocks occurs with walking, running, or climbing stairs. Symptoms are often relieved by flexing at the spine or sitting. Conversely, lying prone or in any position that extends the lumbar spine exacerbates the symptoms, presumably because of ventral infolding of the ligamentum flavum in a canal already significantly narrowed by degenerative osseous changes. Middle-aged patients and the elderly are most commonly affected.

Disease onset is usually insidious; early symptoms may be mild and slowly progress to become disabling. Typically, the earliest complaint is nonspecific back pain; patients then often experience leg fatigue, pain, numbness, and weakness, sometimes several months to years after the back pain was first noticed. Once the leg pain begins, it is most commonly bilateral, involving the buttocks and thighs, and spreading distally toward the feet, typically with the onset and progression of leg exercise. In some patients, the pain, paresthesia, and/or weakness are limited to the lower legs and feet, remaining present until movement ceases. The lower extremity symptoms are almost always described as burning, cramping, numbness, tingling, or dull fatigue in the thighs and legs.

Symptom severity does not always correlate with the degree of lumbar canal narrowing. Causes include osteoarthritis, spondylosis, spondylolisthesis with associated edema in the area of the cauda equina, and Paget disease affecting the lower spine.

Spinal stenosis may be difficult to distinguish from claudication; however, with spinal stenosis, there are usually neurologic deficits present and peripheral pulses are normal. Magnetic resonance imaging is the preferred modality for establishing a diagnosis and excluding other conditions. Treatment for symptomatic lumbar stenosis is usually surgical decompression. Medical treatment alternatives such as bed rest, pain management, and physical therapy should be reserved for use in debilitated patients or patients whose surgical risk is prohibitive as a result of concomitant medical conditions.

Additional Reading: Spinal stenosis. In: Domino F, ed. *The 5-Minute Clinical Consult*. Lippincott Williams & Wilkins; 2022.
Category: Neurologic system

45. A 31-year-old man is brought to the emergency department after being severely injured in a motor vehicle crash while riding his motorcycle. A dipstick urinalysis shows hemoglobin. However, microscopic examination fails to show red blood cells (RBCs) or white blood cells. The most likely diagnosis for this presentation is which one of the following conditions?

A) A laboratory error
B) Renal trauma
C) Rhabdomyolysis
D) Urethral rupture
E) Urinary tract infection

The answer is C: Myoglobinuria is a condition that results when there is massive muscle destruction known as rhabdomyolysis. The condition occurs because of severe infection, toxic insult, inflammation, or metabolic or traumatic damage to the muscles. Laboratory findings include elevated creatine kinase, lactate dehydrogenase, aspartate aminotransferase, alanine aminotransferase, and a positive urine test for hemoglobin, but with the absence of RBCs. Specific tests for the detection of myoglobinuria are performed with immunoassays. Treatment involves correcting the underlying causative factor and administering fluids. Renal failure may require further treatment.

Additional Reading: Clinical manifestations and diagnosis of rhabdomyolysis. In: *UpToDate*. 2022.
Category: Nephrologic system

46. A young patient is being evaluated for a cut on his face. Before repairing any facial laceration, it is important to ensure that the five branches of the facial nerve were not affected. Asking the patient to do which one of the following maneuvers would test the function of the zygomatic branch of the facial nerve?

A) Contract the forehead and elevate the eyebrows.
B) Contract the platysma (neck) muscles.
C) Frown.
D) Open and shut eyes.
E) Smile.

The answer is D: When repairing a facial laceration, the facial nerve function should be tested in all five branches as follows:

Temporal: Contract the forehead and elevate the eyebrow.
Cervical: Contract the platysma muscle.
Mandibular: Frown.
Zygomatic: Open and shut eyes.
Buccal: Smile.

Additional Reading: Assessment and management of facial lacerations. In: *UpToDate*. 2022.
Category: Special sensory systems

47. A young child presents with his mother, who is concerned that he has put something into his right ear. On examination, you detect a foreign body and consider removal using plain water irrigation; however, which one of the following should not be removed using this method?

A) A BB gun pellet
B) A dried pea
C) A metal part from a matchbox car
D) A plastic bead
E) A small pebble

The answer is B: Most ear and nose foreign bodies can be removed in the office utilizing various methods, which include the use of forceps, water irrigation, and suction catheter. Small, inorganic objects can be removed from the external auditory canal by irrigation. The irrigation solution should be at body temperature, and the stream of water should be directed along the superior margin of the external ear canal and should deliver an adequate volume of water with brisk flow. This volume can be achieved using a 20 to 50 mL syringe attached to a flexible catheter or plastic tubing from a butterfly needle. This technique is contraindicated if the tympanic membrane is perforated or the foreign body is vegetable matter or an alkaline button battery. Organic matter swells as it absorbs water, leading to further obstruction. Irrigation of the button battery enhances leakage and potential for liquefaction necrosis.

Additional Reading: Foreign bodies in the ear, nose, and throat. *Am Fam Physician*. 2007;76(8):1185-1189.
Category: Special sensory systems

48. Which one of the following conditions is associated with a positive Tinel sign?

A) Carpal tunnel syndrome
B) de Quervain tenosynovitis
C) Gamekeeper's thumb
D) Raynaud phenomenon
E) Scaphoid fracture

The answer is A: Carpal tunnel syndrome occurs when there is an entrapment of the median nerve at the level of the wrist. Symptoms include pain, numbness, and paresthesia in the distribution of the median nerve, including the palmar surface of the first three fingers. Symptoms characteristically occur at night and may awaken the patient. Symptoms may also involve the forearm or shoulder. Women are more frequently affected than men, and the condition can involve one or both hands. Percussion of the median nerve at the area of the carpal tunnel (Tinel sign), sustained flexion of the wrist (Phalen sign), or extension of the wrist (reverse Phalen sign) reproduces symptoms. Other clinical findings include weakness of the thumb and thenar atrophy. Carpal tunnel syndrome is associated with continuous repetitive flexion of the wrist, pregnancy (most cases resolve after delivery), acromegaly, rheumatoid arthritis, and myxedema. Nerve conduction tests are used to help make the diagnosis but are not always necessary. Treatment includes anti-inflammatory agents, wrist braces, and steroid injections; surgery is indicated in severe cases that are unresponsive to conservative therapy.

Additional Reading: Carpal tunnel syndrome. In: Domino F, ed. *The 5-Minute Clinical Consult*. Lippincott Williams & Wilkins; 2022.
Category: Musculoskeletal system

49. A young woman calls for advice because she sustained a minor burn while taking a cooking class. You tell her to do which one of the following measures immediately after a minor burn?

A) Apply cool butter.
B) Rapidly cool the area with ice.
C) Cool the area with room temperature water.
D) Firmly wash the area to remove any particulate matter.
E) Immediately seek medical treatment to debride nonviable skin.

The answer is C: Initial treatment of minor thermal injuries consist mainly of cooling (with room temperature water, not with ice), simple gentle cleansing with mild soap and water, and appropriate dressing. Pain management and tetanus prophylaxis are important.

Extensive debridement is generally not immediately necessary and may be deferred until the initial follow-up visit.

Additional Reading: Burns. In: Domino F, ed. *The 5-Minute Clinical Consult*. Lippincott Williams & Wilkins; 2022.
Category: Integumentary system

50. A young high school football player is shaken from a tough tackle during a game for which you are providing medical coverage. Although he was not unconscious, he felt like his vision was "fussy" for a brief period. Now, he is doing well and wants to get back into the game. The results of his examination are normal. The most appropriate action at this time is which one of the following?

A) Keep him out of the game for a full quarter; if he remains normal, he may return to play.
B) Prohibit him from returning to play during this game.
C) Prohibit him from returning to play for the rest of the season.
D) Transfer him to a local emergency department.

The answer is B: Any athlete with a suspected concussion should not be allowed to return to play on the same day. Return-to-play decisions for athletes should be individually graded and not made without a follow-up evaluation. These include the following:

- Taking complete rest until free of symptoms
- Then beginning gradual reintroduction of activity as long as free of symptoms
- Doing each of the following steps generally 24 hours apart: light aerobic exercise, sport-specific exercise, noncontact training drills, full-contact training, and game play
- Stopping all activities until again asymptomatic for 24 hours if any signs or symptoms recur (ie, exertional headache, visual disturbance, or disequilibrium) and restarting return-to-play plan at the last step when the patient is asymptomatic

Athletes who are high risk for more prolonged recovery include pediatric athletes, athletes with mood disorders, athletes with learning disabilities, and athletes with migraine headaches. These athletes should have a slower return-to-play progression and may require a more intensive evaluation (formal neuropsychologic, balance, and symptoms testing). Athletes with multiple concussions should have slower return to play and may benefit from sports medicine consultation or neurologic referral.

Additional Reading: Concussion. In: Domino F, ed. *The 5-Minute Clinical Consult*. Lippincott Williams & Wilkins; 2022.
Category: Neurologic system

51. A 19-year-old man is brought to the emergency department by ambulance after developing sudden shortness of breath. He had been previously healthy and denies any substance use or recent trauma. A chest radiograph shows a 10% pneumothorax, and he appears stable. Appropriate management at this time is which one of the following?

A) Perform pulmonary function testing.
B) Place a chest tube.
C) Perform a repeat chest radiograph in 4 hours.
D) Place a large-bore needle in the second intercostal space.
E) Prepare for intubation with mechanical ventilation.

The answer is C: Pneumothorax is the accumulation of air within the pleural space. The usual cause of pneumothorax is a penetrating wound such as a stabbing wound, gunshot wound, or deceleration-type injury (eg, as seen in motor vehicle crashes). Spontaneous pneumothorax can also occur and typically affects tall, thin men or smokers (because of a ruptured bleb). Clinical findings include decreased breath sounds on the side affected, shortness of breath, chest pain (the most common symptom), cough, distended neck veins, and hypotension.

A chest radiograph is usually diagnostic, as is bedside ultrasound looking at lung sliding. Ultrasound, however, cannot adequately classify the volume loss, which on a plain radiograph is easily judged by the apex-to-cupola distance. Treatment may require immediate intervention but in many cases depends on the extent of pneumothorax. If pneumothorax involves up to 20% of lung volume, observation is usually the only treatment necessary. However, ensuring that the pneumothorax is stable is paramount, as a small air leak from a ruptured bleb or pleural tear can slowly accumulate, necessitating chest tube placement for tamponade physiology. Repeating a chest radiograph in 4 to 6 hours and the following morning is a reasonable and safe practice to assess stability. Supplemental oxygen is usually administered, and most cases resolve in 10 days. For larger pneumothoraxes, chest tube placement is necessary. Tension pneumothoraxes require emergent decompression with a large-bore needle placed in the second intercostal space of the midclavicular line, followed by chest tube placement. Providing 100% O_2 accelerates the rate of pleural air absorption.

Additional Reading: Pneumothorax. In: Domino F, ed. *The 5-Minute Clinical Consult*. Lippincott Williams & Wilkins; 2022.
Category: Respiratory system

52. You are evaluating a patient with severe sunburn and inform him or her that he or she should use sunscreen to protect the exposed skin to prevent future sunburns. What minimal level of sun protection factor (SPF) is recommended by the American Academy of Dermatology?

A) SPF-8
B) SPF-15
C) SPF-30
D) SPF-45
E) SPF-60

The answer is C: SPF is a measure of the ability of a blocking agent (ie, sunscreen) to prevent erythema in response to sun exposure. The SPF can be multiplied by the time of exposure necessary to produce minimal erythema in an unprotected individual to get the expected time until minimal erythema develops using that protection. As an example, if an unprotected individual develops minimal erythema after 20 minutes of sun exposure, after the use of an SPF-8 sunscreen, minimal erythema would be expected after 160 minutes of exposure. However, the duration of protection with sunscreen may be shorter in many circumstances than what the SPF would indicate.

The American Academy of Dermatology recommends using a broad-spectrum sunscreen that protects against both ultraviolet A and ultraviolet B radiation with an SPF of 30 or greater on exposed skin. Other recommendations include staying out of the sun in the middle of the day (10 AM-4 PM); wearing a wide-brimmed hat, long-sleeve shirt, or long pants; and avoiding tanning beds.

Apply sunscreen generously to all exposed skin 15 to 30 minutes before exposure. Reapply sunscreen after sweating, rubbing the skin, drying off with a towel, or swimming. Reapply sunscreen every 2 or 3 hours.

Additional Reading: Sunscreens revisited. *Med Lett Drugs Ther*. 2011;53(1359):17-18.
Category: Integumentary system

53. You are evaluating a middle-aged alcoholic with a severe headache and suspect that he has a subdural hematoma (SDH). The most appropriate test for the detection of SDH is which one of the following?

A) A computed tomographic (CT) scan of the head without contrast
B) A CT scan of the head with and without contrast
C) A lumbar puncture
D) A skull radiograph series
E) A magnetic resonance imaging (MRI) of the head

The answer is A: An acute SDH is readily visualized on a head CT scan as a high-density crescentic collection across the hemispheric convexity. Subacute and chronic SDHs appear as isodense or hypodense crescent collection-shaped lesions that deform the surface of the brain. An epidural hematoma produces a convex pattern on a CT scan because its collection is limited by firm dural attachments at the cranial sutures. Brain MRI is more sensitive than head CT scanning for the detection of intracranial hemorrhage. MRI is also more sensitive for the detection of small SDH and tentorial and interhemispheric SDH. Brain MRI is used for situations in which there is a suspicion for SDH or other intracranial hemorrhage but no clear evidence of hematoma by CT scanning.

Additional Reading: Subdural hematoma in adults: etiology, clinical features, and diagnosis. In: *UpToDate*. 2022.
Category: Neurologic system

54. A 23-year-old patient with epilepsy is brought to the emergency department in status epilepticus. Which one of the following drugs should you have administered initially?

A) Fosphenytoin
B) Lorazepam
C) Phenytoin
D) Phenobarbital
E) Pentobarbital

The answer is B: Lorazepam should be administered intravenously, and approximately 1 minute is allowed to assess its effect. Diazepam or midazolam may be substituted if lorazepam is not available. If seizures continue at this point, additional doses of lorazepam should be infused and a second intravenous catheter should be placed to begin a concomitant phenytoin (or fosphenytoin) loading infusion. Even if seizures terminate after the initial lorazepam dose, therapy with phenytoin or fosphenytoin is generally indicated to prevent the recurrence of seizures.

Additional Reading: *Status epilepticus in adults*. In: *UpToDate*. 2022.
Category: Neurologic system

55. A young soccer player has been struck by lightning while practicing on an open field. Which one of the following statements is *false* regarding the treatment of lightning strike victims?

A) Airway burns should be excluded.
B) Cardiac monitoring should be maintained after the injury.
C) Cervical spine immobilization and clearance should be performed.
D) Serum creatine kinase, myocardial band (CK-MB) measurements should be measured to assess myocardial injury.
E) Tetanus immunization should be administered.

The answer is D: A patient exposed to a serious electrical burn or lightning strike should be treated as a trauma patient. Resuscitation should begin with a rapid assessment of airway and cardiopulmonary status. Cervical spine immobilization and clearance should be maintained, and tetanus vaccination should be administered. Coexisting smoke inhalation or airway burns should be excluded. Patients can have spontaneous cardiac activity but paralysis of the respiratory muscles. Prompt restoration of a secure airway may prevent secondary cardiac and neurologic dysfunction or death. Coma or neurologic deficit should include brain and/or spine imaging.

An extensive head to toe examination and neurologic examination should be performed. The survivor of high-energy injury should have cardiac and hemodynamic monitoring because of the high incidence of arrhythmia and autonomic dysfunction, especially if there have been arrhythmias in the field or emergency department, loss of consciousness, or if the initial electrocardiogram (ECG) is abnormal. Serum CK-MB measurements and ECG changes are poor measures of myocardial injury. The diagnostic and prognostic values of cardiac troponin levels have not been evaluated in this setting.

Additional Reading: Lightning injuries, emergency medicine. In: Domino F, ed. *The 5-Minute Clinical Consult*. Wolters Kluwer; 2022.
Category: Nonspecific system

56. A teenager with a history of von Willebrand factor (vWF) deficiency is involved in a bicycle collision and presents to the emergency department. There is concern about bleeding; however, he appears stable and has only minor bleeding. Which one of the following would be indicated to help correct the coagulation disorder?

A) Prothrombin complex concentrate
B) Desmopressin (DDAVP)
C) Fresh frozen plasma (FFP)
D) Packed RBCs
E) Platelets

The answer is B: Approaches to treating vWF deficiency include increasing plasma concentration of vWF by releasing endogenous vWF stores through stimulation of endothelial cells with DDAVP; use of vWF concentrates; and promoting hemostasis using hemostatic agents with mechanisms other than increasing vWF.

For minor bleeding and minor surgery, the use of intravenous or intranasal DDAVP is the initial treatment of bleeding or at the time of surgery in patients who have shown a prior response to this agent. For major bleeding or major surgical procedures, it is recommended to use vWF concentrate over DDAVP to reach a target level of approximately 100 IU/dL or vWF ristocetin cofactor activity. The above levels should be maintained for 7 to 14 days or as needed. Cryoprecipitate, used in disseminated intravascular coagulation due to its high concentration of fibrinogen, contains vWF and can be used emergently for vWF deficiency.

Prothrombin complex concentrate is a commercially available product with narrow indications due to its high cost. It is used for reversal of warfarin in bleeding, as it contains vitamin K-dependent coagulation factors.

Packed RBCs can be stored in cold storage for up to 35 days. However, refrigerated temperature causes platelets to degenerate; therefore, banked, packed RBCs contain essentially no functioning platelets. In addition, factors V and VII decrease with refrigeration; however, other factors remain unchanged. Packed RBC transfusion should be used only when time or the clinical situation precludes other therapy.

Platelet transfusions are indicated if patients have thrombocytopenia or platelet dysfunction, or both. Patients are usually administered 6 or 10 units at one time (*6-pack* or *10-pack*). Multiple-unit, single-donor platelets are harvested from one donor using apheresis. Platelets should not be routinely given for bleeding prophylaxis, unless there is evidence of microvascular bleeding or planned surgery and the platelet count is <50,000/mm^3 or <10,000/mm^3 (for prophylaxis against bleeding).

FFP is used to replace labile clotting factors. A unit of FFP contains near-normal levels of all clotting factors, including approximately 400 mg of fibrinogen. A unit of FFP increases clotting factors by approximately 3%. Adequate clotting is usually obtained with factor levels >30%. FFP is used to correct prothrombin time and activated partial thromboplastin time.

Additional Reading: Diagnosis and management of von Willebrand disease: guidelines for primary care. *Am Fam Physician*. 2009;80(11):1261-1268.
Category: Hematologic system

57. A young child is being evaluated with a high fever and somnolence. There is concern that she has meningitis, and a positive Brudzinski sign is noted on examination. Which one of the following describes a positive Brudzinski sign?

A) The patient dorsiflexes the feet when the head is flexed forward.
B) The patient involuntarily flexes the hips with flexion of the neck.
C) The patient involuntarily blinks after gentle tapping on the forehead.
D) The patient shows resistance when the legs are extended from a flexed position.
E) The patient shows extension-type posturing when the arms are flexed.

The answer is B: Symptoms of bacterial meningitis include high-pitched crying, fever, anorexia, irritability, obtundation, lethargy, nausea, vomiting, neck stiffness, and a full fontanel (in infants). In neonates, clinical clues to the presence of meningitis include temperature instability (hypothermia or hyperthermia), listlessness, high-pitched crying, fretfulness, lethargy, refusal to eat, a weak sucking response, irritability, vomiting, diarrhea, and respiratory distress. Because neonates usually do not have meningismus, a change in the child's affect or state of alertness is one of the most important signs. A bulging fontanel may occur late in the course of the disease in one-third of neonates. About 30% of neonates have seizures. Meningeal signs and fever are not always present in infants; however, meningeal signs are more reliable in older children and include the following:

- Brudzinski sign: Flexion of neck with the patient supine causes involuntary flexion at the hips.
- Kernig sign: Attempts to extend the knees from a flexed position are met with resistance.

Among US children, there has been a substantial decrease in deaths and hospitalization from *H influenzae* meningitis but not *Streptococcus pneumoniae* or *Neisseria meningitidis* meningitis in the years after *H influenzae* type B conjugate vaccine licensure. The most common sequelae after meningitis include hearing loss and seizure disorders.

Additional Reading: Diagnosis, initial management, and prevention of meningitis. *Am Fam Physician*. 2010;82(12):1491-1498.
Category: Neurologic system

58. A middle-aged alcoholic presents with abdominal pain that is radiating to his back; and there is concern that he is suffering the effects of acute pancreatitis. Which one of the following statements regarding acute pancreatitis is true?

A) All patients should receive nasogastric suction to maintain strict bowel rest.
B) Anticholinergics are useful in the treatment of acute pancreatitis.
C) Amylase is the most sensitive and specific test for the detection of acute pancreatitis.
D) Enteral feedings (distal to the ligament of Treitz) can be beneficial after 48 hours for severe cases.
E) Nausea and vomiting are rarely present.

The answer is D: Acute pancreatitis usually results from alcohol abuse, bile duct obstruction, or severe hypertriglyceridemia. Patients with acute pancreatitis present with mild to severe epigastric pain with radiation to the flank, back, or both. Classically, the pain is characterized as constant, dull, and boring, and is worse when the patient is supine. The discomfort may lessen when the patient assumes a sitting or fetal position. A heavy meal or drinking binge often triggers the pain. Nausea and vomiting are present in the vast majority of patients.

Serum amylase and lipase (the most sensitive and specific laboratory indicator for pancreatitis) levels are used to confirm the diagnosis of acute pancreatitis. Computed tomographic (CT) scanning will confirm the diagnosis, assess severity, establish a baseline, and rule out other possibilities. A CT scan with intravenous (IV) contrast at day 3 can assess the degree of necrosis when necrotizing pancreatitis is suspected (O_2 saturation <90%, systolic BP <90 mm Hg, worsening symptoms).

IV rehydration should usually be aggressive, with close attention to blood pressure and cardiac and pulmonary status. Withholding food by mouth does reduce pain; however, the use of a nasogastric tube with suction is indicated only for intractable emesis. In mild pancreatitis, oral intake should be withheld until the nausea and vomiting subside.

Total enteral feeding beyond the ligament of Treitz is considered after 48 hours, if oral feeding will not be possible within 5 to 7 days. Multiple randomized control trials support the use of enteral feeds over total parenteral nutrition in acute pancreatitis for improving survival. Nutrition in pancreatitis is an area of active investigation with new treatment paradigms emerging; recent studies show (1) that feeds within 48 hours in mild to moderate pancreatitis likely improves outcomes, and (2) there may be no difference in outcomes between nasojejunal (postpyloric) and nasogastric (prepyloric) feeds in this patient group. Until these trials are replicated in larger data sets, waiting 48 hours to feed postpyloric is a safe practice.

Systemic antibiotics remain controversial.

Additional Reading: Acute pancreatitis. *Am Fam Physician*. 2014;90(9):632-639.
Category: Gastroenterology system

59. A 73-year-old woman presents to your office complaining of anorexia, nausea, and abdominal pain. Lately, she has been more fatigued and states that her muscles seem "weak." Laboratory tests show an elevated calcium level. The most likely diagnosis for this presentation is which one of the following conditions?

A) Chronic fatigue syndrome
B) Hyperparathyroidism
C) Myasthenia gravis
D) Osteoporosis
E) Paget disease

The answer is B: Hyperparathyroidism is a common cause of hypercalcemia. The incidence of hyperparathyroidism increases with age.

Women are more commonly affected. Most patients are asymptomatic because symptoms are vague and often similar to symptoms of depression, irritable bowel syndrome, fibromyalgia, or stress reaction. Some combination of headaches, fatigue, anorexia, nausea, paresthesias, muscular weakness, pain in the extremities, and abdominal pain is the most common presentation of primary hyperparathyroidism. The hypercalcemia usually is discovered during a routine serum chemistry profile.

Primary hyperparathyroidism results from excessive secretion of parathyroid hormone (PTH) with a lack of response feedback inhibition by elevated calcium. Secondary hyperparathyroidism with excessive secretion of PTH from the parathyroid gland occurs in response to hypocalcemia, which usually can be caused by vitamin D deficiency or renal failure. Tertiary hyperparathyroidism results from autonomous hyperfunction of the parathyroid gland in the setting of long-standing secondary PTH.

In most cases, primary hyperparathyroidism is the result of an adenoma in a single parathyroid gland. The incidence of hyperparathyroidism is higher in patients with type I and type II multiple endocrine neoplasia syndromes, in patients with familial hyperparathyroidism, and in patients who received radiation therapy to the head and neck area for benign diseases during childhood. Complications of primary hyperparathyroidism include peptic ulcers, nephrolithiasis, pancreatitis, dehydration, and nephrocalcinosis.

IV hydration is the most critical treatment for a patient with an acute presentation of hyperparathyroidism and hypercalcemia. The addition of furosemide (Lasix) increases urinary calcium loss. Such patients can be treated with bisphosphonates (alendronate) to reduce bone turnover and maintain bone density. When medical management is used, routine monitoring for clinical deterioration is recommended. Critical hypercalcemia requires IV fluid rehydration, IV bisphosphonate therapy, and calcitonin (4 U/kg every 12 hours) for severe symptoms. Surgical management is indicated in cases of hyperparathyroidism, associated with nephrolithiasis, nephrocalcinosis, and/or osteitis fibrosa.

Additional Reading: Hyperparathyroidism. In: Domino F, ed. *The 5-Minute Clinical Consult*. Lippincott Williams & Wilkins; 2022.
Category: Endocrine system

60. Scuba divers should wait before flying because of the risk of decompression illness that occurs with sudden changes in atmospheric pressure. What is the minimal amount of time that a patient should wait after scuba diving before traveling by air?

A) No wait necessary
B) 12 hours
C) 24 hours
D) 72 hours
E) 1 week

The answer is B: Patients who travel by air soon after scuba diving are at increased risk for developing decompression sickness in flight. Such a passenger should be advised to wait 12 hours before flying if he or she has been making only 1 dive per day. Individuals who have participated in multiple dives or those requiring decompression stops on surfacing should consider waiting up to 48 hours before flying.

Additional Reading: Decompression sickness. In: Domino F, ed. *The 5-Minute Clinical Consult*. Lippincott Williams & Wilkins; 2022.
Category: Nonspecific system

61. The mother of a 9-year-old child calls to report that her child was bitten by a pet hamster and she is worried about rabies. Which one of the following is the appropriate management for this situation?

A) Administer human diploid cell vaccine.
B) Administer rabies immune globulin.
C) Hospitalize and observe the child for abnormal behaviors.
D) Reassure the mother that no treatment other than local wound care is necessary.
E) Transport the hamster to the health department for evaluation.

The answer is D: Bites of rodents such as squirrels, opossums, rats, mice, guinea pigs, gerbils, hamsters, rabbits, and hares rarely, if ever, require rabies prophylaxis. Local wound care is all that is necessary for the majority of such bites. The disease is usually found in wild animals such as skunks, foxes, coyotes, raccoons, bobcats, and bats but is also seen in domestic dogs and cats. Other animals affected include livestock.

The rabies virus affects the central nervous system, and the presence of intracytoplasmic Negri bodies seen microscopically is pathognomonic for the infection. Symptoms affecting humans include depression, difficulty with concentration, malaise, fever, extreme restlessness with excessive salivation, painful laryngeal and pharyngeal muscle spasms, and convulsions. Although patients often experience extreme thirst, they are hydrophobic because drinking can often precipitate pharyngeal spasms. Death usually occurs secondary to exhaustion and asphyxia with generalized paralysis.

Treatment of those bitten includes confining the animal for at least 10 days to look for abnormal behavior. If no changes are seen, the patient usually does not need treatment. Animals with abnormal behavior should be humanely killed and examined pathologically for rabies infection. If the animal cannot be caught or if the animal exhibits abnormal behavior and has evidence of rabies infection, the patient should be treated with human diploid cell vaccine or rabies vaccine, which is administered intramuscularly at the time of presentation and then at days 3, 7, 14, and 28 for a total of five doses.

In addition, to bridge the gap of time it takes for the patient to develop antibodies to the rabies vaccine, rabies immune globulin is given, with much of the dose administered at the site of the bite and the rest administered at a distant site from vaccine inoculation intramuscularly. In most cases, the wound should not be sutured.

Prophylaxis for rabies should be considered for high-risk populations such as veterinarians, animal handlers, technicians in laboratories in which rabies is present, and travelers spending a month or more in countries in which rabies is common.

Additional Reading: *Rabies*. www.cdc.gov/rabies/specific_groups/doctors/index.html
Category: Nonspecific system

62. A 17-year-old student presents complaining of a sore throat pain, difficulty swallowing, and now trouble opening his mouth. On examination, you detect erythema and enlargement of the left tonsillar pillar. In addition, the patient tends to hold her head to the left side and has muffled speech. The most likely diagnosis to account for this presentation is which one of the following conditions?

A) Epiglottitis
B) Peritonsillar abscess
C) Retropharyngeal abscess
D) Streptococcal pharyngitis
E) Tonsillar cancer

The answer is B: Peritonsillar abscess (also known as *quinsy*) is the most common ear, nose, and throat abscess. It is seen most commonly in teenagers and young adults and is rare in children below the age of 5 years. The condition occurs when an abscess develops between the tonsil and the superior constrictor muscle.

Symptoms include worsening throat pain, muffled speech (hot potato voice), trismus (spasm of the jaw muscles), and difficulty swallowing. The patient often holds his or her head toward the side that the abscess affects. If the abscess is large, airway compromise may occur.

Ultrasonography or computed tomographic scanning can help distinguish between cellulitis and abscess formation. Treatment of peritonsillar abscess is accomplished by lancing a fluctuant area, if present, with an 18-gauge needle (making certain not to go deeper than 1 cm where the internal carotid artery passes!) and prescribing penicillin-containing antibiotics. The fluid should be cultured before initiation of antibiotics. Common infecting organisms include group A *Streptococcus* and anaerobes. Recurrent episodes necessitate tonsillectomy.

Additional Reading: Peritonsillar abscess. *Am Fam Physician.* 2017;95(8):501-506.
Category: Nonspecific system

63. A boy who plays little league baseball presents with "locking" and swelling of his elbow. On examination, you detect swelling over the medial elbow and elicit pain with valgus and varus stress while flexing and extending the elbow. His plain radiograph films show the presence of loose bodies. The most likely diagnosis to account for this presentation is which one of the following conditions?

A) Chondromalacia
B) Nursemaid's elbow
C) Osteochondritis dissecans
D) Tennis elbow

The answer is C: Little league elbow is an overuse injury caused by compressive forces at the radiocapitellar joint and opposite pulling forces at the medial aspect of the elbow. These injuries usually occur in adolescents who use motions such as overhand pitching in sports such as baseball. The repetitive forces may lead to damage of the articular surface of the capitellum, ligamentous injury of the medial elbow, and ulnar nerve dysfunction. In severe cases, osteochondritis dissecans of the capitellum with the formation of loose bodies can occur and result in locking of the elbow joint. Other symptoms include pain with valgus and varus stress while flexing and extending the elbow.

For most cases, treatment involves rest (no throwing for 4-6 weeks), ice, elevation, and nonsteroidal anti-inflammatory drugs. However, if there are signs of osteochondritis dissecans, orthopedic referral for possible surgical intervention is necessary.

Additional Reading: Busconi BD, Stevenson JH. Approach to the athlete with little league elbow. *Sports Medicine Consult: A Problem-Based Approach to Sports Medicine for the Primary Care Physician.* Lippincott Williams & Wilkins; 2009.
Category: Musculoskeletal system

64. A newborn is brought to the emergency department with respiratory distress and is diagnosed with aspiration pneumonia. Given this presentation, he should be evaluated for which one of the following conditions?

A) Cystic fibrosis
B) Hypothyroidism
C) Human immunodeficiency virus
D) Tetralogy of Fallot
E) Tracheoesophageal fistula

The answer is E: Tracheoesophageal fistula is a congenital defect seen in newborns. The incidence occurs in 1 in 3500 live births. Boys and girls are equally affected. The condition is commonly associated with esophageal atresia. Polyhydramnios occurs in approximately two-thirds of pregnancies. Symptoms include excessive secretions with coughing and aspiration after feeding. Complications include the development of cyanosis and aspiration pneumonia.

Diagnosis can be established by the inability to pass a red rubber catheter or nasogastric tube into the stomach further than approximately 10 to 15 cm. Anteroposterior radiographs confirm catheter curled in the upper esophageal pouch. If gas is noted below the diaphragm, then an associated fistula is present. If not, the patient most likely is affected with esophageal atresia alone. Care must be taken to avoid aspiration of dye during diagnostic tests.

Additional Reading: Tracheoesophageal fistula and esophageal atresia, pediatric. In: Domino F, ed. *The 5-Minute Clinical Consult.* Wolters Kluwer; 2022.
Category: Gastroenterology system

65. Various objects can be ingested and may lodge into the esophagus. Blunt objects in the esophagus (with the exception of button batteries) may be observed for up to how long before performing an endoscopy for removal?

A) 4 hours
B) 24 hours
C) 3 days
D) 1 week
E) 10 days

The answer is B: Blunt objects (with the exception of button batteries) in the esophagus may be observed for up to 24 hours. If the object fails to pass into the stomach by that time, it should be removed or possibly pushed into the stomach. Objects that have been lodged in the esophagus for more than 24 hours or for an unknown duration should be removed endoscopically. If the object has been lodged in the esophagus for more than 2 weeks, there is significant risk of erosion into surrounding structures, and surgical consultation should be obtained before attempting removal. Early intervention is indicated for patients who have swallowed button or disc batteries because of the potential for voltage burns and direct corrosive effects. These burns can occur as early as 4 hours after ingestion.

Additional Reading: Body ingestion in children. *Am Fam Physician.* 2005;72(2):287-291.
Category: Gastroenterology system

66. A 65-year-old retired secretary presents with a painful bump that is associated with the medial first metatarsal joint. She reports that the bump has slowly developed over the past few years. The most likely diagnosis for her presentation is which one of the following conditions?

A) A bunionette
B) Gout
C) Hallux valgus
D) Morton neuroma
E) Metatarsalgia

The answer is C: Hallux valgus (bunions) is more common in women than in men. Symptoms include a painless or painful bump (exostosis) that forms on the medial aspect of the first metatarsal joint. Contributing physical factors include hyperelasticity syndromes, metatarsus varus, short first metatarsal joint, and pes valgus.

Other factors include a family history of bunions and the prolonged use of narrow high-heeled shoes.

Conservative treatment is usually all that is needed and includes wide shoes, the use of bunion pads, ice, rest, and anti-inflammatory agents for acute pain. Most cases referred for surgery have intermetatarsal angles greater than 10° or fail to improve with conservative measures. Absolute contraindications for surgery include peripheral vascular disease and local tissue infections, whereas relative contraindications include narcissistic personality disorders, painless cosmetic bunions, and age 65 years or older. A bunionette is a bony prominence on the lateral aspect of the fifth metatarsal head.

Additional Reading: Hallux valgus deformity. In: *UpToDate*. 2022.
Category: Musculoskeletal system

Section II. Surgical Care

Each of the following questions or incomplete statements is followed by suggested answers or completions. Select the ONE BEST ANSWER in each case.

1. A 37-year-old white woman has been diagnosed with cholecystitis and is scheduled for surgery. All of the following statements regarding cholecystectomy surgery are true, except which one?

A) Around 5% of patients undergoing elective laparoscopic cholecystectomy require conversion to an open procedure.
B) A common reason for conversion to an open procedure is failure to identify the anatomy.
C) Laparoscopic cholecystectomy is safer than an open procedure.
D) Laparoscopic cholecystectomy has a lower rate of common bile duct injury.
E) Common bile duct injuries are extremely difficult to repair.

The answer is D: The overall incidence of laparoscopic cholecystectomy bile duct injuries ranges from 1.7% in the first case to 0.17% at the 50th case (0.4-0.6). The incidence is four times higher than that with an open cholecystectomy. There is evidence that the rate of bile duct injuries has decreased over time as the standard of care changed to a laparoscopic approach, but the levels have not yet gotten as low as rates from the era of open cholecystectomy. The incidence of conversion-to-open rates has also dropped substantially as laparoscopic cholecystectomy replaced open cholecystectomy universally as the standard of care. Around 5% patients undergoing elective laparoscopic cholecystectomy require conversion to an open procedure. A common reason for conversion is the inability to clearly identify the biliary anatomy.

Additional Reading: Cholelithiasis. In: Domino F, ed. *The 5-Minute Clinical Consult*. Lippincott Williams & Wilkins; 2022.
Category: Gastroenterology system

2. A 47-year-old man presents with a skin lesion that has been changing in size and shape. On examination, she is found to have a 7-mm, asymmetric, darkly pigmented lesion with some color variegation and irregular borders. Which one of the following skin biopsy techniques is most appropriate for confirming the diagnosis?

A) A shave biopsy
B) Electrodesiccation and curettage
C) Elliptical excision
D) Mohs surgery

The answer is C: This lesion is suspicious for melanoma, on the basis of the asymmetry, irregular border, color variegation, and size larger than 6 mm. In addition, a history of evolution of the lesion, with changes in size, shape, or color, has been shown in some studies to be the most specific clinical finding for melanoma. The preferred method of biopsy for any lesion suspicious for melanoma is complete elliptical excision with a small margin of normal-appearing skin, taken to the depth of the subcutaneous tissue. The depth of the lesion is crucial to staging and prognosis; therefore, shave biopsies are inadequate. A punch biopsy of the most suspicious-appearing area is appropriate if the location or size of the lesion makes full excision inappropriate or impractical, but a single punch biopsy is unlikely to capture the entire malignant portion in larger lesions. The punch biopsy should be at least 4 mm to get adequate tissue and should be performed in the thickest part of the lesion. Multiple punch biopsies can and should be taken on large lesions. Electrodesiccation and curettage is not an appropriate treatment for melanoma. Mohs surgery is sometimes used to treat melanomas but is not used for the initial diagnosis.

Additional Reading: Cutaneous malignant melanoma: a primary care perspective. *Am Fam Physician*. 2012;85(2):161.
Category: Integumentary system

3. A patient with biopsy-proven breast cancer presents to discuss her treatment options with you after her surgeon had recommended a mastectomy. Which one of the following is *not* a contraindication for breast conservative therapy?

A) Estrogen/progesterone receptor–positive tumor.
B) Two tumors are located in different quadrants.
C) Diffuse microcalcifications that appear malignant.
D) History of prior therapeutic radiotherapy that included a portion of the affected breast.
E) Negative resection surgical margins.

The answer is A: When there are two or more primary tumors located in different quadrants of the breast or when there are associated diffuse microcalcifications that appear malignant, breast-conserving therapy is not considered appropriate. Additionally, a woman with previous breast irradiation is also not a candidate for breast conservation treatment. Breast irradiation cannot be given during pregnancy, but it may be possible to perform breast-conserving surgery in the third trimester and administer irradiation after delivery. Positive surgical margins are also an absolute contraindication.

Additional Reading: Treatment of breast cancer. *Am Fam Physician*. 2010;81(11):1339-1346.
Category: Integumentary system

4. Which of the following antibiotics given alone is adequate for prophylaxis when performing an appendectomy?

A) Cephalexin
B) Ceftriaxone
C) Cefotaxime
D) Metronidazole
E) Cefoxitin

The answer is E: Antibiotic prophylaxis is warranted in the setting of uncomplicated appendicitis. Reasonable regimens include a cephalosporin with anaerobic activity: cefoxitin or cefotetan. Ceftriaxone, when combined with metronidazole, is an appropriate alternative but ceftriaxone alone has poor anaerobic coverage. Complicated appendicitis consists of perforated or gangrenous appendicitis, including peritonitis or abscess formation.

Additional Reading: Clinical practice guidelines for antimicrobial prophylaxis in surgery. *Surg Infect*. 2013;14(1):73.
Category: Gastroenterology system

➔ While appendectomy remains the choice for most patients with uncomplicated acute appendicitis, those undergoing nonoperative treatment should receive IV antibiotics in hospital for 24 to 72 hours to monitor for worsening pain or clinical deterioration. A common regimen is IV ceftriaxone for 24 hours followed by 5 to 10 days of ciprofloxacin and metronidazole.

5. Which one of the following supplements may have an antiplatelet activity and should be stopped before surgery?

A) Ephedra
B) Ginseng
C) Kava
D) St. John's wort
E) Valerian

The answer is B: Ginseng is touted to protect the body against stress. Pharmacologically, ginseng lowers blood glucose levels (even in patients without diabetes mellitus) and, therefore, may cause intraoperative complications, especially in patients who fasted before surgery. Ginseng may also have a platelet inhibitory effect, and this effect may be irreversible. It should be discontinued at least 7 days before surgery.

Additional Reading: *Asian Ginseng*. National Center for Complementary and Alternative Medicine (NCCAM). https://www.nccih.nih.gov/health/asian-ginseng
Category: Nonspecific system

6. A patient has undergone an elective hip replacement for severe osteoarthritis and is on deep vein thrombosis (DVT) prophylaxis. How long should he be maintained on DVT prophylaxis after his hip surgery?

A) 24 hours
B) 3 days
C) 10 days
D) 1 month
E) Indefinitely

The answer is C: The 2012 American College of Chest Physicians anticoagulation guidelines recommend starting low-molecular-weight heparin either 12 hours before or 12 hours after surgery. Thromboembolic prophylaxis should be continued until the patient is fully ambulatory or for at least 10 to 14 days post operation. Patients at high risk for DVT may require a longer course of anticoagulation. Patients at increased risk include those with a history of thromboembolism or who experienced prolonged immobility or delayed surgery.

Additional Reading: Prevention of VTE in orthopedic surgery patients: antithrombotic therapy and prevention of thrombosis, 9th ed. American College of Chest Physician Evidence-Based Clinical Practice Guidelines. *Chest*. 2012;141(suppl 2):e278S.
Category: Cardiovascular system

7. A general surgeon contacts you regarding preoperative clearance for an otherwise healthy 38-year-old patient scheduled for an appendectomy. He is concerned about the need for coagulation studies because none had been performed. The patient has no history of excessive bleeding, has no family history of bleeding disorders, and is on no medications. A correct response to his concern is that:

A) a bleeding time is sufficient for assessing the risk of bleeding before his surgery.
B) a prothrombin time (PT) and partial thromboplastin time (PTT) test must be performed before the patient has surgery.
C) a normal PT and PTT test performed within the past year is sufficient to clear this patient for surgery.
D) no further testing is necessary to clear this patient for surgery.

The answer is D: Coagulation times are not routinely indicated in patients undergoing surgery. Studies have shown that the yield is very low and that abnormal results are expected or do not significantly affect management. Coagulation studies would be indicated if the patient is receiving anticoagulant therapy, has a family or personal history that suggests a bleeding disorder, or has evidence of liver disease.

Additional Reading: Preoperative testing before noncardiac surgery: guidelines and recommendations. *Am Fam Physician*. 2013;87(6):414-418.
Category: Hematologic system

8. All of the following are considered indications for performing Mohs micrographic surgery when treating worrisome skin finding, except which one?

A) The biopsy had indistinct margins.
B) The biopsy is consistent with an actinic keratosis.
C) The lesion is near the nose.
D) The lesion is >2 cm in diameter.
E) The lesion has recurred.

The answer is B: Patients with nonmelanoma skin cancer measuring >2 cm; lesions with indistinct margins, recurrent lesions, and those close to important structures, including the eyes, nose, and mouth; more invasive histologic subtypes (micronodular, infiltrative, and morpheaform); or tumors with high risk of recurrence should be considered for referral for complete excision via Mohs micrographic surgery.

The Mohs surgeon can confirm the complete removal of the lesion by immediately reviewing the pathology during a staged excision, which, in these high-risk settings, can require removal of much more tissue than might have been clinically apparent initially. The recurrence rate for tumors treated with Mohs micrographic surgery is approximately 1% at 5 years, whereas standard surgical excision has an approximately 5% of recurrence rate at 5 years.

Additional Reading: Diagnosis and treatment of basal cell and squamous cell carcinoma. *Am Fam Physician*. 2012;86(2):161-168.
Category: Integumentary system

9. A middle-aged man who has been diagnosed with a renal stone is inquiring about lithotripsy. Which one of the following statements about extracorporeal shock wave therapy for renal stones is true?

A) An optimal result is rarely achieved.
B) It is most effective for stones less than 2 cm in diameter.
C) Less energy is required to fragment calcium oxalate and cystine stones.
D) Repeated treatments are rarely required, regardless of stone size.
E) Stones must be present in the renal pelvis to be effective.

The answer is B: Lithotripsy has been used to fragment and remove renal and ureteral stones. The procedure involves placing the patient on a lithotripsy gantry so that the calculus overlies a circular window in the table containing the water bath, which is focused on the calculus. The procedure is most effective for stones less than 2 cm in diameter. Calcium oxalate and cystine stones are usually dense and require increased energy. Alternative modes of stone removal should be considered for large or hard calculi, stones in a calyceal diverticulum, or in patients with complex renal anatomy. Percutaneous nephrolithotomy and extracorporeal shock wave lithotripsy may reduce the need for further invasive surgery, but the risks and benefits should be weighed carefully in asymptomatic persons.

Additional Reading:
1. Treatment and prevention of kidney stones: an update. *Am Fam Physician*. 2011;84(11):1234-1242.
2. Clinical evidence kidney stones. *Am Fam Physician*. 2013;87(6):441-443.

Category: Nephrologic system

10. Topical lidocaine is used in addition to which one of the following medications to treat chronic anal fissures?

A) Mupirocin
B) Nifedipine
C) Nystatin
D) Sildenafil

The answer is B: Topical nifedipine in addition to lidocaine gel is effective and well tolerated in the treatment of chronic anal fissures. Treatment with nifedipine has been shown to be superior to topical nitroglycerin with respect to both healing and less side effects as a supportive measure in treating anal fissures.

Additional Reading: Hemorrhoids. *Am Fam Physician*. 2011;84(2):204-210.
Category: Gastroenterology system

11. A 24-year-old woman presents to your office. She is concerned that she is bleeding internally, because her stools have been dark, tarry black. Additionally, she reports that she was also having episodes of diarrhea, but these have resolved with the use of Pepto-Bismol. She denies abdominal pain, light-headedness, nausea, vomiting, or fevers. The most likely cause of her dark stools is which one of the following?

A) An upper gastrointestinal (GI) bleeding source
B) A lower GI bleeding source
C) Bismuth ingestion
D) Rectal outlet bleeding
E) None of the above

The answer is C: Melena is the passage of black tarry stools, which is secondary to GI bleeding. In most cases, the source is located in the upper GI tract; however, a source in the proximal right colon or small intestine can also cause melena. Approximately 100 to 200 mL of blood loss is needed to cause melena. Other causes for black stools that are often confused with melena include iron, bismuth, licorice, blueberries, and lead. Beets and tomatoes can sometimes make stools appear reddish.

Additional Reading: Diagnosis and management of upper gastrointestinal bleeding. *Am Fam Physician*. 2012;85(5):469-476.
Category: Gastroenterology system

12. Various local anesthetics are often used in combination with epinephrine for minor skin procedures. Which one of the following agents has the longest duration of action?

A) Bupivacaine (Marcaine).
B) Lidocaine (Xylocaine).
C) Mepivacaine (Carbocaine).
D) Procaine (Novocaine).
E) All have about the same duration of action.

The answer is A: The longest-acting anesthetic is bupivacaine, and it is useful for nerve blocks; epinephrine should be used cautiously or avoided altogether in areas such as the fingers, nose, penis, and toes or other distal appendages. The vasoconstrictive effect can lead to ischemic necrosis. The most common reason for inadequate anesthesia is not allowing enough time for the anesthetic to take effect. Bupivacaine has a longer onset of action (5 minutes) compared to lidocaine (2 minutes). Mixing 50/50 bupivacaine and lidocaine is a practice that allows for fast onset and long duration of the local anesthetic.

- Lidocaine and mepivacaine 1 to 3 hours depending on whether it is mixed with epinephrine
- Bupivacaine duration 4 to 8 hours
- Procaine duration 1.5 hours

Additional Reading: Subcutaneous Infiltration of local anesthetics. In: *UpToDate*. 2022.
Category: Integumentary system

13. Which of the following statements regarding preoperative evaluations is correct?

A) A baseline renal function study should be carried out for all surgical candidates.
B) A patient with a previous coronary bypass graft 2 years earlier should undergo cardiac stress testing before clearance, regardless of the presence of cardiac symptoms.
C) A urine pregnancy testing should be considered for women of childbearing age.
D) Coagulation studies should be included in the assessment of all surgical candidates.
E) Patients who have had angioplasty within 6 months are not required to have further cardiology assessment.

The answer is C: Before elective surgery, a review of the patient's history is necessary. Routine preoperative laboratory tests (complete blood count, hemoglobin, platelets, electrolytes, glucose, coagulation, and liver test) have not been shown to improve outcomes for otherwise healthy patients.

Hemoglobin measurement should be considered for patients older than 65 years undergoing major surgery and for younger patients undergoing surgery that is expected to result in significant blood loss. Creatinine is indicated for patients older than 50 years undergoing intermediate or high-risk surgery and for younger patients suspected of having renal disease, when hypotension is likely to happen during surgery or when nephrotoxic medications will be used. A urine pregnancy test should be considered for women of childbearing age.

Coagulation studies would be indicated if the patient is receiving anticoagulant therapy, has a family or personal history that suggests a bleeding disorder, or has evidence of liver disease. An electrocardiogram is indicated for vascular surgical procedures, for patients with preexisting cardiovascular disease who are undergoing intermediate-risk surgery, and in severely obese patients with poor effort tolerance or at least one additional cardiovascular risk.

Chest x-rays or pulmonary function tests are not ordered for a healthy patient but is indicated for those with cardiopulmonary disease and those older than 50 years who are undergoing abdominal aortic aneurysm surgery or upper abdominal/thoracic surgery. In general, patients in whom cardiac stress testing was normal within the previous 2 years or who have had coronary bypass surgery within the previous 5 years and are without symptoms require no further assessment. Clinically stable patients who have undergone angioplasty between 6 months and 5 years previously require no further assessment. However, patients who have had angioplasty within the previous 6 months may require cardiac reevaluation and/or consultation with a cardiologist before surgery.

Patients at high risk for complications usually warrant cardiology consultation and possibly angiography. Cardiac stress testing should be performed in patients at intermediate risk and with poor functional capacity or who are undergoing high-risk procedures such as vascular surgery. Among patients with minor clinical predictors, only patients who have poor functional capacity and are undergoing high-risk procedures require stress testing. Patients with a positive stress test result warrant cardiology consultation before proceeding with surgery.

Assessment of left ventricular function is not routinely indicated for preoperative evaluation whether the patient has cardiac disease. The preoperative assessment guideline from the American College of Physicians notes that radionuclide or echocardiographic assessment of left ventricular function does not appear to improve the risk prediction provided by the clinical examination alone.

In summary, recommendations do not call for preoperative cardiac testing in all patients. The need for further cardiac evaluation before surgery is determined by the clinical risk predictors identified from the patient's history, physical examination, electrocardiography, and functional status, along with the risk associated with the operation itself. Pulmonary function testing may be helpful in diagnosing and assessing disease severity. Baseline chest radiographs may be helpful in at-risk patients. Preoperative guidelines do not define the degree of pulmonary function impairment that would prohibit surgery other than that for lung resection.

Additional Reading: Preoperative testing before noncardiac surgery: guidelines and recommendations. *Am Fam Physician*. 2013;87(6):414-418.
Category: Nonspecific system

14. When utilizing a local anesthetic such as lidocaine for an injection, in which one of the following locations should the additional use of epinephrine be avoided?

A) An ear lobe
B) The back
C) The forehead
D) The lip
E) The scalp

The answer is A: Epinephrine administration should be avoided in the following areas: nose, ear lobes, or tip of the penis. It is also avoided near the terminal arterial branches in the digits. Epinephrine is contraindicated for digital anesthesia in patients with peripheral artery disease and in patients with periorbital infiltration with narrow-angle glaucoma and for large wounds in patients with underlying conditions (eg, hyperthyroidism, pheochromocytoma, severe hypertension, and coronary artery disease) that may be exacerbated by epinephrine effect.

Epinephrine infiltration with local anesthetics should be avoided in patients receiving β-blockers, monoamine oxidase inhibitors, phenothiazines, or tricyclic antidepressants and in patients with catecholamine sensitivity.

Additional Reading: Myth of not using lidocaine with epinephrine in the digits. *Am Fam Physician*. 2010;81(10):1188.
Category: Integumentary system

15. Which of the following is the standard prophylaxis treatment for subacute bacterial endocarditis for dental procedures in low-risk adult patients?

A) Amoxicillin: 1 g given intravenously at the time of the procedure.
B) Amoxicillin: 2 g given orally 1 hour before the procedure.
C) Ampicillin: 2 g given intravenously plus gentamicin (1.5 mg/kg intravenously) 30 minutes before the procedure; dose repeated 8 hours after the procedure.
D) Ampicillin: 500 mg given orally 1 hour before the procedure and 250 mg given 6 hours after the procedure.
E) No antibiotics are necessary.

The answer is E: Antibiotic prophylaxis (amoxicillin 2 g orally 30-60 minutes before the procedure) is recommended for patients who have high-risk cardiac conditions, which include the following:

- Prosthetic cardiac valve
- History of infective endocarditis
- Unrepaired cyanotic congenital heart disease; a completely repaired congenital heart defect with prosthetic material, during the first 6 months after the procedure; or a repaired congenital heart defect with residual defects at the site or adjacent to the site of a prosthetic patch or prosthetic device (which inhibits endothelialization)
- Cardiac transplantation recipients with cardiac valvular disease

The guidelines suggest preventive treatment for high-risk cardiac patients, not for all dental procedures but only for those that involve manipulation of gingival tissue (around bone and teeth) or the periapical region of teeth (tip of the tooth root). The guidelines do not recommend antibiotics for routine anesthetic injections through noninfected tissue, placement or adjustment of orthodontic appliances, shedding of baby teeth, or bleeding from trauma to the lips or inside of the mouth.

Furthermore, the American Heart Association guidelines no longer consider any gastrointestinal (colonoscopy or esophagogastroduodenoscopy) or genitourinary procedures high risk and therefore do not recommend routine use of endocarditis prophylaxis even in patients with the highest risk cardiac conditions.

Vaginal or cesarean delivery is not an indication for routine antibiotic prophylaxis.

Additional Reading: AHA releases updated guidelines on the prevention of infective endocarditis. *Am Fam Physician*. 2008;77(4):538-545.
Category: Cardiovascular system

16. All of the following suture materials are absorbable, except which one?

A) Catgut
B) Vicryl
C) Polypropylene
D) Polydioxanone suture (PDS)
E) Chromic catgut

The answer is C: The goal of suturing is to approximate the skin and eliminate unnecessary dead space. Tension at the wound site should be minimized. To achieve maximal cosmetic result, a suture is chosen based on the clinical situation. Monofilament sutures have significantly lowered the incidence of infection compared with multifilament sutures that can harbor bacteria. Nonabsorbable sutures (ie, nylon, silk, polypropylene [Prolene], braided polyester [Mersilene/Surgidac, Ethibond/Ti-Cron], and polybutester) are usually used to close the superficial layer of skin.

Absorbable sutures (i.e., catgut, chromic catgut, polycaprolate [Dexon II], PDS, Maxon, and polyglactin 10 [Vicryl], poliglecaprone [PDSII], and Caprosyn) are used to close deep layers of skin.

Additional Reading: Essentials of skin laceration repair. *Am Fam Physician*. 2008;78(8):945-951.
Category: Nonspecific system

17. Total parenteral nutrition (TPN) is indicated for those patients who require nutritional support but for whom enteral feeding is contraindicated or not tolerated. Which one of the following statements is true about administering TPN?

A) Because glucose is delivered in standard amounts at predetermined rates, there is little need to follow glucose on a regular basis.
B) Electrolytes should be monitored closely until stable.
C) Equivalent amounts of calories can be delivered via a central or peripheral access.
D) In most cases, TPN is administered through peripheral access.
E) Lipid emulsions can lead to fatty emboli and are not added to TPN solutions.

The answer is B: Central venous access is usually required to administer TPN, given that it has high osmotic load. TPN requires water (30-40 mL/kg per day), carbohydrate as dextrose 70% (3.4 kcal/g), amino acids 10% (4 kcal/g), and fat 20% (9 kcal/g), depending on the degree of catabolism. Indications include malnourished patients scheduled for surgery, chemotherapy, or radiation. Patients with severe burns, anorexia, coma, Crohn disease, ulcerative colitis, or pancreatitis may benefit from TPN.

The following parameters are monitored daily: weight, plasma urea, and glucose level (several times daily until stable), complete blood cell count, liver function tests, accurate fluid balance, 24-hour urine, and electrolytes. When the patient becomes stable, the frequency of these tests can be reduced. Liver function tests should be performed, and plasma proteins, prothrombin time; plasma and urine osmolality; and calcium, magnesium, and phosphate should be measured.

Additional Reading: Nutrition support in critically ill patients: parenteral nutrition. In: *UpToDate*. 2022.
Category: Nonspecific system

18. Appendicitis during pregnancy is more difficult to diagnose than in the nongravid state. Which one of the following factors makes appendicitis during pregnancy difficult to diagnose?

A) Location of the appendix
B) Absence of fever
C) Presence of pyuria
D) Rebound tenderness

The answer is A: Appendicitis during pregnancy may be difficult to diagnose. The white blood cell count is mildly elevated during a normal pregnancy, making it difficult to distinguish the leukocytosis seen with infection. In addition, as pregnancy progresses, the position of the appendix migrates superiorly (usually above the iliac crest in patients at more than 5 months' gestation). Therefore, there is a greater risk for perforation in those with appendicitis as pregnancy progresses. In addition, there is a greater risk of perinatal mortality when the appendix is perforated. The complications involved with appendectomy include premature labor and infection.

The differential diagnosis of abdominal pain during pregnancy is extensive and includes gastroenteritis, inflammatory bowel disease, cholecystitis, intestinal obstruction, pancreatitis, pyelonephritis, nephrolithiasis, spontaneous abortion, round ligament pain, ectopic pregnancy, uterine contractions, placental abruption, and pelvic infections.

Additional Reading: Acute Appendicitis: Efficient Diagnosis and Management. *Am Fam Physician*. 2018;98(1):25-33.
Category: Gastroenterology system

19. Elective hip arthroplasty is usually performed for elderly patients with severe degenerative arthritis. Relief of hip pain after such a hip replacement usually occurs at what time interval after surgery?

A) Almost immediately
B) After 3 months
C) After 6 months
D) Usually after 1 year
E) Rarely; hip replacement mostly improves functionality

The answer is A: Hip arthroplasty is usually reserved for elderly patients with severe degenerative or rheumatoid arthritis. Indications include intractable pain or severe limitation of motion that interferes with the patient's activity level. Those patients with rheumatoid arthritis have longer and more lasting improvement than those with osteoarthritis.

Complications include bleeding, infection, and the major immediate complication of thromboembolism. Bone resorption is a major complication that may affect the life of the prosthesis. Long-term complications include loosening of the prosthesis, which may require further surgery. In most cases, relief is immediate after hip replacement, and 90% of hip replacements are never revised.

Additional Reading: Osteoarthritis management: updated guidelines from the American College of Rheumatology and Arthritis Foundation. *Am Fam Physician*. 2021;103(2):120-121.
Category: Musculoskeletal system

20. Your 67-year-old mildly obese diabetic patient is recovering from knee replacement surgery, and you have been asked to assist with her postoperative management. You have been prescribing metformin (Glucophage), 1000 mg twice daily to control her blood glucose. She is now awake and has been able to eat dinner. Her examination is normal except for edema of her right leg. A complete blood count and chemistry profile were normal except for an elevated glucose (210 mg/dL). Her hemoglobin A1c level, which is the result of the test performed a month ago, was 6.8%. Which one of the following would be the best management for her diabetes at this time?

A) Stop her usual medications and begin a sliding-scale insulin regimen.
B) Initiate an insulin drip to maintain glucose levels of 80 to 120 mg/dL.
C) Decrease the dose of metformin.
D) Continue with her usual medication regimen.

The answer is D: The use of a "sliding-scale" insulin regimen to control glucose in hospitalized diabetics is inadequate, and although postoperative patients using an insulin drip to maintain control have a decreased risk of sepsis, there is no mortality benefit. Metformin should be stopped if the serum creatinine level is greater than 1.5 mg/dL in men or 1.4 mg/dL in women, or if an imaging procedure requiring contrast is needed. In patients who have not had their hemoglobin A1c level measured in the past 30 days, this could be performed to provide a better indication of glucose control. If adequate control has been demonstrated and no contraindications are noted, the patient's usual medication regimen should be continued.

Additional Reading: Glycemic control in hospitalized patients. *Am Fam Physician*. 2017;96(10):648-654.
Category: Endocrine system

21. Decubitus ulcers occur when there is prolonged pressure of skin against an external object such as a bed or a wheelchair. Which one of the following measures can impede, rather than assist, with the healing of decubitus ulcers?

A) Air-fluidized mattresses
B) Debridement of nonviable tissue
C) Doughnut cushions
D) Frequent position changes
E) Wet to dry dressing changes

The answer is C: Decubitus ulcers occur most often in patients who are debilitated and have impaired sensory function. The sacrum, ischia, greater trochanters, external malleoli, and heels are at particular risk for tissue breakdown. There are four stages in the development of decubitus ulcers:

- *Stage 1*—nonblanchable erythema of intact skin
- *Stage 2*—partial-thickness dermal or epidermal loss causing a blister, shallow crater, or abrasion
- *Stage 3*—full-thickness necrosis causing a deep crater down to fascia
- *Stage 4*—full-thickness destruction of muscle, bone, or supporting structures

Intrinsic and extrinsic factors play a role in the development of pressure ulcers. Intrinsic factors include loss of pain and pressure sensations (which ordinarily prompt the patient to shift position and relieve the pressure) and minimal fat and muscle padding between bony weight-bearing prominences and skin. Disuse atrophy, malnutrition, anemia, and infection also contribute. In a paralyzed patient, loss of vasomotor control leads to lowered tone in the vascular bed and lowered circulatory rate. Spasticity, especially in patients with spinal cord injuries, can place a shearing force on the blood vessels to further compromise circulation.

Extrinsic factors include pressure due to infrequent shifting of the patient's position; friction, irritation, and pulling of the skin from ill-adjusted supports or wrinkled bedding or clothing also contribute. In an immobilized patient, severe pressure can impair local circulation in fewer than 3 hours, causing local tissue anoxia that, if unrelieved, progresses to necrosis of the skin and subcutaneous tissues. Moisture (eg, from perspiration or incontinence) leads to tissue maceration and predisposes to pressure sores.

The treatment of decubitus ulcers includes wet to dry dressing changes and the use of air-fluidized beds, particularly for large ulcers. Ulcers that have not advanced beyond stage 3 may heal spontaneously if the pressure is removed and the area is small. Hydrophilic gels and hydrocolloid dressings speed healing.

Stage 4 ulcers require debridement or more extensive surgery. When the ulcers are filled with pus or necrotic debris, dextranomer beads or newer hydrophilic polymers may hasten debridement without surgery. Conservative debridement of necrotic tissue with forceps and scissors should be instituted. Some ulcers may be debrided by cleansing them with hydrogen peroxide. Whirlpool baths may also assist debridement.

The use of egg crate mattresses, sheepskins, and doughnut cushions is not adequate to prevent ulcers; doughnut cushions can actually decrease the blood flow to the area of the body in the center of the cushion, thereby impeding the healing process. The use of antibiotics is unnecessary, unless cellulitis, osteomyelitis, or systemic infection is present. The use of topical antiseptics and antibiotics may also impede the healing process by damaging fibroblasts, which are needed for healing. Compared with standard hospital mattresses, pressure-reducing devices decrease the incidence of pressure ulcers.

Additional Reading: Chronic Wounds: Evaluation and Management. *Am Fam Physician*. 2020;101(3):159-166.
Category: Integumentary system

22. A 72-year-old man complains that he cannot void the day after his knee replacement surgery. He has not voided in the past 12 hours. A urethral catheter is placed and 500 mL of urine is removed from his bladder. Which one of the following is most likely to improve the success rate of a voiding trial?

A) Inserting a specialized catheter instead of a standard catheter
B) Immediately removing the catheter
C) Leaving the catheter in place for at least 2 weeks
D) Starting tamsulosin (Flomax), 0.4 mg daily, at the time of catheter insertion
E) Starting antibiotic prophylaxis at the time of catheter insertion

The answer is D: Urinary retention is a common problem in hospitalized patients, especially following certain types of surgery. Starting an α-blocker (such as tamsulosin) at the time of insertion of the urethral catheter has been shown to increase the success of a voiding trial. Voiding trial success rates have not been shown to be improved by immediate removal of the catheter or by leaving the catheter in for 2 weeks. Specialized catheters, such as a coudé catheter that is designed with a curved tip that makes it easier to pass through the curvature of the prostatic urethra, have not been shown to make a difference. Antibiotic prophylaxis has no impact on urinary retention.

Additional Reading: Urinary retention in adults: diagnosis and initial management. *Am Fam Physician*. 2008;77(5):643-650.
Category: Nephrologic system

23. A patient is being seen after a colonoscopy and he is concerned because two hyperplastic polyps were resected. You inform him that which of the following types of polyps is associated with the greatest risk for malignant transformation?

A) Distal hyperplastic polyp.
B) Mixed tubulovillous adenoma.
C) Tubular adenoma.
D) Villous adenoma.
E) All of the above have equal risk.

The answer is D: The development of colon polyps has been associated with a high-fat, low-fiber diet. They also occur more frequently in patients with a positive family history (two to four times more common than in the healthy population). Villous histology, increasing size of polyps, and high-grade dysplasia are risk factors for focal cancer within an individual adenoma. Adenomatous polyps greater than 1 cm in diameter are a risk factor for colorectal cancer. Older age is also associated with high-grade dysplasia within an adenoma, independent of size or histology. The number of adenomas, particularly three or more, is a risk factor for development of metachronic adenomas with advanced pathologic features. Polyps are divided into differing histologic types:

- Hyperplasic polyps: Distal small hyperplastic polyps rarely develop into cancer.
- Tubular adenoma: 5% chance of cancer development.
- Mixed tubulovillous adenoma: 22% chance of cancer development.
- Villous adenoma: 40% chance of cancer development.

Additional Reading: Colonic polyps. In: Domino F, ed. *The 5-Minute Clinical Consult*. Wolters Kluwer; 2022.
Category: Gastroenterology system

24. A 39-year-old woman is found to have chronic cholestasis and she asks about her prognosis. You inform her that the most serious complication associated with this diagnosis is which one of the following conditions?

A) Cholelithiasis
B) Chronic urticaria
C) Hypercholesterolemia
D) Intractable hiccups
E) Primary biliary cirrhosis

The answer is E: Primary biliary cirrhosis is a condition that is characterized by chronic cholestasis, which can damage the liver and ultimately result in the development of cirrhosis. The cause is unknown but may be associated with an underlying autoimmune disorder. The condition typically affects women between 35 and 70 years of age; the condition can also occur in men. The disease usually involves four stages:

1. Bile duct inflammation
2. Periportal fibrosis
3. Progressive scarring
4. Cirrhosis

Symptoms include itching secondary to elevations of bilirubin, fatigue, and jaundice. Physical findings include hepatosplenomegaly, skin xanthomas (especially around the eyelids and involving the tendons), clubbing, and jaundice. Laboratory tests show elevated alkaline phosphatase, bilirubin, γ-glutamyl transferase, aspartate transaminase, and alanine transaminase. Serum cholesterol is also usually elevated.

Diagnostic procedures include ultrasonography, endoscopic retrograde cholangiopancreatography, and liver biopsy. Unfortunately, no specific treatment is available; however, those affected may be candidates for liver transplantation if they develop cirrhosis with hepatic failure. Cholestyramine may be beneficial for the pruritus. Those affected have a variable prognosis, depending on the severity of the disease. Those with slow progression may be minimally affected. Chronic urticaria may be associated with underlying urticarial vasculitis and is diagnosed by skin biopsy.

Additional Reading: Clinical manifestations, diagnosis, and natural history of primary biliary cirrhosis. In: *UpToDate*. 2022.
Category: Gastroenterology system

25. A 50-year-old patient is asking about the diverticulosis that was seen on his recent screening colonoscopy. You inform him that diverticulosis is a condition associated with which one of the following?

A) An increased risk for developing colon cancer
B) Development of herniations of the bowel mucosa and submucosa through the muscular layers of the bowel wall
C) Development of inflammatory bowel disease
D) Diverticulitis in most patients

The answer is B: Diverticulosis, an outpouching of the bowel wall, increases in frequency after 40 years of age. Acquired diverticular disease affects approximately 5% to 10% of the Western population older than 45 years and approximately 80% of persons older than 85 years. It is more common in the sigmoid and distal colon. Colonic diverticula are related primarily to two factors: increased intraluminal pressure and a weakening of the bowel wall. Patients with known diverticula have been found to have elevated resting colonic pressures. The Western diet, which tends to be low in dietary fiber and high in refined carbohydrates, is also believed to be a contributing factor. The condition occurs when there is herniation of bowel mucosa and submucosa through muscular layers of the colon.

Inflammation of the small herniations, referred to as *diverticulitis*, occurs in 10% to 20% of patients with diverticulosis and more commonly in men. Most patients with diverticulosis remain asymptomatic. Symptoms of diverticulitis include lower abdominal pain usually located on the left that may be steady or cramping and is sometimes relieved with a bowel movement, anorexia, nausea, vomiting, and constipation. Physical examination usually shows abdominal tenderness and guarding and, occasionally, a palpable abdominal or rectal mass with abscess formation. Occult blood is present in approximately 20% of patients. Diverticular hemorrhage occurs in 3% to 5% of patients with diverticular disease. Fever and an increased white blood cell count may also be present. Computed tomographic scanning is the diagnostic procedure of choice.

Treatment of diverticulitis can take place on an outpatient basis for a patient with a mild first attack who is able to tolerate oral hydration and an antibiotic. Recent level 1 evidence shows that select patients with uncomplicated diverticulitis can be treated without antibiotics, and this is now recommended by the American Society of Colon and Rectal Surgeons in their clinical practice guidelines. For patients with multiple comorbidities, signs of systemic infection (eg, fever), or immunosuppression, antibiotics are still recommended for uncomplicated diverticulitis. Regardless of whether antibiotics are given, treatment consists of a liquid diet until the patients abdominal pain improves. Those receiving antibiotics should receive 7 to 10 days of therapy with broad-spectrum antimicrobials such as metronidazole and ciprofloxacin. Patients with severe illness, or those who cannot tolerate oral hydration or who have pain severe enough to require narcotic analgesia, should be hospitalized. Because feeding increases intracolonic pressure, patients should receive nothing by mouth and should be treated with intravenous triple therapy consisting of ampicillin, gentamicin, and metronidazole. Alternative monotherapy includes piperacillin or tazobactam. If narcotics are required for pain control, meperidine is recommended because morphine sulfate causes colonic spasm. If the pain, fever, and leukocytosis do not resolve within 3 days, further imaging studies are indicated. If an abscess is uncovered and is >5 cm in size, computed tomography-guided drainage and adequate antibiotic coverage should be considered. Approximately 20% of patients with diverticulitis require surgery.

Indications for emergent surgery include peritonitis, uncontrolled sepsis, visceral perforation, colonic obstruction, or acute deterioration. Bowel resection is usually recommended for recurrent episodes of diverticulitis or if fistulas are present.

Additional Reading: Diverticular disease. In: Domino F, ed. *The 5-Minute Clinical Consult*. Wolters Kluwer; 2022.
The American Society of Colon and Rectal Surgeons Clinical Practice Guidelines for the treatment of left-sided colonic diverticulitis. *Dis Colon Rectum*. 2020;63: 728-747.
Category: Gastroenterology system

26. A patient is using patient-controlled analgesia (PCA) after his operation. Which one of the following statements is true regarding this form of pain control?

A) Administration of PCA is labor-intensive.
B) Oversedation can usually be avoided with PCA.
C) PCA basal infusion rates should be routinely used.
D) Patient response is not a good indicator of PCA effectiveness.
E) The PCA delivery system can usually increase the time interval between patient demand and delivery of the medication.

The answer is B: All postoperative patients should have their pain managed with a multimodal approach that includes a narcotic. Using multimodal therapy minimizes narcotics and provides superior pain relief than relying on one medication alone. This can be important when working with patients at high risk for delirium where mind- and mood-altering medications need to be limited. In addition to low-dose opioids, options include acetaminophen, nonsteroidal anti-inflammatory drugs when bleeding is not a risk, gabapentin, lidocaine patches, epidurals or long-acting field blocks with liposomal bupivacaine (72 hours duration), abdominal binders, and ice/warm packs.

PCA is the preferred mode of administering opioids for moderate to severe postoperative pain. The benefits include easier access for patients to pain medication, reduced chance of medication error, and ready titration. PCA pumps avoid the lag period between when the patient senses pain and initiates the call for medication and actual delivery by a nurse. It can also reduce the amount of work of drawing up and delivering multiple doses of medication by the nursing staff. PCA pumps can also deliver a constant rate of medication per hour whether or not the patient hits the demand button. Compared with conventional parenteral analgesia, PCA provides better pain control and results in greater patient satisfaction.

Morphine, hydromorphone, and fentanyl can be administered via the PCA pump. The pump is discontinued when the patient can tolerate oral analgesics. A fentanyl PCA may be used for patients with allergies or intolerances to morphine and hydromorphone but is less desirable in most patients because of its short duration of action. Fentanyl may be easier to titrate in patients with renal and hepatic insufficiency. Alternatively, hydromorphone can be used in patients with renal insufficiency.

Importantly, dosing is titrated and patients can be locked out from receiving too much narcotic. With electronic health records, calculating daily doses of intravenous narcotic can easily be performed, and this allows one to convert a patient to oral narcotics on a matched dose as the patient progresses toward discharge.

Additional Reading: Management of postoperative pain. In: *UpToDate*. 2022.
Category: Nonspecific system

27. A 48-year-old woman presents with questions about her mammogram. Which one of the following statements about breast cancer is true?

A) Cystic lesions found on screening are usually benign.
B) Early menopause is a risk factor for breast cancer.
C) Mammograms can be used to determine whether a mass is benign.
D) Mammogram screening should begin at 35 years of age to obtain a baseline reading.
E) Mammograms have less than a 5% false-negative rate.

The answer is A: A breast mass requires a thorough evaluation to rule out a possible malignancy. Risk factors for breast cancer include increased age, early menarche, late menopause, *BRCA* gene mutation, being nulliparous, having a first-degree relative with breast cancer, or having cancer in the contralateral breast.

A palpable mass can be evaluated with fine-needle or excisional biopsy. It is important to remember that mammograms have a 10% to 15% false-negative rate; therefore, a palpable solid mass should, in most cases, be biopsied despite a negative mammogram. In addition, a solid lesion is more worrisome for malignancy than a cystic lesion, and ultrasonography may be used to differentiate between the two. If the mass is cystic, it can be watched closely with serial ultrasonographies or aspirated. The screening guidelines for the diagnosis of breast cancer are continually changing. The U.S. Preventive Services Task Force (USPSTF) and the American College of Physicians recommend beginning routine screening at the age of 50 years; however, many other organizations recommend starting at the age of 40 years. These include the American Cancer Society, American College of Radiology, American Medical Association, the National Cancer Institute, the American College of Obstetricians and Gynecologists, and the National Comprehensive Cancer Network.

Additional Reading: *Recommendation: Breast Cancer – Screening | United States Preventive Services Taskforce*. (uspreventiveservicestaskforce.org)
Category: Integumentary system

The USPSTF recommends biennial screening mammography for women aged 50 to 74 years (grade B recommendation).

28. A 69-year-old hospitalized patient underwent a bowel resection last week and has been unable to tolerate oral feedings. He is now receiving total parenteral nutrition (TPN), and as you review his laboratory work, you note that he has developed a mild elevation in his liver function tests. The most appropriate approach at this time is to take which one of the following actions?

A) Continue monitoring and observation.
B) Discontinue the parenteral nutrition.
C) Obtain a liver biopsy.
D) Order an ultrasonography of the liver, pancreas, and gallbladder.
E) Refer for an exploratory laparoscopy.

The answer is A: TPN is the administration of a patient's daily nutritional requirements intravenously. Generally, the concentrated solution is given through central venous access. Patients who may be candidates for TPN include burn victims, malnourished patients in the perioperative period, or patients who have severe trauma or are in a comatose state. Formulations include daily nutritional requirements, including vitamin supplementation.

Patients should be monitored closely with laboratory tests, daily weights, and accurate intakes and outputs. Complications involve metabolic, nutritional deficiencies, administration complications (eg, infection of intravenous sites), and refeeding syndrome. Laboratory abnormalities may include elevated liver function tests, hepatosplenomegaly, thrombocytopenia, or hyperlipidemia.

Hepatic dysfunction is a common manifestation of long-term TPN support, and liver function tests should be monitored. Steatosis is associated with mild elevations of the transaminases, alkaline phosphate, and bilirubin. Cholecystitis, particularly the acalculous type, may occur in patients who receive TPN for extended periods.

Additional Reading: Nutrition support in critically ill patients: parenteral nutrition. In: *UpToDate*. 2022.
Category: Nonspecific system

29. A 33-year-old father of two children comes in to discuss having a vasectomy. You inform him that which one of the following statements is true regarding vasectomies?

A) Patients may resume unprotected intercourse after one sperm-free semen analysis.
B) Sperm antibodies develop in <1% of men after a vasectomy.
C) Sperm antibodies are related to the future development of coronary artery disease.
D) The failure rate is less than 1%.
E) Vasectomy raises the incidence of testicular cancer.

The answer is D: Vasectomies are performed to provide sterilization for men. Complications include bleeding, hematoma, infection, sperm granuloma (15%-40%), and postvasectomy pain syndrome. The patient should be monitored with a sperm count after vasectomy, and if motile sperm are confirmed on two samples 1 month apart (after 20 ejaculates), it is likely the vasectomy has failed. The patient should be advised to have a second procedure and use alternative contraception. Vasectomy offers a safe, effective, and permanent method of male contraception, with an overall failure rate of less than 1%. Failure can be due to technical errors, recanalization, or unprotected intercourse before azoospermia is documented.

As many as 60% to 80% of patients develop sperm antibodies after vasectomy; however, there is no association between anti-sperm antibodies and other immune-mediated diseases, such as lupus erythematosus, scleroderma, or rheumatoid arthritis. Additionally, there is no increased risk of cardiovascular disease, prostate cancer, or testicular cancer with vasectomy.

Additional Reading: Common questions about vasectomy. *Am Fam Physician*. 2013;88(11):757-761.
Category: Reproductive system

30. You are evaluating a retired 67-year-old accountant, who is asking about a knee replacement, because he is having increased problems with his right knee and it is affecting his golf game. You inform him that the primary indication for joint replacement surgery in patients with osteoarthritis is which one of the following?

A) Intractable pain
B) Joint laxity
C) Limited range of motion
D) Recurrent subluxation

The answer is A: Osteoarthritis of the knees is a common disabling condition that affects a third of those older than 65 years, and a quarter of those affected cannot perform major activities of daily living. Osteoarthritis is a degenerative disease characterized by erosion of the articular cartilage, hypertrophy of bone at the margins (osteophytes), and subchondral sclerosis. Exercise, weight loss, physical therapy, intra-articular corticosteroid injections, and the use of nonsteroidal anti-inflammatory drugs, along with braces or heel wedges, decrease pain and improve function. All those with symptomatic knee osteoarthritis should also participate in self-management programs, strengthening, low-impact aerobic exercise, and neuromuscular education.

Total joint arthroplasty of the knee should be considered when conservative symptomatic management is ineffective. According to the American Academy of Orthopedic Surgeons, the main indication for total knee arthroplasty is relief of pain, which is almost always relieved by the surgery. Joint replacement may also be appropriate for patients with significant limitations of joint function or with altered limb alignment. Range of motion, joint laxity, and recurrent subluxations relate to musculotendinous function and are not reliably improved by joint replacement. Arthroscopic surgery is not an appropriate treatment for knee osteoarthritis, unless there is evidence of loose bodies or mechanical symptoms such as locking, giving way, or catching.

Additional Reading: Osteoarthritis management: updated guidelines from the American College of Rheumatology and Arthritis Foundation *Am Fam Physician*. 2014;89(11):918-920.
Category: Musculoskeletal system

Acupuncture, glucosamine, chondroitin, and hyaluronic acid injections are not recommended therapies for knee osteoarthritis. Evidence to support corticosteroid injections is inconclusive.

31. Latex allergy has become a significant problem since the widespread adoption of universal precautions against infection. Which one of the following statements is false regarding latex allergies?

A) Latex is not found in catheters.
B) Many consumer products contain latex.
C) Persons allergic to latex also may be sensitive to fruits such as bananas, kiwis, pears, pineapples, grapes, and papayas.
D) Ten percent of health care workers experience some form of allergic reaction to latex.

The answer is A: The incidence of latex allergy is 1% to 2% in the general population, but as many as 17% of health care workers experience some form of allergic reaction to latex; however, not all are anaphylaxis. Recognizing latex allergy is crucial because physicians may inadvertently expose the patient to more latex during treatment. Latex is in gloves, catheters, and numerous other medical supplies (bandages, blood pressure cuffs, condoms, dental dams, diaphragms, tourniquets, stethoscope tubing, pacifiers, gutta-percha, and gutta balata [to seal root canals]), as well as consumer products.

Persons allergic to latex also may be sensitive to fruits such as bananas, kiwis, pears, pineapples, grapes, and papayas. Reactions to latex allergy can range from type IV delayed hypersensitivity (contact dermatitis) to type I immediate hypersensitivity (urticaria, bronchospasm, anaphylaxis).

Occupations in which latex allergy are commonly used include health care workers; food handlers/restaurant workers; domestic workers; hairdressers; security personnel; construction workers; greenhouse workers; gardeners; painters; funeral home workers; and first responders such as police officers, firefighters, and ambulance attendants.

Main risk factors for latex allergy are occupational exposure and an atopic tendency. The most reliable indicator of allergy is a strong clinical history, associating exposure with the symptoms. Skin testing with extracts prepared from latex C-serum is a safe and effective diagnostic procedure when extracts are standardized in terms of their allergen content and stability.

Additional Reading: Latex allergy. *Am Fam Physician*. 2009;80(12);1413-1418.
Category: Nonspecific system

32. A 50-year-old patient presents for a preventive medicine visit and is asking if he really needs a colonoscopy as his wife has suggested. The major risk factors for colon cancer include all of the following conditions, except which one?

A) A diet high in red meat
B) A family history of breast cancer
C) A personal history of villous polyps
D) A personal history of inflammatory bowel disease
E) Peutz-Jeghers syndrome

The answer is B: Of cancers that affect both men and women, colorectal cancer (CRC) is the second leading cause of cancer-related deaths in the United States (lung cancer is the number one) and the third most common cancer in men and women. The major factors that increase the risk of colon cancer include the following:

- Age: More than 90% of people diagnosed with CRC are older than 50 years.
- A personal history of colorectal polyps: Risk increases with multiple polyps, villous polyps, and larger polyps.
- A personal history of cancer: Rectal cancer has a higher incidence of local recurrence than proximal cancer (20%-30% vs 2%-4%); childhood cancer requiring abdominal radiation therapy also increases the risk.
- A personal history of inflammatory bowel disease: Those with ulcerative colitis and Crohn disease have a prevalence of ~3%, with a cumulative risk of CRC of 18% at 30 years.
- A family history of CRC: CRC is present in 10% of adults and about 25% of cases. Individuals with one or more first-degree or two or more second-degree relatives with CRC are at higher lifetime risk of developing CRC, which ranges from twofold to sixfold.

Certain genetic syndromes are clearly associated with CRC as well. The more common syndromes include the following:

- Lynch syndrome (hereditary nonpolyposis colorectal cancer): a 2% to 3% risk of developing CRC and also an increased risk for endometrial, stomach, ovarian, pancreas, ureter and kidney, biliary tract, and brain cancers.
- Familial adenomatous polyposis: tumors begin in the 20s, and nearly all will develop CRC, usually before the age of 50 years.
- Peutz-Jeghers syndrome: individuals often have freckles in the mouth, hands, and feet and large polyps in gastrointestinal tract.

Race and ethnicity issues are related to CRC risk as well:

- African Americans: highest CRC incidence and mortality rates in the United States.
- Ashkenazi Jews: Various associated gene mutations have been identified.

Epidemiologic data now show a strong association between diets high in red meat and CRC (as well as other cancers), though the exact mechanism is still being debated.

Additional Reading: Colorectal cancer. In: Domino F, ed. *The 5-Minute Clinical Consult*. Wolters Kluwer; 2022.
Category: Gastroenterology system

33. You are assessing a newborn who has been experiencing projectile vomiting after his first few feedings. You are suspicious for duodenal obstruction and would expect to see which one of the following radiographic signs with this condition?

A) Bird's beak sign
B) Hampton hump
C) Double bubble sign
D) Kerley B lines
E) Scalloping of the diaphragm

The answer is C: Duodenal obstruction is a congenital abnormality that can be caused by several different abnormalities, including duodenal atresia, duodenal stenosis, and malrotation of the intestine. In neonates, malrotation can also present as duodenal obstruction. The obstruction may be caused by Ladd bands or associated duodenal atresia. Infants with Down syndrome are at increased risk. Symptoms include projectile vomiting after the first few feedings. Polyhydramnios may also be present during pregnancy and is caused by a failure of absorption of amniotic fluid in the distal intestine.

Diagnosis is usually made radiographically. Plain abdominal radiographs show the characteristic "double bubble" sign—one large bubble in the stomach with a smaller adjacent bubble that represents the duodenum. Upper gastrointestinal (GI) contrast series is the best examination to visualize the duodenum. If atresia is present, no abdominal gas is seen in the distal bowel; however, if stenosis is present, a small amount of gas may be present. A barium swallow helps localize the site of obstruction. Treatment involves nasogastric suction to decompress the stomach and surgery to correct the obstruction.

The bird's beak sign is a descriptor for GI tract findings by barium studies, which have been likened to a bird's beak. Conditions include volvulus of the sigmoid colon (barium enema) and achalasia of the esophagus seen on a barium swallow.

Hampton hump refers to a soft tissue density seen on a chest x-ray as a manifestation of pulmonary infarction, due to a pulmonary embolism. Kerley B lines are peripheral septal lines seen primarily in the lung bases also on a chest x-ray, due to edema or fibrosis. Scalloping of the diaphragm is a normal anatomic variant seen on chest x-ray.

Additional Reading: Approach to the infant or child with nausea and vomiting. In: *UpToDate*. 2022.
Category: Gastroenterology system

34. A man has long-standing gynecomastia and asks about treatment. He reports that he has this problem for a dozen years and denies an associated galactorrhea. A careful drug history and physical examination, along with an endocrine and malignancy workup, are negative. Which one of the following is the treatment of choice?

A) Prescribe clomiphene (Clomid, Serophene).
B) Prescribe danazol.
C) Prescribe tamoxifen (Soltamox).
D) Prescribe topical testosterone (AndroGel).
E) Refer for surgery.

The answer is E: Surgery is indicated to treat long-standing gynecomastia because the initial glandular hyperplasia has transformed into a progressive fibrotic state. Medical management is most useful when the onset is recent or to prevent the initial development of the problem. The listed drugs have been tried with varying success in this context, but their clinical usefulness is not established.

Additional Reading: Gynecomastia. *Am Fam Physician*. 2012;85(7):716-722.
Category: Integumentary system

35. A young woman is being seen for a routine Papanicolaou test and is asking about how to perform regular breast self-examinations (BSEs). You inform her that using BSE to screen for breast cancer is associated with which one of the following?

A) An increase in the number of breast biopsies performed.
B) A reduction in mortality due to breast cancer.
C) A reduction in all-cause mortality in women.
D) Regular BSE is not recommended by the U.S. Preventive Services Task Force (USPSTF).

The answer is D: Performance of regular BSEs, even by trained women, does not reduce breast cancer–specific mortality or all-cause mortality. The USPSTF breast cancer screening recommendations recommend against teaching BSE. The rationale for this "D" recommendation is that there is moderate certainty that the harms outweigh the benefits. Trials have demonstrated that more additional imaging procedures and biopsies are performed on women who performed BSE than for controls, with no gains in breast cancer detection or reduction in breast cancer–related mortality.

Additional Reading: *Recommendation: Breast Cancer – Screening | United States Preventive Services Taskforce* (uspreventiveservicestaskforce.org)
Category: Integumentary system

36. You are seeing a 52-year-old woman who is considering silicone breast augmentation and has questions about her subsequent health risks. Which one of the following statements is true regarding silicone breast implants?

A) They are associated with a higher incidence of connective tissue disease.
B) They are associated with a higher incidence of breast cancer.
C) They should no longer be used according to the U.S. Food and Drug Administration.
D) Mammography with Eklund views can be helpful in assessing breast lumps after augmentation.
E) Magnetic resonance imaging (MRI) is not useful to detect implant rupture.

The answer is D: Women who have undergone augmentation mammoplasty with silicone gel or other implants may present for routine breast cancer screening with palpable breast lumps. Standard imaging technique in women with breast implant involves four views, rather than the usual two views per breast. Standard cranial-caudal and mediolateral oblique projections of each breast are obtained with the implant included. The Eklund technique consists of posterosuperior displacement of the implants simultaneously to an anterior traction of the breast, pushing the implants toward the chest wall up to flatten. These additional views permit evaluation of the implant as well as the deep breast tissues. MRI is the most accurate imaging examination for detecting rupture of breast implants.

Numerous meta-analyses have concluded that there is no evidence of an increased risk of any specific connective tissue diseases or other autoimmune conditions associated with the use of breast implants, including nonsilicone and silicone implants. There is no increased risk of breast cancer.

Additional Reading: Coombs DM, Grover R, Prassinos A, Gurunluoglu R. Breast augmentation surgery: clinical considerations. *Cleve Clin J Med*. 2019;86(2):111-122. doi:10.3949/ccjm.86a.18017.
Category: Integumentary system

37. Bariatric surgery procedures are proving useful in the management of obesity and its comorbid complications. Individuals who have a body mass index (BMI) that exceeds which threshold should be considered for such a procedure?

A) 10 kg/mm^2
B) 20 kg/mm^2
C) 30 kg/mm^2
D) 40 kg/mm^2
E) 50 kg/mm^2

The answer is D: A BMI of greater than 40 kg/m^2 or a BMI of 35 kg/m^2 with an obesity-related comorbidity (eg, diabetes and hypertension) is an indication of bariatric surgery. Additionally, the patient must be able to adhere to postoperative care plans.

Exclusion criteria include cardiopulmonary disease that would make the risk prohibitive; current drug or alcohol abuse; lack of comprehension of risks, benefits, expected outcomes, alternatives, and required lifestyle changes; reversible endocrine or other disorders that can cause obesity; and uncontrolled severe psychiatric illness.

Bariatric surgery procedures, including laparoscopic sleeve gastrectomy and Roux-en-Y bypass, result in an average weight loss of 50% of excess body weight. Laparoscopic banding is falling out of favor due to higher complication rates, including erosion and band slippage. Remission of diabetes mellitus occurs in approximately 80% of patient after Roux-en-Y bypass. Other obesity-related comorbidities are greatly reduced, and health-related quality of life improves.

The Obesity Surgery Mortality Risk Score identifies patients with increased risk from bariatric surgery. The Roux-en-Y procedure carries an increased risk of malabsorption sequelae but leads to the greatest weight loss (up to 10 lb [4.5 kg] per month) during the first one to two postsurgical years, followed by laparoscopic sleeve gastrectomy and laparoscopic adjustable gastric banding. After bariatric surgery, many patients maintain a long-term (8-10 years) weight loss of greater than 50% of excess body weight. Hyperlipidemia, hypertension, diabetes, and most other obesity-related conditions significantly improve after bariatric surgery. Overall, these procedures have a mortality risk of less than 0.5%.

Additional Reading: Treatment of adults obesity with bariatric surgery. *Am Fam Physician*. 2016;93(1):31-37.
Category: Endocrine system

➔ **BMI is the weight (in kilograms) divided by the height (in centimeters) squared.**

37. You are seeing a 47-year-old man for a "check-up." He is in excellent health, although his cholesterol is borderline high. His family history includes adult-onset diabetes. He is up to date on his immunizations. His wife was telling him to get a screening colonoscopy now that he is getting older. Which one of the following statements about the U.S. Preventive Services Task Force (USPSTF) recommendations for colorectal cancer (CRC) is false?

A) The USPSTF recommends screening for colorectal cancer in adults aged 45 to 49 years.
B) The USPSTF recommends screening for colorectal cancer in adults aged 50 to 75 years
C) The USPSTF recommends that screening be discontinued after 75 years of age.
D) The USPSTF recommends that screening be discontinued after 85 years of age.

The answer is C: Of cancers that affect both men and women, CRC is the second leading cause of cancer-related deaths in the United States (lung cancer is the number one) and the third most common cancer in men and women. The USPSTF recently lowered the age for screening to 45 years of age (B recommendation), while maintaining an A recommendation for screening between 50 and 75 years of age. The change was based on an assessment of the available empirical, modeling, and epidemiologic data—they found adequate evidence that screening this younger age group provided a moderate net benefit. The USPSTF recommends that clinicians selectively offer screening between 76 and 85 years of age. Evidence indicates that the net benefit of screening all persons in this age group is small. In determining whether this service is appropriate in individual cases, patients and clinicians should consider the patient's overall health, prior screening history, and individual preferences (C recommendation). The USPSTF recommends that screening be discontinued after 85 years of age. While several screening tests were recommended, they added language to the "Practice Considerations" section that colonoscopy to follow up an abnormal noncolonoscopy screening test result should be considered part of screening.

Additional Reading: *Recommendation: Colorectal Cancer – Screening | United States Preventive Services Taskforce* (uspreventiveservicestaskforce.org)
Category: Gastroenterology system

38. You are seeing a 43-year-old woman who underwent a laparoscopic Roux-en-Y gastric bypass for morbid obesity 2 years ago. She is in your office for a routine physical. You are reviewing her home medications. Which regimen below is necessary to prevent long-term complications of this surgery?

A) Niacin, B12, pancrelipase (CREON), iron, multivitamin
B) Multivitamin, B12, antacid, thiamine, iron
C) Pancrelipase (CREON), iron, daily aspirin (81 mg), antacid
D) Folic acid, copper, iron, prednisone
E) B12 and antacid alone

The answer is B: Bariatric surgery is becoming more common with rates of morbid obesity increasing overtime, and you will likely encounter these patients in your clinic. It is important to recognize that these patients require micronutrient supplementation for life, with a focus on vitamins affected by foregut metabolism. B12 requires intrinsic factor and an acidic environment for absorption, both of which are lacking in the small residual gastric pouch. Iron and thiamine (B1) are absorbed mostly in the duodenum and first portion of the jejunum, which are bypassed by the new anatomic arrangement. Clinically significant thiamine deficiency may manifest as Wernicke encephalopathy, which may be permanent. Multivitamins provide many necessary micronutrients but do not contain enough thiamine, iron, and B12 alone and so these are supplemented separately. All bypass patients should be on an antacid for life, either a proton pump inhibitor or an H2 receptor antagonist, to prevent marginal ulcer formation at the gastrojejunostomy anastomosis. These medications are often managed by a nutritionist early in a patient's course, but patients may be lost to follow-up and be seen in the primary care setting with nutritional deficiencies. Smoking cessation and avoidance of nonsteroidal anti-inflammatory drugs are also important for these patients to prevent marginal ulcer formation.

Pancrelipase is not indicated as pancreatic enzymes are still produced and sent down the pancreaticobiliary limb. Aspirin should be avoided in these patients. Prednisone is not indicated.

Additional reading: Bariatric Surgery: postoperative nutritional management. In: *UpToDate*. 2022.
Category: Gastroenterology system

39. A 62-year-old man with a 10 pack-year history of smoking cigarettes and social history significant for three alcoholic beverages per night presents with new-onset postprandial epigastric pain at night when lying down. He complains of a chronic cough, globus sensation in the back of his throat, and hypersalivation when these symptoms come on. Which feature of this patient's presumed gastroesophageal reflux disease (GERD) symptoms is considered an "alarm feature" that would necessitate endoscopy before a trial of a proton pump inhibitor (PPI)?

A) Age of 62 years
B) Hypersalivation with symptoms
C) Globus sensation
D) Tobacco use
E) Chronic cough

The answer is A: New-onset dyspepsia in persons greater than 60 years of age is considered an alarm feature of presumed reflux that should trigger a referral for endoscopy instead of empirically trialing a PPI. Other alarm features include evidence of GI bleeding, iron deficiency anemia, anorexia, weight loss, dysphagia, odynophagia, persistent vomiting, and having a first-degree relative with a gastrointestinal malignancy. All of these are concerning for esophageal or gastric malignancy. While alcoholism and tobacco use are risk factors for esophageal malignancy, neither is considered an alarm feature of newly diagnosed esophageal malignancy. Tobacco use alone would prompt the need for endoscopy in an individual with a 5- to 10-year history of GERD symptoms, as this is a risk factor for Barrett esophagus, a pathology that takes years to develop after the onset of GERD. Chronic cough, globus sensation, and water brash (hypersalivation) are atypical symptoms of GERD but are frequently seen nonetheless.

Additional reading: Clinical manifestations and diagnosis of gastroesophageal reflux in adults. In: *UpToDate*. 2022.
Category: Gastroenterology system

40. The parents of a 1-year-old, otherwise healthy, infant girl comes to your office concerned about bulging at her umbilicus. The patient is meeting all her growth metrics and has no signs of intermittent obstructive symptoms or incarceration of this umbilical hernia. You examine the child and find that the hernia feels about 1 cm in size. What is the next best step?

A) Bring the patient to the emergency room to have this seen by the on-call surgeon, as the risk of incarceration is extremely high after the age of 6 months.
B) Refer the parents to a pediatric surgeon within 1 to 2 weeks so that this can be repaired in a semiurgent fashion.
C) Reassure the parents that, unless she develops symptoms from this hernia, she is safe watching this hernia until age 2, when it should be repaired.
D) Reassure the patient that, unless she develops symptoms from this hernia, she is safe watching this hernia until age 5, when it should be repaired.
E) Reassure the parents that the natural history of umbilical hernias is that they nearly all close by age 2, and only rarely do they require repair during early adulthood.

The answer is D: Eighty percent of umbilical hernias will close by age 5, after which, operative repair is indicated. Exceptions that require early surgical consultation are there are signs or symptoms of incarceration, the umbilical hernia is >2 cm, the hernia is rapidly enlarging, or the proboscis is larger than 3 cm. Hernias larger than 2 cm rarely close spontaneously.

Additional reading: Chung DH. (2017). Pediatric surgery. In: Townsend CM, Evers BM, Beauchamp RD, Mattox KL, *Sabiston's Textbook of Surgery*. 20th ed. Elsevier; 2017:1884.
Category: Gastroenterology system

41. You are seeing a patient with a medical history of morbid obesity, chronic back pain, and hypertension who presents with abdominal pain. He has a surgical history of lumbar discectomy, appendectomy, and Roux-en-Y gastric bypass. He confides in you that he is going through a divorce and has picked up smoking and drinking again. He is taking his home medications but states that he misses them on some days. He reports that his stomach hurts all the time because he is overeating and "stretching out his small stomach pouch." He says when he eats, the pain gets better, but then it comes back. He also states that he is not exercising anymore, and his back pain is worse because of it, so he is now taking Tylenol around the clock. What is the likely cause of this man's abdominal pain?

A) Overeating
B) Around-the-clock Tylenol
C) Smoking
D) Drinking alcohol
E) Referred pain

The answer is C: Patients with a history of Roux-en-Y gastric bypass have a stomach-jejunal anastomosis (gastrojejunostomy), which is at risk of forming an ulcer due to the intestinal mucosa being adjacent to the acid-producing gastric mucosa. This is called a marginal ulcer. Patients who have undergone a Roux-en-Y gastric bypass require lifelong acid suppression with a proton pump inhibitor (PPI) or H2 receptor antagonist to prevent these ulcers. Risk factors for marginal ulceration include tobacco and chronic nonsteroidal anti-inflammatory drug (NSAID) use. As such, patients must quit smoking before being considered candidates for this operation. This patient resumed smoking, and although he was having chronic back pain, he was not using an NSAID. The clue that this was an ulcer is also that his pain was made better by eating. He should increase his PPI to bid dosing, get tested for *Helicobacter pylori*, and receive an upper endoscopy by his bariatric surgeon.

Additional reading: Late complications of bariatric surgical operations. In: *UpToDate*. 2022.
Category: Gastroenterology system

42. You have just admitted a 65-year-old man directly from clinic after a same-day computed tomographic (CT) scan–confirmed sigmoid diverticulitis with a phlegmon, requiring intravenous antibiotics and bowel rest. Once he is discharged from the hospital, he should:

A) be referred to a colorectal surgeon because he needs a sigmoid resection.
B) avoid nuts and seeds for the rest of his life.
C) start a low-fiber diet and drink at least 4 liters of water daily.
D) do daily sitz baths.
E) undergo a colonoscopy.

The answer is E: Patients who present with diverticulitis need to have a colonoscopy 6-8 weeks after resolution of their episode to ensure that there is no malignancy in the area. Many people have diverticuli, and a microperforation from a colon cancer in the sigmoid colon can easily masquerade as an episode of diverticulitis on a CT scan. It will similarly resolve with antibiotics. The decision for having a colectomy after an episode of diverticulitis is a mutual decision between the patient and a surgeon, and many people elect to not have surgery for their diverticulitis. Data show that the first episode is usually the worst or the same as subsequent episodes. Avoiding nuts and seeds will not prevent diverticulitis. Patients should be counseled on taking a high-fiber diet with plenty of fluid intake.

Additional reading: Acute colonic diverticulitis: medical management. In: *UpToDate*. 2022.
Category: Gastroenterology system

43. A 49-year-old man presents to your office with a new groin bulge. He states that he noticed it in the shower and that it occasionally aches when he is on his feet for a long time. He is able to do work at his job as a computer programmer unimpeded and go jogging without issue. You perform an exam and note a small right-sided inguinal hernia when the patient does Valsalva maneuvers. He is very afraid of surgery but is concerned because his uncle needed an emergency operation with a small bowel resection for an inguinal hernia. You tell him the risk of incarceration from a minimally symptomatic inguinal hernia that goes unrepaired is:

A) 15% in the next 4 years
B) 60% in the next 10 years
C) <1% in the next 4 years
D) 25% in the next 10 years
E) 5% annually

The answer is C: All inguinal hernias can be repaired if the patient desires, even if asymptomatic. The risk of incarceration over 4 years is around 0.6% if left untreated, as described in the "Watchful Waiting" trial (citation below). This randomized controlled trial demonstrated the safety of watchful waiting in minimally symptomatic or asymptomatic patients who do not desire surgery. This patient may be an ideal candidate for watchful waiting given his minimal symptoms and fear of surgery. He should be counseled on the signs of incarceration and bowel obstruction, though he should be reassured that the risk of this is, again, very low. If he changes his mind at any point, he can be referred to a general surgeon for repair.

Additional Reading: Fitzgibbons RJ Jr., Giobbie-Hurder A, Gibbs JO, et al. Watchful waiting vs repair of inguinal hernia in minimally symptomatic men: a randomized clinical trial. *JAMA*. 2006;295(3):285-292.
Category: Gastroenterology system

44. You are seeing a 65-year-old woman with a long-term history of gastroesophageal reflux disease who recently moved to the area. You see that she underwent an endoscopy for worsening symptoms 6 months prior, and the report reads, "short segment of Barrett esophagus with low-grade dysplasia." She has not followed up with any providers about this and cannot remember what her last doctor said because she was in the process of moving around the time of her last visit. What is your recommendation?

A) Referral to a thoracic surgeon for distal esophagectomy
B) Repeat the upper endoscopy 2 years from the last endoscopy
C) Repeat the upper endoscopy now
D) Only repeat the endoscopy if her symptoms get worse
E) Refer her for staging positron emission tomographic/computed tomographic scan

The answer is C: Barrett esophagus is caused by metaplastic changes of the esophageal mucosa, changing from stratified squamous epithelium to intestinal and gastric-type columnar epithelium. The overall risk of progression to esophageal cancer from Barrett esophagus without dysplasia is low, but patients with Barrett esophagus with *high-grade dysplasia* have 40X risk of developing esophageal cancer. Because of this, there is a tiered approach to surveillance and treatment in these patients.

Patients without dysplasia undergo surveillance every 2 years if there is a short-segment Barrett esophagus, and annually if there is a long-segment Barrett esophagus.

Patients with low-grade dysplasia should have surveillance endoscopies every 6 months or endomucosal ablation or resection. Patients with high-grade dysplasia should be referred for endoscopic resection, ablation, or occasionally esophagectomy. This patient's last endoscopy was 6 months prior, and she should therefore receive a repeat endoscopy.

Additional reading: Barrett's esophagus: Surveillance and management. In: *UpToDate*. 2022.
Category: Gastroenterology system

Care of the Elderly Patient

CHAPTER 6

In addition to general questions about geriatric care, this chapter is subdivided into sections focused on common areas of concern (neurologic, cardiovascular, musculoskeletal and integumentary, special sensory, and the urologic and reproductive systems) to help focus your American Board of Family Medicine study preparation.

Section I. General Geriatric Considerations

Each of the following questions or incomplete statements is followed by suggested answers or completions. Select the ONE BEST ANSWER in each case.

1. An elderly patient is brought in by her daughter because she has been confused over the past week; she notes that she does not have fever but that because she has gotten older, her temperature seems to "run low." All of the following statements about temperature variations in the elderly are true, except which one?

A) Norms for fever are adjusted on the basis of the patient's age after 75 years of age.
B) Serious infections may not be accompanied by comparable elevations in the patient's temperature.
C) Temperature in the elderly may not accurately reflect their health status.
D) The elderly tend to have disturbances of temperature regulation compared with younger patients.

The answer is A: Norms for fever or hypothermia are not adjusted for age; however, elderly patients do have a tendency toward disturbances of temperature regulation (hypothermia or hyperthermia) compared with younger individuals. It is possible that some elderly patients may present with serious infections that do not produce much temperature increase. There are suggested alternative fever definitions for *frail* older adults (one read over 100.0 or persistent reads over 99.0), but there is no standard age at which fever guidelines change.

Additional Reading: Approach to infection in the older adult. In: *UpToDate*. 2022.

2. Unfortunately, hospitalization often leads to a loss of independence in doing some basic activities of daily living for many elderly patients. Approximately what percent of elderly patients lose independence in performing one or more of the basic activities of daily living after discharge from a hospitalization for an acute illness?

A) Up to 15%
B) 15% to 25%
C) 25% to 35%
D) More than 35%

The answer is C: After a hospital admission, 25% to 35% of elderly patients lose independence in one or more of the basic activities of daily living by the time of discharge. The loss of independent functioning during hospitalization is associated with important complications including prolonged length of hospital stay, greater risk of institutionalization, and higher mortality rates.

Additional Reading: Geriatric Assessment: An office-based approach. *Am Fam Physician*. 2018;97(12):776-784.

3. In considering medication prescribing in the elderly, it is important to understand common changes in pharmacokinetics that occur with aging. Which one of the following statements about pharmacokinetics in the elderly is not true?

A) Body fat stores increase with aging; thus, fat-soluble medications have increased distribution and longer half-lives.
B) The glomerular filtration rate (GFR) is reduced in the elderly, which can lead to a decreased clearance of medication and an increased risk for toxicity.
C) The volume of body water is decreased in the elderly, which may require decreased dosages of water-soluble medications.
D) Accumulation of active metabolites does not occur in the elderly secondary to rapid clearance.
E) Hepatic metabolism of drugs decreases as patients age.

The answer is D: Changes that occur in the elderly often affect the pharmacokinetics of medications that are administered to them. As patients age, they increase their body stores of fat. Because of this, fat-soluble medications have increased distribution and a longer half-life in the body. Although expression of drug-metabolizing enzymes in the cytochrome P450 systems does not appear to decline with age, the overall hepatic metabolism of many drugs by these enzymes is reduced. The GFR in the elderly is also reduced, which can lead to a decreased clearance of medications and an increased risk for toxicity. The volume of body water is also reduced in the elderly, and the administration of water-soluble medications can lead to toxicity with some medications.

Increased sensitivity with aging must be considered when drugs that can have serious adverse effects are used. These drugs include morphine, pentazocine, warfarin, angiotensin-converting enzyme inhibitors, diazepam (especially when given parenterally), and levodopa. The effects of some drugs are reduced with aging (eg, glyburide and β-blockers), and such drugs should also be used with caution because serious dose-related toxicity can still occur and signs of toxicity may be delayed.

Many drugs produce active metabolites in clinically relevant concentrations. Examples are some benzodiazepines (eg, diazepam and chlordiazepoxide), tertiary amine antidepressants (eg, amitriptyline and imipramine), antipsychotics (eg, chlorpromazine and thioridazine; not haloperidol), and opioid analgesics (eg, morphine, meperidine, and propoxyphene). The accumulation of active metabolites (eg, *N*-acetylprocainamide and morphine-6-glucuronide) can cause toxicity in the elderly as a result of age-related decreases in renal clearance; toxicity is likely to be severe in those with renal disease.

Additional Reading: Reducing the risk of adverse drug events in older adults. *Am Fam Physician.* 2013;87(5):331-336.

4. The elderly are frequently seen in the emergency department with disease exacerbations; however, injuries are also seen. The leading cause of these injury-related visits in elderly patients (older than 65 years) to the emergency department in the United States is the consequences of which one of the following?

A) Depression and suicide gestures and/or attempts
B) Elder abuse
C) Exposure to extremes of temperature (hot or cold)
D) Falls
E) Motor vehicle crashes

The answer is D: Falls affecting the elderly are a major cause of morbidity and are the leading cause of injury-related visits to the emergency department in the United States and the primary cause of accidental deaths in persons older than 65 years. They may result in severe injury, including hip or other bone fractures, bruises, and subdural hematomas, as well as dehydration and hypothermia if the patient is not found early enough after a fall.

Many factors are related to the cause of falls, including muscle weakness, lack of coordination, poor vision, joint stiffness, autonomic dysfunction, increased reaction time, dementia, delirium, and medications. However, the physician should always search for precipitating medical causes such as stroke, cardiac arrhythmias, hypoglycemia, and orthostasis, in addition to environmental causes.

Preventive approaches include exercise interventions, proper lighting, short-pile carpet (avoiding throw rugs), railings, shower chairs, and walkers or canes for those with gait disorders. A visit to the patient's home or living environment may be helpful in identifying dangerous conditions, and patients at high risk for falls can benefit from a referral to a falls prevention program.

Additional Reading: The U.S. Preventive Services Task Force (USPSTF) recommendations on prevention of falls in community-dwelling older adults. https://www.uspreventiveservicestaskforce.org/uspstf/document/RecommendationStatementFinal/falls-prevention-in-older-adults-interventions#bootstrap-panel--6

5. Many changes in metabolic functioning are observed during aging, which can be reflected in changes in commonly obtained laboratory tests. All of the following laboratory findings would be expected, except which one?

A) A decrease in the creatinine clearance
B) An increase in alkaline phosphatase levels
C) A higher likelihood of false-positive rapid plasma reagin tests
D) A decrease in fasting serum glucose levels

The answer is D: For the most part, many laboratory normal values, including electrolytes, serum creatinine, and liver function tests, usually remain the same for elderly patients. However, there are some exceptions. With increasing age, there is usually:

- a decline in renal function, as is evident by a 10% decrease in creatinine clearance per 10 years after 40 years of age;
- an increase in fasting blood glucose levels (1 mg/dL for every 10 years); however, most patients remain within the normal limit values;
- an increase in alkaline phosphatase, an enzyme found in many organs, with the highest concentration from liver and bone;
- an increased incidence of false-positive rapid plasma reagin tests for syphilis.

Additional Reading: *Wallach's Interpretation of Laboratory Tests.* 11th ed. Lippincott Williams & Wilkins; 2020.

6. A 69-year-old white woman presents with a vesicular rash on her trunk, which you diagnose as a herpes zoster (shingles) infection. Which one of the following statements about herpes zoster is true?

A) The virus remains dormant in the muscle fibers and can be reactivated by stress.
B) The rash is usually vesicular and bilateral, and typically affects the face.
C) The virus can lead to chronic, debilitating pain for an extended period after resolution of the rash.
D) Steroids are the mainstay of treatment.
E) Exposure to patients with varicella (chickenpox) can cause a herpes zoster outbreak.

The answer is C: Herpes zoster, also known as *shingles*, is caused by a reactivation of the virus that causes varicella (chickenpox). The virus remains dormant in the nerve endings and reactivates itself, in some cases, as a result of stress or infection. There have been studies of adults who had chickenpox as children and were later exposed to children who had chickenpox. Interestingly, that exposure apparently boosted the adult's immunity, which actually helped them avoid getting shingles later in life, and there is no evidence that such exposure causes a zoster outbreak.

The elderly are most frequently affected. Areas of involvement usually include the trunk; however, it may occur on the face (in the distribution of the trigeminal nerve). In most cases, a vesicular, painful rash develops in a single, unilateral, dermatomal pattern. Herpes zoster typically presents with a prodrome consisting of hyperesthesias, paresthesias, burning dysesthesias, or pruritus along the affected dermatome(s). Other symptoms include fatigue, fever, and headache. The prodrome generally lasts 1 to 2 days but may precede the appearance of skin lesions by up to 3 weeks. After the resolution of the rash, many patients develop postherpetic neuralgia, which can be chronic and debilitating.

For acute herpes zoster, antivirals such as acyclovir (Zovirax), valacyclovir (Valtrex), and famciclovir (Famvir) are useful for treatment, particularly if administered early in the course of the disease. If the use of orally administered prednisone is not contraindicated, adjunctive treatment with this agent is justified based on its effects in reducing pain, despite questionable evidence for its benefits in decreasing the incidence of postherpetic neuralgia. Given the theoretic risk of immunosuppression with corticosteroids, some investigators believe that these agents should be used only in patients older than 50 years because they are at greater risk of developing postherpetic neuralgia, and prednisone may be beneficial.

Treatment of postherpetic neuralgia consists of topical capsaicin and amitriptyline. Pregabalin (Lyrica) is also approved for the treatment of postherpetic neuralgia.

SHINGRIX is an U.S. Food and Drug Administration–approved vaccine for the prevention of shingles (herpes zoster) in adults 50 years and older.

Additional Reading: Herpes zoster. In: Domino F, ed. *The 5-Minute Clinical Consult*. Wolters Kluwer; 2022.

7. The perceived misuse and overprescribing of psychotropic medications in the elderly led to the nursing home reform legislation known as the Omnibus Budget Reconciliation Act of 1987 (OBRA-87). This Act mandated freedom for every resident from medically unnecessary "physical or chemical restraints imposed for purposes of discipline or convenience." After institution of this legislated action, which of the following occurred?

A) The use of antipsychotic medications increased.
B) The use of long-acting benzodiazepines (eg, diazepam) increased.
C) The use of neuroleptics did not appreciably decrease.
D) The use of selective serotonin reuptake inhibitors increased.
E) There was no effect noted on physicians' prescribing practices.

The answer is D: Several multiyear, multifacility reviews have examined the impact of OBRA regulations on psychotropic prescribing in nursing homes. These confirm an encouraging trend, including increased awareness of antipsychotic indications and side effects. After OBRA, overall neuroleptic use declined by over a third. However, antidepressant prescribing increased, with significant increases in the use of selective serotonin reuptake inhibitors, nortriptyline, and trazodone, and decreases in amitriptyline and doxepin.

Anxiolytic/hypnotic prescribing patterns are less consistent. A large study documented a 12% increase in anxiolytics but decreases in particular agents (eg, diazepam and diphenhydramine). Two studies identified the implementation of OBRA regulations alone as responsible for decreased neuroleptic dosing.

Additional Reading: Medical care in skilled nursing facilities in the United States. In: *UpToDate*. 2022.

8. Many changes occur within the kidney as a result of increasing age. Aging-associated changes affecting the kidneys include all of the following except which one?

A) A decrease in renal size
B) An increase in serum creatinine
C) A decrease in the glomerular filtration rate (GFR)
D) A decrease in renal blood flow (RBF)
E) An increased threshold for glucose

The answer is C: With aging, there is a gradual decrease in renal size, a decrease in RBF, and, most importantly, a decrease in GFR, which can have a significant effect on drug metabolism. However, in most cases, serum creatinine remains essentially unchanged. In many cases, the doses of renal-metabolized medications need to be reduced in patients with decreased creatinine clearance. Additionally, the renal threshold for glucose increases with increasing age, and there is a decrease in maximal urinary concentration.

Additional Reading: Reducing the risk of adverse drug events in older adults. *Am Fam Physician*. 2013;87(5):331-336.

9. Hyperthyroidism in the elderly is often more difficult to diagnose than in younger patients, and when comparing elderly patients with hyperthyroidism to younger, middle-aged patients with hyperthyroidism, elderly patients are more likely to have which one of the following findings?

A) Atrial fibrillation
B) Goiter
C) Hyperactive appearance
D) Restlessness
E) Weight gain

The answer is A: Hyperthyroidism in the elderly is often more difficult to diagnose than in younger patients. Only 25% of elderly with hyperthyroidism present with symptoms that are typically seen in younger patients, such as restlessness and hyperactive appearance. Instead, elderly patients are more likely to show weight loss, new-onset atrial fibrillation, and withdrawal or depression. Other complications include cardiac failure, angina, myocardial infarction, and osteoporosis with an increased risk of bone fractures.

Behavioral changes in younger patients include anxiety, emotional lability, insomnia, lack of concentration, restlessness, and tremulousness. In contrast, elderly patients show apathy, lethargy, pseudodementia, and depressed moods.

Older patients have a lower incidence of goiter. The most common cause of hyperthyroidism in the elderly is Graves disease or diffuse toxic goiter. Graves disease is an autoimmune disorder resulting from the action of a thyroid-stimulating antibody on thyroid-stimulating hormone receptors. Thyroid-stimulating hormone receptor antibodies are detectable in the serum of approximately 80% to 100% of untreated patients with Graves disease.

Additional Reading: Atrial fibrillation and atrial flutter. In: Domino F, ed. *The 5-Minute Clinical Consult*. Wolters Kluwer; 2022.

10. You are caring for an 83-year-old white man with advanced Alzheimer disease (AD). He has been failing over the past few weeks and you suspect that his death is imminent. You consider contacting his family. All of the following are appropriate considerations, except which one?

A) Inform the family of the physical findings that occur during the dying process.
B) Inform your covering group that death is imminent and that you should be called to contact the family.
C) Discuss an autopsy before or after the death has occurred.
D) Discuss an organ donation before or after the death has occurred.

The answer is D: The family should be thoroughly informed of the changes that the patient's body may exhibit directly before and after death. They should not be surprised by irregular breathing, cool extremities, confusion, a purplish skin color, or somnolence in the last hours.

A discussion about autopsy can occur either before or just after death. Families may have strong feelings, either in favor of or against it. The discussion of autopsy should not be left to a covering physician or house officer who has not had previous contact with the family.

Discussions about organ donation, if appropriate, should take place before death because plans to potentially donate organs or other body parts should be developed before death.

Additional Reading: Palliative care. In: Domino F, ed. *The 5-Minute Clinical Consult*. Wolters Kluwer; 2022.

11. An 87-year-old man is accompanied by his son who is requesting assistance in obtaining a *durable power of attorney* for his father because he is worried that he is exhibiting signs of confusion and having some trouble with his memory. A *durable power of attorney* is defined as which one of the following statements?

A) A written advanced directive that assigns one person as a decision-making proxy should the user become incapacitated.
B) A written advanced directive in which a competent person indicates his or her health care preferences while cognitively and physically intact.
C) A written advanced directive that describes in questionnaire format what type of treatment a person would or would not want in various medical situations.
D) A written document requiring an attorney to manage all of an elderly person's affairs.
E) None of the above.

The answer is A: A *durable power of attorney* is defined as a written advanced directive that assigns one person as a decision-making proxy should the user become incapacitated. A *living will* is a written advanced directive in which a competent person indicates health care preferences while cognitively and physically intact. A *medical directive* is a detailed written directive that describes in questionnaire format what type of treatment a person would or would not want in various medical situations.

Additional Reading: Respecting end-of-life treatment preferences. *Am Fam Physician*. 2005;72(7):1263-1268.

12. A 77-year-old patient is accompanied by her daughter, who is worried about her risk for falling because she is often alone at home. Which one of the following tests can be easily performed in the office to help identify elders who are at an increased risk for falls?

A) Get up and go test
B) One-foot hop test
C) Sit down and stop test
D) Straight line test
E) Two hand–one foot test

The answer is A: Approximately one-third of noninstitutionalized elders fall each year. The annual incidence of falls approaches 50% in patients above 80 years of age. Factors contributing to falls include age-related postural changes, decreased vision, certain medications (particularly anticholinergic, sedative, and diuretic medications), and diseases affecting muscle strength and coordination.

The simple physical examination maneuver called the "get up and go" test can help identify those at risk for falls. In this test, the patient is instructed to arise from a sitting position, walk 10 ft, turn, and return to the chair to sit. If the patient struggles to complete the process in less than 16 seconds or is observed to have postural instability or gait impairment, he or she is considered to be at an increased risk of falling. A number of effective interventions are available for people with a history of falls or who are at risk for falling.

Additional Reading: Falls in older persons: risk factors and patient evaluation. In: *UpToDate*. 2022.

13. You receive a frantic call from the nursing home where you serve as the part-time medical director that an 86-year-old patient with Alzheimer disease is missing. You make all of the following statements regarding the directions for a search, except which one?

A) The hottest and coldest times of the year are associated with the highest risk of death.
B) Most people found alive are found within the first 24 hours of being missing.
C) Of those who die, more than 90% are found in natural areas.
D) The first areas searched should be concentrated on open, populated areas.
E) Night searches are unnecessary because individuals are unlikely to wander after dark.

The answer is E: The issue of wandering and becoming lost, with the possibility of physical harm or death, is one of the concerns that often leads families and caregivers to place demented patients in nursing homes. Caregivers should report the person missing immediately to local authorities. An exhaustive search should begin immediately so that the individual has less time to find a secluded hiding place and has reduced exposure to the environment. Searches should continue through the night because individuals often continue to wander after dark. The initial 6 to 12 hours of the search should cover a 5-mile radius around the location where the lost person was last seen, concentrating on open, populated areas, including the inside of easily accessible buildings. If initial search efforts fail, then subsequent efforts should be devoted to an intensive foot search of natural and sparsely populated areas beginning within a 1-mile radius of the last known location and extending from there. If the person with dementia traveled by car, initial search efforts should focus on locating the vehicle.

Becoming lost appears to be a highly unpredictable event and can occur even when individuals with dementia are in their own homes or are participating in activities they had routinely performed many times in the past without any incident. A review of this issue that analyzed data from several available studies produced the following observations:

- All persons with dementia are at risk of becoming lost, and the risk may be higher for men than women.
- Individuals residing in professional care settings are at risk as well as those at home.
- The risk of becoming lost is increased when persons are unattended. However, about 65% of people with dementia are in the presence of a caregiver at the time they become lost.
- Most individuals who are found alive remain out in the open, populated areas of the community.
- The risk of death is increased if the demented person ends up secluded in natural or sparsely populated areas. About 91% of persons with dementia who died were found in natural areas such as woods, fields, ditches, bodies of water (approximately 20% drowned), or abandoned vehicles.
- The risk of death also appears to be associated with the hottest and coldest times of the year.
- The time it took to search for and locate a missing person with dementia also correlated with the risk of death because most individuals found alive were located within 24 hours and all were found within 4 days.

Locating a person with dementia who becomes lost can be difficult, and this problem is complicated by several factors related to the increased likelihood of abnormal behavior. People with dementia are often unpredictable when lost. The accuracy of the search is usually not enhanced by predictions from families and caregivers. The lost persons rarely call for help or respond to searcher's calls. Search strategies should not be based on the individual characteristics of the missing person because the unpredictable and abnormal behavior is likely to negate any prior individual patterns.

Caregivers, both formal and informal, must be informed that all persons with dementia are at risk of becoming lost, even if the individual has never wandered or exhibited "risky" behavior in the past. Because the risk is highest when persons with dementia are left unattended, every effort should be made to ensure continuous supervision. Community resources, adult day care and respite care facilities, and caregiver support groups may be utilized, if available, to reduce the burden on families and caregivers.

Additional Reading: Behavioral disorders in dementia: Appropriate nondrug interventions and antipsychotic use. *Am Fam Physician*. 2016;94(4):276-282.

14. You are caring for an elderly patient with advanced breast cancer and her family is wondering about hospice services. You inform them that which one of the following is true regarding hospice services?

A) Patients who use hospice must be eligible for Medicare part A.
B) Patients enrolled in hospice must be terminally ill.
C) Patients enrolled are expected to die within 6 months.
D) Patients must sign a statement choosing hospice care instead of routine Medicare benefits for the specified illness.
E) All of the above are true.

The answer is E: Medicare patients may choose to use the Medicare hospice benefit in situations of terminal illness. Terminal illness is defined as a life expectancy of 6 months or less if the condition progresses as expected. Patients who decide to use the hospice benefit must be eligible for Medicare part A, be certified by their physician and hospice medical director as terminally ill, sign a statement choosing hospice care instead of routine Medicare benefits for the specified illness, and receive care for their terminal illness through a Medicare-approved hospice program.

Additional Reading: Hospice: what you should know. *Am Fam Physician*. 2008;77(6):817-818.

15. Medicare requires skilled nursing facilities to complete a "Minimum Data Set" (MDS). This document must contain which one of the following types of information?

A) A list of vital signs for every nursing home resident
B) A description of the activities available to all nursing home residents
C) A set of minimum data that a nursing home has to abide by to receive state certification
D) A group of safety and quality data indicators that are used to rank nursing homes
E) A comprehensive assessment of a nursing home resident and a developed care plan

The answer is E: The MDS is a federally mandated document that is based on a comprehensive resident assessment. Information from the physician's history and physical and progressive notes is used to complete an MDS. The MDS is then used to develop a plan of care for the patient. The MDS is also used to determine Medicare reimbursement for the patient.

Additional Reading: Medical care in skilled nursing facilities in the United States. In: *UpToDate*. 2022.

16. Many family physicians care for patients who reside in a skilled nursing environment. Medicare regulations require that physicians see nursing home patients on which one of the following visit schedules?

A) Weekly for the first month and then monthly thereafter
B) Monthly as long as they reside there
C) Monthly for 3 months and then every 2 months thereafter
D) Monthly for 3 months and then every 3 months (quarterly) thereafter

The answer is C: Medicare regulations require that a physician make monthly visits for the first 3 months of a resident's nursing home stay and then every 2 months thereafter. Obviously, if a patient is acutely ill, more frequent visits can occur.

Additional Reading: Medical care in skilled nursing facilities in the United States. In: *UpToDate*. 2022.

17. You attended an 83-year-old nursing home patient for a corneal abrasion and treated her with antibiotic ophthalmic ointment and an eye patch, with plans to reexamine her in the morning. Later that evening, the nursing home care staff called to report that she had become very confused. The most appropriate action at this time would be to do which one of the following?

A) Advise that the patient be taken to the local emergency department for an acute evaluation.
B) Advise the use of bedrails to protect the patient from injury.
C) Reassure the nursing staff and see the patient the next morning as planned.
D) Remove the eye patch.
E) Prescribe haloperidol.

The answer is D: Sensory deprivation, such as patching an elderly patient's eyes, may lead to an acute case of delirium. Even small alterations in the elderly patient's environment can lead to confusion. In cases of corneal abrasions, an elderly patient should receive topical ophthalmic antibiotics. Additionally, although eye patching has traditionally been recommended in the treatment of corneal abrasions, multiple well-designed studies show that patching does not help and may hinder healing.

The use of bedrails has not been shown to prevent falls, and the use of haloperidol can cause additional problems from side effects.

Additional Reading: Delirium. In: Domino F, ed. *The 5-Minute Clinical Consult*. Wolters Kluwer; 2022.

18. You receive a phone call from the wife of a 71-year-old patient whom you have recently diagnosed with early Alzheimer disease (AD) because she is concerned over his ability to drive. True statements regarding this situation include all of the following, except which one?

A) In the first year after the diagnosis is made, patients with AD have a similar rate of accidents as registered drivers of all ages.
B) The risk of accidents increases as AD patients grow older.
C) The department of transportation is the only group that has a role in the determination of driving skills.
D) The department of motor vehicles often performs roadside testing to determine the ability to drive.

The answer is C: In many situations, one of the first safety issues to be confronted with elderly patients affected with dementia is their driving. In the first year after diagnosis, patients affected with AD have a similar rate of accidents as registered drivers of all ages, although the rate is higher than that for age-matched controls. The risk of motor vehicle crashes increases dramatically in the following years. This increase is likely underrepresented in that the risk per mile driven is much greater because patients substantially reduce their driving.

Discussions of driving cessation are often difficult. Patients are generally unaware of their deficits (particularly their deficits in judgment), and surrendering a license often represents a severe loss of independence. With early diagnosis, many patients will still be able to drive safely for a period, but all will eventually progress to the point where it is no longer safe to drive. Discussions with patients in the intermediate stages of dementia pose the greatest difficulty.

Only a few states require physicians to notify the motor vehicle authorities when a patient is diagnosed with dementia. Although a number of driving safety tests have been suggested, no general guidelines have been broadly instituted. Local programs may exist to evaluate these patients with neuropsychologic and roadside tests. In the absence of these programs, the department of motor vehicles often performs roadside testing, but patients must be informed that even if they pass, they must be retested at regular intervals as their disease progresses.

Families must be warned about the potential liability for accidents. They may need to take possession of car keys, or even the cars, and restrict all driving. The American Academy of Neurology has issued guidelines for driving in patients with AD based on the clinical dementia rating scale.

Additional Reading: AAN updates guidelines on evaluating driving risk in patients with dementia. *Am Fam Physician.* 2010;82(9):1144-1147.

19. Cancer is a leading cause of death for the elderly, and the solid tumor malignancy most frequently diagnosed in elderly men is which one of the following cancers?

A) Lung cancer
B) Colon cancer
C) Prostate cancer
D) Lymphoma
E) Esophageal cancer

The answer is C: In the United States, prostate cancer is the most common solid tumor malignancy in men and is the second leading cause of cancer deaths (lung cancer is the first). African Americans are at higher risk for prostate cancer than whites. The risk increases with age, and 70% of men older than 80 years are affected. Diagnosis is usually made by the detection of a palpable prostate nodule on physical examination followed by a prostate-specific antigen (PSA) determination, which shows an elevated level of PSA. The combination of a digital rectal examination and PSA test is more accurate in diagnosing early prostate cancer than either alone.

However, there is significant controversy over prostate cancer screening, because even though this is a relatively common malignancy, it is the actual cause of death in only a small proportion of patients who have histologic evidence of prostate cancer. Thus, screening asymptomatic patients for prostate cancer is not recommended, as it will likely result in the detection and treatment of many asymptomatic cancers that will have no impact on the length of the patient's life. The decision to offer prostate cancer screening must be made on an individual basis, depending on the patient's age, health status, family history, risk of prostate cancer, and personal health care beliefs. The patient must be informed about the risks and potential benefits of screening. The patient also must be helped to realize that although prostate cancer can grow quickly, it generally grows slowly.

Additional Reading: Localized prostate cancer: treatment options. *Am Fam Physician.* 2018;97(12):798-805.

➜ The U.S. Preventive Services Task Force recommends against PSA-based screening for prostate cancer. This is a "D" recommendation: There is moderate or high certainty that the service has no net benefit or that the harms outweigh the benefits.

20. Advanced directives are being used with increased frequency. Which one of the following statements concerning advanced directives is true?

A) Once recorded, they cannot be changed.
B) Living wills are often easier for patients to complete than designating a health care power of attorney.
C) Advanced directives should be discussed only when life-threatening illnesses are present.
D) Physicians are not required to comply with patients' requests for treatment when they believe such requests are ill-advised, harmful, or futile.
E) There is no need to update advanced directives.

The answer is D: An advanced directive consists of a person's oral and written instructions about his or her future medical care if he or she becomes unable to communicate, becomes incompetent to make health care decisions (during a terminal illness), or is in a persistent vegetative state. There are two types of advanced directives: a health care power of attorney and a living will.

- The health care ("durable") power of attorney, or *health care proxy*, is a document by which the patient appoints a trusted person to make decisions about his or her medical care if he or she cannot make those decisions.
- A *living will* is a written form of advanced directive in which the patient's wishes regarding the administration of medical treatment are delineated in case the patient becomes unable to communicate his or her wishes.

Discussion of advanced directives should take place early on in the care of patients to discuss the patient's wishes should they become debilitated and cannot answer for themselves. The durable power of attorney allows the patient to designate a surrogate to make medical decisions if the patient loses the decision-making capacity. The durable power of attorney is often less emotionally laden than outlining specific treatments to give or withhold.

The five steps identified in the ideal process of advanced care planning are as follows:

1. Raise the topic and give information regarding the advanced directive and health care proxy.
2. Facilitate a structured discussion.
3. Complete a statement, date and record it, and have the patient supply copies to their health care proxy and anyone else deemed appropriate (eg, clergy).
4. Periodically review and update the directive, and initial and date all changes.
5. Implement the plan by following the patient's wishes when the appropriate time comes.

Finally, physicians are not automatically obliged to comply with patients' requests for treatment when they believe such requests are ill-advised, harmful, or futile. Strict adherence to such requests may interfere with the physician's autonomy and ability to provide sound medical care.

Additional Reading: Implementing advance directives in office practice. *Am Fam Physician*. 2012;85(5):461-466.

21. Which one of the following statements regarding home visits is true?

A) They are increasing in frequency.
B) Reimbursement has increased their use.
C) Physicians who perform home visits have increased job satisfaction.
D) Home visits are not effective in managing patients because of a lack of resources.
E) Home visits rarely identify new medical problems but are better suited to manage chronic medical problems.

The answer is C: Years ago, home visit was an essential part of primary care practice, but with the rise of office-based practice, the home visit has been used less frequently. The reason for this decline is the result of many coincident factors, including insufficient physician compensation for such visits, time constraints, perceived limitations of technologic support, concerns about the risk of litigation, lack of physician training and exposure, and corporate and individual attitudinal biases.

Health care providers who have long-established relationships with their patients are more likely to use house calls, and rural practice setting, older patient age, and need for terminal care correlate with an increased frequency of home visits. Studies suggest that home visits can lead to improved medical care through the discovery of undetected health care needs. Home assessment of elderly patients with relatively good health status and function can increase the detection of new medical problems and new intervention recommendations. There is also improved effectiveness of home visits in assessing unexpected problems in patient compliance with therapeutic regimens. Additionally, specific home-based interventions such as adjusting the elderly patient's home environment to prevent falls have also yielded health benefits. Beyond the potential benefit of improved patient care, family physicians who conduct home visits report a higher level of practice satisfaction than those who do not offer this service.

Additional Reading: House Calls. *Am Fam Physician*. 2020;102(4):211-220.

22. The Omnibus Budget Reconciliation Act of 1987 (OBRA-87) mandated freedom for nursing home residents from medically unnecessary "physical or chemical restraints imposed for purposes of discipline or convenience." This included the use of antipsychotic medications. The regulations require that when prescribing any antipsychotic medication to nursing home patients, the orders be reviewed and an attempt to withdraw or taper them be made at what frequency?

A) Monthly
B) Quarterly
C) Semiannually (ie, every 6 months)
D) Annually
E) A regular interval determined and charted by the attending physician, based on the patient's response

The answer is C: OBRA-87 regulations require an attempt to withdraw (or decrease) the dose of medications to manage agitation or psychosis in nursing homes semiannually (every 6 months).

Additional Reading: Medical care in skilled nursing facilities in the United States. In: *UpToDate*. 2022.

23. The Medicare Hospice Benefit covers all of the following expenses for patients in nursing homes except which one?

A) Durable medical equipment rental or purchase
B) Room and board charges
C) Supplies that are ordered by the hospice team
D) Visits by hospice team members

The answer is B: When an elderly patient has developed a life-threatening illness or condition, it is appropriate to plan for end-of-life care. The Medicare Hospice Benefit can help greatly with the many tasks involved in providing palliative management of the dying patient's symptoms, attending to increased hygienic needs, and supplying bereavement services. For eligible terminally ill patients, the Medicare Hospice Benefit supplies an interdisciplinary team with skills in pain management, symptom control, and bereavement assistance. The services of the hospice team supplement usual nursing home care at a time when staff, family members, and the patient are facing the increased and urgent needs associated with the dying process.

The Medicare Hospice Benefit can make it much easier for physicians and nursing home staff to provide comprehensive palliative care for terminally ill patients. When a nursing home resident is referred for care under the Medicare Hospice Benefit, the hospice assumes responsibility for the professional management of many interdisciplinary services that supplement the usual care provided by nursing home staff. All medical treatments should have the goal of symptom control, and they should be consistent with the hospice plan of treatment.

The Medicare Hospice Benefit covers all visits by hospice team members, the rental or purchase of durable medical equipment, and the cost of supplies that are ordered by the hospice team. The hospice also supplies drugs for the palliation and management of the terminal illness, a benefit that is normally not available under the regular Medicare program. For each of these drugs, the beneficiary is only responsible for a small copayment. Thus, hospice care is not an additional expense for many nursing home residents.

However, payment of room and board remains the responsibility of the patient and/or the family. Impoverished patients may be eligible for government assistance programs that cover those costs (eg, under Medicaid). The Medicare Hospice Benefit cannot be provided for nursing home residents who are receiving skilled Medicare coverage if their diagnoses for hospice and nursing home skilled care are the same. Before the Medicare Hospice Benefit can be initiated, these patients may choose to use all their skilled care days, or they may elect to waive their skilled coverage.

Additional Reading: Hospice: what you should know. *Am Fam Physician*. 2008;77(6):817-818.

24. You have just advised your 50-year-old white male patient that he is due for colon cancer screening, and you suggest that he undergo a screening colonoscopy. Interestingly, he notes that his 77-year-old mother, who is also your patient, has not had a colonoscopy and is asking if she too should be screened. Which one of the following responses is consistent with the recommendations of the U.S. Preventive Services Task Force (USPSTF)?

A) It is recommended that she be screened using high-sensitivity fecal occult blood testing.
B) Because of her age, it is recommended that she be screened at more frequent intervals than are younger persons.
C) Regardless of whether she has been screened before, his mother should be screened at the recommended intervals throughout her life.
D) It is recommended that screening for colorectal cancer at her age be an individual decision, because the net benefits of screening after 75 years of age are small.

The answer is D: Although considerations may warrant screening in particular patients, the USPSTF recommends against routine screening in adults 76 to 85 years of age. The recommendations state the following:

- The decision to screen for colorectal cancer in adults aged 76 to 85 years should be an individual one, taking into account the patient's overall health and prior screening history.
- Adults in this age group who have never been screened for colorectal cancer are more likely to benefit.
- Screening would be most appropriate among adults who are healthy enough to undergo treatment if colorectal cancer is detected and do not have comorbid conditions that would significantly limit their life expectancy.

Additional Reading: Colorectal cancer: screening. https://www.uspreventiveservicestaskforce.org/uspstf/recommendation/colorectal-cancer-screening

The USPSTF recommends shared-decision making for colorectal cancer screening in adults aged 76 to 85 years (grade C recommendation), as the net benefit is small.

The USPSTF recommends against screening for colorectal cancer in adults older than 85 years (grade D recommendation).

25. Which one of the following is true regarding respiratory rate in the elderly?

A) Subtle differences in age-adjusted respiratory rate are present and should be adjusted for in the evaluation of the elderly patient.
B) Respiratory rates in the elderly are 5% higher than age-adjusted controls.
C) Respiratory rates and patterns do not change as the patient ages.
D) Elevated respiratory rates do not represent concern in elderly patients.
E) Respiratory rates do not correlate with disease in elderly patients.

The answer is C: Respiratory rate and patterns do not change significantly with age. An elevated respiratory rate may be a subtle clue to a serious medical illness (eg, acidosis, hypoxia, and central nervous system disturbance) and should be detected and evaluated as in any other patient.

Additional Reading: The geriatric assessment. *Am Fam Physician*. 2011;83(1):18-22.

26. Influenza is typically associated with the rapid onset of headache, fever, chills, muscle aches, malaise, cough, and sore throat. However, the elderly are less likely to experience which one of the following symptoms?

A) Headache
B) Fever
C) Muscle aches
D) Fatigue
E) Sore throat

The answer is B: Influenza is a common respiratory tract infection that causes significant morbidity and mortality in older adults. The signs and symptoms of influenza infection in older adults are similar to those occurring in younger patients; however, a febrile response may be absent in older adults. Influenza is typically associated with the rapid onset of headache, fever, chills, muscle aches, malaise, cough, and sore throat. Most people recover fully within 1 week, but older adults may develop a persistent weakness that can last for many weeks and are also at higher risk for developing complications such as pneumonia. Diagnosis is usually made clinically.

There are several influenza tests available that may be used to help make a diagnosis. Rapid influenza diagnostic tests are used to detect the virus in nasal secretions and can be completed in the office or sent to a laboratory, with the results available the same day. This can help differentiate influenza from other viral and bacterial infections with similar symptoms. Rapid flu tests are best used within the first 48 hours of the onset of symptoms to help diagnose influenza and determine whether antiviral drugs are a treatment option.

Rapid tests vary in their ability to detect influenza. Some types can only detect influenza A; others can detect both influenza A and B but not distinguish between the two. Still others can detect and distinguish between influenza A and B. However, none of them are able to differentiate between the strains of influenza A such as H1N1.

The main disadvantage of the rapid influenza antigen test is the high rate of false-negative results. Rapid tests will generally detect 40% to 70% of influenza cases. Therefore, the Centers for Disease Control and Prevention recommends not withholding treatment for patients with suspected influenza, even if they test negative. If someone needs confirmation from a laboratory diagnosis, it would be necessary to follow a negative test with a viral culture or reverse transcriptase–polymerase chain reaction test.

Influenza is responsible for more than $1 billion in annual Medicare expenditures. Of deaths resulting from influenza, the vast majority occur in adults 65 years and older. Older adults are susceptible to severe and potentially fatal complications from this common illness because of coexisting chronic disease and weakened immunity. Older adults can benefit most from vaccination, early detection, and aggressive therapy.

Additional Reading: *Key facts about influenza (Flu)*. Centers for Disease Control and Prevention. www.cdc.gov/flu/keyfacts.htm.

27. Although urinary incontinence is frequent in the elderly, fecal incontinence can also be seen and may not be mentioned over embarrassment. Which one of the following is a risk factor for fecal incontinence in the elderly?

A) A high-fiber diet
B) A history of marathon running
C) A history of multiple childbirths
D) Prolonged sitting

The answer is C: Fecal incontinence is a serious and embarrassing problem that affects up to 5% of the general population and up to 39% of nursing home residents. Providing effective treatment is challenging because of the difficulties in identifying the underlying cause. Risk factors include female sex, older age, physical limitations, and poor health. Previous studies in women have shown that obstetric or iatrogenic surgical injuries damage the internal or external sphincters, and straining or childbirth can injure the pudendal nerves. Anal ultrasonography detects defects in the sphincter complex in up to 87% of incontinent women. Anorectal physiologic studies can identify pudendal nerve injuries in many of the remaining patients.

Fecal incontinence may be associated with other causes, including spinal cord injuries, diabetes, dementia, fecal impaction, tumors, trauma, chronic constipation, or previous rectal surgery. All of these conditions result in a low anal sphincter resting tone.

Physical examination should include a rectal examination to check for adequate anal sphincter tone and sensation. Further tests include electromyographic studies of the pelvic floor and anal manometry.

Treatment involves a strict bowel program to develop predictable bowel movements. Adequate diet with fiber and bulk, proper positioning when defecating, and occasional bowel stimulants can be used to help regulate bowel movements into a regular pattern. For resistant cases, loperamide (Imodium) or diphenoxylate with atropine (Lomotil) may be used to control bowel movements. Other methods to help with rectal incontinence include Kegel exercises to strengthen the pelvic floor muscles and biofeedback; surgery can be considered for resistant cases.

Additional Reading: Fecal incontinence in adults. In: *UpToDate*. 2022.

28. A 66-year-old otherwise healthy man presents to your office for a general examination. He had been given the 23-valent pneumococcal vaccine 1 year ago and inquires whether he needs another one. You correctly answer which one of the following?

A) Further immunizations are not needed.
B) He should receive only one booster 10 years after the first.
C) He should receive a dose of a pneumococcal conjugate vaccine (PCV15 or PCV20).
D) He should receive a booster dose of the 23-valent pneumococcal vaccine now.
E) He should receive boosters every 10 years indefinitely.

The answer is C: The Centers for Disease Control and Prevention (CDC) had recommended that everyone aged 65 years and older get a single-dose of the pneumococcal polysaccharide vaccine 23 (PPSV23) as a standard for many years. The PPSV23 provides protection from 85% to 90% of the serotypes that cause invasive disease in the United States. The vaccine is 56% to 81% effective in preventing invasive bacteremia.

A controlled trial published in 2014 showed that a second vaccine, called pneumococcal conjugate vaccine 13 (PCV13), also provides protection against community-acquired pneumococcal pneumonia and other invasive *Streptococcus pneumoniae* infections.

In 2015, the CDC updated its recommendation from a single dose of PPSV23 to include a second PCV13 immunization for older adults.

In 2021, the Advisory Committee on Immunization Practices changed the guidelines, adding PCV20 and PCV15.

Individuals who have never gotten a pneumonia vaccine should get PCV15 or PCV20 for adults 65 years or older and adults 19 through 64 years old with certain medical conditions or risk factors. If PCV15 is used, this should be followed by a dose of PPSV23.

Those who have already been vaccinated with PPSV23 should get a dose of PCV20 or PCV15 at least a year after the PPSV23 vaccination.

Additional Reading: *Pneumococcal vaccination: what everyone should know*. Centers for Disease Control and Prevention. https://www.cdc.gov/vaccines/vpd/pneumo/public/index.html

29. Aging has several negative effects on men's health and well-being. Which one of the following *increases* as men age?

A) Bone mineral density
B) Muscle mass
C) Muscle strength
D) Serum-free testosterone
E) Sex hormone–binding globulin (SHBG)

The answer is E: Serum SHBG concentrations increase gradually as a function of age. SHBG binds testosterone with high affinity, so that with increasing age, less of the total testosterone is free (ie, biologically active). Because of the increase in SHBG with age, it is not surprising that conversely the serum-free testosterone concentration decreases with increasing age to a greater degree than the total testosterone. No consequences of the decline in serum testosterone with age are known with certainty, but several parallels between the effects of aging and those of hypogonadism suggest that the decline in serum testosterone might be related to decreased frequency of orgasm or intercourse. Men with hypogonadism due to known disease also have a decline in sexual function, as illustrated by an improvement after testosterone treatment.

As men age, their bone mineral density declines. In a study of healthy men who had never had any fractures, the bone mineral density of the femur and, to a lesser extent, the spine declined from the age of 20 to 90 years. Men who are hypogonadal due to disease or whose testosterone has been lowered surgically or medically also have a decline in bone mineral density.

As men age, their muscle mass declines and fat mass increases. Hypogonadal men also have less muscle mass and more fat mass than do normal men; testosterone treatment in men with hypogonadism tends to reverse these changes. Men aged 60 to 79 years have less muscle strength than those aged 20 to 39 years.

The decrease in serum testosterone concentrations, which occurs with aging in men, may be associated with a decline in neuropsychologic function.

Additional Reading: Male reproductive physiology. In: *UpToDate*. 2022.

30. Cancer of the gallbladder is a rare condition that predominantly affects the elderly. Gallbladder carcinoma is associated with all of the following, except which one?

A) A life expectancy of 5 to 10 years
B) A history of chronic cholecystitis
C) Jaundice
D) Metastasis at the time of diagnosis

The answer is A: Cancer of the gallbladder is rare, affects predominantly the elderly, and is very difficult to detect clinically. In most cases, it is found during surgery for presumed cholelithiasis (1% of patients undergoing surgery for cholelithiasis). Unfortunately, it has usually metastasized at the time of diagnosis. Thus, the prognosis is poor with few patients surviving longer than 6 months.

Symptoms, when they are present, include right-upper-quadrant pain that radiates to the back, jaundice, weight loss, and anorexia. A palpable gallbladder with obstructive jaundice usually signifies cancer of the gallbladder. Treatment is limited, and surgery is used only in certain situations to relieve biliary obstruction. Chronic calculus cholecystitis increases the risk for cancer of the gallbladder, and cholecystectomy is recommended.

Additional Reading: Prognosis and adjuvant treatment for localized, resected gallbladder cancer. In: *UpToDate*. Waltham, MA, 2022.

31. You are assessing a 77-year-old white woman with a macrocytic anemia and consider pernicious anemia in your diagnosis. Pernicious anemia is associated with which one of the following conditions?

A) Chronic blood loss
B) Iron deficiency
C) Malignancy
D) Myelofibrosis
E) Vitamin B_{12} malabsorption

The answer is E: Anemia should not be accepted as an unavoidable consequence of aging. A cause is found in approximately 80% of elderly patients. The most common causes of anemia in the elderly are chronic disease and iron deficiency. However, vitamin B_{12} deficiency, folate deficiency, and myelodysplastic syndrome are also causes of anemia in the elderly.

The condition of pernicious anemia is the result of malabsorption or lack of ingestion of vitamin B_{12}. The lack of absorption is usually the result of atrophic gastric mucosa, which fails to produce the intrinsic factor that is required for the absorption of vitamin B_{12}. With pernicious anemia, the lack of intrinsic factor results from destruction of the gastric parietal cells by autoimmune antibodies. Previous gastrectomy, blind loop syndrome, fish tapeworm infections, or thyroid abnormalities may also decrease intrinsic factor secretion. Achlorhydria (lack of acid production) is usually associated with pernicious anemia as well.

The anemia usually develops over time and is associated with macrocytic features (as opposed to microcytosis with iron deficiency), basophilic stippling of red blood cells, and an increased red blood cell distribution width index.

Symptoms of pernicious anemia include anorexia, constipation, diarrhea, and abdominal pain; glossitis; loss of sensation involving the distal extremities; weight loss; and generalized fatigue.

High-dose oral vitamin B_{12} effectively treats the deficiency regardless of the cause. Vitamin B_{12} deficiency is effectively treated with high-dose oral or parenteral vitamin B_{12} supplementation.

Additional Reading: Vitamin B_{12} deficiency: recognition and management. *Am Fam Physician*. 2017;96(6):384-389.

32. You have decided to start giving an oral agent to treat type 2 diabetes mellitus in a 69-year-old obese white female patient whom you have been caring for a number of years. Mindful of the risks of hypoglycemia in the elderly, which one of the following medications is most likely to cause hypoglycemia in such individuals?

A) Glipizide (Glucotrol)
B) Glyburide (Micronase, DiaBeta)
C) Metformin (Glucophage)
D) None of the above

The answer is B: Diabetes and its treatment in the elderly poses some additional concerns. The use of glyburide has shown a twofold relative risk of hypoglycemia when compared with glipizide. Metformin does not cause hypoglycemia with monotherapy. The elderly develop microvascular complications such as diabetic retinopathy and peripheral neuropathy more quickly than do younger patients. Diabetes also represents a major risk factor for the development of atherosclerosis. The renal threshold for glucose is also increased in the elderly, allowing higher levels of blood glucose before glycosuria is seen.

Additional Reading: Hypoglycemia in adults with diabetes mellitus. In: *UpToDate*. 2022.

33. Polypharmacy is an issue for many elderly patients. All of the following statements about medication use in the elderly are true, except which one?

A) Two-thirds of the elderly in the United States take a medication daily.
B) Men take more medications than do women.
C) At any given time, the average older person uses four to five prescription drugs.
D) A typical nursing home resident receives seven or eight drugs.

The answer is B: In the United States, approximately two-thirds of persons aged 65 years or older take prescription and nonprescription (over-the-counter) medications daily. Women take more drugs than men because they are, on average, older, and they use more psychoactive and arthritic drugs. At any given time, an average older person uses 4 to 5 prescription drugs, 2 over-the-counter drugs, and fills 12 to 17 prescriptions a year. The frail elderly take the most medications. Drug use is greater in hospitals and nursing homes than in the community; typically, a nursing home resident receives seven or eight drugs.

Additional Reading: Reducing the risk of adverse drug events in older adults. *Am Fam Physician*. 2013;87(5):331-336.

34. A 71-year-old woman whom you have been caring for comes in for a preoperative evaluation prior to cataract surgery at the request of her ophthalmologist. You have been treating her type 2 diabetes mellitus with metformin 500 mg bid and her hypertension is well controlled on lisinopril 20 mg daily. She is also taking simvastatin, 20 mg daily for hyperlipidemia. Her blood pressure is 132/78 mm Hg, and the laboratory tests from her last routine visit about 3 months ago show a hemoglobin A1c level of 7.3% (4.0-5.6) and a serum creatinine level of 1.9 mg/dL (N 0.6-1.3). She reports feeling well and walks her dog around the block without difficulty.

Which of the following would be most appropriate regarding preoperative medical testing for this patient?

A) A basic metabolic panel
B) A chest x-ray
C) An electrocardiogram
D) All of the above
E) None of the above

The answer is E: Preoperative testing should be based on the patient's medical history and risk factors, the risk associated with planned surgery, and the patient's functional capacity, with an assessment of the risks for undergoing anesthesia and the stress of surgery. Cataract surgery is considered a low-risk procedure, and studies do not demonstrate any benefit from preoperative testing for such patients in their normal state of health.

The American Academy of Ophthalmology recommends against routine medical tests before cataract surgery, although preoperative medical tests can be ordered when indicated by findings on a patient's history or physical examination. The American Heart Association recommends against the use of routine testing in asymptomatic patients undergoing low-risk procedures such as cataract surgery because the cardiac risk associated with low-risk procedures is generally less than 1%.

Additional Reading: Preoperative testing for patients undergoing cataract surgery. *Am Fam Physician*. 2009;80(11):1228.

35. A 69-year-old man has obvious gynecomastia that has been present for the past several years. A physical examination is otherwise benign, and he has not had any galactorrhea. An endocrine and malignancy workup is unrevealing, but he is embarrassed and would like treatment to decrease the size of his breasts.

Which one of the following is the treatment of choice?

A) Prescribe an estrogen receptor modulator (eg, clomiphene, tamoxifen)
B) Prescribe an antiestrogen (eg, danazol)
C) Prescribe a topical testosterone (eg, AndroGel)
D) Refer for surgery

The answer is D: Medical management is most useful with recent onset of the condition. Estrogen receptor modulators, antiestrogens, and topical testosterone have been tried with varying success, but none have been shown to have a significant benefit. However, the initial glandular hyperplasia seen with gynecomastia progresses to become a fibrotic tissue, and as such, surgery is the recommended treatment.

Additional Reading: Severe male breast enlargement. *Am Fam Physician*. 2017;95(9):583-584.

36. You are seeing an elderly couple. They have been staying at their lake camp and have felt lousy the last 2 days with nausea, headaches, and light headedness. They do note that they feel better already just coming into the office to see you but worry that they may have eaten some poisoned seafood. Upon further exam, you noted that both individuals appear to have flushed cheeks and you wonder about carbon monoxide (CO) poisoning.

Which test would rule out such a concern?

A) A pulse oxygen saturation level >98%
B) A clear chest x-ray (CXR)
C) A normal arterial blood gas oxygen level
D) A CO level test

The answer is D: CO is an odorless, tasteless, colorless gas produced during the incomplete combustion of carbon-based compounds. If inhaled, CO may cause nonspecific symptoms and is potentially fatal. Exposure is mostly seen during cold weather conditions when people use heaters or stoves in closed quarters to keep warm. Symptoms include headache, nausea, vomiting, and weakness, and symptoms are commonly attributed to viral illnesses. Patients may present with "flushed cheeks," although this tends to be a late finding with severe exposure. CO inhalation results in the formation of carboxyhemoglobin, displacing oxygen. Oxygen-carrying sites are occupied by CO, which has a high affinity for hemoglobin than does oxygen. However, a pulse oximeter will show an oxygen saturation of 100% because the color of carboxyhemoglobin is bright red, which is what the pulse oximeter detects. Thus, pulse oximetry is not reliable in patients with CO poisoning.

Arterial blood gas measurements are based on oxygen gas tension (pO2) and not oxygen content or true oxygen saturation, and this too will be a false reading. The only arterial blood gas abnormality in CO poisoning may be metabolic acidosis, which is a late consequence of inadequate oxygen delivery to the peripheral tissues and is not seen early in CO poisoning. A CXR will not be abnormal. It is necessary to order a CO level test to rule out CO poisoning.

Additional Reading: Carbon monoxide poisoning. In: Domino F, ed. *The 5-Minute Clinical Consult*. Wolters Kluwer; 2022.

37. You are seeing a 73-year-old nursing home patient and note that her conjunctiva and skin appear jaundiced. On exam, you palpate a solitary enlarged left supraclavicular lymph node and a sense of fullness over her gallbladder, which is nontender. You do not detect any other significant physical abnormalities. Other than her baseline confusion, the staff report that she has been eating and moving her bowels as usual without any new complaints. This scenario is most consistent with what diagnosis?

A) Biliary cirrhosis
B) Hepatocellular carcinoma
C) Chronic pancreatitis
D) Pancreatic cancer

The answer is D: The presence of a single enlarged left supraclavicular lymph node (Virchow node) is associated with a gastrointestinal malignancy. When combined with painless jaundice and a palpable nontender gall bladder (Courvoisier sign), pancreatic cancer is the most likely diagnosis. Conjugated hyperbilirubinemia, reflected as an elevated direct bilirubin level, with a negative viral hepatitis panel is reflective of extrahepatic obstruction.

Biliary cirrhosis and hepatocellular carcinoma typically present with pain, fatigue, malaise, hepatomegaly, jaundice, and eventually ascites. The jaundice of biliary cirrhosis is generally accompanied by severe pruritus. In neither condition is a palpably enlarged gall bladder present. Chronic pancreatitis is not typically associated with jaundice.

Additional Reading: Diagnosis and management of pancreatic cancer. *Am Fam Physician*. 2014;89(8):626-632.

Section II. Neurologic Conditions

Each of the following questions or incomplete statements is followed by suggested answers or completions. Select the ONE BEST ANSWER in each case.

1. A 75-year-old man is brought into your office by his wife. She reports that he has not been the same over the past 6 months. He is having more problems remembering things and has become incontinent of urine, often wetting himself during the day, in addition to overnight. She also notes that he has been having more difficulty walking, which seems to be particularly a problem when he starts walking because he seems to have trouble getting started. Which of the following is the most likely diagnosis based on his history?

A) Alzheimer disease
B) Normal pressure hydrocephalus (NPH)
C) Parkinson disease (PD)
D) Pick disease
E) Progressive supranuclear palsy

The answer is B: NPH is a cause of dementia in the elderly. Elderly NPH patients seldom have a history of predisposing disease;

however, it may be due to a previous insult to the brain, such as a subarachnoid hemorrhage or an episode of meningitis. The mechanism of insult is thought to be the result of scarring of the arachnoid villi over the brain convexities where cerebrospinal fluid (CSF) absorption usually occurs, resulting in a buildup of CSF causing hydrocephalus.

NPH classically consists of a triad of findings, namely, dementia, gait instability, and incontinence ("*Wacky, Wobbly, and Wet*"); however, many patients with such symptoms do not have NPH. Typically, tremor, motor weakness, and staggering, which are common in PD, are absent, but initiation of gait is hesitant (described as a "slipping clutch" or "feet stuck to the floor" gait) and walking eventually occurs.

NPH has also been associated with various psychiatric manifestations that are not categorical; however, it should be considered in the differential diagnosis of any new mental status changes in the elderly.

Additional Reading: Normal pressure hydrocephalus. In: *UpToDate*, 2022.

2. Lewy body dementia is the result of Lewy body (α-synuclein protein) deposits in the brain, whereas Alzheimer disease (AD) is thought to be secondary to amyloid deposits. Although each of these disorders results in progressive dementia, which one of the following is more commonly seen in patients with Lewy body dementia when compared with AD?

A) Emotional lability
B) Hallucinations
C) Lip smacking
D) Repetitive behavior
E) Tremor

The answer is B: Lewy body dementia is a progressive dementia that is the result of Lewy body (α-synuclein protein) deposits in the nuclei of the neurons in areas of the brain that control memory and motor control. It is the second most common dementia after AD. Although the signs and symptoms of Lewy body dementia resemble those of AD, hallucinations (mainly visual) are more common, and patients appear to have an exquisite sensitivity to antipsychotic-induced extrapyramidal adverse effects.

Lewy bodies are also the hallmark lesions of degenerating substantia nigra neurons in PD. However, in Lewy body dementia the α-synuclein protein deposits are more widespread, and individuals may or may not have coexisting features of PD with their dementia. An autopsy (or a brain biopsy) is the only way to confirm the diagnosis of Lewy body dementia.

Additional Reading: Clinical features and diagnosis of dementia with Lewy bodies. In: *UpToDate*, 2022.

3. A patient with Pick disease is brought in by his daughter. She is his main caregiver and notes that although he is increasingly apathetic, she has noticed that he is exhibiting more sexually inappropriate behaviors and seems to be smacking his lips more frequently over time. You suspect that he is suffering from the effects of which one of the following conditions?

A) Chronic hypoxia
B) Elder abuse
C) Klüver-Bucy syndrome
D) Medication side effects
E) Toxin exposure

The answer is C: Pick disease (frontotemporal dementia) is a less common form of dementia than Alzheimer disease. The disease predominantly involves the frontal and temporal lobes, and patients will present with apathy and memory disturbances. They often show increased carelessness, poor personal hygiene, and a decreased attention span. Although the clinical presentation and computed tomographic findings in Pick disease are fairly distinctive, definitive diagnosis is possible only at autopsy.

The Klüver-Bucy syndrome is associated with Pick disease and can occur early in the course of the disease, with emotional blunting, hypersexual activity, hyperorality (bulimia and sucking and smacking of lips), and visual agnosia.

Additional Reading: Frontotemporal dementia: clinical features and diagnosis. In: *UpToDate*. 2022.

4. A 69-year-old white man presents with his wife to discuss problems that he has been having with his memory. It has been slowly progressing over the past couple of years, but he had chalked it up to "old age." However, over the past couple of months, he has been having some problems with his gait because he feels like he may fall backward, and his wife notes that he has also been complaining that his vision is blurry and that he should get new glasses. Which one of the following conditions is he most likely to be developing?

A) Normal-pressure glaucoma
B) Normal pressure hydrocephalus
C) Parkinson disease
D) Pick disease
E) Progressive supranuclear palsy (PSP)

The answer is E: PSP (also known as the Steele-Richardson-Olszewski syndrome, after the physicians who described it in 1963) is a neurodegenerative disease whose signs include a vertical gaze dysfunction accompanied by extrapyramidal gait disturbances and cognitive dysfunction.

The characteristic signs and symptoms of PSP include a loss of balance while walking, with a tendency to fall backward, along with visual difficulties. Patients will often have problems looking downward, which they can experience as blurry or doubled vision. The disease usually develops after the sixth decade of life, and the diagnosis is made on clinical grounds.

Supranuclear refers to the region of the spinal tract above the level of the motor neurons for the spinal or cranial nerves. Thus, supranuclear palsies are movement disorders caused by destruction or impairment of brain structures other than the motor neurons, such as the motor cortex, pyramidal tract, or striate body. Supranuclear palsy is distinguished from nuclear (lower motor neuron) paralysis that results from destruction or impairment of the motor neurons or their axons.

Additional Reading: Progressive supranuclear palsy (PSP): clinical features and diagnosis. In: *UpToDate*, 2022.

5. You have been called to assess an elderly patient who was admitted to the hospital with pneumonia. She has become delirious, accusing the nurses of trying to poison her food. Factors known to precipitate delirium in elderly hospitalized patients include all of the following, except which one?

A) A recent computed tomographic scan utilizing contrast media
B) Malnutrition
C) Taking three or more medications
D) The placement of a bladder catheter
E) The use of restraints

The answer is A: Delirium is found at admission or during the hospitalization in a quarter of all elderly patients admitted for an acute medical illness. Those elderly with baseline dementia and severe systemic illness are predisposed to delirium, and dementia is the main known predisposing factor for delirium in these situations.

Additional Reading: Delirium. In: Domino F, ed. *The 5-Minute Clinical Consult*. Wolters Kluwer; 2022.

Other factors known to precipitate delirium include the use of physical restraints, the addition of more than three medications to the regimen, the use of a bladder catheter, and malnutrition.

6. A 65-year-old man presents to your office complaining of a tremor that seems to be affecting his right hand. The patient reports the tremor is worse with sustained positions and stressful situations. Surprisingly, a shot of scotch makes the tremor better. He also reports a positive family history for tremors because his father had a tremor and he seems to recall that his grandfather did as well. There are no signs of bradykinesia or rigidity on your neurologic examination. The most likely diagnosis for this patient's presentation is which one of the following conditions?

A) Alcohol withdrawal
B) Caffeine withdrawal
C) Essential tremor
D) Huntington disease
E) Parkinson disease (PD)

The answer is C: A tremor is an involuntary contraction and relaxation of a muscle, resulting in oscillations or twitching movements of the affected body part. Essential tremor is the most common movement disorder and is characterized by a rapid, fine tremor that is made worse with sustained positions. The frequency of essential tremor is 4 to 11 Hz, depending on which body segment is affected. Hz refers to hertz, the number of cycles (tremors) per second that are counted. Essential tremor usually affects patients older than 50 years, but it can be seen anywhere between the second and sixth decades of life, with an increasing prevalence with age.

A postural tremor (also called an action tremor) describes the involuntary movement occurring when an individual holds a physical position against gravity. An essential tremor is typically a postural tremor, but it may also occur at rest (eg, while the hands are resting in the lap) in severe and advanced cases. It most commonly affects the hands but can also affect the head, voice, tongue, and legs.

The tremor may be intensified by stress, anxiety, fatigue, drugs (eg, caffeine, alcohol withdrawal, and steroids) or thyroid disorders. In many cases, the patient may report relief with alcohol use and a positive family history for tremors.

Treatment of essential tremors involves the treatment of the underlying disorder and the use of propranolol (Inderal), or primidone (Mysoline). Second-line agents include gabapentin (Neurontin) or topiramate (Topamax), along with two other β-blockers—atenolol (Tenormin) or sotalol (Betapace). If not effective, benzodiazepine alprazolam (Xanax) is recommended.

Patients who have a very low-amplitude rapid tremor are generally more responsive to these agents than those who have a slower tremor with greater amplitude. Patients who have a tremor of the head and voice may also be more resistant to treatment than do patients with an essential tremor of the hands. In severe cases, surgery may be considered.

Huntington disease is a genetic degenerative neurologic disorder. Abnormal movements include facial grimaces, turning the head to shift eye position, and an unsteady gait. Tremors are not usually seen; however, abnormal choreiform movements with quick, sudden jerking actions of the arms, legs, or other body parts are seen.

PD is differentiated by the presence of a pill-rolling tremor at rest, masked face, bradykinesias, and rigidity. PD also shows a favorable response to the administration of L-dopamine and does not improve with the use of alcohol.

Additional Reading: Tremor: sorting through the differential diagnosis. *Am Fam Physician*. 2018;97(3):180-186.

Essential tremor is the most common movement disorder and is characterized by a rapid, fine tremor that is made worse with sustained positions.

7. An 80-year-old man is brought in by his wife. She notes that her husband has had a noticeable change in his personality, with increasing impulsivity and exhibiting inappropriate behaviors at times. Although he has difficulty naming objects, his memory, ability to calculate, and his visuospatial skills appear to be intact. The most likely diagnosis is which one of the following?

A) Alzheimer disease (AD)
B) Lewy body dementia
C) Parkinson disease (PD)
D) Pick disease
E) Wilson disease

The answer is D: Pick disease and other frontotemporal dementias (FTDs) are a heterogeneous group of disorders that share several clinical features with AD such as the rate of progression and duration. Many FTD patients are also aphasic but maintain their motor integrity. The language disturbance characteristic of Pick disease initially includes anomia (a form of aphasia in which the patient is unable to recall the names of everyday objects), but there is a more stereotyped and perseverative verbal output than that found in AD.

Unlike AD, in the early stages of FTDs, memory, calculation, and visuospatial function are relatively well preserved. The most striking feature of this disorder is an extravagant change in the patient's personality, including disinhibition, impulsivity, inappropriate jocularity, and intrusiveness.

Patients with PD with dementia typically show deficits on tests of executive function, visuospatial abilities, and verbal fluency.

Symptoms in Wilson disease usually appear between 6 and 20 years of age, and although cases in older people have been described, psychiatric symptoms are accompanied by neurologic symptoms.

Lewy body dementia is often accompanied by delirium.

Additional Reading: Frontotemporal dementia: clinical features and diagnosis. In: *UpToDate*. 2022.

8. One must consider whether a patient has delirium or dementia when completing an evaluation of a patient with mental status changes; which one of the following features can usually distinguish delirium from dementia?

A) There is a lack of long-term memory loss with delirium.
B) The time span over which symptoms develop differs.
C) There is an absence of long-term memory loss with dementia.
D) There is a loss of orientation with delirium.
E) None of the above are helpful in distinguishing delirium from dementia.

The answer is B: Delirium is a condition that usually develops in an acute situation (over a period of hours to days) and is characterized by confusion, agitation, loss of orientation, lack of attention, hallucinations, paranoia, disturbed sleep-wake cycles, and loss of perception. The condition is a transient global disorder of cognition and consciousness. The delirious patient may also have psychomotor and emotional disturbances.

In most patients, delirium due to a medical disease is reversible with treatment of the underlying condition. The symptoms of delirium tend to fluctuate in their course. The etiology may be related to toxin exposure, withdrawal from narcotics or alcohol, medications, vitamin deficiencies, infection, trauma, or structural abnormalities affecting the brain (eg, tumor and abscess). The best treatment is to correct the underlying cause.

Dementia is a slow, progressive condition that may take months to years to develop.

Additional Reading: Delirium. In: Domino F, ed. *The 5-Minute Clinical Consult*. Wolters Kluwer; 2022.

9. An 87-year-old white woman is brought in by her husband. She has been diagnosed with Alzheimer disease (AD) and he is asking if any medications will help with her memory loss. You decide to prescribe a medication from which one of the following drug classes because they have shown to have a modest improvement in cognitive symptoms associated with AD?

A) Cholinesterase inhibitors
B) Dopamine agonists
C) Norepinephrine antagonists
D) Serotonin reuptake inhibitors
E) None of the above

The answer is A: Treatment with cholinesterase inhibitors can provide mild improvement of symptoms, temporary stabilization of cognition, or reduction in the rate of cognitive decline in some patients with mild to moderate AD. Approximately 20% to 35% of patients treated with these agents exhibit a 7-point improvement on neuropsychologic tests (equivalent to 1 year's decline and representing a 5% to 15% benefit over placebo). Before treatment is started, it is important to inform the family of the expected, modest benefits of cholinesterase inhibitors. Some cholinesterase inhibitors include donepezil (Aricept), rivastigmine (Exelon), galantamine (Reminyl), and tacrine (Cognex). These agents raise acetylcholine levels in the brain by inhibiting acetylcholinesterase.

Dopamine agonists are used to treat the motor dysfunction associated with PD, and many antidepressants contain norepinephrine antagonists and/or serotonin reuptake inhibitors.

Additional Reading: Alzheimer disease: pharmacologic and nonpharmacologic therapies for cognitive and functional symptoms. *Am Fam Physician*. 2017;95(12):771-778.

10. Dementia is a slow, progressive condition that develops over time. Which one of the following symptoms is the predominant component in dementia?

A) Anxiety
B) Confusion
C) Depression
D) Memory loss
E) Paranoia

The answer is D: Dementia is a condition characterized by the loss of intellectual abilities and the impairment of usually short-term memory. Memory deficit is the predominant component of dementia, and the deterioration of intellectual functioning may occur over months to years. Most patients are older than 65 years, and the course is usually slow and progressive. The condition is characterized by a decline in intellectual functioning to the extent that the patient is unable to perform the usual activities of daily living. Confusion and loss of orientation at night in unfamiliar surroundings ("sundowning") is also common.

Commonly seen dementing diseases in the elderly include Alzheimer disease and vascular dementia (previously called multi-infarct dementia), along with other disorders. The precise mechanisms of the dementias are generally unclear, and no effective cures are available. There is usually no history of prior psychiatric illness, and patients affected typically perform poorly on cognitive tests.

As many as 15% of dementias are reversible; thus, physiologic causes must be ruled out. Treatable causes include medication side effects, depression, hypothyroidism, dehydration, infection, schizophrenia, Wernicke-Korsakoff syndrome, liver or kidney failure, electrolyte abnormalities, hypoglycemia, vitamin deficiency (eg, vitamin B_{12}), subdural hematoma, normal pressure hydrocephalus, neoplasm, and stroke. The workup should be individualized but in many cases consists of electrolytes, complete blood count, thyroid-stimulating hormone, vitamin B_{12}, Venereal Disease Research Laboratory and liver function tests, erythrocyte sedimentation rate, urine and plasma heavy metal screens, electrocardiogram, computed tomographic scan or magnetic resonance imaging of the head, chest x-ray, electroencephalogram, O_2 saturation, and lumbar puncture.

Additional Reading: Evaluation of cognitive impairment and dementia. In: *UpToDate*, 2022.

11. There are many causes of dementia, including all of the following conditions. Which one is considered to be the most common cause of cognitive impairment in elderly patients?

A) Alcohol-induced encephalopathy
B) Alzheimer disease (AD)
C) Multi-infarct dementia
D) Parkinson disease–associated dementia
E) Pick disease

The answer is B: Although all of the listed conditions are associated with cognitive impairment in the elderly, AD is the most common, with an incidence that doubles every 5 years after the age of 60 years. This disease afflicts approximately 4 million Americans and is estimated to cost the US economy $60 billion annually.

Additional Reading: Evaluation of cognitive impairment and dementia. In: *UpToDate*. 2022.

12. Lewy body deposits in the brain are associated with dementia and various other neurologic signs. Lewy body dementia is associated with all of the following signs, except which one?

A) Bradykinesia
B) Delirium
C) Tremor
D) Visual hallucinations

The answer is C: A Lewy body is a build-up of the protein alpha-synuclein associated with a variety of brain disorders, depending on where the bodies are located. Parkinson disease (PD) is caused by Lewy bodies deposited in the neurons of the substantia nigra. The deposits cause destruction of dopaminergic neurons, resulting in PD with its characteristic tremor and movement difficulties. Lewy body dementia is due to the deposits occurring in many other areas of the brain, and in addition to dementia, delirium and visual hallucinations are common. Parkinsonian signs are also seen, including bradykinesia and rigidity, but tremor is often absent in dementia due to Lewy bodies.

Additional Reading: Clinical features and diagnosis of dementia with Lewy bodies. In: *UpToDate*, 2022.

Dementia with Lewy bodies is the second most common type of degenerative dementia after AD.

13. An elderly patient complains of problems sleeping for several months. In considering insomnia in the elderly, you tell him that chronic insomnia:

A) does not lead to nursing home placement.
B) is relatively rare in the elderly.
C) is a natural progression of aging and has little effect on the well-being of elderly individuals.
D) is an independent risk factor for cognitive decline in elderly men.

The answer is D: Chronic insomnia is an independent risk factor for cognitive decline in patients 65 years of age and older, especially in men. Insomnia is often associated with dependence on sleep medications, chronic fatigue, and increased risk of falls. Chronic sleep disturbances may lead to nursing home placement.

Additional Reading: Primary insomnia in older persons. *Am Fam Physician*. 2018;98(5):319-322.

14. You are considering rehabilitation orders for your 74-year-old patient who is now stable following a right-sided stroke 2 days ago. Which one of the following statements about rehabilitation after a stroke is true?

A) Physical therapy should be instituted for stretching and strengthening once supporting muscles are strong enough to support appropriate loads.
B) Tennis ball exercises can be used to strengthen the hand muscles.
C) Most motor function improvement occurs more than 6 months after a cerebral vascular accident.
D) A walking cane used on the affected side can help with ambulation and balance.
E) Bladder or bowel incontinence has no effect on prognosis after stroke.

The answer is A: Rehabilitation after a stroke is often a difficult and lengthy process. Most improvement in motor function occurs in the first 6 to 12 weeks after a stroke; speech may continue to improve significantly after this period. Stretching and strengthening exercises should be instituted when the supporting muscles are capable of supporting the appropriate loads. Gait training should take place as soon as the hip musculature is capable of supporting the patient's weight. In many cases, the patient can use a cane in the hand opposite to the side the stroke affected to help support the weaker side. Squeezing a tennis ball as a hand exercise should be discouraged because it favors finger flexors over extensors and can lead to contractures.

Using a team approach with a physical therapist, occupational therapist, speech therapist, and social workers is often beneficial. The outcome after a stroke is most likely to be positive when patients have bladder and bowel continence, are able to feed themselves, and have a healthy and caring spouse. Stroke rehabilitation must include the prevention or early diagnosis of medical complications, as well as patient and family education concerning the prevention of recurrent stroke.

Additional Reading: Stroke rehabilitation. In: Domino F, ed. *The 5-Minute Clinical Consult*. Wolters Kluwer; 2022.

15. Alzheimer disease (AD) is the most common cause of dementia. AD is associated with which one of the following?

A) Microscopic senile plaques and neurofibrillary tangles in the brain
B) Birth trauma
C) Reversibility
D) Tremors, ataxia, and muscle rigidity

The answer is A: AD is a progressive, irreversible cause of dementia. Symptoms include memory difficulties, disorientation, impaired judgment, aphasia, and apraxia. Histopathologic changes seen in the brain with AD include microscopic senile plaques, neurofibrillary tangles, and granulovacuolar degeneration of neurons. A computed tomographic scan usually shows cerebral cortical atrophy and ventricular dilation.

There is no identifiable cause, and other causes for dementia must be ruled out before a diagnosis of AD is made. It is important to remember that 5% to 15% of non-AD dementias are reversible and may be caused by factors such as meningiomas, subdural hematomas, systemic illnesses, deficiency states and endocrinopathies, heavy metal and drug poisonings, and infections.

Treatment is supportive. Efforts should be made to provide regular accustomed routines for the patient. The mainstay of medication options is acetylcholinesterase inhibitors, which increase the duration of acetylcholine action in synapses. Tacrine, the earliest drug in this group, has only limited benefit and a poor side effect profile, including hepatotoxicity. Donepezil is a highly selective acetylcholinesterase inhibitor that improved cognitive scores with a better side effect profile. Rivastigmine has a good side effect profile but requires more time for dose titration than does donepezil.

Estrogen therapy increases acetylcholine concentrations and has antioxidant activity, but the proof of its ability to reduce the risk of AD has not been shown. Anti-inflammatory drugs are under investigation. Antioxidants, including selegiline and *Ginkgo biloba*, have demonstrated some benefits in improving cognition and delaying progression of the disease, but the outcome measures used have been variable, making treatment recommendations difficult.

Additional Reading: Evaluation of cognitive impairment and dementia. In: *UpToDate*, 2022.

16. You have recently diagnosed an elderly man with Parkinson disease (PD) and inform him that which one of the following statements associated with this condition is true?

A) The condition is associated with neurofibrillary tangles found in the substantia nigra.
B) The carbidopa component of Sinemet blocks peripheral DOPA decarboxylase.
C) Amantadine is an antagonist of levodopa.
D) Benztropine (Cogentin) is helpful for the bradykinesia late in the course of PD.
E) Surgery for PD has not been shown to be beneficial.

The answer is B: PD is a progressive neurologic disorder that is associated with the loss of dopamine-containing neurons in the substantia nigra. It usually affects older patients, and there is usually no family history. The diagnosis is usually made clinically. Symptoms include a resting, pill-rolling tremor, bradykinesia (the most common complaint), and cogwheel or lead-pipe rigidity. Other manifestations include infrequent blinking, a distinguishing blank stare, festinating gait (shuffling gait with a rapid initiation and the inability to stop once started), and increased salivation. The patient may also show signs of depression or dementia.

Dopamine replacement is considered the most efficacious treatment for PD. Because dopamine itself does not cross the blood-brain barrier, it is administered as the precursor levodopa in combination with carbidopa (Sinemet). Carbidopa blocks peripheral DOPA decarboxylase, the enzyme that converts levodopa to dopamine within the blood-brain barrier. With the levodopa-carbidopa combination, more levodopa reaches the brain and is converted to dopamine.

Dopamine receptor agonists are used as adjuncts to levodopa therapy to help control the motor fluctuations that occur in patients with PD. The dopamine agonists available for the treatment of PD in the United States include bromocriptine (Parlodel), pergolide (Permax), pramipexole (Mirapex), and ropinirole (Requip). Dopamine enhancement through the inhibition of dopamine breakdown in the central nervous system was the mechanism behind the development of selegiline (Eldepryl), a monoamine oxidase B inhibitor. This agent is used as an adjunct to levodopa therapy. Theoretically, it allows levodopa to be administered less often, but this has not been observed in practice. Although selegiline has antioxidant properties, no evidence supports the earlier notion that the drug is neuroprotective and delays the natural progression of PD.

Trihexyphenidyl (Artane) or benztropine may be prescribed as an adjunctive therapy to levodopa. Either of these anticholinergic drugs may be helpful in managing significant tremor early in the course of PD. Anticholinergic agents have been used with mixed results in patients with essential tremor, dystonias, and certain dyskinesias. Elderly patients are often unable to tolerate the side effects of these drugs, which include cognitive impairment, dry mouth, and urinary retention.

Surgery is considered an option even in elderly patients as long as they meet medical screening criteria, including failure to respond to available medications and absence of cardiopulmonary risk factors for surgery. Thalamotomy effectively reduces tremor and sometimes rigidity on the contralateral side. Thalamic stimulation can reproduce the benefits of thalamotomy without the risk of irreversible tissue loss because no physical lesion is created. Pallidotomy is a procedure in which a portion of the globus pallidus is treated permanently. The procedure has significant associated risks, including visual field deficits and hemiparesis (because of the proximity of the medial pallidum to the optic tracts and internal capsule).

Additional adjunctive therapies include physical therapy, nutritional counseling, and techniques to help patients manage emotional and cognitive changes related to the disease.

Additional Reading: Parkinson's disease. In: Domino F, ed. *The 5-Minute Clinical Consult*. Wolters Kluwer; 2022.

➔ **Dopamine replacement is considered the most efficacious treatment for PD.**

17. A patient's brother had joined the "ice bucket challenge" to raise money for amyotrophic lateral sclerosis (ALS) and he is asking what symptoms are typically associated with this condition. You note that the most commonly presenting symptom seen with ALS is which one of the following?

A) Loss of peripheral sensation
B) Dizziness and vertigo
C) Atrophy of the muscles and fasciculations
D) Double vision
E) A resting hand tremor

The answer is C: ALS, also known as Lou Gehrig disease, affects upper and lower motor neurons. Two-thirds of patients present with symptoms associated with the limbs, and 25% have bulbar symptoms. Bulbar relates to the medulla and symptoms are a result of disease affecting the lower cranial nerves (VII-XII). A speech deficit and dysphagia occurs due to paralysis or weakness of the muscles of articulation, which are supplied by these cranial nerves. Atrophy of the limb muscles and motor fasciculations are common as well. ALS does not affect sensory, cerebellar, or extraocular muscle function. Men are more commonly affected. Most cases occur between the ages of 40 and 70 years.

Rapidly fatal disease is associated with increasing age and bulbar symptoms. Electromyographic studies show muscle denervation with preserved nerve conduction velocities. Treatment is primarily symptomatic. Attention should be focused on emotional support and "end-of-life" issues.

ALS is also known as Lou Gehrig disease, named after the famous New York Yankee slugger who died from the condition in 1935. Recently, other athletes have taken up fundraising for a cure with a program known as the ice bucket challenge.

Additional Reading: Amyotrophic lateral sclerosis. In: Domino F, ed. *The 5-Minute Clinical Consult*. Wolters Kluwer; 2022.

18. A 73-year-old white man who is on warfarin for a history of atrial fibrillation is being evaluated because of new-onset left-sided hemiparesis and a change in personality noted by his wife. She reports that he had a minor fall 2 weeks ago, but he did not seem to have injured himself. You send him to the emergency department where a head computed tomographic (CT) scan shows a small illuminated crescentic collection of fluid that is located adjacent to the convexity of the hemisphere. The most likely diagnosis is which one of the following conditions?

A) Brain tumor
B) Epidural hematoma
C) Subarachnoid hemorrhage
D) Subdural abscess
E) Subdural hematoma

The answer is E: Subdural hematomas are associated with rupturing of the bridging veins beneath the dura. The elderly and those taking anticoagulants are at increased risk. Acute subdural hematomas become symptomatic within minutes to hours after the injury. Patients may report a unilateral headache, and the examination shows a slightly enlarged pupil on the side affected. Stupor, coma, hemiparesis, and unilateral papillary enlargement are typical signs of larger hematomas. Pupillary dilation is contralateral in 5% to 10%.

For the patient with a rapidly declining course, burr holes or emergency craniotomy is indicated to reduce intracerebral pressure from an expanding lesion. Most subdural hematomas appear as crescentic collections over the convexity of the hemisphere and are located in the frontotemporal region.

Chronic subdural hematomas may develop as a result of mild trauma and manifest as chronic headaches, slowed thinking, change in personality, seizures, or a mild hemiparesis that develops weeks to months after the injury. Many are bilateral.

Symptoms may resemble a cerebrovascular accident or transient ischemic attack. Epidural hematomas develop more quickly than subdural hematomas and are more dangerous. They occur as a result of arterial bleeding between the dura mater and skull, and are less common in the elderly. Most patients are comatose when first seen. The epidural hematoma forms a lenticular-shaped clot, which is seen on CT. Treatment is surgical evacuation.

Additional Reading: Subdural hematoma in adults. In: *UpToDate*, 2022.

19. You are examining a 69-year-old white woman who is complaining of problems with her memory. You decide to perform a Mini-Mental State Examination and need to adjust scoring based on which of her following characteristics?

A) Her age and sex
B) Her age and level of education
C) Her need for a supported living arrangement
D) Her height and weight
E) No adjustments are needed

The answer is B: The Mini-Mental State Examination is a 30-point tool that tests orientation, immediate recall, delayed recall, concentration/calculation, and language and visuospatial domains. As a general guideline scores >26 are normal, scores of 24 to 26 may indicate mild cognitive impairment, and a score of <24 is consistent with dementia. Adjustments are made for age and level of education; for example, 70-year-olds with a high school education have a mean score of 27, but those with a college education score higher with a mean of 28.

Additional Reading: Mini-mental state examination for the detection of dementia in older patients. *Am Fam Physician*. 2016;94(11):880-881.

20. A 65-year-old retired professor is asking whether there is any blood testing, which can be obtained to assess his risk for developing Alzheimer disease (AD), because his father developed AD just 3 years after retiring at the same age. Which one of the following blood tests has been correlated with an increased risk of AD?

A) Apolipoprotein E—E4
B) Apolipoprotein E—E2
C) C-reactive protein
D) Homocysteine

The answer is A: The association between apolipoprotein E and AD is well established. The presence of one E4 allele increases the risk of AD about two to three times, whereas the E2 allele may be protective. The absence of an E4 allele does not rule out the diagnosis, nor does the presence of homozygous E4/E4 rule it in. The test is considered controversial and not routinely obtained.

Additional Reading: Alzheimer disease. In: Domino F, ed. *The 5-Minute Clinical Consult*. Wolters Kluwer; 2022.

21. Acetylcholinesterase inhibitors are frequently prescribed for elderly with Alzheimer dementia; however, side effects can limit their use. The most common side effect that results in the discontinuing of acetylcholinesterase inhibitors is which one of the following?

A) Cataracts
B) Gastrointestinal side effects
C) Headache
D) Hepatotoxicity
E) Rash

The answer is B: Gastrointestinal side effects, including nausea, vomiting, and diarrhea, are a class effect and are the most common reason for discontinuation of acetylcholinesterase inhibitors (donepezil, rivastigmine, and galantamine). These can usually be minimized by slowly titrating the dose of the medication upward over a 2- to 3-month period.

Additional Reading: Alzheimer disease. In: Domino F, ed. *The 5-Minute Clinical Consult*. Wolters Kluwer; 2022.

22. Normal pressure hydrocephalus (NPH) is a cause of dementia and has several associated findings, including which one of the following?

A) Macrocephaly
B) Small ventricles
C) Short stature
D) Tremor
E) Urinary incontinence

The answer is E: NPH is a rare disorder characterized by the following classic triad: dementia, gait ataxia, and urinary incontinence. Lumbar cerebrospinal fluid (CSF) pressure must be normal, and there is usually ventricular dilation noted on the computed tomographic or magnetic resonance imaging (MRI) examination that is disproportionate to cortical atrophy. The cause is unknown, but there appears to be inadequate absorption of CSF, which leads to hydrocephalus. It may follow head injury, subarachnoid hemorrhage, or meningoencephalitis; however, in many cases, there are no preceding conditions. The patient shows no weakness but has a stuttering gait in which the initiation of gait is hesitant but gives way to walking. In addition, the patient may show lower extremity spasticity and upgoing toes on neurologic examination.

Computed tomography or MRI and a lumbar puncture are necessary for the diagnosis. On scanning the ventricles are dilated; however, CSF pressure measured by a lumbar puncture is normal. A limited improvement after removing about 50 mL of CSF indicates a better prognosis with shunting. Radiographic or pressure measurements alone do not seem to predict response to shunting. Shunting CSF from the dilated ventricles sometimes results in clinical improvement, but the longer the disease has been present, the less likely the shunting will be curative.

Additional Reading: Normal pressure hydrocephalus. In: Domino F, ed. *The 5-Minute Clinical Consult*. Wolters Kluwer; 2022.

23. You are seeing a frail elderly white man with a history of cardiac conduction abnormalities who is asking for medication to address his chronic neuropathic pain. Given this situation, which one of the following medications would be the best choice for this patient?

A) Amitriptyline (Elavil)
B) Cyclobenzaprine (Flexeril)
C) Fluoxetine (Prozac)
D) Gabapentin (Neurontin)
E) Phenytoin (Dilantin)

The answer is D: Gabapentin (Neurontin) is preferred if the patient cannot tolerate the side effects of tricyclic antidepressants, has cardiac contraindications to the use of tricyclic antidepressants (eg, conduction abnormalities and recent cardiac events), or is a "frail elder." It has proven efficacy in several neuropathic pain conditions.

Treatment with gabapentin should be initiated at a low dose with gradual increases until pain relief, dose-limiting adverse effects, or 3600 mg/d in three divided doses is achieved. An adequate trial of treatment with gabapentin can require 2 months or more.

Additional Reading: Nonopioid drugs for pain. *Treatment Guidelines from The Medical Letter*. 2022.

24. Elderly patients frequently complain of trouble sleeping. All of the following statements are true regarding insomnia in the elderly, except which one?

A) Women are more commonly affected than men.
B) The condition is associated with inadequate tryptophan levels.
C) Exercise before bedtime can help relieve symptoms of insomnia.
D) Low-dose trazodone (Desyrel) is recommended for treating insomnia.
E) Small doses of alcohol given at bedtime can be used to treat insomnia.

The answer is E: Elderly patients often sleep more than younger patients; however, some elderly patients suffer great difficulty with sleep patterns, such that the number of those patients sleeping less than 5 hours a night dramatically increases as patients grow older. Interestingly, women are more commonly affected than men. Patients with insomnia may experience one or more of the following problems: difficulty falling asleep, difficulty maintaining sleep, waking up too early in the morning, and nonrefreshing sleep. In addition, daytime consequences such as fatigue, lack of energy, difficulty concentrating, and irritability are often present.

Behavior and pharmacologic therapies are used in treating insomnia. Behavior approaches take a few weeks to improve sleep but continue to provide relief even after training sessions have ended. Patients should be encouraged to keep a sleep diary for several weeks. Sleep diaries usually record bedtime, total sleep time, time until sleep onset, number of awakenings, use of sleep medications, time out of bed in the morning, and a rating of the quality of sleep and daytime symptoms. The sleep diary provides a nightly record of the patient's sleep schedule and perception of sleep. Moreover, it may serve as a baseline for assessment of other treatment effects.

Treatment involves attention to contributing factors for insomnia, including depression, caffeine use, tobacco use, or alcohol use. Medications include tricyclic antidepressants or trazodone given in low doses 1 hour before bed. Zolpidem (Ambien) has less tendency for rebound and habituation, and may be a suitable alternative to other medications. Other medications that are used include eszopiclone (Lunesta) and zaleplon (Sonata) and the melatonin receptor agonist ramelteon (Rozerem).

Additional Reading: Treatment of insomnia. In: *UpToDate*, 2022.

Section III. Cardiovascular Conditions

Each of the following questions or incomplete statements is followed by suggested answers or completions. Select the ONE BEST ANSWER in each case.

1. You are seeing a 79-year-old sedentary African American woman who presents with complaints that she has not been feeling well over the past couple of hours. Her medical history is remarkable for hypertension and hyperlipidemia for which she is on current treatment. She has a history of tobacco abuse, having smoked for 30 pack-years before quitting on her 65th birthday. You consider that she likely has coronary artery disease. Which one of the following symptoms is more likely than chest pain to represent myocardial ischemia in older patients, such as this individual?

A) Back pain
B) Diaphoresis
C) Dyspnea
D) Jaw pain

The answer is C: Instead of chest pain, ischemia may be more commonly manifested as dyspnea in elderly patients. Although exertional angina (chest pain) is the most common manifestation of myocardial ischemia in young and middle-age persons, it is a less likely presentation in an elderly patient. Whether this is because the elderly tend to lead a sedentary lifestyle or the result of pathophysiology differences related to aging is unknown. Some elderly patients with coronary artery disease are asymptomatic; however, silent ischemia may be demonstrated by stress testing.

Additional Reading: Evaluation of the adult with dyspnea in the emergency department. In: *UpToDate*, 2022.

2. An 81-year-old white man has presented to the emergency department with signs and symptoms consistent with an acute coronary syndrome. Which one of the following statements is true about thrombolytic therapy in treating myocardial infarctions (MIs) in elderly patients?

A) Elderly patients are frequently overtreated with thrombolytics.
B) Elderly patients with non–Q-wave MIs should receive thrombolytics.
C) Tissue plasminogen activator (tPA) is associated with a higher risk of hemorrhagic stroke when compared with streptokinase in elderly patients.
D) Up to 75% of elderly patients have absolute contraindications to thrombolytics.

The answer is C: Despite the evidence in support of thrombolytic treatment for elderly patients presenting with an acute MI, such therapy is often not used in this age group. The reasons include a time delay by the patient in seeking medical assistance, misdiagnoses due to atypical presentations, increased contraindications in the elderly, and a higher prevalence of non–Q-wave MIs, for which repeated studies have demonstrated that thrombolytic therapy has no benefits regardless of age.

Physicians are often reluctant to use thrombolytics in the elderly population for fear of hemorrhage; however, most studies show that intracerebral hemorrhage is not significantly increased in elderly MI patients who receive thrombolytics. However, when considering the choice for a specific thrombolytic agent, initial studies comparing streptokinase to tPA found that both drugs increased the survival rate equally. The Global Utilization of Streptokinase and Tissue Plasminogen Activator for Occluded Coronary Arteries (GUSTO) trial, which was designed specifically to compare thrombolytic agents, reported a significant advantage with tPA for the overall study population. Patients above the age of 75 years, however, had a significantly higher risk of hemorrhagic stroke when treated with tPA than with streptokinase, and the incidence of death or nonfatal disabling stroke was not significantly different between the two therapies in this age group. Therefore, streptokinase may be appropriate in patients above the age of 75 years.

Although elderly have more contraindications to thrombolytic therapy than younger adults, only about a third of elderly patients presenting with acute MI have an actual contraindication to thrombolytic therapy and less than 5% have absolute contraindications.

Additional Reading: Coronary reperfusion for acute myocardial infarction in older adults. In: *UpToDate*, 2022.

3. A 76-year-old white man whom you have cared for over the years presents today with slowly worsening weakness along with complaints of dyspnea on exertion over the past few weeks. On auscultation of his heart, you hear a high-pitched, blowing diastolic murmur and a wide pulse pressure with bounding pulses. The most likely diagnosis is which one of the following?

A) Aortic insufficiency
B) Aortic stenosis
C) Coarctation of the aorta
D) Mitral stenosis
E) Mitral insufficiency

The answer is A: Aortic insufficiency with accompanying symptoms of aortic regurgitation increases with age. Symptoms of aortic valve insufficiency are the same in older and younger persons. Usually, the main symptoms are related to heart failure, with exertional dyspnea and weakness as common symptoms. In some elderly patients, symptoms of dyspnea and palpitations may be paradoxically more common at rest than with exertion. Nocturnal angina pectoris, often accompanied by flushing, diaphoresis, and palpitations, may also occur; this is thought to be related to the slowing of the heart rate and the drop of arterial diastolic pressure.

The classic findings of a high-pitched, blowing diastolic murmur and a wide pulse pressure with an abruptly rising and collapsing pulse should make the diagnosis of aortic valve insufficiency easily recognized in elderly patients.

Chronic aortic insufficiency may be caused by aortic root disease secondary to systemic hypertension and autoimmune diseases such as ankylosing spondylitis, rheumatoid arthritis (RA), Reiter disease, and systemic lupus erythematosus. It is also associated with some genetic disorders such as Ehlers-Danlos syndrome.

Chronic aortic insufficiency can also be caused by valve leaflet disease, including rheumatic heart disease, congenital heart disease, RA, ankylosing spondylitis, or myxomatous degeneration. Myxomatous degeneration refers to deterioration of connective tissue and is most often used in the context of mitral valve prolapse.

Acute aortic insufficiency may be due to infective endocarditis, aortic dissection, trauma, or rupture of the sinus of Valsalva.

Additional Reading: Adult aortic regurgitation. In: Domino F, ed. *The 5-Minute Clinical Consult*. Wolters Kluwer; 2022.

4. You are seeing an 83-year-old white man who has been diagnosed with aortic stenosis. He is reluctant to consider a valve replacement and asks about his prognosis if he does not undergo surgery. You inform him that without intervention, once symptoms develop, the survival in elderly patients with aortic stenosis is approximately how long?

A) Less than a year
B) 1 to 3 years
C) 3 to 5 years
D) 5 to 7 years
E) Greater than 7 years

The answer is B: Once symptoms develop in patients with critical aortic valve stenosis, symptoms and left ventricular dysfunction progress rapidly with the average survival being only for 1 to 3 years. Surgical treatment is recommended and should be considered.

Additional Reading: Aortic stenosis. In: Domino F, ed. *The 5-Minute Clinical Consult*. Wolters Kluwer; 2022.

5. A 67-year-old African American woman presents with orthopnea and dyspnea on exertion. She notes that her ankles have been a lot more swollen over the past 3 days. She has otherwise been feeling well. You suspect congestive heart failure. Appropriate first-line medication includes which of the following?

A) Diltiazem
B) Hydralazine
C) Lisinopril
D) Nitroglycerin
E) Verapamil

The answer is C: This patient is experiencing symptoms related to volume overload with fluid retention, and a diuretic would be beneficial in improving her symptoms. Angiotensin-converting enzyme (ACE) inhibitors (eg, lisinopril) have been shown to be beneficial in relieving symptoms and preventing progressive ventricular deterioration; thus, they are recommended for the initial therapy in treating patients with heart failure. Although a diuretic is not one of the listed choices, it should be prescribed along with the ACE inhibitor because the use of ACE inhibitors alone has not been found to be successful in relieving the signs and symptoms of volume overload. However, ACE inhibitors are beneficial in improving symptoms and prolonging survival in symptomatic patients with left ventricular systolic dysfunction.

ACE inhibitors appear to be beneficial and well tolerated in symptomatic elderly patients; however, their use in asymptomatic elderly patients with depressed left ventricular systolic dysfunction is somewhat controversial. ACE inhibitors have been found to be beneficial in improving long-term survival and reducing the development of heart failure and recurrent myocardial infarction (MI) in patients with reduced left ventricular systolic function following an acute MI, regardless of the patient's age.

Additional Reading: Ace inhibitors in heart failure due to systolic dysfunction: therapeutic use. In: *UpToDate*, 2022.

6. A 79-year-old retired schoolteacher presents for a renewal of her hypertensive medication. You note that she has had a slow increase in her systolic readings over time; however, her diastolic blood pressure has remained normal. In the elderly, an increase in the systolic blood pressure with no change in the diastolic blood pressure, like in this patient, most likely suggests which one of the following conditions?

A) Anemia
B) Aortic insufficiency
C) Atherosclerosis
D) White coat hypertension
E) None of the above

The answer is C: Atherosclerosis with stiffened blood vessels impacts blood pressure readings in later life. Systolic blood pressure increases throughout life in Western populations, whereas diastolic pressure peaks and plateaus in middle age and later life. "Normal" blood pressure has been defined by determining the cardiovascular risk associated with a given blood pressure. The presence of an isolated increase in the systolic pressure without a diastolic increase (isolated systolic hypertension) is fairly unique to older patients and, unlike younger patients, does not necessarily imply anemia, thyrotoxicosis, or aortic insufficiency, which can cause a bounding pulse and wide pulse pressure in the young.

Additional Reading: Treatment of hypertension in the elderly patient, particularly isolated systolic hypertension. In: *UpToDate*, 2022.

Isolated systolic hypertension is defined as a systolic blood pressure greater than 140 mm Hg and a diastolic blood pressure less than 90 mm Hg.

7. A 73-year-old African American man presents complaining of light-headedness whenever he stands up. He has not fallen and the sensation passes after a few moments. He denies feeling dizzy, but he is worried that he will pass out. You suspect orthostatic hypotension, which you confirm when documenting a drop in his blood pressure when he stands. Causes for orthostatic hypotension in the elderly include all of the following except which one?

A) Declining baroreceptor sensitivity
B) Decreased arterial compliance
C) Decreased renal sodium conservation
D) Increased venous tortuosity
E) Increased plasma volume

The answer is E: Determination of orthostatic hypotension should be routinely performed in geriatric patients. Although several factors such as declining baroreceptor sensitivity, diminished arterial compliance, decreased renal sodium conservation, increased venous tortuosity, and diminished plasma volume are all related to orthostatic blood pressure among older patients, there is no clear evidence that the pressure drops solely as a function of age. However, a blood pressure drop when changing from the supine to the upright position is common among geriatric patients (possibly as many as 30% of unselected patients may experience a 20 mm Hg or more drop in systolic pressure on standing).

Diseases and medications that cause the problem are common offenders, and one should carefully review medications that the patient has been prescribed that may be contributing to the condition.

Additional Reading: Orthostatic hypotension. In: Domino F, ed. *The 5-Minute Clinical Consult*. Wolters Kluwer; 2022.

8. Which one of the following statements is true according to the U.S. Preventive Services Task Force (USPSTF) report on screening for abdominal aortic aneurysms (AAAs)?

A) All women and men who are 65 years or older should be screened once for AAAs utilizing computed tomographic scanning.
B) All men who are 65 years or older should be screened once for AAAs utilizing an ultrasonography.
C) All men who are 65 years or older who have a history of smoking should be screened once for AAAs utilizing an ultrasonography.
D) Screening for AAAs has not been shown to be cost-effective.

The answer is C: The USPSTF guideline recommends one-time screening with an ultrasonography for an AAA in men aged 65 to 75 years who have ever smoked. This recommendation is to screen for AAAs in patients who have a relatively high risk of dying from an aneurysm. Major risk factors include age 65 years or older, male sex, and smoking at least 100 cigarettes in a lifetime. No recommendation was made for or against screening in men aged 65 to 75 years who have never smoked, and it recommended against screening women.

Ultrasonography is the standard imaging tool for the detection of an AAA. In experienced hands, it has a sensitivity and specificity approaching 100% and 96%, respectively, for the detection of AAAs. Men with a strong family history of AAAs should be counseled about the risks and benefits of screening as they approach 65 years of age.

Additional Reading: *Screening for abdominal aortic aneurysm*. US Preventive Service Task Force. https://www.uspreventiveservicestaskforce.org/uspstf/recommendation/abdominal-aortic-aneurysm-screening

9. You are following a 73-year-old man who was diagnosed with an abdominal aortic aneurysm (AAA) 4 years ago. A follow-up abdominal ultrasonography has shown that the diameter of his aneurysm is slowly increasing. You advise him that the threshold to refer for an elective repair of his AAA is when it has reached a diameter of how many centimeters (cm)?

A) 4.5 cm
B) 5.5 cm
C) 6.5 cm
D) 7.5 cm

The answer is B: Patients with an AAA that has increased to a diameter of 5.5 cm should be considered for elective repair. The 1-year incidence of rupture slowly increases at that diameter—9% for aneurysms 5.5 to 6.0 cm in diameter and 10% for aneurysms 6.0 to 6.9 cm, with a significant risk (about 33%) for AAAs of 7.0 cm or more. Patients with an aneurysm <5.5 cm in diameter should have follow-up serial ultrasonographies. Smoking is the biggest risk factor for the development of aneurysms.

Additional Reading: Abdominal aortic aneurysm. *Am Fam Physician*. 2015;91(8):538-543.

10. An 84-year-old white man presents for his annual wellness visit. He is healthy and has no history of coronary artery disease. He reports being active, walking in the park several times a week. He is wondering about taking a medication for his elevated cholesterol in addition to the hydrochlorothiazide that he takes for his mild hypertension. Which one of the following statements is true regarding treatment of his elevated cholesterol?

A) Based on his advanced age, he does not qualify for treatment of his hyperlipidemia.
B) Only lifestyle measures should be used to treat his cholesterol because of the risk of medication use.
C) Treatment of hyperlipidemia should be individualized on the basis of the patient's chronologic and physiologic age and life expectancy.
D) The decision to treat hyperlipidemia in the elderly should not be influenced by a patient's terminal diagnosis.

The answer is C: The decision whether to treat high or high-normal serum cholesterol in an elderly individual must be individualized and based on both chronologic and physiologic age of the patient. As an example, a patient with a limited life span from a concomitant illness (eg, metastatic cancer and dementia) is probably not a candidate for drug therapy. However, an otherwise healthy elderly individual should not be denied drug therapy simply on the basis of age alone.

Additional Reading: Treatment of dyslipidemia in the elderly. In: *UpToDate*, 2022.

11. When considering treatment of hypertension in elderly patients, which one of the following statements regarding expected changes in physiology is false?

A) Elderly patients will experience a physiologic decrease in renal blood flow.
B) Elderly patients will experience an increase in diastolic blood pressure.
C) Elderly patients will experience an increase in systolic blood pressure.
D) Elderly patients will experience a physiologic increase in peripheral resistance.
E) Elderly patients will experience a physiologic widening of the pulse pressure.

The answer is B: Physiologic changes related to aging include decreased cardiac output and renal blood flow, with an increase in peripheral resistance. This results in a decrease in diastolic blood pressure, but an increase in systolic blood pressure, with a widening of the pulse pressure. The pulse pressure is a measure of vascular stiffness and is a risk factor for cardiac events. With increasing age, the strongest predictor of coronary artery disease shifts from diastolic to systolic blood pressure and then to pulse pressure.

Additional Reading: Normal aging. In: *UpToDate*, 2022.

Section IV. Musculoskeletal/Integumentary Problems

Each of the following questions or incomplete statements is followed by suggested answers or completions. Select the ONE BEST ANSWER in each case.

1. A 77-year-old white woman presents with morning stiffness and complaints of severe shoulder and hip pain that has been worsening over the past few months. She also notes low-grade fevers and weight loss. She has no headache or visual disturbances but just has not been feeling well. You obtained some laboratory test results and note that she has a normocytic-normochromic anemia and her erythrocyte sedimentation rate (ESR) was found to be 60 mm/h. Appropriate management at this time includes which one of the following?

A) Perform a joint injection.
B) Prescribe a nonsteroidal anti-inflammatory drug (NSAID).
C) Prescribe prednisone.
D) Refer for a temporal artery biopsy.
E) Refer for physical therapy.

The answer is C: This patient is likely suffering from polymyalgia rheumatica (PMR), which usually occurs in patients older than 60 years, with a female-to-male ratio of 2:1. Onset may be acute or subacute and is characterized by severe pain and stiffness of the neck, shoulders, and hips; morning stiffness; stiffness after inactivity; and systemic complaints, such as malaise, fever, depression, and weight loss.

PMR usually responds dramatically to prednisone initiated at doses of at least 15 mg/d. If temporal arteritis is suspected, treatment should be started immediately, with 60 mg/d to prevent blindness. As symptoms subside, corticosteroids are tapered to the lowest effective dose, regardless of ESR. Some patients are able to discontinue corticosteroids in less than 2 years, whereas others require small amounts for years. Rarely do patients respond adequately to salicylates or other NSAIDs.

On laboratory test results, normochromic-normocytic anemia may be present. In most patients, the ESR is dramatically elevated, usually greater than 50 mm/h and often more than 100 mm/h. C-reactive protein levels are usually elevated (above 0.7 mg/dL) and may be a more sensitive marker of disease activity in certain patients than ESR. If obtained, there is no selective muscle weakness or evidence of muscle disease on electromyography (EMG) or muscle biopsy.

In some patients, the condition is a manifestation of underlying temporal arteritis. Although most patients are not at significant risk for the complications of temporal arteritis, they should be warned of the possibility and should immediately report symptoms such as headache, visual disturbance, and jaw muscle pain on chewing.

PMR is distinguished from rheumatoid arthritis by the usual absence of small joint synovitis (although some joint swelling may be present), erosive or destructive disease, rheumatoid factor, or rheumatoid nodules.

PMR is differentiated from polymyositis by usually normal muscle enzymes, EMG, and muscle biopsy, as well as by the prominence of pain over weakness. PMR is differentiated from myeloma by the absence of monoclonal gammopathy and from fibromyalgia by the systemic features and elevated ESR.

Additional Reading: Polymyalgia rheumatica. In: Domino F, ed. *The 5-Minute Clinical Consult*. Wolters Kluwer; 2022.

3. You have been called that a 79-year-old nursing home patient has a serious methicillin-resistant *Staphylococcus aureus* (MRSA) infection on her right thigh. The drug of choice to treat a serious MRSA infection is which one of the following antibiotics?

A) Ceftazidime
B) Imipenem
C) Metronidazole
D) Penicillin
E) Vancomycin

The answer is E: MRSA is a major problem for elderly patients, especially those in institutional settings. An active serious infection with MRSA is treated with vancomycin as the preferred antibiotic. Older adults may require dosage adjustment based on renal function. Other regimens include vancomycin plus gentamicin (Garamycin) or rifampin (Rifadin), sulfamethoxazole-trimethoprim (Sulfa), doxycycline, minocycline, and clindamycin. Elderly also have a higher risk of death because of resistance to typical antibiotics.

Nursing homes and other institutional settings must be especially careful to prevent the spread of infection caused by this organism. Poor functional status is associated with being an MRSA carrier, and patients colonized with MRSA are also at an increased risk of developing an MRSA infection. Hand washing, isolation of infected patients, and proper handling of body secretions are essential to prevent the spread of MRSA. The most common reservoirs for MRSA colonization are the nasal mucosa and oropharynx. Skin contamination from persons already colonized in these areas may also be a source for MRSA infection.

Although colonization by MRSA does not require systemic treatment, attempts to identify the original infected person (source case) should be made by swabbing the nasopharynx of patients and staff near to the outbreak and treating those found to have MRSA infection. Staff and patients who are MRSA carriers should be isolated, and some authorities recommend treatment with topical mupirocin

(Bactroban), which is applied twice daily for 2 weeks to the nares or other areas of skin carriage (eg, wounds) to reduce the shedding of MRSA. Colonization recurs in approximately one-half of treated subjects.

Additional Reading: IDSA guidelines on the treatment of MRSA infections in adults and children. *Am Fam Physician*. 2011;84(4):455-463.

4. When assessing a hospitalized elderly patient for the development of pressure ulcers, which one of the following is considered to put them at an increased risk?

A) An elevated lymphocyte count (lymphocytosis)
B) Increased body weight
C) Moist skin
D) Skin with blanchable erythema
E) None of the above conditions

The answer is E: None of these conditions are associated with an increased risk for the development of decubitus ulcers. Rather, pressure ulcers occur more often in patients who have nonblanchable erythema, lymphocytopenia, immobility, dry skin, and decreased body weight. Patients with such risk factors need aggressive skin care and mobilization to avoid developing pressure sores.

Additional Reading: Pressure ulcers. In: Domino F, ed. *The 5-Minute Clinical Consult*. Wolters Kluwer; 2022.

5. A 67-year-old white woman has recently retired and is now on Medicare. She is asking about a test for osteoporosis because an older friend fell down and broke her hip, and she is worried about her risk for such a fracture. Which one of the following statements regarding osteoporosis in this situation is true?

A) Dual-energy x-ray absorptiometry (DEXA) scans result in more radiation exposure than qualitative computed tomography (CT).
B) Medicare will not pay for bone density examination.
C) Plain x-rays are a good diagnostic test for assessment of osteoporosis.
D) Routine screening of women older than 65 years is not recommended.
E) T scores are used to diagnose osteoporosis.

The answer is E: Osteoporosis afflicts 75 million persons in the United States, Europe, and Japan, and results in more than 1.3 million fractures annually in the United States. Osteoporosis is defined as the loss of bone below the density for mechanical support. It occurs when there is a loss of bony matrix and mineral composition of the bone, which is defined as osteopenia. Those most commonly affected are white and Asian postmenopausal women. Bones typically affected include vertebrae, wrist, and hip.

Risk factors include menopausal state, positive family history, small bone structure, decreased calcium intake, lack of exercise, smoking, excessive alcohol use, and long-term steroid use. Physicians should recommend bone mineral density testing to all women at the age of 65 years, postmenopausal women who present with fractures, and women aged 60 years and older who have multiple risk factors.

The most widely used techniques of assessing bone mineral density are DEXA and quantitative CT. Of these methods, DEXA is the most precise and the diagnostic measure of choice. Quantitative CT is the most sensitive method but results in substantially greater radiation exposure than DEXA. Bone densitometry reports provide a T score (the number of standard deviations above or below the mean bone mineral density for sex- and race-matched young controls) or a Z score (comparing the patient with a population adjusted for age, sex, and race).

Osteoporosis is the classification for a T score of more than 2.5 standard deviations below the gender-adjusted mean for normal young adults at peak bone mass. A T score of −1.0 to −2.5 represents osteopenia. Z scores are not used for the diagnosis. Medicare pays for bone density examination at the age of 65 years for initial diagnosis and for follow-up after 24 months.

Additional Reading: Osteoporosis. In: Domino F, ed. *The 5-Minute Clinical Consult*. Wolters Kluwer; 2022.

6. You are caring for an elderly patient who has become bedridden following a recent stroke. She was admitted to a local nursing home, and her daughter calls you concerned that she has developed a bedsore. On examination, you discover that she has a break in the skin with surrounding erythema and induration on her sacrum. These findings are classified as a ____ pressure ulcer.

A) stage 1
B) stage 2
C) stage 3
D) stage 4

The answer is B: Pressure ulcers are common in elderly debilitated patients, particularly if they are bedridden. Between 3% and 11% of nursing home and hospital patients suffer from pressure ulcers, which are classified as follows:

Stage 1: a localized area of nonblanchable, erythematous skin.
Stage 2: a break in the skin with surrounding erythema and induration.
Stage 3: a full-thickness ulcer that extends to the subcutaneous layer but not through the underlying fascia.
Stage 4: ulcer that penetrates the deep fascia exposing bone or underlying muscle.

Precipitating factors include constant pressure, moisture (incontinence), shearing forces, and friction. The ulcers may form as quickly as in 2 to 3 hours if the patient is not repositioned. If patients are placed on their sides, they should be positioned at a 30° angle to avoid excessive pressure over the greater trochanter and lateral malleolus. Soft pillows, padded chairs, and egg crate mattresses can help decrease the risk of ulcer formation but are not a substitute for repositioning. Doughnut-type cushions are not helpful and can cause decreased circulation to the tissue in the center of the doughnut and worsening of any existing ulcers. Alternating air mattresses and waterbeds have been shown to help reduce the incidence of pressure ulcers.

Additional Reading: Common questions about pressure ulcers. *Am Fam Physician*. 2015;92(10):888-894.

7. You have been called to examine an elderly nursing home patient who has developed a decubitus ulcer. On examination, you note a full-thickness ulcer that extends to the subcutaneous layer but not through the underlying fascia. This finding is consistent with a stage III pressure sore. Your treatment should include all of the following therapies, except which one?

A) The area should be kept exposed and kept dry.
B) Repositioning the patient frequently to keep the area free from pressure.
C) Culturing the wound and prescribing an antibiotic based on the culture result.
D) Debridement of any necrotic tissue with forceps and scissors.

The answer is C: Mild pressure sores (stages I and II) require prophylactic measures such as the use of egg crate mattresses and frequent repositioning to prevent necrosis. Stage III ulcers should be kept exposed, free from pressure, and dry. Stimulating the circulation by gentle massage can accelerate healing. Ulcers that have not advanced beyond stage III may heal spontaneously if the pressure is removed and the area is small. Hydrophilic gels and hydrocolloid dressings can speed healing. A culture is generally not helpful in choosing an antibiotic because surface growth is often polymicrobial; however, if there is evidence for surrounding cellulitis, a penicillinase-resistant penicillin or a cephalosporin is necessary.

Conservative debridement of necrotic tissue with forceps and scissors may be necessary. Some ulcers may be debrided by cleansing with 1.5% hydrogen peroxide solution. Whirlpool baths can assist with debridement as well.

Stage IV ulcers require debridement or more extensive surgery. When the ulcers are filled with pus or necrotic debris, dextranomer beads or hydrophilic polymers may hasten debridement without surgery. More advanced ulcers with fat and muscle involvement require surgical debridement and closure.

Additional Reading: Common questions about pressure ulcers. *Am Fam Physician*. 2015;92(10):888-894.

8. You are assessing an elderly patient who has fallen out of her bed and is complaining of severe left hip pain. On examination, the patient's left leg is shorter than the right and is externally rotated. This presentation is most consistent with which type of fracture?

A) A left fibula-tibia fracture
B) A dislocated patella
C) A stable left hip fracture
D) An unstable left hip fracture
E) An unstable right hip fracture

The answer is D: Hip fractures represent significant morbidity and mortality for the elderly. Fractures of the femoral neck are classified as being stable or unstable. Stable fractures include stress or impacted fractures. Patients usually report minimal pain and may be able to walk with only mild groin pain and perhaps a limp. The physical examination is unremarkable. Unstable fractures include displaced and comminuted fractures, and most patients report considerable pain with any movement of the hip. The physical examination usually shows the affected extremity to be externally rotated and shorter in length than the unaffected side. Thus, this patient's presentation is consistent with an unstable left-sided hip fracture.

Unstable fractures require surgical reduction and internal fixation followed by traction, but stable fractures, whether stress or impacted, may be treated conservatively; however, impacted fractures are at an increased risk to become displaced and are, therefore, usually corrected with internal fixation to stabilize a reduction and allow earlier weight-bearing.

Patients who are demented, nonambulatory, or poor surgical candidates should be treated by nonsurgical means. Conservative measures to protect the injured extremity, to prevent decubitus ulcers, and to avoid pneumonia should be instituted.

Additional Reading: Hip fracture. In: Domino F, ed. *The 5-Minute Clinical Consult*. Wolters Kluwer; 2022.

9. You are assessing a 73-year-old African American woman with osteoporosis who has had a recent fall. All of the following statements about hip fractures associated with osteoporosis are true, except which one?

A) African Americans have a higher incidence of osteoporosis and associated fractures.
B) Bisphosphonates have been found to be beneficial in preventing hip fractures.
C) Most fractures result from falling laterally rather than from compression-type injuries.
D) More than 10% of persons with hip fractures die from complications.
E) The affected leg in a hip fracture is usually shortened, abducted, and externally rotated.

The answer is A: Hip fractures because of osteoporosis represent a major morbidity for the elderly. Other fracture sites include the spine (compression type), wrist, humerus, and tibia. The risk is greatest for postmenopausal women who suffer from osteoporosis. Whites have a higher incidence of osteoporosis and associated fractures than do African Americans. Most hip fractures occur because of falling sideways and not from compression. This mechanism of injury has a direct impact on the greater trochanter at the proximal femur. Most hip fractures present with the affected leg shortened, abducted, and externally rotated.

Elderly persons often suffer from a loss of independence associated with fractures. Six months after a hip fracture, many older persons still require assistance with the activities of daily living. More than 10% of persons with hip fractures die of complications, and in the United States alone, hip fractures are responsible for more than 31,000 deaths each year.

The use of bisphosphonates, such as alendronate (Fosamax); risedronate (Actonel); etidronate (Didronel); once-monthly ibandronate (Boniva); calcitonin (Miacalcin); or raloxifene (Evista), a selective estrogen receptor modulator, can be beneficial in preventing further bone loss. Hip protectors may also help prevent hip fractures; however, evidence is controversial.

Additional Reading: Hip fractures. In: Domino F, ed. *The 5-Minute Clinical Consult*. Wolters Kluwer; 2022.

10. Elderly patients are frequently seen as outpatients with gait disturbances by the primary care physician. In this setting, which one of the following is most commonly identified as the underlying disorder?

A) Myelopathic conditions
B) Osteoarthritis
C) Parkinson disease
D) Sensory ataxias
E) Stroke syndrome

The answer is B: Unfortunately, problems with gait increase with advancing age and are usually the result of various individual or combined disease processes. Findings may be subtle initially, making it difficult to make an accurate diagnosis, and knowing the relative frequencies of primary causes may be useful for management. A cautious gait (broadened base, slight forward leaning of the trunk, and reduced arm swing) may be the first manifestation of many diseases, or it may just be somewhat physiologic if not excessive. In the past, a problematic gait abnormality in an elderly person was generally termed a senile gait if there was no clear diagnosis; it is more accurate, however, to describe this as an undifferentiated gait problem secondary to subclinical disease.

From the long list of potential causes, arthritic joint disease is by far the most likely to be seen in the family physician's office, accounting for more than 40% of total cases. It most frequently causes an antalgic ("against pain") gait characterized by a reduced range of motion. The patient favors affected joints by limping or taking short, slow steps.

Additional Reading: Gait and balance disorders in older adults. *Am Fam Physician*. 2010;82(1):61-68.

11. Although elderly patients are at risk for falls, many conditions increase this risk. Which of the following is considered a risk factor for falls?

A) Anemia
B) Addison disease
C) Hypothyroidism
D) Vitamin D deficiency
E) All of the above

The answer is E: Many conditions that affect the elderly can increase the risk for falls. Hypothyroidism, anemia, Addison disease, vitamin B_{12} deficiency, and vitamin D deficiency are some notable causes that should be ruled out when assessing an elderly patient after a fall.

Additional Reading: Preventing falls in older persons. *Am Fam Physician*. 2017;96(4):240-247.

12. Based on the results of the Women's Health Initiative study, the long-term use of estrogens (primarily for osteoporosis prevention/treatment) is no longer recommended, because of which finding compared with the control group?

A) Those taking estrogens combined with medroxyprogesterone had an increased risk of breast cancer alone.
B) Those taking estrogens combined with medroxyprogesterone had an increased risk of coronary artery disease alone.
C) Those taking estrogens combined with medroxyprogesterone had an increased risk of stroke and pulmonary embolism alone.
D) Those taking estrogens combined with medroxyprogesterone had an increased risk of breast cancer, coronary artery disease, stroke, and pulmonary embolism.

The answer is D: The conjugated estrogen/medroxyprogesterone acetate arm of the Women's Health Initiative study was terminated early because the combined estrogen/progestin treatment group had an increased risk of breast cancer, coronary heart disease, stroke, and pulmonary embolism, which outweighed the evidence of a benefit in preventing colorectal cancer and fractures.

Additional Reading: Long-term follow-up after the women's health initiative study. *Am Fam Physician*. 2012;85(7):727-728.

13. A 73-year-old man presents with a second flare of his gout within the last 6 months, which presents with a painful left great toe. He has swelling and erythema of his first metatarsophalangeal joint, and his labs reveal a uric acid level of 8.7 mg/dL (N 3.1-7.0) and a 24-hour urine uric acid excretion of 920 mg (N 250-800). His basic metabolic panel and glomerular filtration rate are normal. Which one of the following would be best for lowering his uric acid level?

A) Allopurinol (Zyloprim)
B) Chlorthalidone
C) Colchicine (Colcrys)
D) Probenecid

The answer is A: Allopurinol, a xanthine oxidase inhibitor, has the best effect on lowering uric acid levels and is recommended as the medication of choice for initial urate-lowering therapy in patients with no contraindications to its use. The American College of Rheumatology guidelines for the management of gout suggests a serum uric acid value of 6 mg/dL. Chlorthalidone, a thiazide diuretic, increases serum uric acid levels and should not be prescribed for patients with gout. Colchicine appears to predominantly act as an anti-inflammatory agent and is used in the initial treatment of gout and to reduce flares, but it does not seem to lower the uric acid level directly. Probenecid is a second-line agent and would be used if a xanthine oxidase inhibitor is contraindicated.

Additional Reading: Gout: rapid evidence review. *Am Fam Physician*. 2020;102(9):533-538.

Section V. Special Sensory Conditions

Each of the following questions or incomplete statements is followed by suggested answers or completions. Select the ONE BEST ANSWER in each case.

1. A 71-year-old white man presents for a routine visit for hypertension management and his wife accompanies him today. She is attending the visit, because she wants to inform you that he seems to be having trouble with his hearing, which he mostly dismisses. He blames her for talking too softly and feels that in general he has no issues. You suspect that he is suffering from presbycusis. Which one of the following statements about presbycusis is true?

A) Low-frequency tones are affected first.
B) The condition cannot be treated with amplification.
C) The condition can lead to depression.
D) The condition does not affect the ability to interpret speech.
E) Women are more commonly affected than are men.

The answer is C: Presbycusis, a progressive, high-frequency hearing loss, is the most common cause of hearing impairment in geriatric patients, and men are more commonly affected than women. Presbycusis usually begins after 20 years of age and affects the high-frequency tones first (18-20 kHz). Softer women's voices can be particularly troublesome, and patients often report trouble hearing normal conversations in crowds. This type of sensorineural hearing loss decreases the ability to interpret speech, which can lead to a decreased ability to communicate and a subsequent increased risk for social isolation and depression. Hearing loss in the elderly can also adversely affect physical, emotional, and cognitive well-being.

Questionnaires such as the Hearing Handicap Inventory for the Elderly—Screening Version have been shown to accurately identify persons with hearing impairment. The reference standard for establishing hearing impairment, however, remains pure tone audiometry, which can be performed in the physician's office. Combining the Hearing Handicap Inventory for the Elderly—Screening Version questionnaire with pure tone audiometry has been shown to improve screening effectiveness.

Exposure to loud noises and genetic factors play a role in the etiology of this condition, and periodic screening to provide early detection of hearing impairment should be considered. The avoidance of ototoxic drugs (in addition to avoiding loud noises) and providing support for obtaining and continued use of hearing aids are also important interventions to recommend.

Additional Reading: Presbycusis. In: Domino F, ed. *The 5-Minute Clinical Consult*. Wolters Kluwer; 2022.

2. A 67-year-old mechanic presents with concerns about his vision. A younger coworker was recently diagnosed with a retinal detachment after he strained himself removing a truck tire, and he wonders whether he is at such risk, as he has been having some pain in his right eye over the past week. You tell him that his work should not be a risk factor but advise him that which one of the following would be associated with the typical signs and symptoms for a retinal detachment?

A) Conjunctival injection
B) Excessive tearing
C) Pain associated with the eye
D) Photophobia
E) Seeing flashes of light

The answer is E: Retinal detachment usually affects individuals older than 50 years. It does not cause pain or erythema of the eye. Warning symptoms include floaters, flashes of light (photopsia), or blurred vision. As detachment progresses, the patient may report a "curtain or shade coming down" phenomenon.

Retinal detachment can be caused by retinal tears, retinal holes, or other causes, including ocular melanoma and metastatic tumors. Macular involvement leads to central visual loss and a worse prognosis. Bilateral spontaneous detachments are present in as much as 25% of those affected.

Patients suspected of retinal detachment should undergo emergent ophthalmologic evaluation. Prognosis is best if there is no macular involvement. Without treatment, total detachment usually occurs within 6 months. Treatment of retinal tears or holes is accomplished with laser photocoagulation, cryotherapy, or a scleral buckle. Uncomplicated retinal detachment can be repaired in up to 90% of cases.

Additional Reading: Retinal detachment. In: Domino F, ed. *The 5-Minute Clinical Consult*. Wolters Kluwer; 2022.

3. True statements concerning cataracts include all of the following statements except which one?

A) They are usually bilateral.
B) Asymptomatic lens opacities should be removed because of risk to the retina.
C) Ultraviolet light exposure may contribute to the progression of cataract formation.
D) Most cataracts can be visualized with a handheld ophthalmoscope.
E) Cataract surgery is the most common surgical procedure covered by Medicare.

The answer is B: Cataracts are lens opacities that result in a painless loss of vision in patients usually older than 60 years. The prevalence of cataracts is approximately 50% in those 75 years of age and older. Cataracts are usually bilateral and develop gradually over many years. Exposure to ultraviolet light may contribute to the progression of cataract formation.

Typical symptoms related to cataracts include decreased visual acuity, particularly at night, with excessive glare in bright light or sunlight. Most cataracts can be visualized with a handheld ophthalmoscope; however, slit lamp examination may be more revealing.

Cataract surgery is the most common surgical procedure covered by Medicare, with more than 1 million procedures performed annually. This surgery should be considered when the cataract reduces vision function to a level that interferes with everyday activities. The mere presence of lens opacities—that is, lens opacities not associated with decreased visual function—is not an indication for surgery in most instances.

Cataract surgery is an outpatient procedure performed under local or topical anesthesia. More than 90% of patients undergoing cataract surgery experience visual improvement and improved quality of life if there is no ocular comorbidity. Complications of cataract surgery are unusual and occur in less than 1% of surgical procedures. Potentially serious complications include glaucoma, bleeding, infection, vitreous loss, retinal detachment, and loss of vision.

Additional Reading: Cataract in adults. In: *UpToDate*. 2022.

4. A 77-year-old African American woman with a history of atherosclerosis and hypertension presents to the local emergency department with complaints of a sudden loss of vision in her left eye on awakening. She reports no pain associated with the eye and has no other symptoms. Funduscopic examination shows disk swelling, extensive retinal hemorrhages, and cotton-wool spots. Which one of the following is the most likely diagnosis?

A) Central retinal vein occlusion
B) Cerebrovascular accident
C) Closed-angle glaucoma
D) Macular degeneration
E) Transient ischemic attack

The answer is A: Central retinal vein occlusion usually affects elderly patients with atherosclerosis. The severity is variable; however, older individuals are usually affected more severely. Predisposing factors include hypertension, diabetes mellitus, glaucoma, increased blood viscosity, and elevated hematocrit. Symptoms include a sudden, dramatic, painless loss of vision usually first noticed on awakening in the morning.

Physical findings include disk swelling, venous dilation, retinal hemorrhages, and cotton-wool spots. Those with poor visual acuity at the onset have the worst prognosis. These patients usually have extensive hemorrhages and cotton-wool spots, indicating retinal ischemia, and they may develop neovascular (rubeotic) glaucoma within 3 months after the initial occlusion. Should this occur, laser photocoagulation should be performed; otherwise, there is no medical therapy available. Underlying predisposing factors should be ruled out and treated appropriately if present. Branch vein occlusions may show varying degrees of visual loss and have a better prognosis than central vein occlusion.

The other causes listed perhaps have associated visual changes but typically do not present as a painless loss of vision. Closed-angle glaucoma often presents with severe eye pain that comes on suddenly, with blurred vision and bright halos appearing around objects. In macular degeneration, the first signs are changes in vision and straight lines appearing distorted. This gradually turns into a loss of central vision, with reports of dark, blurry, or whiteout areas in the center of the patient's vision.

Additional Reading: Retinal vein occlusion: epidemiology, clinical manifestations, and diagnosis. In: *UpToDate*. 2022.

5. You are seeing an elderly white man who is accompanied by his wife. He needed a new pair of glasses and his optometrist said that he was concerned that he had macular degeneration based on his examination findings, and his wife wants to know more about his condition. You note that all of the following statements concerning macular degeneration are true, except which one?

A) Macular degeneration is the leading cause of severe vision loss among the elderly.
B) Peripheral vision is typically spared.
C) Drusen is seen on examination in early disease.
D) The exudative form is the most commonly seen.
E) Vision rehabilitation is often beneficial.

The answer is D: Age-related macular degeneration is the leading cause of severe vision loss among the elderly. In this condition, central vision is lost, but peripheral vision almost always remains intact. Affected persons rarely require canes or guide dogs. However, the loss of central visual acuity can lead to a reduction of daily activities and mobility in the elderly and increases the risks of falls, fractures, and depression in this population. Patients with age-related macular degeneration may complain of acute loss of vision, blurred vision, scotomas (areas of lost vision), or chronic distortion of vision. All patients with vision loss should be referred to an ophthalmologist; those with acute loss of vision should be referred immediately.

The diagnosis of age-related macular degeneration is based on symptoms and ophthalmoscopic findings. The disease is usually classified as early or late. In early disease, the macula shows yellowish subretinal deposits called *drusen*, which are thought to be by-products of retinal pigment epithelium dysfunction. In most eyes with early disease, visual acuity remains stable for many years, and loss of vision is usually gradual.

Late disease can be divided into atrophic (dry) and exudative (wet) forms, which can lead to significant loss of vision. Exudative disease occurs in only 10% of patients with age-related macular degeneration, but it is responsible for most cases of severe vision loss related to the disease. In atrophic (dry) disease, the macula usually shows areas of depigmentation. In the exudative (wet) form, fluid can accumulate underneath the retina, resulting in epithelial detachments or subretinal neovascularization, and loss of vision is usually sudden. Fluorescein angiography can be used to help determine whether a patient has the atrophic or exudative form of the disease.

The two currently proven treatments are laser photocoagulation and photodynamic therapy, but these measures are effective in only a small fraction of eyes with the exudative form of macular degeneration.

A study by the National Eye Institute of the National Institutes of Health, called Age-Related Eye Disease Study, demonstrated vision benefit from a supplement formula containing vitamins C and E, β-carotene, zinc, and copper for those with intermediate to advanced dry disease. An updated Age-Related Eye Disease Study 2 formula added lutein, zeaxanthin, and omega-3 fatty acids and removed β-carotene, which might be safer for smokers.

Vision rehabilitation can help patients maximize their remaining vision and adapt so that they can perform activities of daily living. Families need encouragement in providing support and helping patients adjust to being partially sighted.

Additional Reading: Age related macular degeneration. In: Domino F, ed. *The 5-Minute Clinical Consult*. Wolters Kluwer; 2022.

Section VI. Urologic/Reproductive Systems

Each of the following questions or incomplete statements is followed by suggested answers or completions. Select the ONE BEST ANSWER in each case.

1. A healthy 65-year-old white woman is being seen for her annual wellness visit and she has requested a Papanicolaou test. Her examination is normal, although you are able to palpate what feels like a right ovary on her pelvic examination. The most likely diagnosis is which one of the following?

A) Cecal fecalith
B) Fibroid tumor
C) Normal variant
D) Ovarian carcinoma
E) Polycystic ovary syndrome

The answer is D: The presence of a palpable ovary in an elderly patient is of concern and raises a suspicion for a pathologic condition, including ovarian carcinoma. Given that this patient has enlarged ovary, it is likely that she has ovarian carcinoma, which often starts silently, not showing signs until later stages. The average age of diagnosis is about 63 years.

Polycystic ovary syndrome would include other findings (eg, acne, hirsutism, menstrual irregularities, and infertility) and is typically diagnosed at a much younger age. Fecaliths are often associated with acute illnesses such as appendicitis, intussusception, and diverticulitis.

Additional Reading: Ovarian cancer. In: Domino F, ed. *The 5-Minute Clinical Consult*. Wolters Kluwer; 2022.

2. A 67-year-old African American woman, who is otherwise well, presents complaining of urinary incontinence, which has become problematic over the past couple of months. This is a new complaint for her and you decide to obtain which one of the following in the initial workup of her urinary incontinence?

A) A renal ultrasonography
B) A urine cytology
C) A voiding and bowel history
D) An intravenous pyelogram
E) Urodynamic studies

The answer is C: Urinary incontinence is often seen in the elderly. In most cases, the evaluation of urinary incontinence requires only a history (including frequency of urination and bowel movements, fluid and caffeine intake, and medication review), a physical examination, urinalysis, and culture. If no cause is easily identified, a postvoid residual urine measurement should also be obtained.

The initial purpose of the evaluation for incontinence is to detect and treat reversible causes that may be present (eg, urinary tract infection) and to identify conditions requiring referral or more specialized workup. Causes may include infection, atrophic urethritis, pelvic floor weakness (usually related to previous childbirth), medications (eg, diuretics), altered mental status, or overflow incontinence related to obstruction (eg, fecal impaction and prostatic hypertrophy). If reversible cause is not identified, the next step is to categorize the patient's symptoms as typical of urge or stress incontinence and treat the patient accordingly.

Urge incontinence results from bladder contractions that overwhelm the ability of the cerebral centers to inhibit them. These uncontrollable contractions can occur because of inflammation or irritation within the bladder resulting from calculi, malignancy, infection, or atrophic vaginitis-urethritis. They can also occur when the brain centers that inhibit bladder contractions are impaired by neurologic conditions such as stroke, Parkinson disease, or dementia; drugs such as hypnotics or narcotics; or metabolic disorders such as hypoxemia and encephalopathy.

Stress incontinence is caused by a malfunction of the urethral sphincter that causes urine to leak from the bladder when intra-abdominal pressure increases, such as during coughing or sneezing. Classic or genuine stress incontinence is caused by pelvic prolapse, urethral hypermobility, or displacement of the urethra and bladder neck from their normal anatomic alignment. Stress incontinence can also occur as a result of intrinsic sphincter deficiency in which the sphincter is weak because of a congenital condition or denervation resulting from α-adrenergic-blocking drugs, surgical trauma, or radiation damage. Treatment involves the strengthening of pelvic floor muscles with Kegel exercises, voiding schedules, and biofeedback.

Tolterodine (Detrol) and extended-release oxybutynin chloride (Ditropan XL) are used as a first-line treatment option for overactive bladder. A trial of therapy may be attempted before formal urodynamic studies are ordered. If treatment fails or a presumptive diagnosis of urge or stress incontinence cannot be reached, the final step would be to perform more sophisticated tests or refer the patient for testing to define the cause and determine the best treatment.

Additional Reading: Incontinence, urinary adult female. In: Domino F, ed. *The 5-Minute Clinical Consult*. Wolters Kluwer; 2022.

3. A postvoid residual (PVR) of 74 mL is obtained as part of your workup in an elderly patient with new-onset incontinence. When assessing a patient for urinary retention, which one of the following PVR volumes represents the *threshold* volume for an abnormal finding?

A) 25 mL
B) 50 mL
C) 100 mL
D) 200 mL
E) 500 mL

The answer is B: A PVR is obtained by asking a patient to void, fully emptying their bladder. Once voiding is completed, the remaining volume of urine is then assessed. This can be done by an ultrasonography measurement or by straight-cathing the patient and recording the PVR volume. In general, a patient should be able to empty 80% of the total bladder volume and have a PVR volume of less than 50 mL immediately after emptying their bladder; thus PVR volumes greater than 50 mL are considered abnormal. High PVR volumes are suggestive of either detrusor weakness or obstruction.

Additional Reading: Urodynamic evaluation of women with incontinence. In: *UpToDate*, 2022.

4. Benign prostatic hypertrophy (BPH) is a common condition in older men, and various medications have been found to improve symptoms. Which one of the following medications used in the treatment of BPH works by inhibiting the transformation of testosterone to dihydrotestosterone?

A) Doxazosin (Cardura)
B) Finasteride (Proscar)
C) Prazosin (Minipress)
D) Tamsulosin (Flomax)
E) Terazosin (Hytrin)

The answer is B: BPH refers to the condition associated with enlargement of the prostate gland that gives rise to obstructive urinary symptoms. The condition affects men older than 50 years and is characterized as adenomatous hyperplasia. Enlargement of the gland is usually asymptomatic until bladder outlet obstruction occurs. Symptoms reported by patients include decreased force and caliber of the urinary stream, incomplete voiding, hesitancy, frequency, overflow incontinence, retention, nocturia, and dribbling after urination.

Various medications are available for such symptoms and include the following classes of drugs:

- 5α-Reductase inhibitors (finasteride or dutasteride) work to shrink the prostate by blocking the transformation of testosterone to dihydrotestosterone. However, these inhibitors often require several months to work before the patient will experience significant relief of their symptoms. Additionally, regrowth of the prostate occurs after discontinuation of the medication.
- α-Adrenergic blockers (prazosin, doxazosin, and terazosin) have been used in the treatment of hypertension. Tamsulosin (Flomax) is a newer selective α-adrenergic blocker that does not significantly affect blood pressure. These medications relax the muscles of the prostate and bladder neck, which allows urine to flow more easily.
- Anticholinergic agents (oxybutynin, solifenacin) are used primarily for patients with predominantly irritative symptoms.

Physical examination consistent with BPH shows an enlarged bladder and an enlarged prostate, which is usually firm and symmetrical. The median furrow may be absent. Hard nodules found within the gland are more worrisome for cancer. Laboratory findings with BPH may show an elevated prostate-specific antigen, usually <10 ng/dL, and elevated creatine when there is obstruction severe enough to lead to renal impairment. Postvoid residual (PVR) volumes are usually large and may predispose to infection. The most common cause of hematuria in older men is BPH.

Acute urinary retention may be precipitated by prolonged attempts to retain urine, immobilization, exposure to cold, anesthetics, anticholinergic and sympathomimetic drugs, or ingestion of alcohol.

Definitive therapy is surgical. Although sexual potency and continence are usually retained, approximately 5% to 10% of patients experience some postsurgical problems. Transurethral resection of the prostate is preferred. Larger prostates (usually >75 g) may require open surgery using the suprapubic or retropubic approach, permitting enucleation of the adenomatous tissue from within the surgical capsule. The incidence of impotence and incontinence is much higher than that after transurethral resection of the prostate. Alternative surgical approaches include intraurethral stents, microwave thermotherapy, high-intensity focused ultrasound thermotherapy, laser ablation, electrovaporization, and radiofrequency vaporization.

Additional Reading: Common questions about the diagnosis and management of benign prostatic hyperplasia. *Am Fam Physician*. 2014; 90(11):769-774.

5. A female patient is being seen with complaints of hot flushes and wants to know if she is going through menopause because she has not had a period in several months. Which one of the following is necessary to diagnose menopause?

A) Estrogen levels <30 mg/dL
B) Follicle-stimulating hormone (FSH) level >35 mg/dL
C) An abnormal progesterone challenge test
D) The absence of menses for 6 months

The answer is D: Menopause is defined as the absence of menses for 6 months. The average age of onset is 51 years. Symptoms of menopause are common and include hot flashes, night sweats, mood swings with emotional lability and irritability, depression, insomnia, vaginal dryness, dyspareunia, dysuria, and urinary incontinence. Hormone replacement therapy (estrogen with or without progestin) was the primary treatment for the symptoms and long-term risks associated with menopause; however, concerns over associated adverse effects have limited its use.

Menopause can be confirmed by measuring FSH levels; however, this is not necessary for the diagnosis. FSH levels >35 mg/dL support a menopausal state. In addition, a progesterone challenge test (10 days of progestin) resulting in no withdrawal bleeding after the medication has been administered indicates a lack of estrogen and the menopausal state.

Additional Reading: Clinical manifestations and diagnosis of menopause. In: *UpToDate*. 2022.

6. A 68-year-old white woman is being seen in a routine follow-up for her hypertension. She has a new complaint today that she has been wearing a pad because she is losing some urine when she coughs or sneezes, which she finds embarrassing. The most likely diagnosis to explain her condition is which one of the following?

A) Interstitial cystitis
B) Neurogenic bladder
C) Stress incontinence
D) Urinary tract infection
E) Urge incontinence

The answer is C: Stress urinary incontinence is defined as bladder outlet incompetence and the loss of urine with coughing, sneezing, straining, lifting, or any activity that requires a Valsalva maneuver and associated increased abdominal pressure. In women, the usual cause is a loss in the normal posterior ureterovesical angle because of pelvic floor muscle laxity. Pelvic floor weakness is a common result of aging and multiparity.

Treatment may involve the use of Kegel exercises (multiple contractions of the pelvic floor muscles as if the patient were shutting off the flow of urine). Estrogens may also be effective in treating women with stress incontinence. The presence of estrogen receptors in high concentrations throughout the lower urinary tract makes it possible to treat women with stress incontinence by localized estrogen replacement therapy. Estrogen replacement therapy causes engorgement of the periurethral blood supply and subsequent thickening of the urethral mucosa. Localized estrogen replacement therapy can be given in the form of estrogen cream or an estradiol-impregnated vaginal ring (Estring).

Surgery may be considered if the condition is severe and refractive to medication. Another minimally invasive procedure for the treatment of stress incontinence is periurethral injection. This procedure involves injection of material at the bladder neck just under the urothelium and is performed in an office setting under local anesthesia. In some cases, the use of a pessary may be beneficial.

Urge incontinence is manifested by difficulty holding the urine when patients first sense the "urge" to go, and patients will complain of urinary leakage if they cannot quickly find a bathroom to relieve themselves.

A neurogenic bladder refers to bladder spasticity and results in incontinence as well.

Patients with interstitial cystitis have urgency and frequency, like those suffering from an infection in the urinary tract.

Additional Reading: Urinary incontinence. In: Domino F, ed. *The 5-Minute Clinical Consult*. Wolters Kluwer; 2022.

7. You are evaluating an elderly woman with new complaints of incontinence. Your initial evaluation could include all of the following tests, except which one?

A) Blood glucose levels
B) Urinalysis
C) Urine culture
D) Urodynamic testing
E) Vitamin B_{12} levels

The answer is D: Physicians should initiate a discussion of voiding symptoms because at least one-half of incontinent individuals do not report the problem to their providers. If not recorded recently, it is necessary to measure renal function, glucose, and, in older people, vitamin B_{12} levels. A urinalysis should be obtained in all patients, and a urine culture should be obtained if infection is suspected. Routine urodynamic testing is not recommended as part of the initial evaluation.

A physical examination for incontinence should be completed, and for individuals with symptoms of stress incontinence, a clinical stress test may be performed by having the patient (who should have a full bladder) give a single vigorous cough while standing and maintaining a relaxed perineum. Instantaneous leakage suggests stress incontinence, whereas a delay of several seconds before leakage suggests stress-induced detrusor overactivity. If urinary retention is suspected, it is important to consider postvoid residual testing, either by catheterization or ultrasonography.

Additional Reading: Clinical presentation and diagnosis of urinary incontinence. In: *UpToDate*. 2022.

8. A 65-year-old otherwise healthy woman presents to your office complaining of pain with intercourse. On a pelvic examination, you note a pale-pink vaginal mucosa, with loss of rugae and a friable cervix. The most appropriate treatment at this time is which one of the following?

A) Apply cryotherapy to her cervix.
B) Apply trichloroacetic acid vaginally.
C) Consider psychotherapy.
D) Prescribe estrogen vaginal cream.
E) Refer for vaginal dilation.

The answer is D: Atrophic vaginitis is the result of a lack of estrogen on the vaginal tissue. Up to 40% of postmenopausal women have symptoms of atrophic vaginitis. Related to estrogen deficiency, the condition may occur in premenopausal women who take antiestrogenic medications (medroxyprogesterone [Provera], tamoxifen [Nolvadex], danazol [Danocrine], leuprolide [Lupron], and nafarelin [Synarel]) or who have medical or surgical conditions that result in decreased levels of estrogen.

The thinned endometrium and increased vaginal pH level induced by estrogen deficiency predispose the vagina and urinary tract to infection and mechanical weakness. The earliest symptoms are decreased vaginal lubrication, followed by other vaginal and urinary symptoms that may be exacerbated by superimposed infection. Patients often report vaginal pruritus, burning, discharge, and excessive dryness with dyspareunia. Urethritis with urinary incontinence, dysuria, and frequency may also occur.

Physical findings include a pale-pink vaginal mucosa with friable or atrophic cervix.

Once other causes of symptoms have been eliminated, treatment usually depends on estrogen administration. Estrogen replacement therapy may be provided systemically or locally (preferred), but the dosage and delivery method must be individualized. Vaginal moisturizers and lubricants, and participation in coitus may also be beneficial in the treatment of women with atrophic vaginitis.

Additional Reading: Atrophic vaginitis. In: Domino F, ed. *The 5-Minute Clinical Consult*. Wolters Kluwer; 2022.

9. A 69-year-old woman presents complaining that she has frequent episodes with a sudden desire to void that causes her to leak urine while she is trying to reach the bathroom. She also reports occasional urinary frequency and waking up once or twice a night to urinate.

Which one of the following would you recommend as the first-line treatment for her complaints?

A) Anticholinergic drugs such as oxybutynin or solifenacin (Vesicare)
B) β-Adrenergic agonists such as mirabegron (Myrbetriq)
C) Bladder training
D) Duloxetine (Cymbalta)

The answer is C: Half of all older women in the United States suffer from bothersome urinary symptoms. Chronic incontinence can be classified as stress, urge, mixed, overflow, or functional. This patient has urge urinary incontinence, defined as the loss of urine accompanied or preceded by a strong impulse to void. It may be accompanied by frequency and nocturia, and is common in older adults. Bladder training and lifestyle modification are the recommended first-line treatment for both stress and urge urinary incontinence. If ineffective, any of the listed medications can be prescribed depending on patient preferences, although all have associated side effects that often limit their use. Solifenacin and mirabegron are used to treat overactive bladder conditions as an antispasmodic. Duloxetine is a serotonin-norepinephrine reuptake inhibitor that has been used to address stress incontinence.

Additional Reading: Clinical presentation and diagnosis of urinary incontinence. In: *UpToDate*. 2022.

10. You are seeing a 67-year-old woman for her annual wellness visit and your medical assistant (MA) has obtained a urine dip test prior to you seeing her. The MA reports that the urine dip test is positive for blood. The patient has not noticed any blood in her urine and has not had any vaginal bleeding. Although she has been smoking since she was a teenager, she is relatively healthy. You obtain a complete urinalysis (UA) which is only remarkable for a few red blood cells, consistent with microscopic hematuria, and a urine culture is negative. Her blood urea nitrogen level is 9 mg/dL (6-24 mg/dL) and serum creatinine level 1.0 mg/dL (N 0.6-1.3). The best next step would be to:

A) Obtain a urine cytology.
B) Refer for a cystoscopy.
C) Refer to nephrology.
D) Repeat a complete UA in 6 weeks.

The answer is B: Microscopic hematuria should be assessed for benign causes such as urinary tract infections or renal disease. A complete UA and renal function tests can be helpful in this regard. If the results are negative, imaging may be considered depending on the risk factors of the patient, and cystoscopy should be performed.

Urine cytology is less sensitive than cystoscopy for bladder cancer and should not be done. This patient has normal renal function and no signs of renal disease on the UA other than hematuria, so a nephrology consultation is not necessary at this time. Performing a repeat UA is indicated by some guidelines in some very low–risk, generally younger patients with minimal red blood cells, before proceeding with the workup. In those situations, the UA needs to be repeated periodically to ensure no further progression. This patient is older and has a history of smoking, so she would not be considered a low risk for urinary tract cancer.

Additional Reading: Hematuria. In: Domino F, ed. *The 5-Minute Clinical Consult*. Wolters Kluwer; 2022.

Pictorial Atlas

CHAPTER 7

There are a few images on the American Board of Family Medicine examination. Usually, you will see a couple of radiographs, a cardiac tracing or two, and some common physical exam findings and skin conditions. We have included some images here for you to consider as you prepare for the examination. The first section covers skin findings, and the second section covers common exam findings and other diagnostic tests.

Section I. Skin Findings

Each of the following questions or incomplete statements is followed by suggested answers or completions. Select the ONE BEST ANSWER in each case.

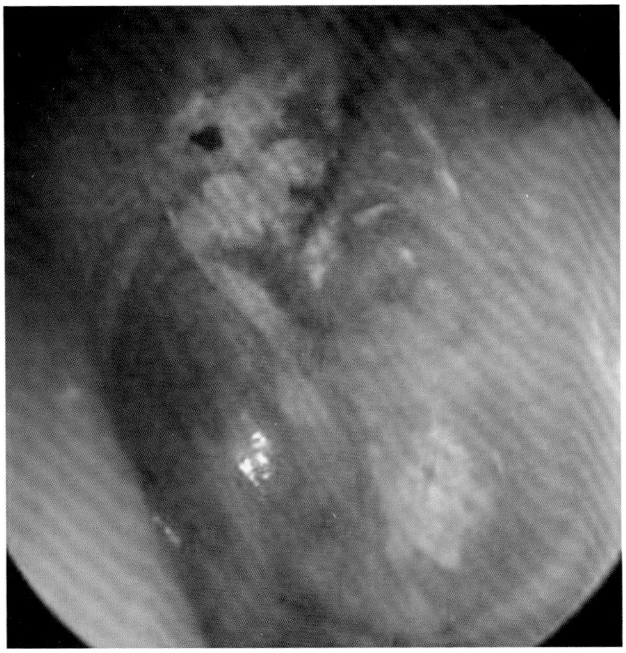

Used with permission of Thieme, from Sanna M, Russo A, DeDonato G, et al. *Color Atlas of Otoscopy: From Diagnosis to Surgery*. 2nd ed. 2002; permission conveyed through Copyright Clearance Center, Inc.

1. A 37-year-old man presents with problems hearing out of his right ear over the past few months. He is otherwise healthy and reports no family history of deafness. When you examine his right ear, you observe this abnormality through your otoscope. What would be the most appropriate treatment for this condition?

A) Hearing aids
B) Topical otic antibiotic drops
C) Topical otic decongestant drops
D) Topical otic corticosteroid drops
E) Tympanomastoidectomy

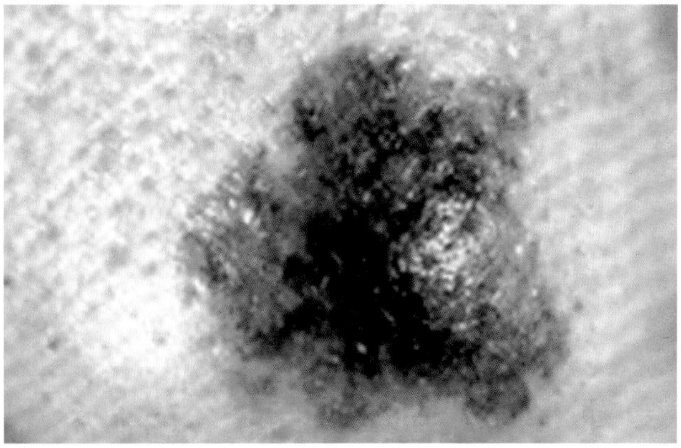

2. A 44-year-old woman presents with a mole on the back of her leg that has been slowly enlarging (see figure). She has no significant medical problems and otherwise feels well. Appropriate initial management of this skin lesion is which one of the following approaches?

A) Shave biopsy
B) Electrodesiccation and curettage
C) Complete excision with wide margins
D) Complete excision with normal margins
E) Observation and removal if bleeding or further change occurs

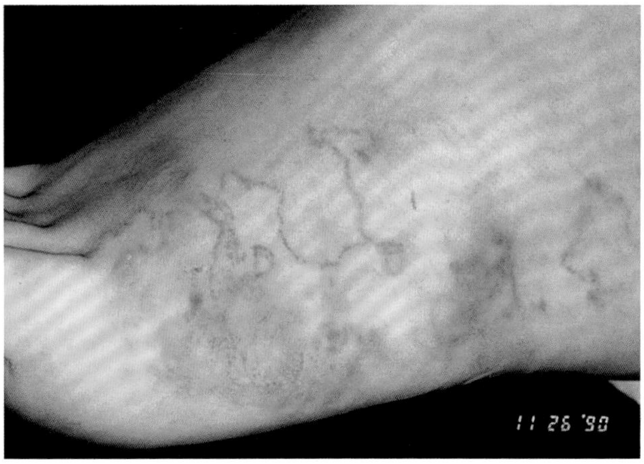

Reproduced with permission from Fleisher GR, Ludwig S, Baskin MN. *Atlas of Pediatric Emergency Medicine*. Lippincott Williams & Wilkins; 2004.

3. A 23-year-old diver presents with an itchy rash on his foot. He reports that it developed after a recent diving trip and is slowly enlarging. The most likely diagnosis for this rash is which one of the following conditions?

A) Bathing suit dermatitis
B) Cutaneous larva migrans
C) Jellyfish sting
D) Swimming pool granuloma

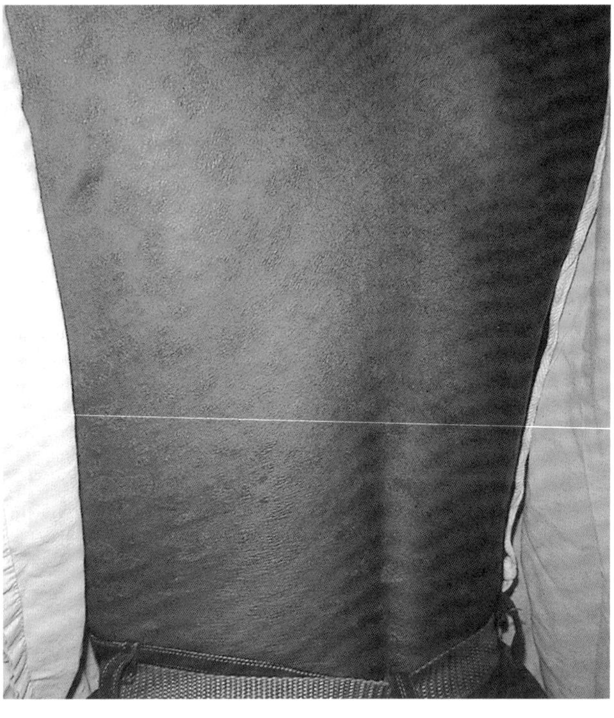

4. A 21-year-old student presents with a rash. He states the rash developed over the past week and is not very bothersome, but it seems to be spreading. He reports a mild viruslike illness just before it started, and he thinks it began as a patch on his chest. The most likely diagnosis to account for his presentation is which one of the following?

A) Coccidioidomycosis
B) Pityriasis rosea
C) Psoriasis
D) Tinea versicolor
E) Varicella

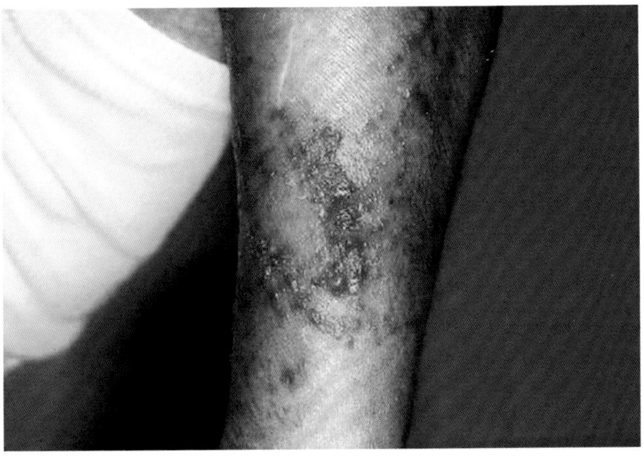

Reproduced with permission from Goodheart H. *Goodheart's Photoguide to Common Pediatric and Adult Skin Disorders*. 3rd ed. Wolters Kluwer; 2009.

5. A 12-year-old boy is brought into your office by his father after a weekend camping trip. He complains of a very itchy rash that has developed over the past 24 hours. The most likely diagnosis for this rash is which one of the following?

A) Rhus dermatitis
B) Herpes zoster
C) Lichen sclerosis
D) Erythema multiforme
E) Varicella

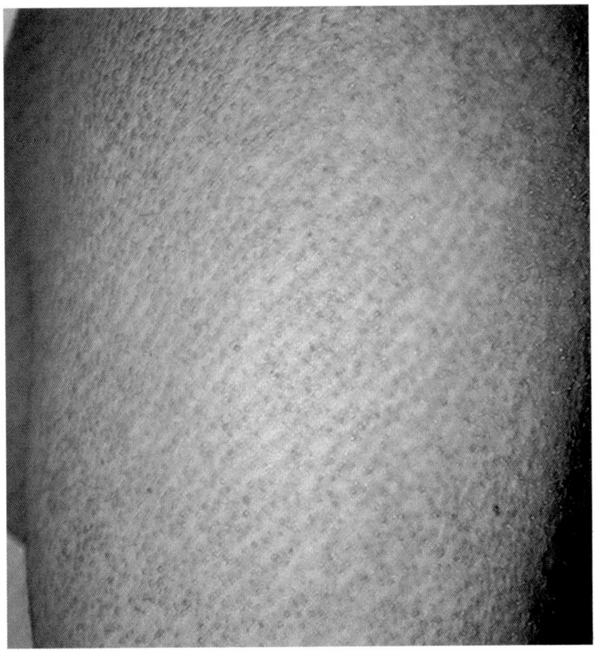

Reproduced with permission from Hall JC, Hall BJ. *Sauer's Manual of Skin Diseases*. 11th ed. Lippincott Williams & Wilkins; 2018.

6. A 23-year-old man presents complaining of sandpaperlike rash that affects his upper outer arms. He is otherwise healthy, the rash does not itch, and he has no other symptoms. The most likely diagnosis for this presentation is which one of the following conditions?

A) Keratosis pilaris
B) Psoriasis
C) Rheumatic fever
D) Scarlet fever
E) Seborrheic dermatitis

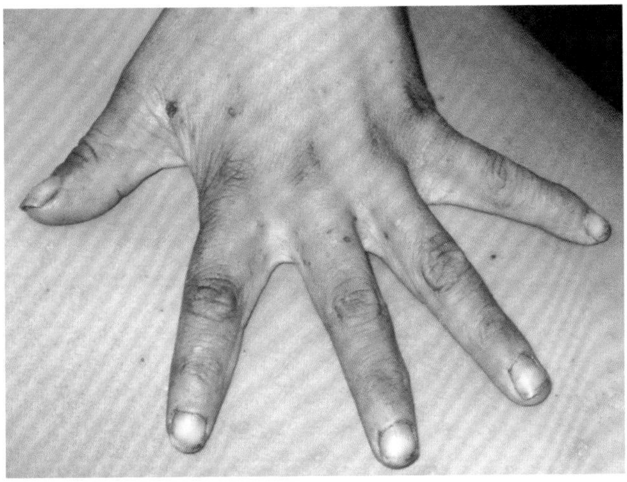

Reproduced with permission from Berg D, Worzala K. *Atlas of Adult Physical Diagnosis*. Lippincott Williams & Wilkins; 2006.

7. A 27-year-old woman presents with an itchy rash on her fingers that she has for the past couple of weeks, which looks like the image shown. She is otherwise healthy and reports no new soaps or lotions. She works at a daycare, and although there have been some children out with fevers, she does not recall any with rashes. The itch is worse at night, and she has been using topical over-the-counter hydrocortisone creams, but they do not help much. She is worried that she has a fungal infection. The likely diagnosis is which one of the following conditions?

A) Dyshidrotic eczema
B) Poison ivy
C) Psoriasis
D) Scabies
E) Tinea corporis

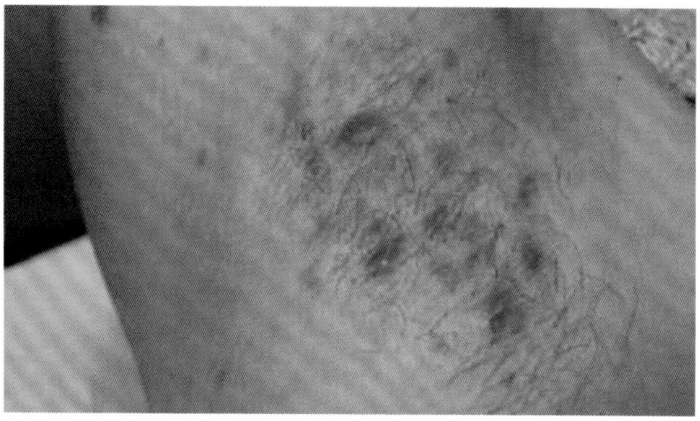

Reproduced with permission from *Stedman's Illustrated Guide of Dermatology Eponyms*. Wolters Kluwer; 2004.

8. A 31-year-old woman presents with complaints of a recurrent rash under her right arm. The rash will develop into painful pimples that drain pus, and she notes that they heal as hard bumps. The most likely diagnosis for the condition seen above is which one of the following?

A) Antiperspirant dermatitis
B) Hidradenitis suppurativa
C) Impetigo
D) Scrofuloderma
E) Tinea corporis

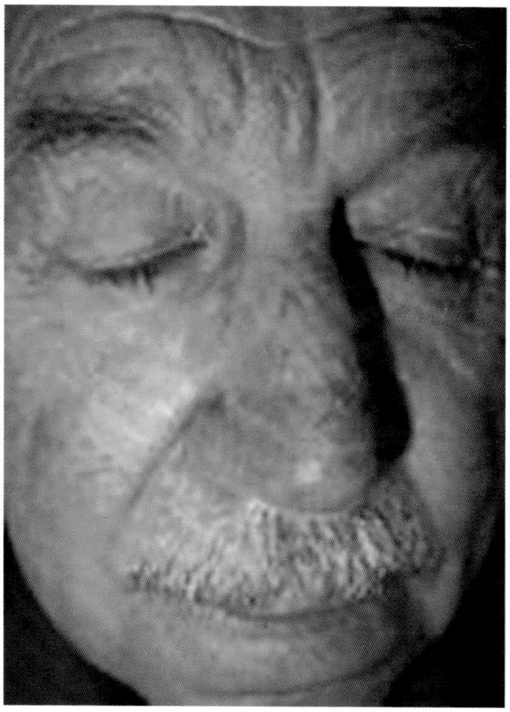

Reproduced with permission from *Stedman's Illustrated Guide of Dermatology Eponyms*. Wolters Kluwer; 2004.

9. A 72-year-old man presents to your office complaining of an area of redness around his nose. He states that the rash is often worse in the summer because sunlight exposure makes it worse. Appropriate treatment of this condition would be to prescribe which one of the following agents?

A) Acyclovir ointment
B) Hydrocortisone cream
C) Metronidazole cream
D) Mupirocin ointment
E) Tretinoin gel

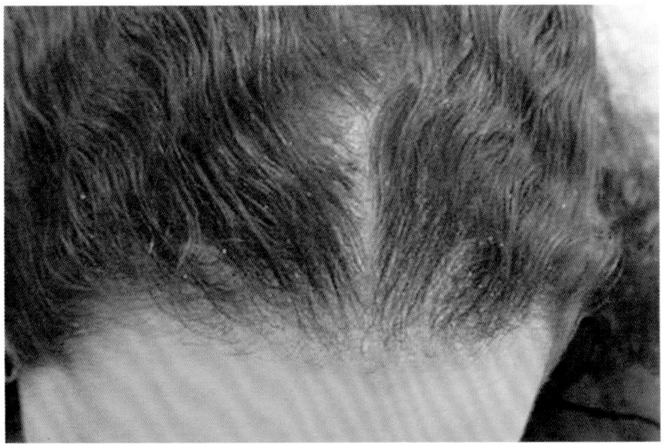

Reproduced with permission from Domino FJ, Baldor RA, Barry KA, Golding J, Stephens MB. *The 5-Minute Clinical Consult 2023*. 31st ed. Wolters Kluwer; 2023.

10. A 41-year-old woman presents with a localized area of erythematous scaly patches that typically affect her head along the scalp line as seen here. She also will have outbreaks on her elbows as well. The likely diagnosis for her condition is which one of the following?

A) Mycosis fungoides
B) Nummular eczema
C) Pityriasis rosea
D) Psoriasis
E) Tinea corporis

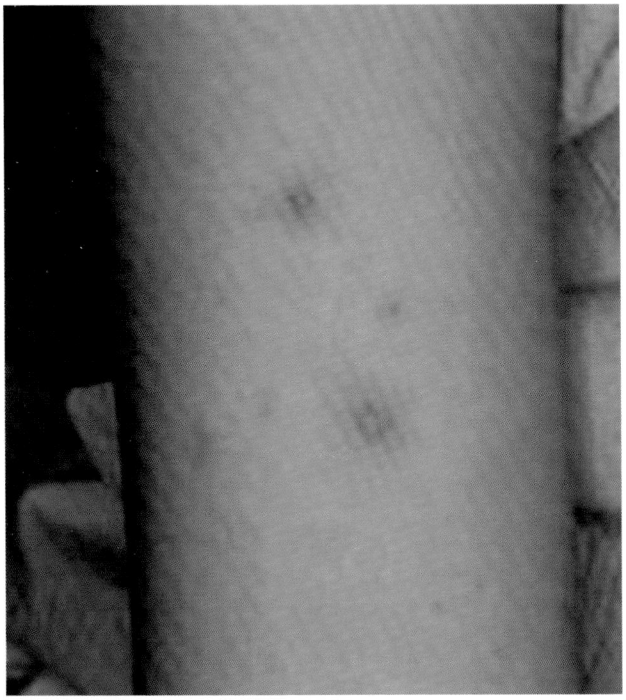

11. A 36-month-old immigrant child is brought in by his mother with a sore throat and an erythematous, pruritic rash that has developed over the past 24 hours. The most likely diagnosis for the rash, which consists of a vesicular eruption on an inflamed base, as shown, is which one of the following infections?

A) Fifth disease
B) Measles
C) Rocky Mountain spotted fever
D) Scarlatina
E) Varicella zoster

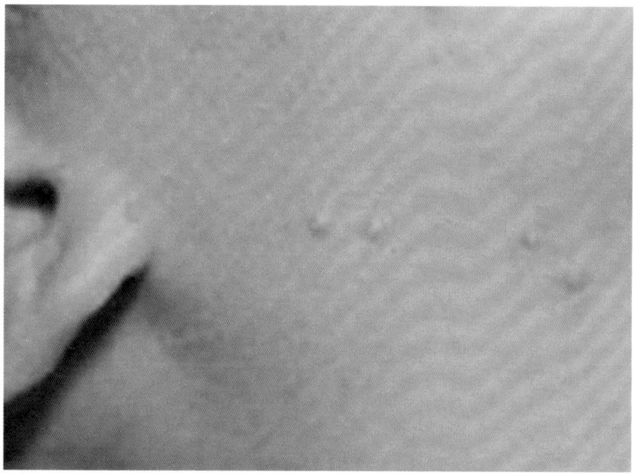

12. A 4-year-old preschooler presents with the papular skin lesions shown. The lesions have been present over the past month, and the child has reported no symptoms associated with them. The most likely diagnosis for these lesions is which one of the following?

A) Molluscum contagiosum
B) Rhus dermatitis
C) Scabies
D) Herpes zoster
E) Varicella zoster

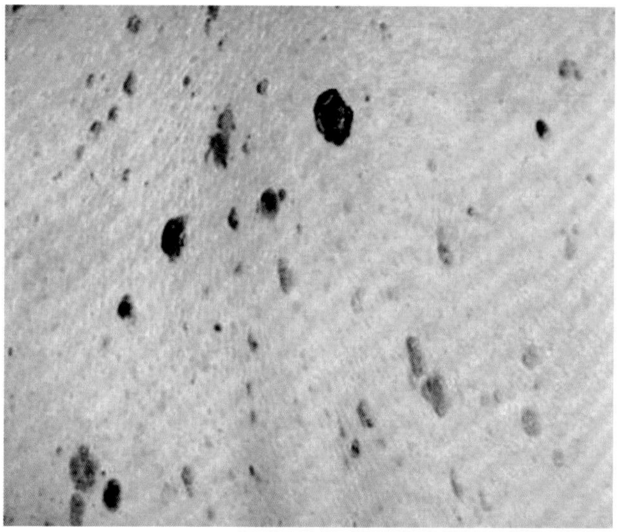

Reproduced with permission from Goodheart H. *Goodheart's Photoguide to Common Pediatric and Adult Skin Disorders*. 3rd ed. Wolters Kluwer; 2009.

13. An 86-year-old patient is brought in by her daughter who is concerned about dark lesions that she had seen on her mother's back when helping her to bathe. The patient has several lesions that look like those seen above. Appropriate management would include which one of the following?

A) Perform a punch biopsy.
B) Prescribe topical 5-fluorouracil cream.
C) Prescribe topical hydrocortisone cream.
D) Treat with cryotherapy.
E) Offer reassurance and observation.

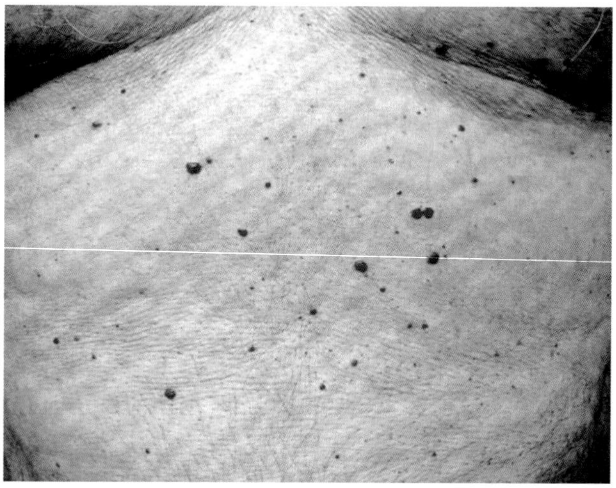

Reproduced with permission from Goodheart H. *Goodheart's Photoguide of Common Skin Disorders*. 2nd ed. Lippincott Williams & Wilkins; 2004.

14. A middle-aged man presents for a routine examination and is worried about red lesions that have formed on his chest and abdomen over the past few months, like the ones shown. The most likely diagnosis for this condition is which one of the following?

A) Cherry angiomas
B) Chigger bites
C) Erythroderma
D) Granuloma annulare
E) Scabies

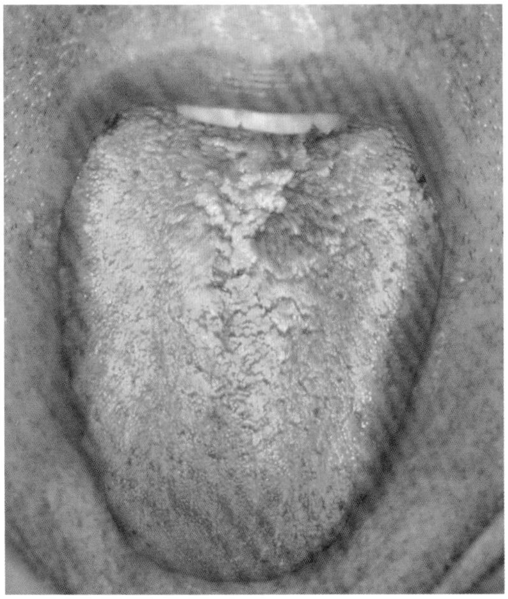

Reproduced with permission from DeLong L, Burkhart N. *General and Oral Pathology for the Dental Hygienist*. Lippincott Williams & Wilkins; 2008.

15. A patient arrives with concern over his tongue, which he states has been turning black. His girlfriend has told him that it looks like he is growing a beard on his tongue, and he is quite concerned. You tell him that "hairy tongue" is associated with which one of the following conditions?

A) Addison disease
B) Chronic gastroesophageal reflux
C) Malignant melanoma
D) Smoking
E) Sjögren syndrome

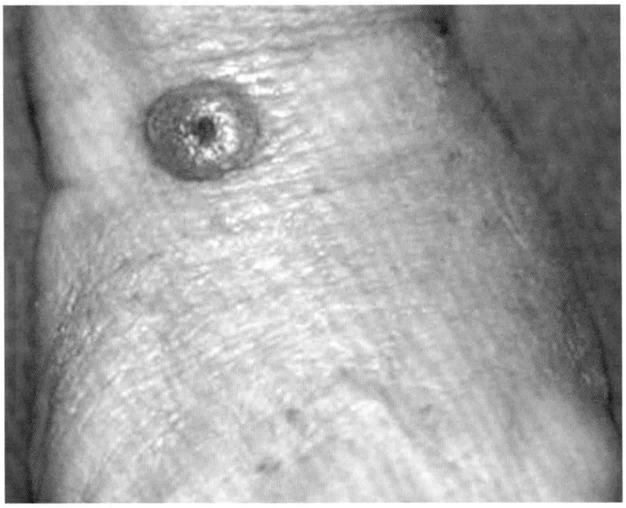

Reproduced with permission from McConnell TH. *Nature of Disease*. Wolters Kluwer; 2013.

16. A 67-year-old man presents with concern over a lump on the back of his right hand that has just developed over the past few weeks. The lesion is rapidly becoming larger. The most likely diagnosis for this finding is which one of the following?

A) Basal cell carcinoma
B) Actinic keratosis
C) Keratoacanthoma
D) Seborrheic keratosis
E) Squamous cell carcinoma

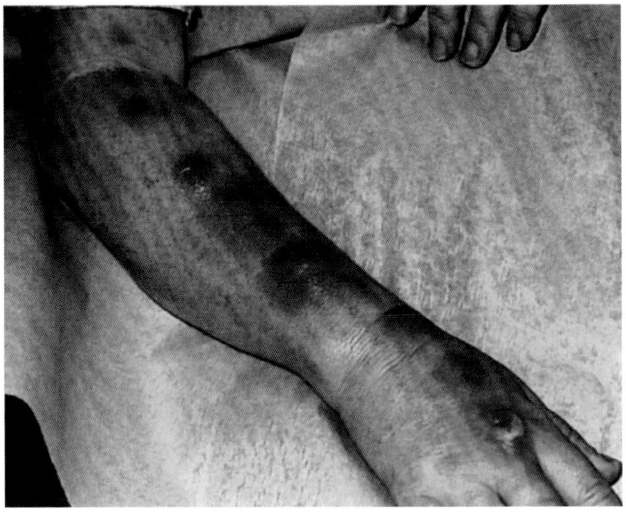

Reproduced with permission from Elder DE. *Atlas of Dermatopathology*. 4th ed. Lippincott Williams & Wilkins; 2020.

17. A 47-year-old gardener presents complaining of the lesion shown. He is growing flowers and had been pruning his roses earlier this spring and recalls removing a thorn from the area a couple of weeks before the lesion developed. It started as a small painless lump that now has crusted over. The most likely diagnosis for this presentation is which of the following infections?

A) Blastomycosis
B) Coccidioidomycosis
C) Histoplasmosis
D) Lyme disease
E) Sporotrichosis

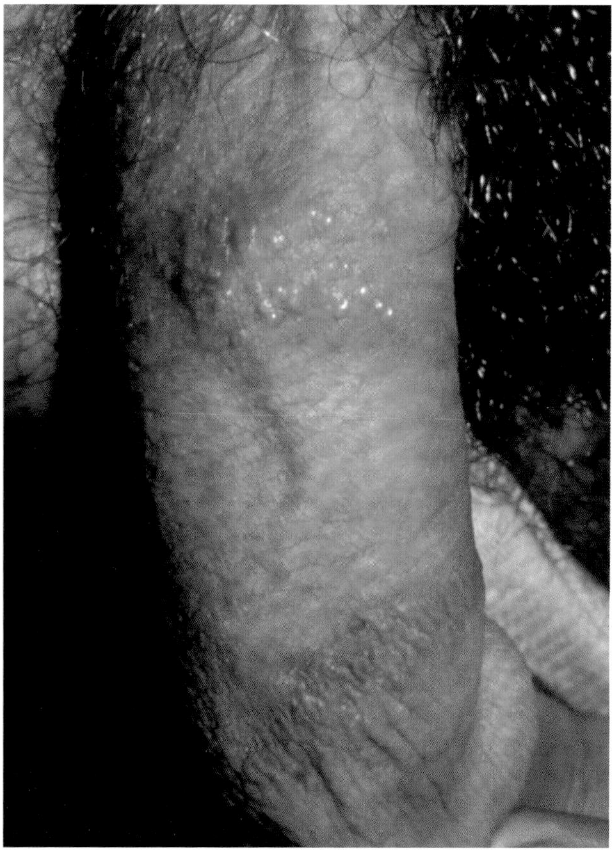

Reproduced with permission from Craft N, Fox LP, Goldsmith LA, et al. *VisualDX: Essential Adult Dermatology*. Lippincott Williams & Wilkins; 2011.

18. A 21-year-old college student is seen in the college health clinic with the recurrent lesion shown here on his penis. He reports pain and discomfort associated with the lesion but no difficulty with urination. The likely cause for this presentation is which of the following conditions?

A) Chancroid
B) Gonorrhea
C) Herpes simplex
D) Molluscum contagiosum
E) Syphilis

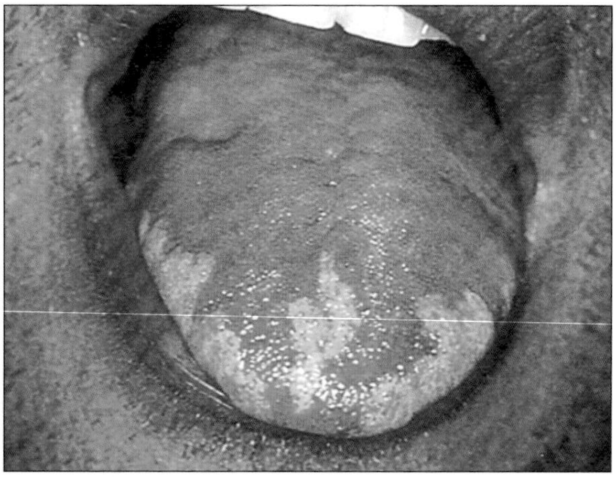

Reproduced with permission from Neville BW, Damm DD, White DK. *Color Atlas of Clinical Oral Pathology*. 2nd ed. Williams & Wilkins; 1998.

19. Which of the following conditions is associated with the tongue finding shown here?

A) Gastroesophageal reflux
B) Hypothyroidism
C) Human immunodeficiency syndrome
D) Periodontitis
E) Vitamin B_{12} deficiency

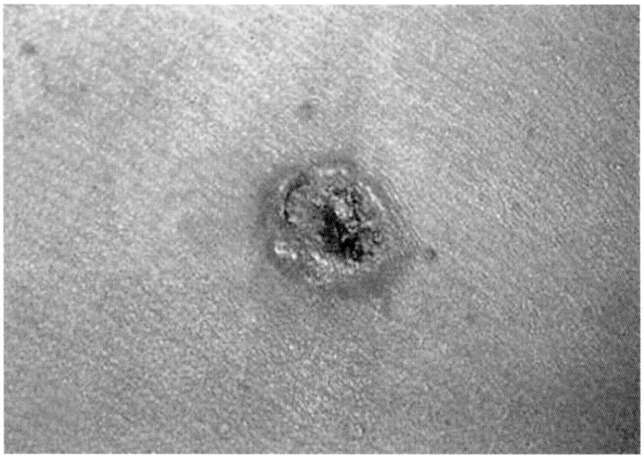

Reproduced with permission from Domino FJ, Baldor RA, Barry KA, Golding J, Stephens MB. *The 5-Minute Clinical Consult 2023*. 31st ed. Wolters Kluwer; 2023.

20. An older gentleman presents concern over the lesion pictured, which has developed on his neck. He has been putting a topical antibacterial ointment on it for the past couple of months, but it seems to be slowly enlarging. The most likely diagnosis is which one of the following?

A) Basal cell carcinoma
B) Dermatofibroma
C) Keratoacanthoma
D) Melanoma
E) Molluscum contagiosum

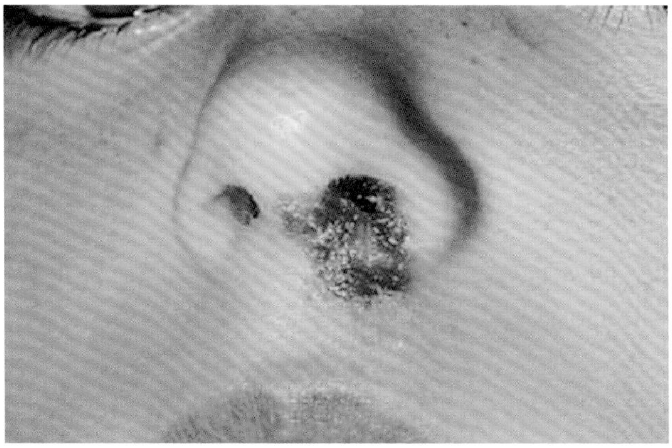

Reproduced with permission from Smeltzer SC, Bare BG. *Brunner & Suddarth's Textbook of Medical-Surgical Nursing*. 9th ed. Lippincott Williams & Wilkins; 2000.

21. A young boy is brought in by his mother with a crusted honey-brown lesion that affects his nose as shown above. The best treatment for this condition is which one of the following?

A) Intramuscular ceftriaxone
B) Oral ciprofloxacin
C) Oral acyclovir
D) Topical hydrocortisone cream
E) Topical mupirocin ointment

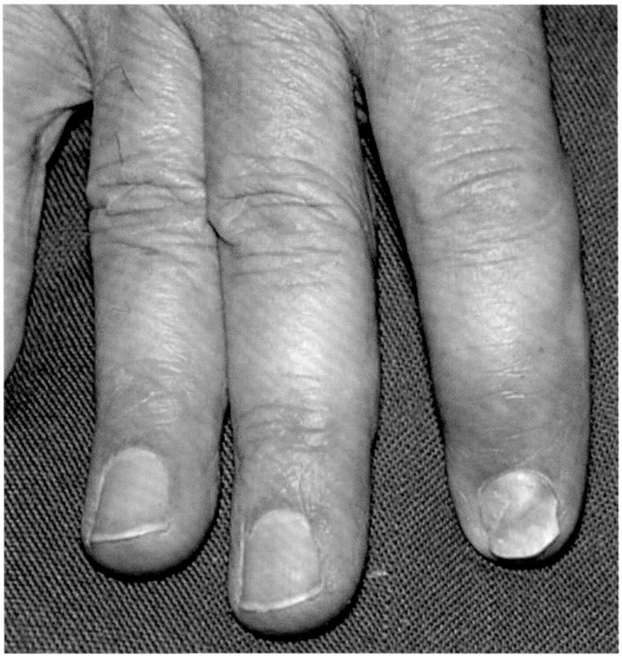

Reproduced with permission from Goodheart H. *Goodheart's Photoguide to Common Pediatric and Adult Skin Disorders*. 3rd ed. Wolters Kluwer; 2009.

22. A 43-year-old woman reports that she has had to use nail polish to cover her fingernails over the past couple of years because they look like those pictured above. The most likely diagnosis to account for this change in her nails is which one of the following conditions?

A) Chronic obstructive pulmonary disease
B) Onychomycosis
C) Psoriasis
D) Scleroderma

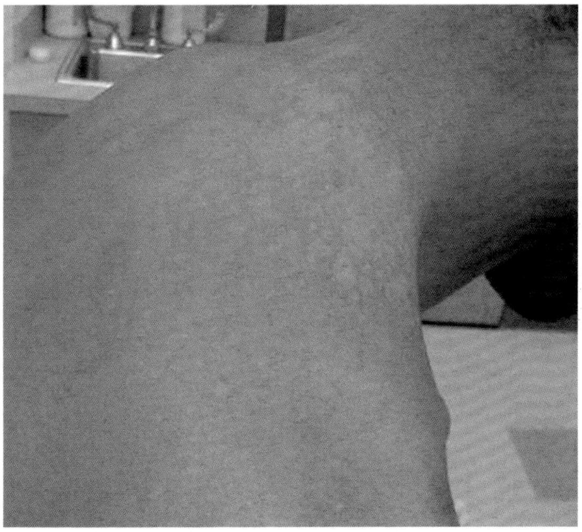

Reproduced with permission from Domino FJ, Baldor RA, Barry KA, Golding J, Stephens MB. *The 5-Minute Clinical Consult 2023*. 31st ed. Wolters Kluwer; 2023.

23. A 21-year-old lifeguard presents with a concern over his skin, as seen above. The most likely diagnosis for this finding is which one of the following conditions?

A) Eczema
B) Pityriasis rosea
C) Secondary syphilis
D) Seborrheic dermatitis
E) Tinea versicolor

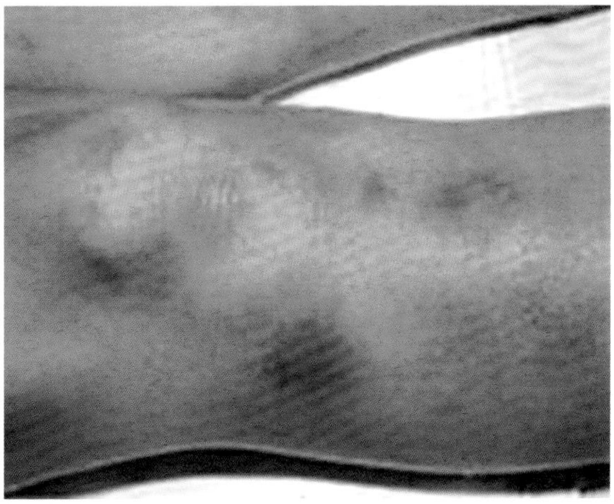

24. A 23-year-old teacher presents complaining of tender nodules that have developed on her lower legs. She is otherwise healthy and has no other symptoms. She denies any fevers and has no history of recent trauma. She takes an oral contraceptive but has not started any new medications. The likely diagnosis to explain her presentation is which one of the following conditions?

A) Erythema multiforme
B) Erythema nodosum
C) Lyme disease
D) Pyoderma gangrenosum
E) Rheumatoid arthritis

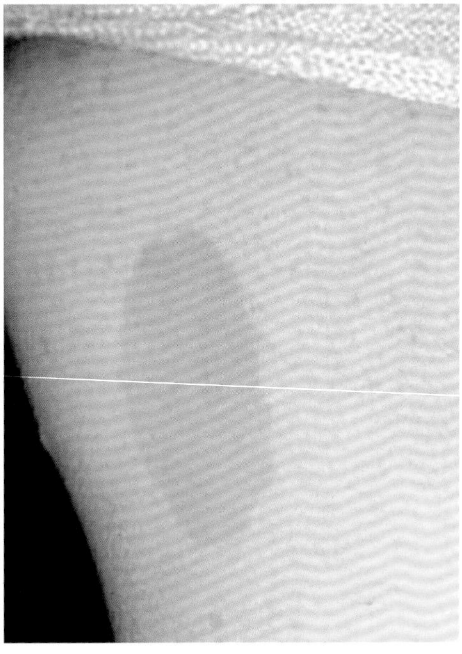

Reproduced with permission from Nelson LB, Olitsky SE. *Harley's Pediatric Ophthalmology*. Lippincott Williams & Wilkins; 2014.

25. A 19-year-old student is seen with complaints of a cough. As you listen to his lungs with your stethoscope, you notice the lesion shown above. When you ask if he has seen a dermatologist, he states that his father has similar lesions, and he was taken to see a specialist when he was a child. The differential diagnosis for this finding would include which of the following conditions?

A) Addison disease
B) Gardner syndrome
C) Hypothyroidism
D) Multiple sclerosis
E) Neurofibromatosis

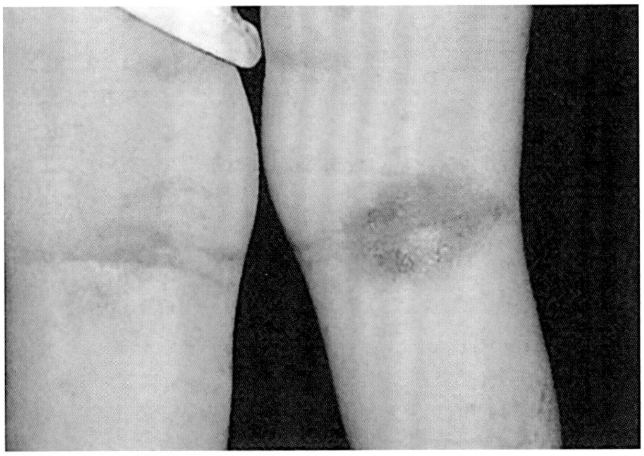

Reproduced with permission from Goodheart H. *Goodheart's Photoguide to Common Pediatric and Adult Skin Disorders*. 3rd ed. Wolters Kluwer; 2009.

26. A 3-year-old child is brought in by his mother, who is concerned about an itchy rash behind his knees that has been getting worse over the winter. The most likely diagnosis for this presentation is which of the following?

A) Atopic dermatitis
B) Dyshidrotic eczema
C) Ichthyosis vulgaris
D) Scabies
E) Tinea corporis

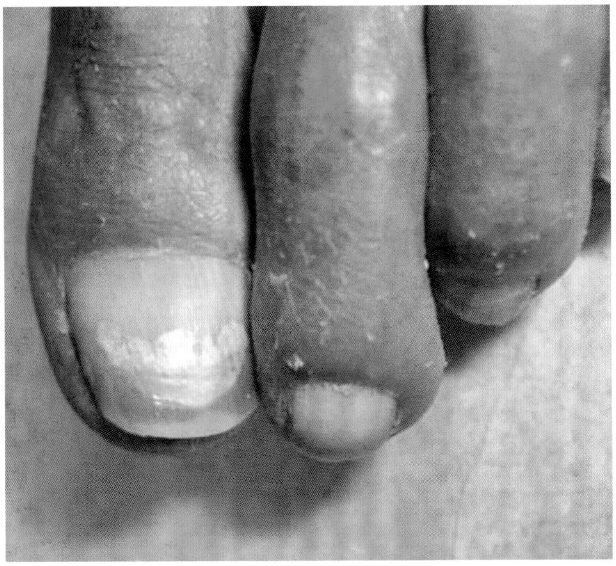

Reproduced with permission from *Stedman's Illustrated Guide of Dermatology Eponyms*. Wolters Kluwer; 2004.

27. A 47-year-old runner presents with concern over the condition of his toenails, which is slowly worsening, as seen above. The most common infectious agent that gives rise to this condition is which one of the following?

A) *Aspergillus flavus*
B) *Candida glabrata*
C) *Candida albicans*
D) *Epidermophyton floccosum*
E) *Trichophyton rubrum*

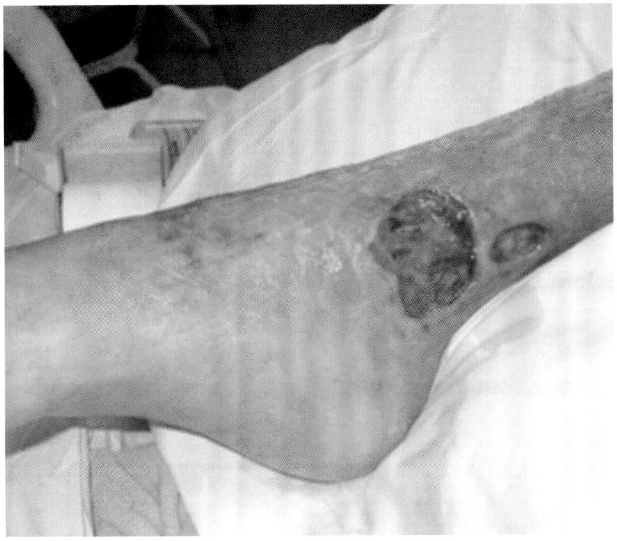

Reproduced with permission from McNichol LL, Ratliff C, Yates S. *Wound, Ostomy and Continence Nurses Society® Core Curriculum: Wound Management*. 2nd ed. Lippincott Williams & Wilkins; 2021.

28. A 67-year-old man with a history of coronary artery disease and atrial fibrillation presents complaining of a painful lesion on his foot. He reports that, in addition, he has been experiencing pain in his lower legs when walking even short distances over the past year. The most likely diagnosis for this lesion is which one of the following?

A) Arterial ulcer
B) Basal cell carcinoma
C) Diabetic foot ulcer
D) Livedo reticularis
E) Venous stasis ulcer

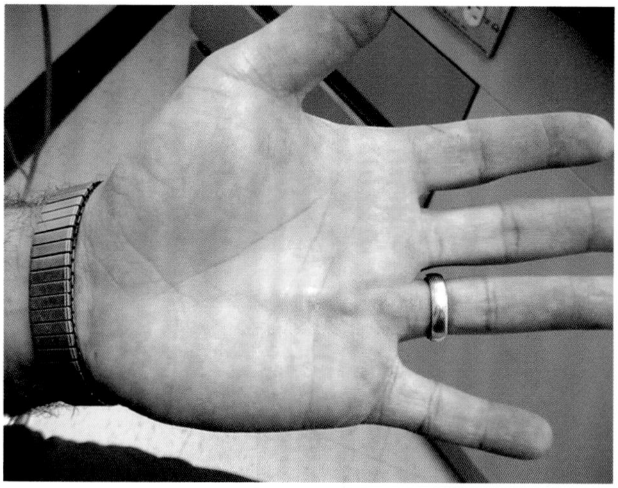

Reproduced with permission from Weisel SW. *Operative Techniques in Orthopaedic Surgery*. 2nd ed. Wolters Kluwer; 2015.

29. A 44-year-old carpenter presents complaining of painful lumps that have developed on the palm of his left hand, as shown. He denies any injury and although he works as a carpenter, he holds his hammer and most tools in his right hand. The lumps seem to be slowly enlarging, and he is now having some trouble fully opening his hand. This condition is most consistent with:

A) Ganglion cysts
B) Trigger finger
C) Dupuytren contracture
D) Camptodactyly

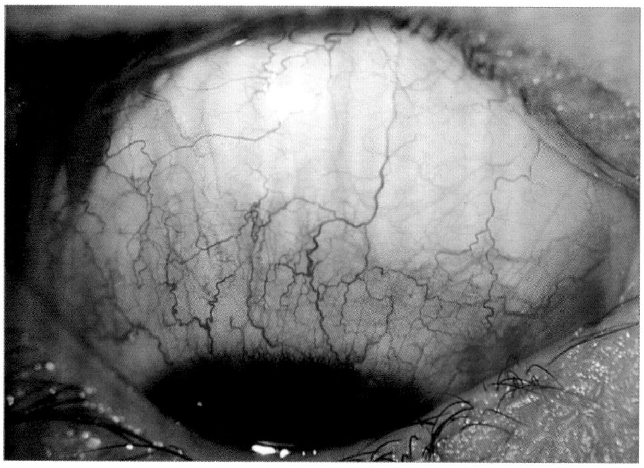

Reproduced with permission from Tasman W, Jaeger E. *The Wills Eye Hospital Atlas of Clinical Ophthalmology*. 2nd ed. Lippincott Williams & Wilkins; 2001. Figure 1.60A.

30. A 37-year-old schoolteacher presents with complaints of an itchy red right eye as shown. She thinks that she has gotten "pink-eye" from one of her students. Her eye is itchy, but she has not had any discharge and no issues with her vision. You advise treatment with which of the following:

A) Topical antibacterial eye drops
B) Topical moisturizing eye drops
C) Topical antibacterial ointment
D) Topical ophthalmic steroid drops

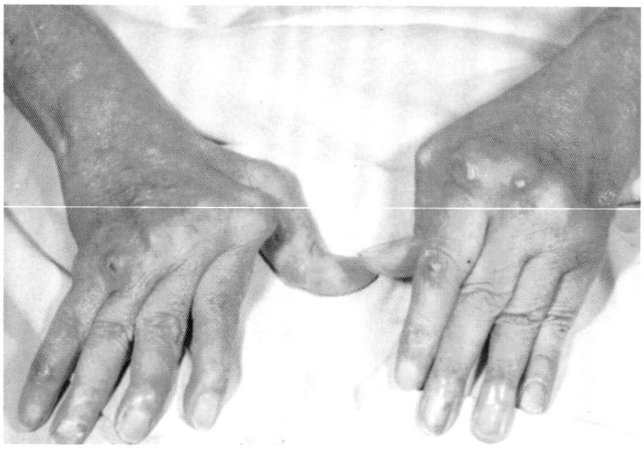

Reproduced with permission from Rubin E, Reisner HM. *Principles of Rubin's Pathology*. 7th ed. Wolters Kluwer, 2018.

31. A 57-year-old administrative assistant presents with her husband as she is having more trouble with her hands and is asking about being on disability as she struggles to complete her work and now even has trouble getting dressed in the morning. Her hands have always been bumpy, but they have been getting worse over the past few years as shown. After examining her hands, you diagnose her with which of the following conditions?

A) Osteoarthritis
B) Sjögren syndrome
C) Rheumatoid arthritis
D) Tophaceous gout

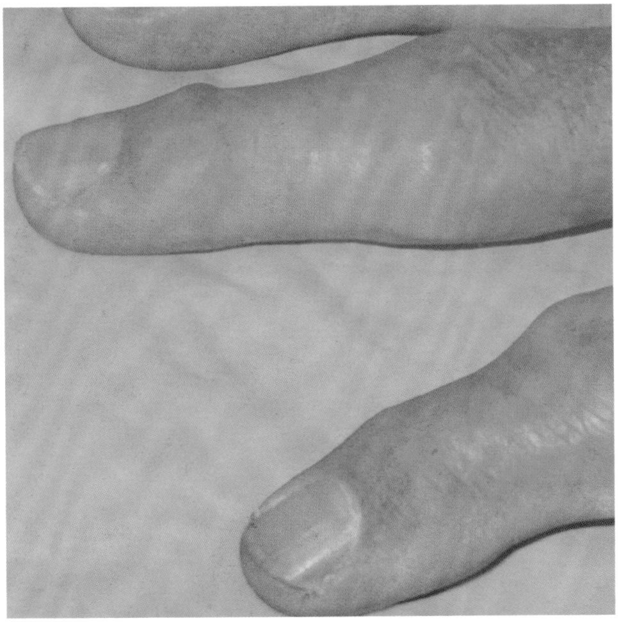

Reproduced with permission from Berg D, Worzala K. *Atlas of Adult Physical Diagnosis*. Lippincott Williams & Wilkins; 2006. Figure 14.60.

32. A 49-year-old mechanic presents complaining of hard lumps that have been slowly growing on his fingers over the past couple of years, as shown. They do not hurt, but he is worried that he may be developing a bone cancer and wanted to have them checked out. After an examination, you reassure him of the benign nature of these lumps and inform him that these lesions are called:

A) Bony exostosis
B) Ganglion cysts
C) Heberden nodules
D) Tophi

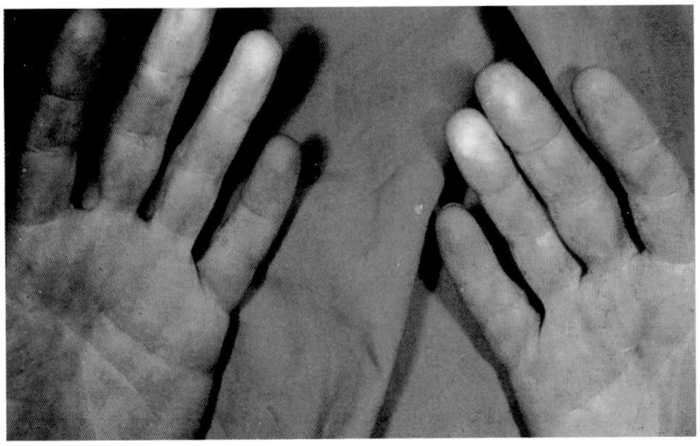

Reproduced with permission from Rubin E, Reisner HM. *Principles of Rubin's Pathology*. 7th ed. Wolters Kluwer; 2018.

33. A 32-year-old nurse presents complaining that her fingers turn white and become painful when she forgets to wear her mittens during the cold weather, as seen here. This seems to be getting worse and she is worried that she has frost bite. She is otherwise healthy and does not smoke. She takes an oral contraceptive daily, otherwise no other medications. After her exam, you advise that she should have which of the following diagnostic tests?

A) Upper extremity arteriogram
B) Upper extremity EMG
C) Venous duplex scan
D) Antinuclear antibody titer

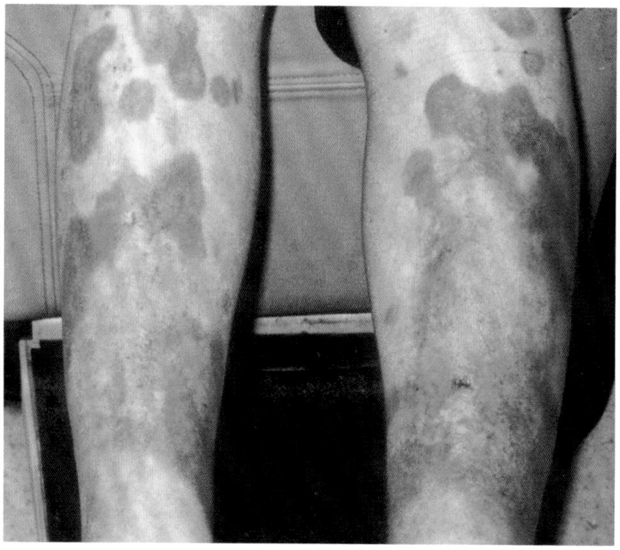

Reproduced with permission from Berg D, Worzala K. *Atlas of Adult Physical Diagnosis*. Lippincott Williams & Wilkins; 2006. Figure 10.27.

34. Louise, a 45-year-old patient of yours, has struggled with her diabetes care for years. First diagnosed at the age of 19, she is on daily insulin and checks her blood sugar levels frequently. She is always worried about passing out from low blood sugar levels, which happened to her once a few years back. Her hemoglobin A1c levels tend to run around 8. Today she is concerned over a rash that has slowly developed on her legs as seen here. This finding is known as:

A) Acanthosis nigricans
B) Bullosis diabeticorum
C) Necrobiosis lipoidica
D) Diabetic dermopathy

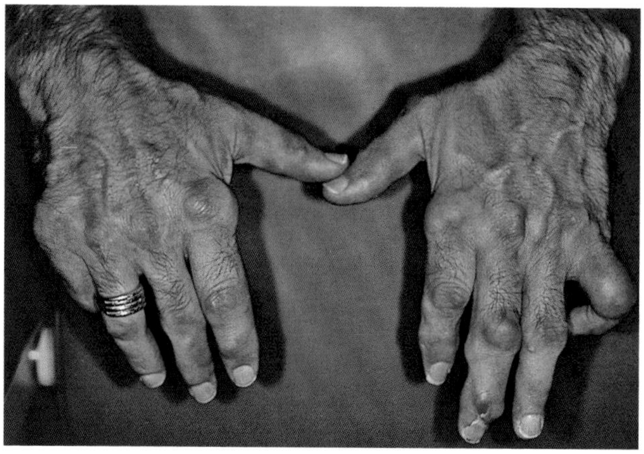

Reproduced with permission from Gold DH, Weingeist TA. *Color Atlas of the Eye in Systemic Disease*. Lippincott Williams & Wilkins; 2001. Figure 91.1.

35. A 53-year-old truck driver presents complaining of painful lumps that have been developing on his fingers over the past year, as shown. They have become red and swollen over the past couple of days and he is worried that he has an infection as he was on a fishing trip with his buddies this past weekend with his "drinking buddies" and stuck himself with a fishing hook. He admits to drinking beer frequently, but other than some "arthritis" in his left knee, he thinks he is healthy. After an examination, you note that it is unlikely that he has an infection and inform him that these lesions are called:

A) Bony exostosis
B) Ganglion cysts
C) Heberden nodules
D) Tophi

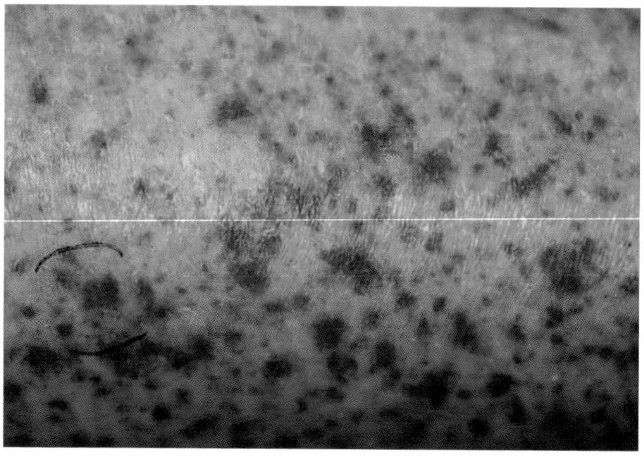

Reproduced with permission from Schalock PC, Hsu JT, Arndt KA. *Lippincott's Primary Care Dermatology*. Lippincott Williams & Wilkins; 2010.

36. You are seeing a 64-year-old painter who comes in with a rash on his lower legs. He has been healthy, although he takes a statin for high cholesterol and was recently treated with an antibiotic for a methicillin-resistant *Staphylococcus aureus* infection. Looking at his legs you observe this rash. You would use which of the following descriptors in your call to the local dermatologist for advice, stating he has a rash consisting of:

A) Petechiae and purpura
B) Pustules and papules
C) Erythematous plaques
D) Macular/papular eruptions

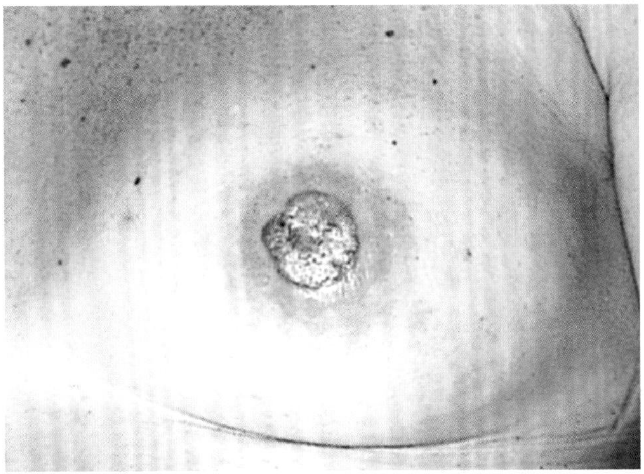

Reproduced with permission from Weber J, Kelley J. *Health Assessment in Nursing*. 2nd ed. Lippincott Williams & Wilkins; 2003.

37. Louise, a 63-year-old schoolteacher, comes in with concern over an "itchy nipple." She has type 2 diabetes mellitus and takes metformin daily. She is prone to yeast infections under her breast and thought she now had an infection on her nipple. She has been applying an over-the-counter antifungal ointment for the past few weeks, but it is not any better and she is requesting a prescription antifungal medication. You exam the breasts and see this lesion on her nipple. You inform her that the diagnosis is most likely which one of the following?

A) Eczema/atopic dermatitis
B) Psoriasis
C) Bowen disease
D) Paget disease
E) Lichen simplex chronicus

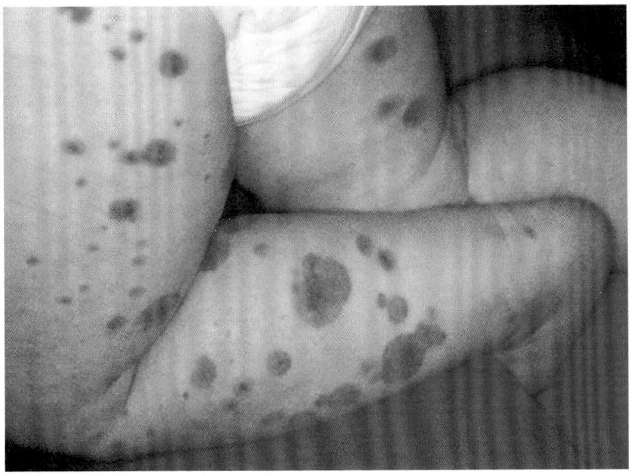

Reproduced with permission from Fleisher GR, Ludwig W, Baskin MN. *Atlas of Pediatric Emergency Medicine*. Lippincott Williams & Wilkins; 2004.

38. A mother brings her 3-year-old son in to be seen with complaint of a rash. He had a cold a week ago, but recovered without incident but developed the rash last evening and this morning complained of a stomachache and did not want to eat any breakfast. He has been drinking ok and has not had a fever. The rash looks like tiny, raised bruises as shown. This rash finding is most consistent with which one of the following conditions?

A) Meningococcemia
B) Rocky Mountain spotted fever
C) Henoch-Schönlein purpura
D) Rheumatic fever
E) Kawasaki disease

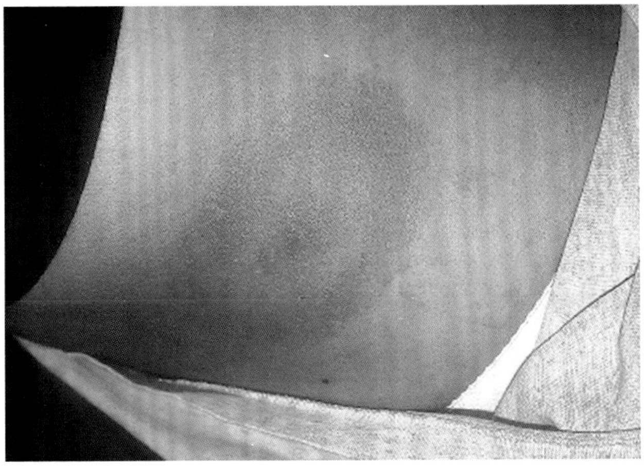

Reproduced with permission from Harpavat S, Nissim S. *Lippincott Microcards: Microbiology Flash Cards*. 4th ed. Wolters Kluwer; 2015.

39. A 37-year-old landscaper comes to see you as she has a rash that developed overnight on her side. She thinks she may have gotten a bug bite but does not remember actually getting bitten. She was trimming an overgrown hedge last week and thinks that she was rubbing up against some poison ivy. She feels fine, and denies fever or any constitutional complaints. She has no known allergies. You decide to treat her with which one of the following?

A) Doxycycline 200 mg once
B) Doxycycline 100 mg BID for 10 days
C) Azithromycin 500 mg QD for 10 days
D) Amoxicillin 500 mg TID for 28 days

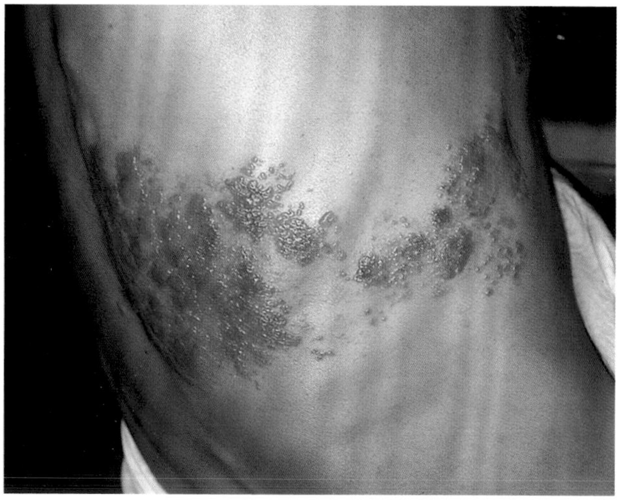

Reproduced with permission from Hogan-Quigley B, Palm ML. *Bates' Nursing Guide to Physical Examination and History Taking*. 3rd ed. Wolters Kluwer; 2021.

40. You are seeing a 53-year-old patient who complains of an irritated rash on his side as shown here. It is red and irritated and somewhat painful. You have been treating him for hypertension and type 2 diabetes mellitus, both of which have been well controlled. He denies fever and has no joint complaints. You decide to treat him with which one of the following?

A) Valacyclovir: 1000 mg TID for 7 days
B) Prednisone 50 mg tapering over 7 days
C) Oxycodone 5 mg QID PRN until gone
D) Sulfamethoxazole 800 mg/trimethoprim 160 mg BID for 7 days

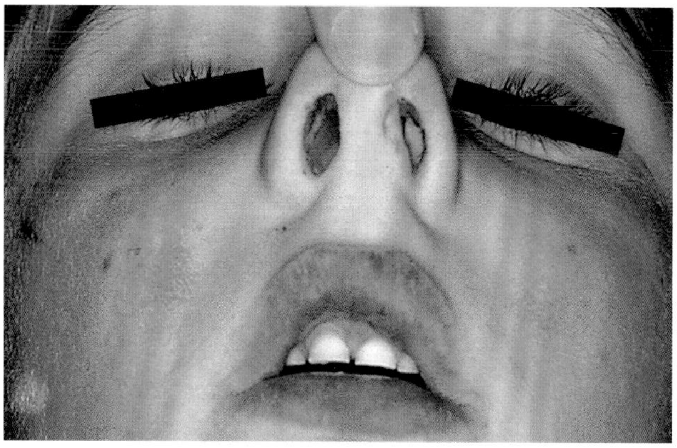

Reproduced with permission from Fleisher GR, Ludwig W, Baskin MN. *Atlas of Pediatric Emergency Medicine*. Lippincott Williams & Wilkins; 2004.

41. A mother brings her 5-year-old daughter in to be seen as she has been sneezing a lot and she thinks that there is something stuck in her nose. She is relatively healthy but tends to be an "allergic kid." She has been treated for eczema in the past and had an episode of wheezing this past winter when she had a bad cold. You examine the child and decide on which of the following?

A) Reassure the mother as nasal polyps are often seen with allergic conditions
B) Send to ENT for a biopsy
C) Obtain a sweat test
D) Prescribe a nasal steroid inhaler to be used BID × 1 month

Answer and Explanations to Section I

1. The answer is E: The image is of a cholesteatoma, a keratinized mass in the middle ear or mastoid, which can occur either as a primary lesion or secondary to tympanic membrane perforation. Cholesteatomas may result in erosion of the ossicles in the middle ear and consequent hearing loss. In rare cases, they can erode directly into the inner ear.

Cholesteatoma removal is typically performed in conjunction with tympanoplasty and, if the lesion extends superiorly or posteriorly, mastoidectomy (tympanomastoidectomy).

Additional Reading: Chronic otitis media, cholesteatoma, and mastoiditis in adults. In: Basow DS, ed. *UpToDate*. UpToDate; 2022.

2. The answer is D: A complete excision with normal skin margins is preferable as an excisional biopsy for any pigmented lesions suspicious for a melanoma. The treatment and prognosis is based on the depth of the lesion, and the patient may require a larger re-excision following the biopsy results. Shave biopsies should be avoided because they may not allow for accurate depth measurement. Lesions that are less than 0.76 mm thick are not associated with metastatic disease and have a 99.5% 10-year survival. Treatment recommendations include the following:

Depth of Invasion	Surgical Margin	Other Considerations
<0.5 mm deep	1 cm	
0.5-1 mm deep	1 to 2 cm	
>1 mm deep	3 cm with underlying fat/fascia	Sentinel node biopsy

Additional Reading: Cutaneous malignant melanoma: a primary care perspective. *Am Fam Physician*. 2012;85(2):161-168.

3. The answer is B: Cutaneous larva migrans is also called the creeping eruption. The causative agent is a hookworm (*Ancylostoma duodenale* and *Necator americanus*). The organisms are found in the feces of dogs, cats, cattle, and monkeys. The larvae penetrate human skin (usually the feet after walking barefoot). The condition is more common in gardeners, sea bathers, plumbers, and farmers. The lesion presents as a thin erythematous, serpiginous, raised tunnel-like lesion. The larvae die in 4 to 6 weeks; thus, the eruption is typically benign and self-limited. Treatment consists of topical steroids, topical or oral thiabendazole, albendazole, or liquid nitrogen.

Bathing suit dermatitis is also known as cercarial dermatitis, which is an allergic reaction to a schistosome infection from swimming in contaminated water. The bumpy, red rash usually occurs on areas not covered by a bathing suit.

Jellyfish stings cause instant pain and inflamed marks on the skin, from microscopic, barbed stingers on their tentacles. Most get better over a few days with home (vinegar compresses) treatment. In rare cases, they cause life-threatening reactions.

Swimming pool granuloma appears as a reddish to purple papule that slowly enlarges to become a painful nodule. This is a chronic skin infection caused by the bacteria *Mycobacterium marinum*, from swimming in contaminated water or contact with fish tanks.

Additional Reading: Acute pruritic rash on the foot. *Am Fam Physician*. 2010;81(2):203-204.

4. The answer is B: Pityriasis rosea is a self-limited, exanthematous skin disease that develops acutely and is characterized by the appearance of slightly inflammatory, oval, papulosquamous lesions on the trunk and proximal areas of the extremities. Pityriasis rosea is largely a disease of older children and young adults. It is more common in women than in men. A prodrome of headache, malaise, and pharyngitis may occur in a small number of cases, but except for mild itching, the condition is usually asymptomatic. The eruption commonly begins with a "herald patch": a single round or oval, sharply demarcated pink or salmon-colored lesion on the chest, neck, or back, 2 to 5 cm in diameter. The lesion soon becomes scaly and begins to clear centrally, leaving the free edge of the scaly lesion directed inward toward the center. A few days or a week or two later, oval lesions similar in appearance to the herald patch, but smaller, appear in crops on the trunk and proximal areas of the extremities. The long axes of these oval lesions tend to be oriented along the lines of cleavage of the skin. This characteristic "Christmas-tree" pattern is most evident on the back, where it is emphasized by the oblique direction of the cleavage lines in that location.

Most cases of pityriasis rosea need no treatment other than reassurance and proper patient education. Topical steroids with moderate potency are helpful in the control of itching. They can be applied to the pruritic areas two or three times daily.

Coccidioidomycosis is a fungal infection that is also known as San Joaquin Valley fever or Valley fever. It occurs in the western United States, Mexico, and Central and South America. It primarily affects the lungs and presents as a respiratory condition. Skin changes may include papules, nodules, pustules, abscesses, ulcers, and scars.

Psoriasis presents with inflamed scaly patches that are covered with thick, silvery scales.

Tinea versicolor presents as flaky discolored patches on the trunk and shoulders. It is due to a superficial skin infection with *Malassezia* yeast.

Varicella is also known as chickenpox, a highly contagious disease caused by the varicella-zoster virus. It causes an itchy, blisterlike rash (characterized as a "dew drop on a rose petal"), accompanied by a fever. The rash first appears on the chest, back, and face, and then spreads over the entire body.

Additional Reading: Pityriasis rosea. In: Domino F, ed. *The 5-Minute Clinical Consult*. Wolters Kluwer; 2022.

5. The answer is A: Poison ivy or poison oak is also referred to as rhus dermatitis. The condition is associated with intensely pruritic vesicles, papules, and blisters often arranged in characteristic linear or streaklike patterns where the plant has made contact with the skin. The plant contains a resinous oil that gives rise to the allergic response.

Symptoms of poison ivy in sensitized individuals generally develop within 4 to 96 hours after exposure and peak between 1 and 14 days after exposure. New lesions can present up to 21 days after exposure in previously unexposed individuals. Lesions may occur at different points in time depending on the degree of exposure to different points on the skin and the thickness of the exposed skin. This may give the impression that the poison ivy is spreading from one region to another. Blister fluid is not antigenic and is not responsible for spreading the rash.

Without treatment, poison ivy dermatitis usually resolves in 1 to 3 weeks. High-potency topical steroids or oral corticosteroids are often necessary for treatment, particularly if poison ivy dermatitis is on the face. The most common complication of poison ivy dermatitis is secondary bacterial infection of the skin with *S aureus* or β-hemolytic group A *Streptococcus*. Bacterial infections can be polymicrobial.

Herpes zoster is also known as shingles and produces an erythematous eruption that is seen in a dermatomal distribution, due to reactivation of the virus years after the original infection.

Lichen sclerosis is an uncommon condition that creates patchy, white skin usually affecting the genital and anal areas. Anyone can get lichen sclerosis, but postmenopausal women are at higher risk.

Erythema multiforme comes on suddenly and develops over a few days. It typically starts as small red spots on the hands or feet, before spreading to the limbs, upper body, and face. The spots become raised patches that look like a target lesion with a darker center that may blister or crust.

Varicella is also known as chickenpox, a highly contagious disease caused by the varicella-zoster virus. It causes an itchy, blisterlike rash (characterized as a "dew drop on a rose petal"), accompanied by a fever. The rash first appears on the chest, back, and face, and then spreads over the entire body.

Additional Reading: Diagnosis and management of contact dermatitis. *Am Fam Physician*. 2010; 82(3):249-255.

6. The answer is A: Keratosis pilaris presents as hyperkeratotic follicular papules on the extensor surface of the upper arms or upper anterior thighs and occasionally on the malar area of the face. It may be associated with atopy and dry skin. A sandpaperlike feel is noted in these isolated areas. The condition is considered benign and is treated with topical lactic acid cream or lotion. Lesions that are associated with the face typically resolve at puberty.

Psoriasis presents with inflamed scaly patches that are covered with thick, silvery scales. Rheumatic fever is an inflammatory disease that can develop after an infection with *Streptococcus* bacteria. Although strep throat is common, rheumatic fever is rare in the United States. The skin sign of acute rheumatic fever is erythema marginatum, which occasionally presents with a characteristic annular erythema on the trunk and upper arms and legs, but almost never on the face, palms, or soles. The rash appears as pink, red macules or papules, which spread outward in a circular shape. As the lesions advance, the edges become raised and red, and the center clears. The lesions can fade and reappear within hours, often unnoticed by the patient, and may persist intermittently for weeks after treatment.

Scarlet fever, also known as scarlatina, develops in some children with a strep throat. Such patients will typically have a high fever with a bright red rash that looks like a sunburn and feels like sandpaper. It typically begins on the face or neck and spreads to the rest of the body with an associated "strawberry tongue."

Seborrheic dermatitis is a relatively common skin condition that mainly affects the scalp, resulting in dandruff. However, it also presents as scaly, red patches on oily areas of the face and chest.

Additional Reading: The generalized rash: Part II. Diagnostic approach. *Am Fam Physician*. 2010;81(6):735-739.

7. The answer is D: Scabies is associated with intense pruritus that is noted predominantly at night. The lesions are brownish and often form irregular burrow lines that may be marked with scaling at one end and a vesicle at the other end. The lesions are typically found in intertriginous areas and warm, protected areas such as the finger webs, inframammary areas, and axilla. The mite *Sarcoptes scabiei* is responsible. Scabies is contracted by being in close contact with an infected individual. The most common way scabies is acquired in the United States is via children in daycare settings. Scrapings of the lesion are treated with 10% potassium hydroxide (KOH) solution and studied under light microscopy. The mite is often identified. Treatment consists of permethrin cream 5% applied from head to toes and left in place for 12 hours before being washed off. Lindane can also be used as an alternative, but not in infants or in pregnant women.

Dyshidrotic eczema and scabies both cause small blisters on the skin. Dyshidrotic eczema blisters usually appear as a sudden rash on the sides of fingers and toes. The blisters tend to clear over 2 to 3 weeks, leaving the skin cracked, dry, and red. Many patients also have other types of eczema such as contact or atopic dermatitis.

Poison ivy (rhus dermatitis) causes a blistery, itchy rash seen in a geographic distribution where the plant leaves have come in contact with the skin.

Psoriasis presents with inflamed scaly patches that are covered with thick, silvery scales.

Tinea corporis, also known as ringworm, is a common fungal infection that presents as a red or silvery ringlike rash anywhere on the body. It is most commonly cause by *T rubrum*, a dermatophyte that lives off keratin. It has nothing to do with a worm.

Additional Reading: Scabies. In: Domino F, ed. *The 5-Minute Clinical Consult*. Wolters Kluwer; 2022.

8. The answer is B: Hidradenitis suppurativa is a painful, erythematous, and nodular condition that affects the axilla, genitalia, and perianal areas. Hallmarks for the disease include open comedones, enlarged follicular orifices, and scarring. Nodules become inflamed and pus-filled, rupture, drain pus and blood, and then cause scarring. Sinus tracts can form. The disease often waxes and wanes. *Staphylococcus* bacteria are frequently the causative agent. Treatment consists of appropriate antibacterial agents based on culture and sensitivities. Intralesional corticosteroids can also be used to reduce the inflammatory response. For severe cases, excision and skin grafting may be necessary. The condition may regress as the patient approaches middle age.

Antiperspirant dermatitis is an erythematous rash that develops because of either an allergic or irritant contact dermatitis.

Impetigo is a superficial skin infection mainly seen in young children. Staphylococci are usually implicated in the infection, which appears as reddish blisters on the face, especially around the nose and mouth and on the hands and feet. As the blisters burst, they leave honey-colored crusts.

Scrofuloderma presents as firm, painless, subcutaneous, red-brown nodules that occur as a direct extension from an underlying focus of tuberculous infection. The neck, axillae, and groin are often involved. The nodules evolve, ulcerating and developing sinus tracts.

Tinea corporis, also known as ringworm, is a common fungal infection that presents as a red or silvery ringlike rash anywhere on the body. It is most commonly caused by *T rubrum*, a dermatophyte that lives off keratin. It has nothing to do with a worm.

Additional Reading: Hidradenitis suppurativa. In: Domino F, ed. *The 5-Minute Clinical Consult*. Lippincott Williams & Wilkins; 2022.

9. The answer is C: Rosacea is associated with areas of erythema and telangiectasia on the face. It is exacerbated by sunlight, hot or spicy foods, and alcohol. Pronounced rosacea may appear as acneiform papules, pustules, or ruddiness. Northern Europeans and those of Celtic descent are most commonly affected. Treatment involves oral tetracycline or doxycycline. Topical metronidazole is also effective for milder cases.

Additional Reading: Acne rosacea. In: Domino F, ed. *The 5-Minute Clinical Consult*. Wolters Kluwer; 2022.

10. The answer is D: Psoriasis typically involves the scalp (including the postauricular regions), the extensor surface of the extremities (particularly elbows and knees), the sacral area, buttocks, and penis. The nails, eyebrows, axillae, umbilicus, or anogenital region may also be affected. More severe cases affect multiple areas over the entire body. Typical lesions are well-demarcated, variously pruritic, ovoid or circular, erythematous papules or plaques covered with overlapping thick silver-appearing, slightly opalescent shiny scales. Papules sometimes extend and coalesce to produce large plaques in annular patterns. The lesions heal without scarring, and hair growth is usually unaltered. The condition appears to be hereditary. Diagnosis is usually based on clinical findings. Skin biopsy may be helpful for definitive diagnosis. Treatment consists of topical steroids, intralesional steroids, tar preparations, anthralin, tazarotene, and calcipotriene.

Mycosis fungoides is a cutaneous type of non-Hodgkin T-cell lymphoma that occurs in the skin. Skin changes are variable from flat, to thicker, raised, scaly patches that can be mistaken for eczema. Tumors develop as papules or nodules, which may or may not ulcerate.

Nummular eczema, also known as discoid eczema, presents as scattered circular patches anywhere on the skin. This is named after the Latin word for "coin," as the spots appear coin-shaped on the skin.

Pityriasis rosacea develops acutely and is characterized by the appearance of slightly inflammatory, oval, papulosquamous lesions on the trunk and proximal areas of the extremities. The eruption commonly begins with a "herald patch": a single round or oval, sharply demarcated pink or salmon-colored lesion.

Tinea corporis, also known as ringworm, is a common fungal infection that presents as a red or silvery ringlike rash anywhere on the body. It is most commonly cause by *T rubrum*, a dermatophyte that lives off keratin. It has nothing to do with a worm.

Additional Reading: Psoriasis. In: Domino F, ed. *The 5-Minute Clinical Consult*. Wolters Kluwer; 2022.

11. The answer is E: Varicella generally develops 10 to 14 days after an exposure and typically includes a prodrome of fever, malaise, or pharyngitis, followed by the development of a generalized vesicular rash, usually within 24 hours. The lesions are commonly pruritic and appear as groups of vesicles over a 3- to 4-day period. The classic description is of a "dew drop on a rose petal," as the vesicles are on an erythematous base. The patient with varicella typically has lesions in different stages of development on the face, trunk, and extremities. New lesion formation generally stops within 4 days, and most lesions have fully crusted by day 6 in normal hosts. The patient remains contagious until all of the lesions have crusted over. Chickenpox is rarely seen in the United States since the widespread administration of the varicella vaccine.

Fifth disease, also called erythema infectiosum, is a mild rash illness caused by parvovirus B19. It got its name because it was fifth in a list of historical classifications of common skin rash illnesses in children. The most recognized feature is a red rash on the face called "slapped cheek" rash. Some develop a second rash a few days later on their chest, back, buttocks, or arms and legs.

Measles, also called rubeola, is relatively rare in the United States. It typically begins with a mild fever, cough, runny nose, sore throat, and conjunctivitis. A papular rash appears on the face, with a splotchy red appearance, then spreads down the arms, chest and back, onto the thighs, legs and feet. At the same time, the fever spikes often as high as 104 to 105 °F (40-41 °C).

Rocky Mountain spotted fever (RMSF) is caused by the tick-borne bacteria *Rickettsia rickettsii*. A rash usually develops 2 to 4 days after a fever. The initial rash presents as small, flat, pink macules on the wrists, forearms, and ankles and spreads to include the trunk and sometimes the palms of hands and soles of feet. The petechial rash of RMSF does not typically appear until day 5 to 6 of illness and is a sign of severe disease.

Scarlatina, also known as scarlet fever, develops in some children with a strep throat. Such patients will typically have a high fever with a bright red rash that looks like a sunburn and feels like sandpaper. It typically begins on the face or neck and spreads to the rest of the body with an associated "strawberry tongue."

Additional Reading: Chickenpox (varicella zoster). In: Domino F, ed. *The 5-Minute Clinical Consult*. Wolters Kluwer; 2022.

12. The answer is A: Molluscum contagiosum is a common, superficial viral infection of the skin that typically occurs in infants and preschoolers. The incidence decreases after the age of 6 to 7 years. The condition can be spread via sexual contact in young adults. The lesions are dome-shaped, waxy, or pearly white papules with a central white core and are 1 to 3 mm in diameter. Frequently, groups of lesions are found. The lesions may resolve spontaneously.

Treatment involves removal with a sharp needle or curette, application of liquid nitrogen, antiwart preparations, electrodesiccation and curettage, or trichloroacetic peels for extensive areas. Typically, infants or young preschool-age children should not be treated aggressively.

Poison ivy (rhus dermatitis) causes a blistery, itchy rash seen in a geographic distribution where the plant leaves have come in contact with the skin.

Scabies is associated with intense pruritus that is noted predominantly at night. The lesions are brownish and often form irregular burrow lines that may be marked with scaling at one end and a vesicle at the other end. The lesions are typically found in intertriginous areas and warm, protected areas such as the finger webs, inframammary areas, and axilla.

Varicella (chickenpox) and herpes zoster (shingles) are caused by the varicella-zoster virus (VZV), a member of the herpesvirus family. The rash of varicella usually begins on the face and scalp and spreads rapidly to the trunk, with relative sparing of the extremities. Lesions are scattered, evolving from rose-colored macules to papules, vesicles, pustules, and crusts. Herpes zoster is characterized by unilateral dermatomal pain and rash that results from reactivation and multiplication of latent VZV that persisted within neurons following varicella.

Additional Reading: Molluscum contagiosum. In: Domino F, ed. *The 5-Minute Clinical Consult*. Wolters Kluwer; 2022.

13. The answer is E: Seborrheic keratoses are common skin lesions that affect the elderly. They tend to be familial. The average diameter is 1 cm, but they can grow up to 3 cm in diameter. The lesions are brown or black, oval in shape, raised, and have a "stuck on" appearance. They most commonly occur on the face, back, neck, and scalp. They may appear suddenly and become pruritic and crusted. Numerous lesions that appear rapidly in younger individuals may signal the development of an underlying malignancy. Treatment is cosmetic and usually reserved for those that are inflamed or causing symptoms. In this instance, reassurance and observation are indicated.

Additional Reading: Seborrheic keratosis. In: Domino F, ed. *The 5-Minute Clinical Consult*. Wolters Kluwer; 2022.

14. The answer is A: Cherry angiomas are common asymptomatic lesions that appear red and blanch with pressure. The diagnosis is clinical. They are more common in elderly patients. They occur more commonly on the trunk and are benign.

Chiggers, also called red bugs, live in grassy wooded areas; they are tiny larvae members of the arachnid family. Bites will generally appear as intensely itchy, inflamed, grouped papules around the ankles, waist, armpits, crotch, or behind the knees.

Erythroderma, also known as exfoliative dermatitis, is an uncommon but serious skin disorder that is the result of a drug reaction or an underlying malignancy. The condition presents as an erythematous pruritic patch, involving the head, trunk, or genital region. These patches spread to cover most of the skin surface, followed by scaling. The palms, soles, and mucous membranes are typically spared and it has also been reported that the nose and paranasal area are spared—called the "nose sign."

Granuloma annulare presents as a painless, raised rash or papules, in a ring pattern, typically affecting the hands and feet. It is not clear what causes granuloma annulare, but it has been seen following insect bites and infections, and has been rarely reported related to cancer, and occasionally associated with diabetes or thyroid disease.

Scabies is associated with intense pruritus that is noted predominantly at night. The lesions are brownish and often form irregular burrow lines that may be marked with scaling at one end and a vesicle at the other end. The lesions are typically found in intertriginous areas and warm, protected areas such as the finger webs, inframammary areas, and axilla.

Additional Reading: Diagnosing common benign skin tumors. *Am Fam Physician*. 2015;92(7):601-607.

15. The answer is D: Black hairy tongue results from hyperplasia of the filiform papillae with deposition of keratin on the surface. The condition causes the tongue to have a dark, velvety, hairlike appearance. Associated conditions include smoking, consumption of coffee, prolonged use of antibiotics, and possibly acquired immunodeficiency syndrome. Treatment involves using a toothbrush to scrape off the excess keratin that forms on the tongue's surface.

Additional Reading: Common oral lesions. *Am Fam Physician*. 2022;105(4):369-376.

16. The answer is C: Keratoacanthomas (KAs) usually develop rapidly over a 2- to 6-week time frame. The lesions are dome-shaped with a central keratin-filled plug. They occur most commonly on sun-exposed areas. KAs are clinically and histologically similar to well-differentiated squamous cell cancer (SCC). The cause of KA is not certain; however, human papillomavirus DNA has been found in some cases. KAs have also occurred in skin soon after radiation therapy. There is controversy regarding whether KAs are malignant or benign. Although they resemble SCCs histologically, most spontaneously regress with scar formation. There have been reported cases of invasive KAs, some with metastases, leading many experts to consider all KAs a form of SCC and treat them as such. Because of the uncertain malignant potential of KAs, most are treated as well-differentiated SCC. Excision is recommended; however, other treatment options include intralesional methotrexate, 5-fluorouracil, interferon, systemic retinoids, or radiation therapy. Complete excision is usually curative; however, recurrences can develop at the site of treated lesions.

Basal cell carcinoma (BCC) presents as a slowly growing nodule on sun-exposed areas of the head. The nodule eventually erodes with a central ulcer and is surrounded by a rolled border with visible telangiectasias.

Actinic keratosis is seen in sun-damaged skin and presents as slowly evolving scaly plaques.

Seborrheic keratoses are brown, waxy-looking plaques that appear "stuck-on" the skin. These benign signs of aging are rare in those less than 40 years of age.

Squamous cell carcinoma, like BCC, is typically seen in sun-exposed areas of the skin. They are scaly nodules, but unlike KAs, they grow slowly, enlarging over time.

Additional Reading: Keratoacanthoma. In: Domino F, ed. *The 5-Minute Clinical Consult*. Wolters Kluwer; 2022.

17. The answer is E: Sporotrichosis is a granulomatous fungal infection that affects the skin. The lesion is caused by *Sporothrix schenckii,* a fungus that grows on wood and in the soil. The lesions typically affect farmers, gardeners (especially those who grow roses), laborers, and miners. A primary chancre occurs at the site of inoculation. The primary lesion is painless and forms a subcutaneous nodule that breaks down to form an ulcer. Within a few weeks, multiple nodules can form along the areas of draining lymphatics and break down to form streaks of ulcers, often affecting the arms or legs. The fluid from unopened ulcers can be cultured and can aid in diagnosis. Treatment consists of saturated solution of potassium iodide, ketoconazole, or itraconazole.

Blastomycosis is a rare fungal infection caused by *Blastomyces dermatitidis*, which grows in wood and soil. The disease mainly affects the lungs with "flu-like" symptoms and may spread to other parts of the body, with the skin most commonly affected. Lesions begin as papules, pustules, or as subcutaneous nodules, typically on the face, neck, and extremities. Over time the lesions ulcerate and form crusty sores, which result in raised wartlike scars.

Coccidioidomycosis is a fungal infection that is also known as San Joaquin Valley fever or Valley fever. It occurs in the western United States, Mexico, Central and South America. Like, blastomycoses, it primarily affects the lungs and presents as a respiratory condition. Skin changes may include papules, nodules, pustules, abscesses, ulcers, and scars.

Histoplasmosis is due to an infection with the fungus *Histoplasma capsulatum* and also presents with respiratory symptoms. Skin findings are typically seen in immunocompromised individuals and may include painless mouth ulcers, pustular nodules all over the skin, and erythema nodosum or erythema multiforme on the lower legs.

Lyme disease is a tick-borne infection and will present with typical mildly inflamed "target" lesions (erythema migrans).

Additional Reading: Sporotrichosis. In: Domino F, ed. *The 5-Minute Clinical Consult*. Wolters Kluwer; 2022.

18. The answer is C: Genital herpes is primarily associated with herpes simplex virus type 2. The symptoms include painful vesicles that occur in clusters, often on the shaft of the penis in men or vulvar areas in women. Patients often report fever, regional lymphadenopathy, and generalized fatigue in association with an outbreak. The lesions last for 2 to 3 days before the top of the vesicles rupture. The remaining ulcers crust over and last for an additional 5 to 7 days. Recurrences are common in the same area. Asymptomatic shedding of the virus can occur once the outbreak has resolved and can infect others. Diagnosis *can* be achieved with the use of Tzanck smears (which detect large bizarre mononucleate and multinucleate giant cells and nuclear changes of ballooning degeneration). Treatment is accomplished with the use of antiviral medications (acyclovir, valacyclovir, famciclovir, and topical penciclovir). Prophylactic therapy may be indicated in recurrent infections.

Chancroid is a bacterial condition causes by *Haemophilus ducreyi*, a rare sexually transmitted disease (STD) in the United States. It causes open sores (ulcers) on the genitals referred to as a chancroid.

Gonorrhea is another STD, but does not present with any skin findings.

Molluscum contagiosum is a common, superficial viral infection of the skin that typically occurs in infants and preschoolers. The lesions are dome-shaped, waxy, or pearly white papules with a central white core and are 1 to 3 mm in diameter.

Syphilis is caused by *Treponema pallidum*; a painless papule (chancre) appears at the site of inoculation associated with regional adenopathy. The lesion resolves in 2-6 weeks without treatment. And a few weeks later the secondary stage develops with low-grade fever, generalized adenopathy, and a mucocutaneous rash.

Additional Reading: Herpes, genital. In: Domino F, ed. *The 5-Minute Clinical Consult*. Wolters Kluwer; 2022.

19. The answer is C: Oral hairy leukoplakia is a marker for human immunodeficiency syndrome and is thought to be caused by the Epstein-Barr virus. The condition appears as white plaques that have the look of corrugated cardboard. The lesions are fixed and not friable and appear on the lateral surface of the tongue. Although the condition rarely causes symptoms, burning of the tongue can occur. Treatment consists of acyclovir, topical tretinoin, or podophyllin. Oral hairy leukoplakia can be distinguished from oral candidiasis by the fact that the latter scrapes off easily with a tongue blade. Oral candidiasis typically affects the dorsal aspect of the tongue and buccal mucosa.

Additional Reading: Leukoplakia, oral. In: Domino F, ed. *The 5-Minute Clinical Consult*. Wolters Kluwer; 2022.

20. The answer is A: Basal cell carcinoma (BCC) is the most common form of skin cancer. The lesions are induced by ultraviolet radiation in susceptible individuals. Risk factors include age above 40 years, light complexion, positive family history, and male sex. The lesion has pearly, raised borders with telangiectasia and a central ulcer that may crust. Sun-exposed areas are most commonly affected. Diagnosis is achieved with shave or excisional biopsy. The clinical presentation of BCC can be divided into the following three groups:

Nodular: This is the most common form of BCC. This typically presents on the face as a pink or flesh-colored papule. The lesion usually has a pearly or translucent quality, and a telangiectatic vessel is frequently seen within the papule. Ulceration is frequent, and the term *rodent ulcer* refers to these ulcerated nodular BCCs.

Superficial: This is the second most common subtype. Men are more likely to be affected, and these lesions are most likely to occur on the trunk of the affected patient. The lesion typically presents as a slightly scaly papule or plaque that is most often pale red; the lesion may be atrophic in the center and is usually surrounded with fine translucent micropapules.

Morpheaform: Also known as sclerosing BCC, this is the least common subtype. These lesions are typically smooth, flesh-colored, or very lightly erythematous papules or plaques that are frequently atrophic; they usually have a firm or indurated quality with ill-defined borders.

Treatment is accomplished with excision, electrodesiccation and curettage, liquid nitrogen application, Mohs surgery, radiation, and topical 5-fluorouracil cream. Almost 50% of patients with BCC will have another within 5 years.

Additional Reading: Basal cell carcinoma. In: Domino F, ed. *The 5-Minute Clinical Consult*. Wolters Kluwer; 2022.

21. The answer is E: Impetigo is caused by group A β-hemolytic streptococci or *S aureus* and typically affects young children. The lesions begin as erythematous papules that expand to form crusted patches with a honey-brown appearance. More severe cases may cause bullae to form. The infection occurs more commonly around the nose and mouth and in the intertriginous areas. There are no constitutional symptoms. Examination is usually made on clinical presentation. Treatment for mild infections includes 2% topical mupirocin ointment. More severe cases respond to dicloxacillin, cephalexin, or erythromycin. Impetigo is highly contagious. Glomerulonephritis is a rare complication of impetigo that is caused by certain strains of *Streptococcus*.

Additional Reading: Impetigo. In: Domino F, ed. *The 5-Minute Clinical Consult*. Wolters Kluwer; 2022.

22. The answer is C: Pitting of the nails is commonly associated with psoriasis. Erythematous scaly plaques are usually noted on other parts of the body. Thirty percent of patients with psoriasis have a positive family history for the condition. Men and women are affected equally. Other conditions that are related to nail pitting include alopecia areata and eczematous dermatitis. Chronic obstructive pulmonary disease is related to clubbing. Subungual hyperkeratosis is associated with onychomycosis.

Chronic obstructive pulmonary disease can result in chronic hypoxia, which is associated with clubbing of the nails.

Onychomycosis is the result of a fungal infection and the nails become thickened and dystrophic.

Scleroderma is a connective tissue disease that presents with hard, thickening, or tight skin. This can range from a single to widespread patches over the body. Nail findings are unusual; typically sores tend to develop on the fingers, where the skin is tightly stretched, resulting in pinhead-sized pitted scars on their fingertips and the sides of their fingers.

Additional Reading: Psoriasis. In: Domino F, ed. *The 5-Minute Clinical Consult*. Wolters Kluwer; 2022.

23. The answer is E: Tinea versicolor is a common skin infection caused by the organism *Pityrosporum orbiculare* (also known as *Malassezia furfur, Pityrosporum ovale,* or *Malassezia ovalis*). The condition usually affects adolescents and young adults in tropical environments. Versicolor refers to the variety and changing shades of colors present in this condition. Lesions can be hypopigmented, light brown, or salmon-colored macules. A fine scale is often noted, especially after scraping. Individual lesions are typically small but frequently coalesce to form larger lesions. Typically, the lesions are limited to the outer skin, most commonly on the upper trunk and extremities, and are less common on the face and intertriginous areas. Most patients are asymptomatic; however, some may complain of mild pruritus. The condition may occur in patients who are immunocompromised. It is most evident in the summer because the organism produces a substance that inhibits pigment transfer to keratinocytes, thus making infected skin more demarcated from uninfected, evenly pigmented skin.

The diagnosis of tinea versicolor is made by microscopic examination of skin samples with 10% KOH. Both hyphae and spores are evident in a pattern that is often described as "spaghetti and meatballs." The differential diagnosis includes seborrhea, eczema, pityriasis rosea, and secondary syphilis.

Antifungal therapy given for 2 weeks is the treatment of choice for patients with mild and limited disease. Patients should be informed that the healing process continues after the treatment is complete. A return to normal pigmentation may take months after the completion of successful treatment. Oral medications are more convenient for patients with extensive disease and may also be more effective in patients with recalcitrant infection. Most oral antifungal agents, with the exception of griseofulvin or terbinafine, may be used. Additionally, ketoconazole 2% shampoo in a single application or daily for 3 days may be considered as an option for treatment, especially with mild infections.

Eczema is a chronic skin condition associated with itchy dry skin.

Pityriasis rosea is a self-limited, exanthematous skin disease that develops acutely and is characterized by the appearance of slightly inflammatory, oval, papulosquamous lesions on the trunk and proximal areas of the extremities.

Secondary syphilis is caused by *T pallidum* and is acquired through sexual intercourse; a painless papule (chancre) appears at the site of inoculation associated with regional adenopathy. The lesion resolves in 2 to 6 weeks without treatment. And a few weeks later the secondary stage develops with low-grade fever, generalized adenopathy, and a mucocutaneous rash. The rash is usually nonpruritic and covers the entire body in a symmetric pattern. The skin is indurated and there is often a superficial scale on the lesions, which may lead to a misdiagnosis of psoriasis.

Seborrheic dermatitis is a relatively common skin condition that mainly affects the scalp, resulting in dandruff. However, it also presents as scaly, red patches on oily areas of the face and chest.

Additional Reading: Tinea versicolor. In: Domino F, ed. *The 5-Minute Clinical Consult*. Wolters Kluwer; 2022.

24. The answer is B: Erythema nodosum is an acute inflammatory reaction of the subcutaneous fat. Women between the ages of 20 and 30 years are most likely to be affected. Causes include the use of oral contraceptives or sulfonamides, pregnancy, sarcoidosis, histoplasmosis, tuberculosis, inflammatory bowel disease, lymphoma, leukemia, Behçet disease, and streptococcal infections. Up to 40% of cases are idiopathic.

Typically, the lesions begin as bright red, tender nodules. The lesions tend to occur bilaterally on the lower extremities and occasionally on the arms. Constitutional symptoms (fever, arthralgias, and malaise) may also be present. The lesions become dark brown or violaceous during the resolution phase. Spontaneous resolution occurs in 3 to 6 weeks after onset regardless of the cause. Treatment consists of symptomatic treatment, nonsteroidal anti-inflammatory drugs, and systemic corticosteroids once an infectious cause is ruled out.

Erythema multiforme comes on suddenly and develops over a few days. It typically starts as small red spots on the hands or feet, before spreading to the limbs, upper body, and face. The spots become raised patches that look like a target lesion with a darker center that may blister or crust.

Lyme disease is a tick-borne infection and will present with typical mildly inflamed "target" lesions (erythema migrans).

Pyoderma gangrenosum is a rare condition that results in large, painful ulcers to develop on the legs. It has been seen with inflammatory bowel disease. The ulcers can develop quickly and can be treated with corticosteroids. Scarring and recurrences are common.

Rheumatoid arthritis is associated with several skin conditions; they reflect the severity of the underlying disease. Subcutaneous nodules are seen in up to 25%, and vasculitis is a long-term complication. Sores can develop on the tips of the fingers and toes, with pitting around the nails and ulcers can be seen in severe cases.

Additional Reading: Erythema nodosum. In: Domino F, ed. *The 5-Minute Clinical Consult*. Wolters Kluwer; 2022.

25. The answer is E: Neurofibromatosis is also referred to as *von Recklinghausen disease*. It is associated with autosomal dominant inheritance and is characterized by multiple, macular, pigmented skin lesions called *café au lait spots* (as they look like coffee lightened with milk) and skin tumors called neurofibromas. Axillary or inguinal freckling (Crowe sign) is considered to be pathognomonic for neurofibromatosis. Ocular lesions (Lisch nodules) are asymptomatic, pigmented iris hamartomas that are seen in 80% of cases.

The disease has been associated with defects on chromosomes 17 and 22. Neurofibromas may cause neurologic symptoms. Seizures, paraplegia, and mental retardation may occur secondary to the condition. Treatment consists of surgical removal of symptomatic or disfiguring lesions. Patients should be monitored for the development of neurofibrosarcomas, optic gliomas, acoustic neuromas, and pheochromocytomas. Those who are affected should also receive genetic counseling.

Addison disease is associated with hyperpigmentation of the skin—referred to as "bronzing."

Gardner syndrome is a subtype of familial adenomatous polyposis, an autosomal dominant inherited condition characterized by the presence of multiple polyps in the colon. Extracolonic tumors can also occur, including epidermoid cysts, visible as subcutaneous nodules.

Hypothyroidism can be associated with a variety of skin changes such as chronic urticaria, vitiligo, alopecia, acne vulgaris, and acne rosacea.

Multiple sclerosis causes paresthesia, but no specific skin findings are seen.

Additional Reading: Neurofibromatosis type 1. In: Domino F, ed. *The 5-Minute Clinical Consult*. Wolters Kluwer; 2022.

26. The answer is A: Atopic dermatitis is also referred to as eczema. The condition is associated with erythematous pruritic areas that occur in association with hay fever, asthma, allergic rhinitis, or allergic sinusitis. The flexor surfaces are commonly involved. The course is variable with flares and remissions. The condition affects children and adults. The diagnosis is made based on history and clinical presentation. Dry conditions such as during the winter heating season can be especially problematic. Treatment consists of topical steroids, antihistamines, tar baths, moisturizing ointments, or Burow solution. Severe cases may require systemic steroids, cyclosporine, or phototherapy.

Dyshidrotic eczema typically presents as itchy vesicles on the sides of the fingers and feet. It is commonly associated with atopic dermatitis.

Ichthyosis vulgaris, also known as fish scale or skin disease, is an inherited skin disorder in which dead skin cells accumulate in thick, dry scales. This typically presents during early childhood, with mild cases going undiagnosed, mistaken for extremely dry skin.

Scabies is associated with intense pruritus that is noted predominantly at night. The lesions are brownish and often form irregular burrow lines that may be marked with scaling at one end and a vesicle at the other end. The lesions are typically found in intertriginous areas and warm, protected areas such as the finger webs, inframammary areas, and axilla.

Tinea corporis, also known as ringworm, is a common fungal infection that presents as a red or silvery ringlike rash anywhere on the body.

Additional Reading: Dermatitis, atopic. In: Domino F, ed. *The 5-Minute Clinical Consult*. Wolters Kluwer; 2022.

27. The answer is E: Onychomycosis is usually caused by *T rubrum*. Diagnosis is generally made by clinical presentation; however, fungal elements can be confirmed with observation under a microscope using KOH 10% preparation of nail plate scales. Nail clippings can also be used for culture.

Additional Reading: Onychomycosis. In: Domino F, ed. *The 5-Minute Clinical Consult*. Wolters Kluwer; 2022.

28. The answer is A: Arterial ulcers are usually caused by atherosclerosis and seen in the elderly. Men are more commonly affected. Pain is common, as is claudication. Distinguishing features of arterial ulcers are their sharply defined borders and round, "punched-out" appearance. Patients may have signs of pallor and cyanosis. They tend to be smaller than venous ulcers and are usually deep enough to expose muscle or tendons. Commonly affected sites include the toes, pretibial areas, and dorsum of the feet. Venous ulcers are often painless and usually found on the inner area of the ankle.

Livedo reticularis, a mottled reticulated vascular pattern that appears as a lacelike purplish discoloration of the skin, is also seen. The legs may feel cold and clammy. Decreased peripheral pulses are commonly noted. Treatment consists of alleviating underlying risk factors. Pentoxifylline can be used in some cases. Surgical evaluation should be considered.

Basal cell carcinoma presents as a slowly growing nodule on sun-exposed areas of the head. The nodule eventually erodes with a central ulcer and is surrounded by a role border with visible telangiectasias.

Diabetic foot ulcers start as painless erythema over a bony area, with eventual skin breakdown, developing into an open sore. Ulcers can develop anywhere on the foot or toes, usually on the bottom of the foot.

Livedo reticularis is due to an underlying vascular condition, usually seen on the lower extremities, and exacerbated be exposure to cold conditions. It presents as a lacelike purplish reticular pattern on the skin.

29. The answer is C: Dupuytren disease presents with small, pitted nodules on the palm. The fibrous tissue of the palmar fascia shortens and thickens, which results in contractures of the fingers. This is typically seen in men older than 40 who smoke, use alcohol, or have diabetes.

Ganglion cysts are oval fluid-filled cysts along the tendons or joints of the wrists and hands that will cause discomfort, but do not result in contractures.

Trigger finger, also called stenosing tenosynovitis, is a result of inflammation narrowing the space within the sheath that surrounds the tendon in the affected finger. If severe, the finger may become locked in a bent position.

Camptodactyly is a condition where a finger is fixed in a bent position at the middle proximal interphalangeal joint and cannot fully straighten.

Additional Reading: Dupuytren's disease: diagnosis and treatment. *Am Fam Physician*. 2007; 76(1):86-89.

30. The answer is B: Episcleritis is inflammation of the episclera, a thin layer of tissue covering the sclera. It is not an infection and will not respond to antibiotics. Usually this self-resolves without treatment within 3 weeks. Topical lubricants may relieve symptoms while awaiting spontaneous resolution. While topical corticosteroids can be used, it is best to reserve such use for refractory cases.

Additional Reading: Episcleritis. In: Domino F, ed. *The 5-Minute Clinical Consult*. Wolters Kluwer; 2022.

31. The answer is C: Rheumatoid arthritis is a chronic inflammatory disease primarily causing synovial inflammation leading to the destruction of bone and cartilage. There is swelling and tenderness of metacarpophalangeal (MCP), proximal interphalangeal, metatarsophalangeal, with sparing of the distal interphalangeal (DIP) joints. With joint destruction there is ulnar deviation, boutonnière deformity, MCP joint subluxation, and radial deviation at the wrist.

Osteoarthritis is also known as degenerative arthritis; hard bony lumps on the DIP joints, known as Heberden nodules, are often seen.

Sjögren syndrome is an autoimmune disorder that is characterized by dry eyes and mouth. This often accompanies other immune disorders, such as rheumatoid arthritis and systemic lupus erythematosus.

Tophaceous gout refers to subcutaneous deposits of uric acid crystals (tophi), which can be seen with chronic gout. Tophi are found as hard nodules around the fingers, big toe, and at the tips of the elbows; however, they can appear anywhere in the body.

Additional Reading: Rheumatoid arthritis. In: Domino F, ed. *The 5-Minute Clinical Consult*. Wolters Kluwer; 2022.

32. The answer is C: Primary osteoarthritis, also known as degenerative joint disease, is due to a progressive loss of articular cartilage with reactive changes at joint margins and in subchondral bone. It is the most common form of arthritis seen and hard bony lumps on the distal interphalangeal joints, known as Heberden nodules, are often seen.

Additional Reading: Osteoarthritis. In: Domino F, ed. *The 5-Minute Clinical Consult*. Wolters Kluwer; 2022.

33. The answer is D: The Raynaud phenomenon presents as intermittent episodes of vasoconstriction of digital arterioles in response to cold, emotional stress, or blunt trauma. The fingers appear white. The condition usually responds to warming, although in chronic cases, calcium channel blockers such as nifedipine can be prescribed. Most cases are idiopathic, but the phenomenon can be seen with an underlying connective tissue disease and an antinuclear antibody titer can be helpful to rule out such situations.

Additional Reading: Raynaud phenomenon. In: Domino F, ed. *The 5-Minute Clinical Consult*. Wolters Kluwer; 2022.

34. The answer is C: Necrobiosis lipoidica is characterized by itchy, sometimes painful, yellowish red or brown patches of swollen, hard skin. This condition occurs in patients with diabetes but can also be associated with rheumatoid arthritis. There is no cure; symptomatic treatment with topical steroids can help.

Acanthosis nigricans typically presents as a dark or velvety plaque in a body crease such as the neck, axilla, or groin, although it can also be seen on the hands, elbows, or knees. Considered a sign of insulin resistance, it is commonly seen in obesity and type 2 diabetes.

Bullosis diabeticorum (diabetic blisters) looks like burn blisters, seen on the lower legs and feet, and occasionally on the arms and hands. They are more likely to develop with uncontrolled diabetes, but are benign and will heal on their own without leaving scars.

Diabetic dermopathy, also known as shin spots, are painless, red or brown round macules or lines in the skin. This is often seen on the shins of diabetics. They are benign and often confused with age spots.

Additional Reading: Diabetes mellitus. In: Domino F, ed. *The 5-Minute Clinical Consult*. Wolters Kluwer; 2022.

35. The answer is D: Gout is an inflammatory arthritis presenting with an acutely inflamed joint. Involvement of the first metatarsophalangeal joint (podagra) is characteristic, with the foot, ankle, and knee being often involved. It is also characterized by deposition of monosodium urate crystals that accumulate in joints and soft tissues, resulting in soft-tissue masses called tophi.

Additional Reading: Gout. In: Domino F, ed. *The 5-Minute Clinical Consult*. Wolters Kluwer; 2022.

36. The answer is A: Petechiae and purpura are signs of extravascular blood under the skin. This is a "nonblanching" condition that does not fade when viewed through a glass slide that is pressed over the lesion. This is commonly seen with vasculitis, an inflammatory disorder of blood vessels that results in destruction of blood vessel walls with subsequent leaking of blood into the surrounding subcutaneous tissues.

Additional Reading: Vasculitis. In: Domino F, ed. *The 5-Minute Clinical Consult*. Wolters Kluwer; 2022.

37. The answer is D: Paget disease is characterized by eczematous changes of the nipple, with erythema, ulceration, crusting, bleeding, and/or itching. Relatively rare, it is typically associated with underlying in situ or invasive carcinoma of the breast.

Eczema (atopic) is a chronic skin condition associated with itchy dry skin, typically seen in the antecubital and popliteal fossa.

Psoriasis presents with inflamed scaly patches that are covered with thick, silvery scales, typically seen on extensor surfaces.

Bowen disease is an inflamed scaly plaque that is considered a precancerous lesion (squamous cell carcinoma in situ).

Lichen simplex chronicus, also known as neurodermatitis, presents as well-demarcated, erythematous patches and plaques of thickened leathery skin. Chronic itching and scratching results in an exaggeration of the normal skin marking creases giving a "criss-cross" pattern.

Additional Reading: Paget disease. In: Domino F, ed. *The 5-Minute Clinical Consult*. Wolters Kluwer; 2022.

38. The answer is C: Henoch-Schönlein purpura (HSP), now known as IgA vasculitis, is a condition that usually causes a rash that looks like tiny raised bruises. Seen in children between the ages of 3 and 15, it can affect adults, too. In addition to the rash, other symptoms of IgA vasculitis can include joint and abdominal pain. The condition usually resolves with symptomatic treatment in 3 to 4 weeks, although in severe cases steroids can be used.

Meningococcemia is due to an infection caused by the bacteria *Neisseria meningitidis*. The most common cutaneous sign of meningococcal disease is localized purpura, most commonly on the extremities.

Rocky Mountain spotted fever (RMSF) presents with an initial rash of small, flat, pink, macules on the wrists, forearms, and ankles and spreads to include the trunk and sometimes the palms of hands and soles of feet. The petechial rash of RMSF does not typically appear until day 5 to 6 of illness and is a sign of severe disease.

Rheumatic fever presents with erythema marginatum, a characteristic annular erythema on the trunk and upper arms and legs, but almost never on the face, palms, or soles. The rash appears as pink, red macules or papules, which spread outward in a circular shape. As the lesions advance, the edges become raised and red, and the center clears. The lesions can fade and reappear within hours, often unnoticed by the patient, and may persist intermittently for weeks after treatment.

Kawasaki disease is an acute febrile illness with an associated vasculitis. The rash may present as a morbilliform (measleslike) or targetlike eruption, with skin peeling in the convalescent stage of the illness. Oral signs include pharyngitis, strawberry tongue, and red, cracked lips. Usually this is self-limiting, with spontaneous resolution over 4 to 6 weeks, but 20% of untreated cases develop coronary artery damage and can suffer a myocardial infarction.

Additional Reading: Henoch-Schönlein purpura. In: Domino F, ed. *The 5-Minute Clinical Consult*. Wolters Kluwer; 2022.

39. The answer is B: Lyme disease is a tick-borne infection caused by *Borrelia* spirochetes and will present with typical mildly inflamed "target" lesions (erythema migrans). Doxycycline 100 mg BID for 10 days is indicated to treat Lyme disease. Doxycycline 200 mg once can be given as a prophylactic antibiotic within 72 hours of removal of an identified high-risk tick bite, but in this case the rash is consistent with infection and requires a 10- to 14-day course of the antibiotic.

Azithromycin 500 mg QD for 10 days can be given to those intolerant of doxycycline, but macrolides have lower efficacy, and patients treated with such agents should be monitored to ensure that symptoms resolve.

Amoxicillin 500 mg TID for 28 days would be appropriate for treating Lyme arthritis.

Additional Reading: Lyme disease. In: Domino F, ed. *The 5-Minute Clinical Consult*. Wolters Kluwer; 2022.

40. The answer is A: Shingles results from reactivation of latent varicella-zoster virus (VZV) (human herpesvirus type 3) infection and usually presents as a painful unilateral vesicular eruption with a dermatomal distribution. Antiviral agents, like valacyclovir 1000 mg TID, help relieve symptoms, speed resolution, and mitigate postherpetic neuralgia (PHN) when initiated within 72 hours of the skin lesion.

Corticosteroids do not prevent PHN but may accelerate resolution of acute neuritis, but are not the mainstay of treatment.

Analgesics such as acetaminophen and nonsteroidal anti-inflammatory drugs are recommended, rather than narcotics like oxycodone.

Sulfamethoxazole/trimethoprim is an antibiotic and not indicated to treat a viral infection.

Additional Reading: Herpes Zoster (Shingles). In: Domino F, ed. *The 5-Minute Clinical Consult*. Wolters Kluwer; 2022.

41. The answer is C: Nasal polyps are often seen with allergic conditions in adults, and can be treated with nasal steroids, but in a child have been associated with cystic fibrosis and a sweat test is indicated to rule out this condition.

Additional Reading: Nasal Polyps. In: Basow DS, ed. *UpToDate*. UpToDate; 2022.

Section II. Exam Findings and Diagnostic Testing

Each of the following questions or incomplete statements is followed by suggested answers or completions. Select the ONE BEST ANSWER in each case.

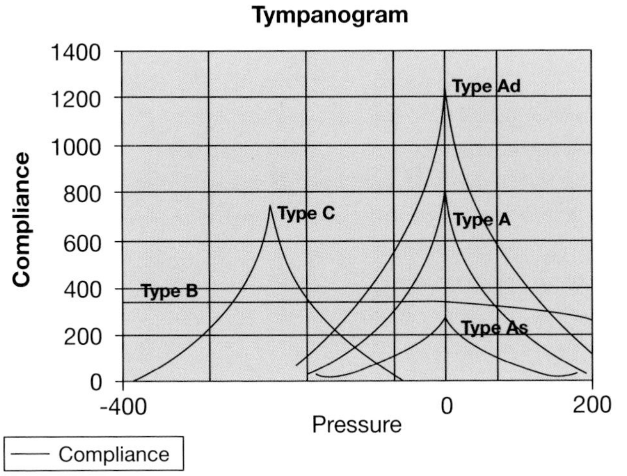

Reproduced with permission from Domino FJ, Baldor RA, Barry KA, Golding J, Stephens MB. *The 5-Minute Clinical Consult 2023*. 31st ed. Wolters Kluwer; 2023.

1. The chart above shows various tympanogram tracings. Which one of these tracings is consistent with a perforated tympanic membrane?

A) Type A
B) Type Ad
C) Type As
D) Type B
E) Type C

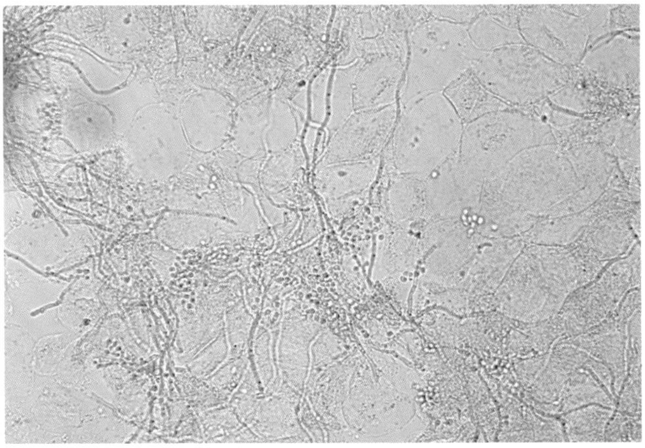

Reproduced with permission from Goodheart H. *Goodheart's Photoguide to Common Pediatric and Adult Skin Disorders*. 3rd ed. Wolters Kluwer; 2009.

2. A young woman presents complaining of an itchy vaginal discharge. She reports being sexually active with a regular partner. You perform a microscopic examination of the discharge, which is pictured above. The most likely diagnosis to explain her presentation is which one of the following conditions?

A) Gonorrhea infection
B) Chlamydia infection
C) Yeast vaginitis
D) *Gardnerella* vaginitis
E) *Trichomonas* vaginitis

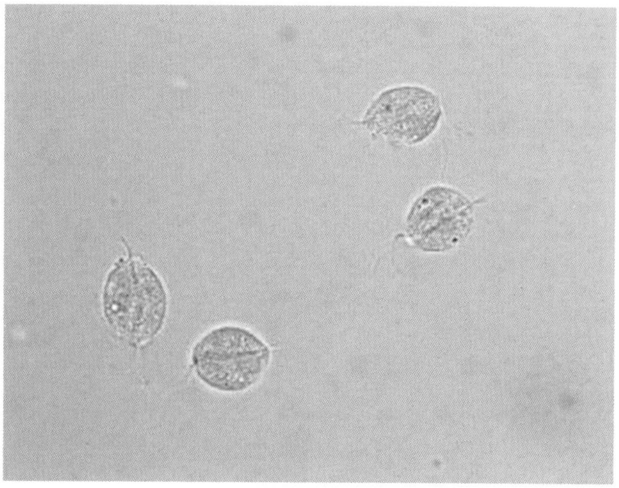

Reproduced with permission from Šoba B, Skvarč M, Matičič M. Trichomoniasis: a brief review of diagnostic methods and our experience with real-time PCR for detecting infection. *Acta Dermatovenerol Alp Pannonica Adriat*. 2015;24:7-10.

3. A young woman presents complaining of an itchy vaginal discharge. She reports being sexually active with a regular partner. You perform a microscopic examination of the discharge, which is pictured above. The most likely diagnosis to explain her presentation is which one of the following conditions?

A) Gonorrhea infection
B) Chlamydia infection
C) Yeast vaginitis
D) *Gardnerella* vaginitis
E) *Trichomonas* vaginitis

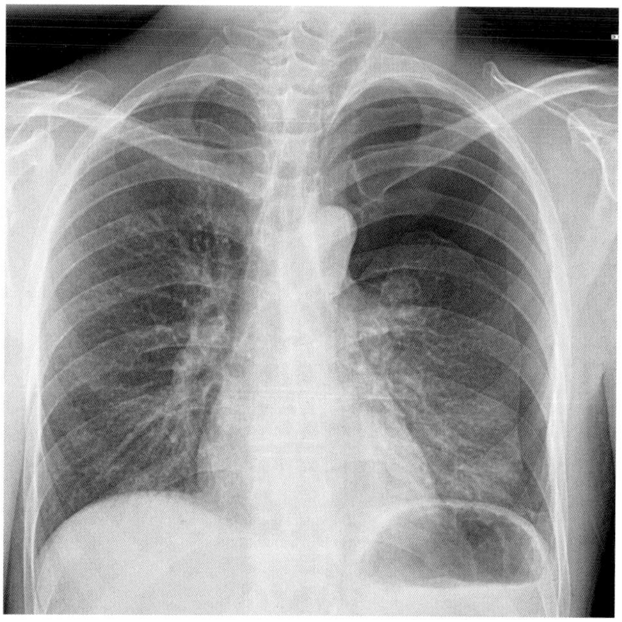

Reproduced with permission from Daffner RH, Hartman M. *Clinical Radiology*. 4th ed. Lippincott Williams & Wilkins; 2014.

4. A 44-year-old truck driver presents to the emergency department complaining of shortness of breath and right-sided chest pain. A chest radiograph is obtained and is shown above. The most likely explanation to his presentation is which one of the following conditions?

A) Congestive heart failure (CHF)
B) Pneumonia
C) Pneumothorax
D) Pulmonary embolism

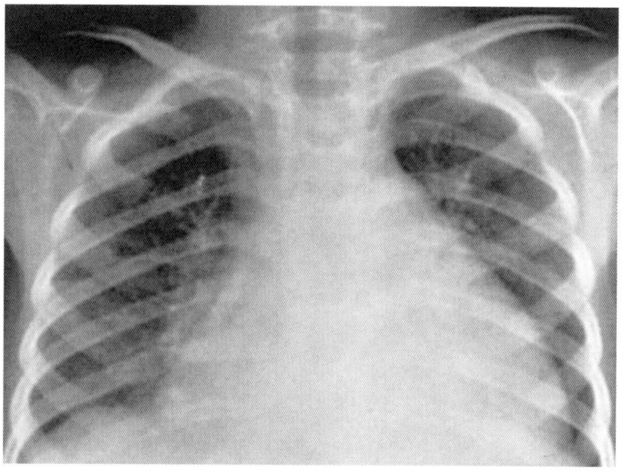

Reproduced with permission from Bachur RG, Shaw KN, Chamberlain J, Lavelle J, Nagler J, Shook JE. *Fleisher & Ludwig's Textbook of Pediatric Emergency Medicine*. 5th ed. Wolters Kluwer; 2020.

5. A 67-year-old retired salesman presents to the emergency department complaining of shortness of breath and a cough. A chest radiograph is obtained and is shown above. The most likely explanation to his presentation is which one of the following conditions?

A) Congestive heart failure (CHF)
B) Pneumonia
C) Pneumothorax
D) Pulmonary embolism

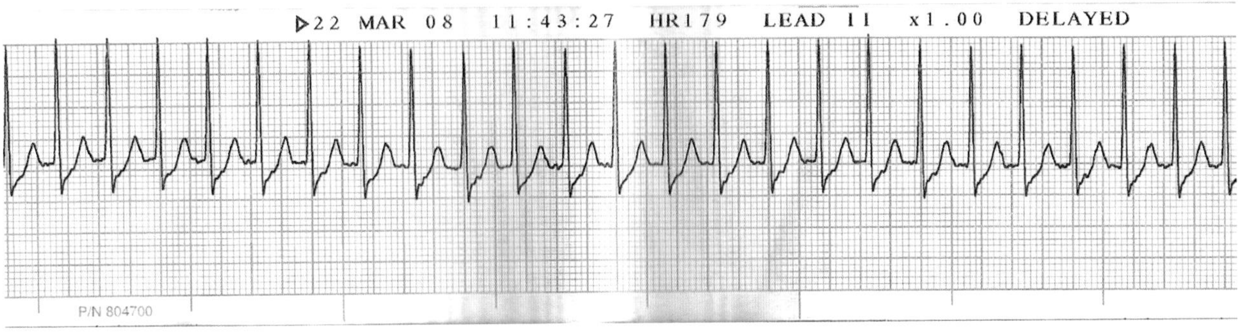

https://commons.wikimedia.org/w/index.php?curid=3986138.

6. A 47-year-old teacher presents to the emergency department complaining of shortness of breath and palpitations. His electrocardiogram (ECG) is shown. Appropriate management at this time includes which one of the following measures?

A) Adenosine IV
B) Lidocaine IV
C) Epinephrine IM
D) Metoprolol PO
E) Cardioversion

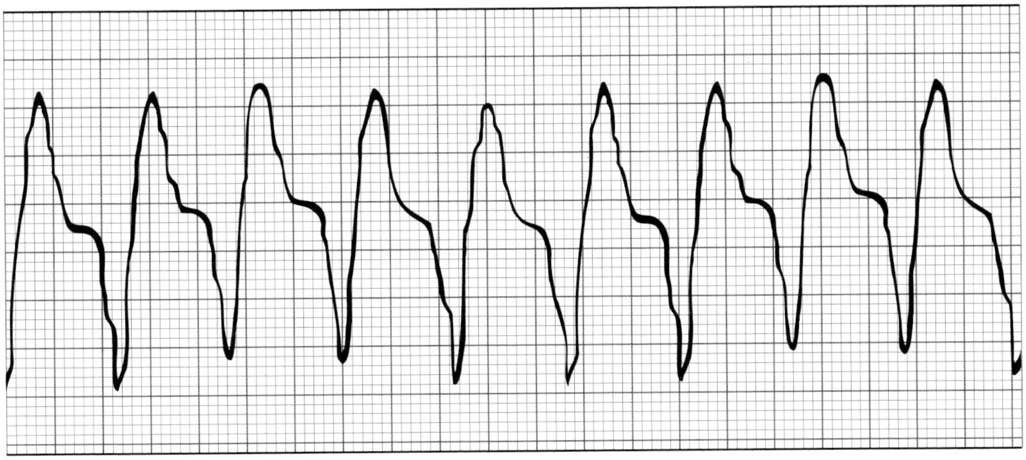

7. A 67-year-old patient collapses in your office, and the above cardiac tracing is obtained on your office ECG. This rhythm is most consistent with which one of the following conditions?

A) Atrioventricular (AV) dissociation
B) Atrial fibrillation
C) Supraventricular tachycardia (SVT)
D) Ventricular fibrillation (V-Fib)
E) Ventricular tachycardia (V-Tach)

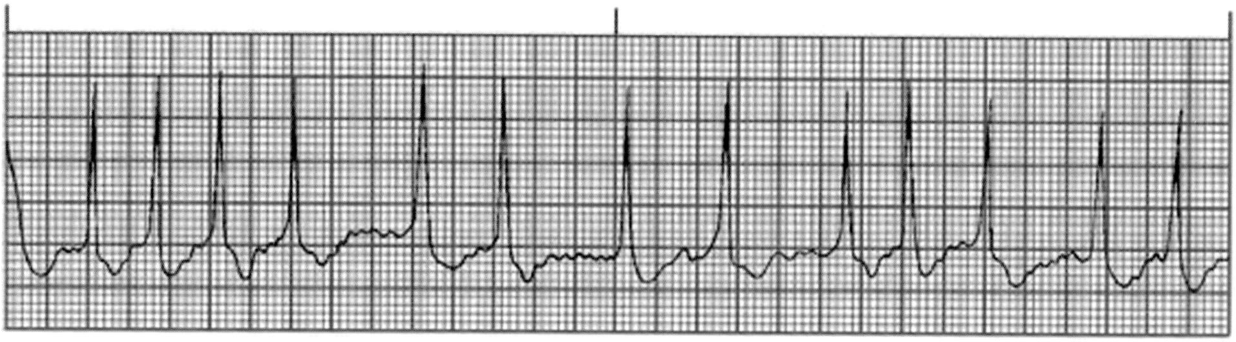

Reproduced with permission from Kline-Tilford AM, Haut C. *Lippincott Certification Review: Pediatric Acute Care Nurse Practitioner*. Lippincott Williams & Wilkins; 2016.

8. A 65-year-old financial analyst presents to your office complaining of palpitations. He has been healthy; however, his blood pressures have been borderline high and he tends to drink heavily on most weekends. You obtain an ECG and his rhythm strip is shown above. His presentation is most likely secondary to which one of the following conditions?

A) Acute myocardial infarction
B) Atrial fibrillation
C) SVT
D) V-Fib
E) V-Tach

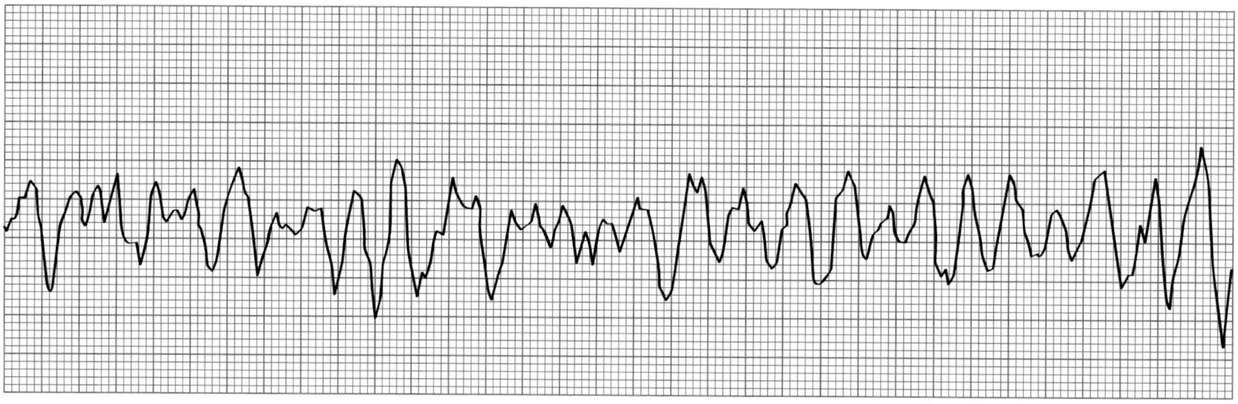

Reproduced with permission from Honan L. *Focus on Adult Health: Medical-Surgical Nursing*. 2nd ed. Lippincott Williams & Wilkins; 2019.

9. A 71-year-old man has slumped over while attending church services and is unresponsive. The paramedics arrive and he is placed on a cardiac monitor, which demonstrates the above tracing. This tracing most likely represents which one of the following conditions?

A) Asystole
B) Atrial ventricular dissociation
C) Sinus tachycardia
D) V-Fib
E) V-Tach

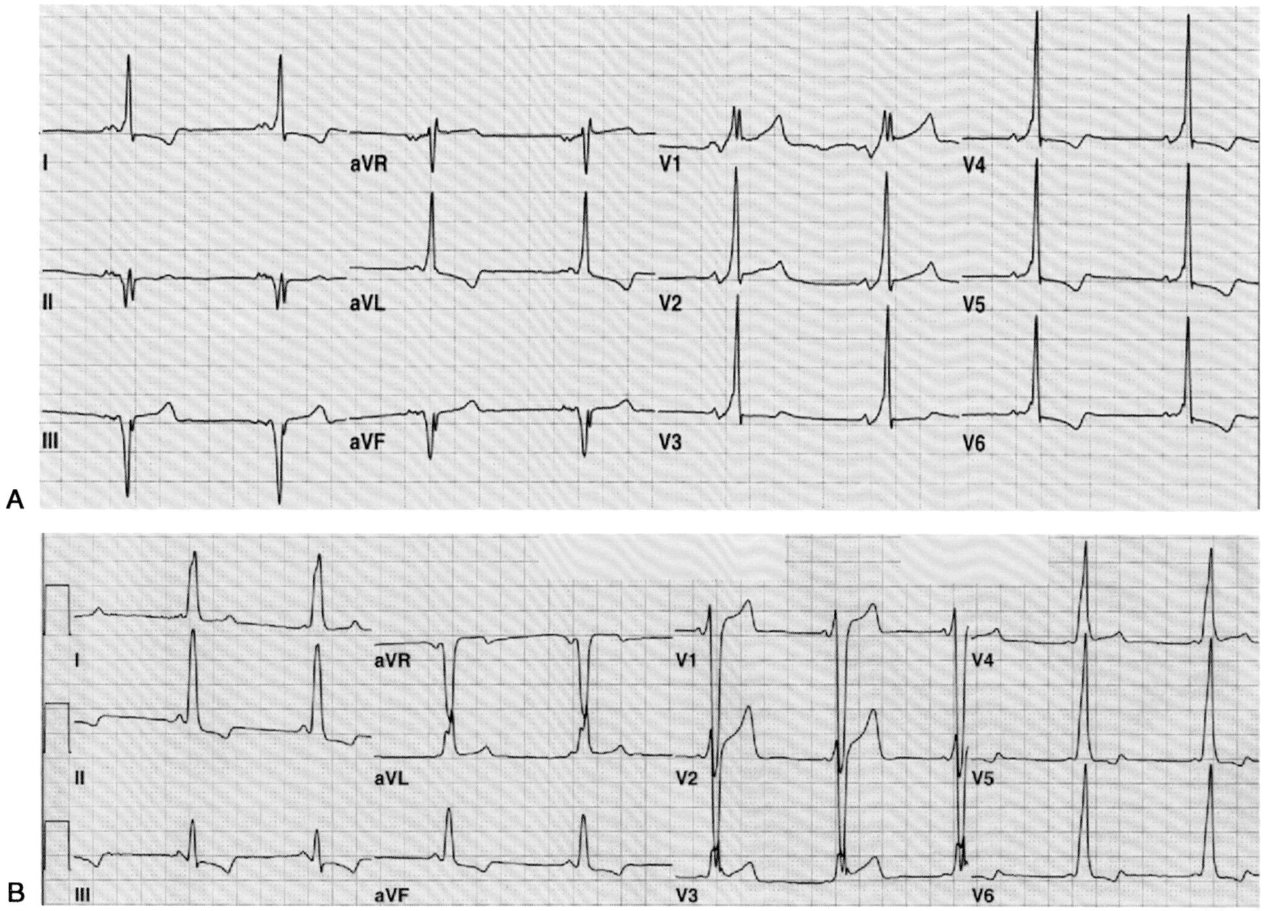

Reproduced with permission from Dunbar C, Saul B. *ECG Interpretation for the Clinical Exercise Physiologist*. 2nd ed. Lippincott Williams and Wilkins; 2022.

10. The ECG rhythm tracing is most likely due to which one of the following conditions?

A) Atrial fibrillation with 3:1 block
B) Hypothermia
C) Inferior myocardial infarction
D) Normal sinus rhythm
E) Wolff-Parkinson-White (WPW) syndrome

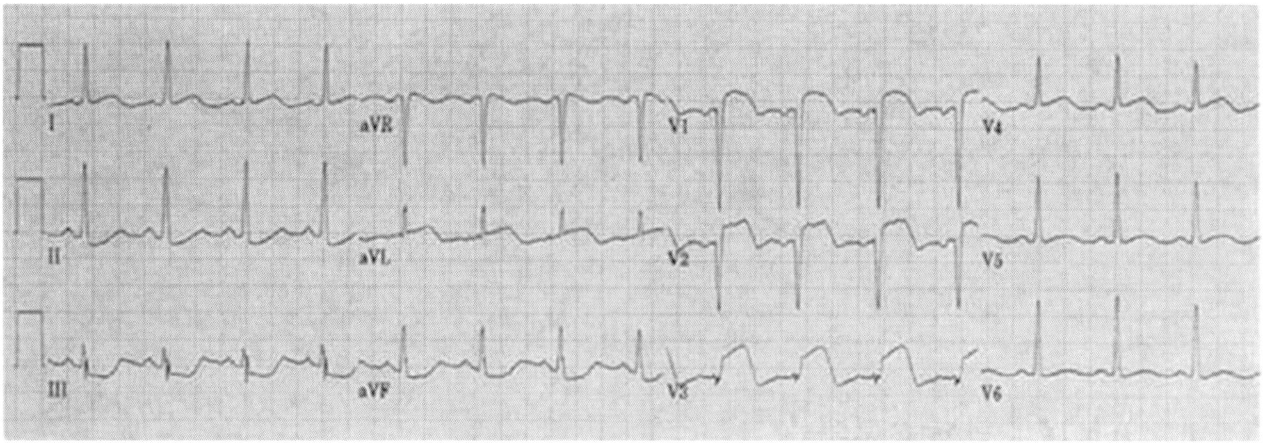

11. A 72-year-old retired farmer presents to the emergency department with complaints of pain and shortness of breath. His medical history is remarkable for hypertension and tobacco abuse. The above tracing is from an urgent ECG. This tracing is most consistent with which one of the following conditions?

A) Acute myocardial infarction
B) Atrial fibrillation
C) SVT
D) V-Fib
E) V-Tach

Answer and Explanations to Section II

1. The answer is D: A common method for describing tympanograms was popularized by Jerger. This description involves three basic types of tympanograms: types A, B, and C.

Type A is a normal tympanogram. Type Ad describes a highly compliant tympanic membrane where there is little impedance. This situation may occur in the face of ossicular discontinuity or scarring of the tympanic membrane in the absence of hearing loss. The type "A" pattern suggests decreased compliance and can be found in cases of ossicular fixations such as otosclerosis.

Type "B" tympanogram describes a flat tympanogram where there is no peak in compliance and little if any change in compliance with changes of pressure. A type B tympanogram would be found in cases of middle ear effusions as in serous otitis media; however, a flat tympanogram associated with a relatively high volume would suggest a tympanic membrane perforation.

Type "C" tympanogram has a compliance peak in the negative pressure range beyond an air pressure of −100 mm H_2O as occurs when there is inadequate ventilation of the middle ear space, which is reflective of eustachian tube dysfunction.

Additional Reading: Tympanometry. In: Domino F, ed. *The 5-Minute Clinical Consult*. Wolters Kluwer; 2022.

2. The answer is C: Yeast vaginitis causes approximately one-third of all vaginal infections. Risk factors include pregnancy, diabetes, use of intrauterine devices, recent antibiotic use, immune deficiency, or corticosteroid use. Diagnosis is made by examination of a vaginal smear under high-power microscopy after KOH has been added (KOH prep) or via a PCR swab. Budding yeast and pseudohyphae are noted. Topical antifungals are effective, as are single-dose oral antifungals (eg, fluconazole).

Additional Reading: Vaginitis: diagnosis and treatment. *Am Fam Physician*. 2018;97(5):321-329.

3. The answer is E: *Trichomonas* vaginitis is a sexually transmitted urogenital infection caused by a pear-shaped, parasitic protozoan. It causes vaginitis/urethritis in women and nongonococcal urethritis in men. Diagnosis has traditionally been made by examination of a vaginal smear under high-power microscopy after a drop of saline has been added (hanging drop). The wet mounts of vaginal or urethral discharge provide direct visualization of motile trichomonads. However, the Centers for Disease Control and Prevention recommends nucleic acid amplification testing for the diagnosis of trichomoniasis in symptomatic or high-risk women as these tests have a higher sensitivity than saline microscopy and can be performed on endocervical, vaginal, or urine specimens, or on liquid-based Pap test samples. Treatment with metronidazole is usually effective.

Gonorrhea and chlamydia infections are often seen with patients complaining of vaginitis, but these sexually transmitted diseases can be asymptomatic or lead to pelvic inflammatory disease. DNA probe testing of vaginal secretions or urine is used for diagnosis.

Gardnerella vaginitis, also known as bacterial vaginitis, has been traditionally diagnosed using the Amsel criteria, which include a thin, homogenous discharge; a positive whiff test; the presence of clue cells on microscopy; and a vaginal pH greater than 4.5. Three out of four criteria are required to make the diagnosis. Testing with a DNA probe for *Gardnerella vaginalis* or detection of vaginal fluid sialidase activity are more sensitive and specific tests.

Additional Reading: Vaginitis: diagnosis and treatment. *Am Fam Physician*. 2018;97(5):321-329.

4. The answer is C: A primary spontaneous pneumothorax is a pneumothorax that occurs without a precipitating event in a person who does not have known lung disease. In actuality, most individuals with primary spontaneous pneumothorax have unrecognized lung disease, with the pneumothorax resulting from rupture of a subpleural bleb.

Additional Reading: *Primary spontaneous pneumothorax in adults*. In: *UpToDate*. UpToDate; 2022.

5. The answer is A: The earliest chest radiograph finding of CHF is cardiomegaly, detected as an increased cardiothoracic ratio (>50%). Normally the veins in the lower lungs appear larger than those in the upper lobes due to gravity; however, in a patient with CHF, the pulmonary capillary wedge pressures increase, and the upper lobe veins dilate and are equal in size or larger than those in the lower lobes (cephalization). As pulmonary capillary pressures increase with worsening CHF, interstitial edema occurs with the appearance of Kerley B lines. Once pulmonary edema develops, the classic perihilar "batwing" density pattern is seen, along with pleural effusions.

Clinical prediction rule can assist with the diagnosis of heart failure. The MICE and Brest scores are best suited for the primary care setting because they do not require blood tests for the initial evaluation. While the Kelder rule is accurate and well validated it requires the N-terminal prohormone BNP test.

Additional Reading: Diagnosis of heart failure with reduced ejection fraction. *Am Fam Physician*. 2020;101(4):230-232.

6. The answer is A: This tracing is consistent with supraventricular tachycardia (SVT), which is often referred to as *narrow complex tachycardia*. The condition is characterized by sustained tachyarrhythmia with a QRS complex that appears normal and has a duration of more than 120 ms. Patients whose condition is unstable should receive immediate synchronized cardioversion. Those who are hemodynamically stable can be treated with vagal maneuvers (Valsalva, cough, carotid massage), adenosine, verapamil, or diltiazem.

Unstable symptoms include hypotension, shortness of breath, shock, decreased level of consciousness, or chest pain suggestive of coronary ischemia.

A SVT with a heart rate of 200 beats per minute may be tolerated by a healthy young patient with no or few symptoms (eg, palpitations). However, a heart rate of 120 beats per minute may precipitate angina in an elderly patient with significant coronary heart disease.

Adenosine is used to manage SVT in which the AV node is involved. The drug is administered by rapid intravenous injection over 1 to 2 seconds at a peripheral site, followed by a normal saline flush. The usual initial dose is 6 mg, with a maximal single dose of 12 mg. The most common side effects of adenosine are facial flushing, palpitations, chest pain, and hypotension. Transient asystole is a rare complication. Another important side effect of adenosine is that it may precipitate atrial fibrillation (AF). In patients with Wolff-Parkinson-White (WPW) syndrome, AF can progress into V-Fib. As a result, caution should be used when giving adenosine if WPW syndrome is a possible mechanism, and emergency resuscitation equipment should be available.

Additional Reading: Diagnosis and management of common types of supraventricular tachycardia. *Am Fam Physician*. 2015;92(9):793-802.

7. The answer is E: V-Tach is defined as three or more successive ventricular complexes, and sustained V-Tach lasts for more than 30 seconds. ECG changes show wide QRS complexes with no discernible P waves. Typically, the rate of V-Tach is greater than 100 beats per minute but may vary significantly. The rhythm is usually regular; however, there may be slight irregularity of the R-R intervals. The width of the QRS complex is generally more than 0.16 seconds.

V-Tach is a potentially life-threatening event. Intravenous procainamide, amiodarone, or lidocaine is used to control the rhythm, although hypotensive V-Tach requires immediate treatment with synchronized direct current shock.

Additional Reading: *ECG tutorial: ventricular arrhythmias*. In: *UpToDate*. 2022.

8. The answer is B: Atrial fibrillation (A-Fib) is a common cardiac arrhythmia. ECG findings include the absence of obvious P waves and the irregular response of QRS complexes. Intra-atrial contractions may show rates of more than 300 beats per minute. The ventricular rate may vary depending on the AV nodal conduction but typically is elevated. Treatment involves the management of underlying causative disorders, control of ventricular rate, restoration of sinus rhythm if possible, and prevention of systemic emboli, with anticoagulation.

Additional Reading: *Overview of atrial fibrillation*. In: *UpToDate*. 2022.

9. The answer is D: V-Fib is a completely disorganized depolarization and contraction of small areas of the ventricle without effective cardiac output. The ECG displays absence of QRS complexes and T waves with the presence of high-frequency, irregular undulations that are variable in both amplitude and periodicity. Early defibrillation of V-Fib is the most important determinant of survival, and each minute without defibrillation reduces survival by 7% to 10%.

Additional Reading: *Ventricular fibrillation, emergency medicine*. In: *The 5-Minute Clinical Consult*. Wolters Kluwer; 2022.

10. The answer is E: WPW syndrome is caused by an accessory pathway that links the atria and ventricles, bypassing the AV node, thereby triggering ventricular excitation before the normal impulse arrives. The most common disturbance in those with WPW syndrome is AV nodal reentrant tachycardia. These patients often present with a heart rate of more than 250 beats per minute, which can result in life-threatening hypotension because of decreased ventricular filling time.

The ECG shows a short PR interval and slurred upstroke at the beginning of the QRS complex known as a delta wave (best seen in V2, V3, and V4). Antegrade and retrograde conduction both occur, causing a reciprocating tachycardia. Direct current cardioversion should be considered when AF is present in the setting of WPW.

Additional Reading: *Epidemiology, clinical manifestations, and diagnosis of the Wolff–Parkinson–White syndrome*. In: *UpToDate*. 2022.

11. The answer is A: Acute coronary syndrome encompasses a spectrum of disease processes including unstable angina pectoris and acute myocardial infarction. In a classic STEMI, there is classic "tombstoning" from ST-segment elevation over the anterior leads. This patient is suffering from an acute anterior MI. In the first few hours after an MI, the ST segments usually begin to increase. Pathologic Q waves may appear within hours or may take greater than 24 hours. The T wave will generally become inverted in the first 24 hours, as the ST elevation begins to resolve. Long-term changes of ECG include persistent Q waves and persistent inverted T waves.

Additional Reading: Acute coronary syndromes: STEMI. In: Domino F, ed. *The 5-Minute Clinical Consult*. Wolters Kluwer; 2022.

Study Grid

		What Type of Test-Taking "Error" Did You Make?			
Category (Approximate Percent of the General Examination Questions)	Wrong Answer	Did Not Read All of the Questions or Choices	Did Not Use Keywords	Lured by a Distractor	Guessed Without Using Partial Knowledge
Cardiovascular system (10%)					
Respiratory system (10%)					
Musculoskeletal system (10%)					
Endocrine system (7%)					
Gastroenterology system (5%)					
Psychogenic disorders (5%)					
Integumentary system (5%)					
Patient-/population-based care (7%)					
Reproductive system (5%)					
Nephrologic system (2%)					
Hematologic system (2%)					
Special sensory systems (2%)					
Neurologic system (2%)					

Index

Note: Page numbers followed by *f* indicate figures.

F